# THERAPEUTIC STRATEGIES IN DEMENTIA

# THERAPEUTIC STRATEGIES IN DEMENTIA

Edited by

C. W. Ritchie, D. Ames, C. L. Masters, J. Cummings

CLINICAL PUBLISHING

OXFORD

**Clinical Publishing**
an imprint of Atlas Medical Publishing Ltd

Oxford Centre for Innovation
Mill Street, Oxford OX2 0JX, UK

Tel: +44 1865 811116
Fax: +44 1865 251550
E-mail: info@clinicalpublishing.co.uk
Web: www.clinicalpublishing.co.uk

**Distributed in USA and Canada by:**

Clinical Publishing
30 Amberwood Parkway
Ashland OH 44805 USA

Tel: 800-247-6553 (toll free within U.S. and Canada)
Fax: 419-281-6883
E-mail: order@bookmasters.com

**Distributed in UK and Rest of World by:**

Marston Book Services Ltd
PO Box 269
Abingdon
Oxon OX14 4YN, UK

Tel: +44 1235 465500
Fax: +44 1235 465555
E-mail: trade.orders@marston.co.uk



First published 2007



A catalogue record for this book is available from the British Library

ISBN 978 1 904392 58 3
ISBN 1 904392 58 X



Project manager: Gavin Smith, GPS Publishing Solutions, Hitchin, Hertfordshire, UK
Typeset by Mizpah Publishing Services Private Limited, Chennai, India
Printed in Spain by T G Hostench s.a., Barcelona, Spain

Cover image provided by Dr Cyril Curtain, Department of Pathology, University of Melbourne, The Mental Health Institute of Victoria and the School of Physics, Monash University, Victoria, Australia

# Contents

# Contributors

**DAVID AMES,** BA, MD, FRCPsych, FRANZCP, Professor of Psychiatry of Old Age, University of Melbourne Academic Unit for Psychiatry of Old Age, St George's Hospital, Kew, Victoria, Australia

**ROBERT BARBER,** MDc, MD, MRCPsych, Consultant Old Age Psychiatrist and Honorary Clinical Senior Lecturer, Institute for Ageing and Health, Newcastle General Hospital, Newcastle upon Tyne, UK

**KAREN BERMAN,** MB BCh, Academic Department for Old Age Psychiatry, School of Psychiatry, Prince of Wales Hospital, Randwick, NSW, Australia

**KONRAD BEYREUTHER,** PhD, Centre for Molecular Biology Heidelberg, (Zentrum für Molekulare Biologie Heidelberg), Heidelberg, Germany

**FRAUKE BODDY,** MRCPsych, Senior Registrar in Old Age Psychiatry, Institute for Ageing and Health, Newcastle General Hospital, Newcastle upon Tyne, UK

**HENRY BRODATY,** MBBS, MD, FRACP, FRANZCP, Professor of Psychogeriatrics, Academic Department for Old Age Psychiatry, School of Psychiatry, University of New South Wales, Sydney, Australia

**ROGER BULLOCK,** MBBS, Director and Principal Investigator, Kingshill Research Centre, Victoria Hospital, Swindon, UK

**JISKA COHEN-MANSFIELD,** PhD, ABPP, Professor/Research Director, Research Institute on Aging, Hebrew Home of Greater Washington, Professor, Department of Health Care Services and of Prevention and Community Health, George Washington University Medical Center and School of Public Health, Washington, DC, USA

**JEFFREY L. CUMMINGS,** MD, Director, UCLA Alzheimer's Disease Center, Department of Neurology, Reed Neurological Research Center, David Geffen School of Medicine at UCLA, Los Angeles, California, USA

**KRISTY DRAPER,** BA (Hons), Research Assistant, Academic Unit for Psychiatry of Old Age, Department of Psychiatry, The University of Melbourne, Melbourne, Australia

**TIMO ERKINJUNTTI,** MD, PhD, Professor in Applied Neurology, Department of Neurology, University of Helsinki, Helsinki, Finland

MARTIN R. FARLOW, MD, Professor and Vice Chairman for Research, Department of Neurology, Indiana University School of Medicine, Indianapolis, Indiana, USA

SERGE GAUTHIER, MD, FRCPC, Director, Alzheimer's Disease & Related Disorders Research Unit, McGill Center for Studies in Aging, Douglas Hospital, Montreal, Canada

YONAS ENDALE GEDA, MD, MSc, Consultant, Department of Psychiatry Mayo Clinic College of Medicine, Mayo Clinic College of Medicine, Alzheimer's Disease Research Centre, Rochester, Minnesota and Department of Psychiatry, Mayo Clinic College of Medicine, Mayo Clinic Jacksonville, Jacksonville, Florida, USA

COLIN GREEN, BA (Hons), MSc, Principal Research Fellow, Southampton Health Technology Assessments Centre (SHTAC), Wessex Institute for Health Research and Development, University of Southampton, Southampton, UK

MANABU IKEDA, MD, PhD, Associate Professor, Department of Neuropsychiatry, Neuroscience, Ehime University Graduate School of Medicine, Ehime, Japan

ROY W. JONES, BSc (Hons), MBBS, Dip Pharm Med, FRCP, FFPM, Professor of Clinical Gerontology and Director, The Research Institute for the Care of the Elderly, St Martin's Hospital, Bath and School for Health, University of Bath, Bath, UK

ANTONIO T. LOPES, MBBS, Senior House Officer in Psychiatry, West London Mental Health NHS Trust, Southall, Middlesex, UK

ALFRED MAELICKE, PhD, Professor and CEO, Galantos Pharma GmbH, Mainz, Germany

COLIN L. MASTERS, MD, Department of Pathology, The University of Melbourne and The Mental Health Research Institute of Victoria, Australia

ROBERT W. MCCARNEY, MPhil, Research Associate, Department of Psychological Medicine, Imperial College, London, UK

SELAMAWIT NEGASH, PhD, Cognitive Neuroscience, Research Fellow, Alzheimer's Disease Research Center, Mayo Clinic College of Medicine, Rochester, Minnesota, USA

AGNETA NORDBERG, MD, PhD, Professor, Karolinska Institutet, Department of Neurobiology, Care Sciences and Society, Division of Molecular Neuropharmacology, Karolinska University, Hospital Huddinge, Stockholm, Sweden

RONALD C. PETERSEN, PhD, MD, Consultant, Department of Neurology, Alzheimer's Disease Research Center, Mayo Clinic College of Medicine, Rochester, Minnesota, USA

CRAIG W. RITCHIE, MB ChB, MRCPsych, MSc, Director of Clinical Trials, Metabolic and Clinical Trials Unit, Department of Mental Health Sciences, Royal Free and University College Medical School, London, UK

**Kenneth Rockwood,** MPA, BSc, MD, FRCPC, Consultant Geriatrician (Geriatrics & Neurology), Department of Medicine, Dalhousie University Centre for Health Care of the Elderly, Halifax, Nova Scotia, Canada

**Elizabeth Sampson,** MBChB, MRCPsych, MD, MSc, MRC Research Fellow, Department of Mental Health Sciences, Royal Free and University College Medical School, London, UK

**Mary Sano,** PhD, Director of the Alzheimer's Disease Research Center, Professor of Psychiatry, Department of Psychiatry, The Mount Sinai Medical Center, New York, Research and Development Program, James J. Peters VA Medical Center, Bronx, New York, USA

**Ajit Shah,** MBChB, MRCPsych, Consultant in Old Age Psychiatry and Honorary Senior Lecturer, West London Mental Health NHS Trust, Southall, Middlesex and Imperial College School of Medicine, London, UK

**Daniel M. Stein,** MD, Research Associate, Department of Psychiatry, The Mount Sinai Medical Center, New York, Research and Development Program, James J. Peters VA Medical Center, Bronx, New York, USA

**Robert Stewart,** MD, MSc, MRCPsych, Clinical Senior Lecturer, King's College London (Institute of Psychiatry), London, UK

**Marie Svedberg,** PhD, Researcher, Karolinska Institutet, Department of Neurobiology, Care Sciences and Society, Division of Molecular Neuropharmacology, Karolinska University, Hospital Huddinge, Stockholm, Sweden

**Alan Thomas,** BSc, MBChB, MRCPsych, PhD, Senior Lecturer and Honorary Consultant in Old Age Psychiatry, Newcastle University and Gateshead Health NHS Foundation Trust, Newcastle upon Tyne, UK

**Christina Unger,** PhD, Researcher, Karolinska Institutet, Department of Neurobiology, Care Sciences and Society, Division of Molecular Neuropharmacology, Karolinska University, Hospital Huddinge, Stockholm, Sweden

**James P. W. Warner,** MD, MRCPsych, Senior Lecturer/Honorary Consultant in Old Age Psychiatry, Department of Psychological Medicine, Imperial College, London, UK

**David Wilkinson,** MB, ChB, MRCGP, FRCPsych, Consultant in Old Age Psychiatry, Memory Assessment and Research Centre, Moorgreen Hospital, University of Southampton Division of Neuroscience, Southampton, UK

**Michael Woodward,** MBBS, FRACP, Associate Professor, Consultant Geriatrician and Medical Director, Aged and Residential Care, Heidelberg Repatriation Hospital, Austin Health, Heidelberg, Victoria, Australia

# Foreword

The explosion in therapeutic opportunities to treat people with progressive cognitive impairment, particularly Alzheimer's disease, over the last decade is one of the success stories of medicine. Based on the established neurochemical abnormalities in Alzheimer's disease, centred largely on the cholinergic system, a group of compounds (the cholinesterase inhibitors) have been firmly established for the treatment of Alzheimer's disease. Clinical observation, neurochemical know-how, clinico-pathological correlations, and clinical trial design methodology have all combined in a synergistic way. The result is an exemplar of experimental medicine. However, there is much more – each of these approaches has spawned (almost) a discipline in itself, which is ultimately for the benefit of patients and their carers.

The range of approaches to therapy in Alzheimer's disease is emphasized by the chapters in this book, which cover a whole range of pathophysiological mechanisms and disease areas. It underscores the scope of possible treatments and summarizes effectively their various roles in the management of dementia and related cognitive disorders. One cannot be anything other than amazed at the breadth of treatments that are available for the management of Alzheimer's disease. Having said that, we have not quite reached, in the public's mind, the level of successful intervention associated with other medical disorders. It may be simply that the question posed, *'will there be a cure for Alzheimer's disease?'* is as naive as the same question relating to a cure for cancer. It may be that the heterogeneity of Alzheimer's disease in itself has not yet been fully appreciated. Matching the array of treatments to the different subtypes of the disease is an achievable and laudable aim.

The editors have put together a very fine compendium and with characteristic thoroughness, clarity of purpose and perspicacity and with the writing skills of their contributors, have achieved a magnificent contribution to the field.

*Professor Alistair Burns*
*Professor of Old Age Psychiatry*
*University of Manchester*
*Manchester, UK, 2006*

# Preface

The global dementia epidemic is among the top three public health challenges to confront humanity at the start of the 21st century, as the number of people who have dementia doubles to 40 million by 2020 and quadruples to 80 million in 2040 [1]. Over the last thirty years much has been learned about the provision of effective health services for people with dementia and their carers, the national Alzheimer associations affiliated to Alzheimer's Disease International have raised public and professional awareness of dementia around the world, behavioural and psychological symptoms of dementia have been recognised as a vital field for research and management, symptomatic treatments for Alzheimer's disease have been developed and marketed, and understanding of the pathophysiology of the common dementias has advanced to a point where effective disease modifying therapies are expected within a few years [2]. However, much remains to be done, and given the rapid expansion of the population of people with dementia and those who look after them, it will be necessary for the providers of healthcare and those who are engaged in research on dementia to run very hard, indeed if we are just to stand still and not be submerged by the rising tide of need. In this book, we and our contributors have attempted to provide an overview of the worldwide effort to cope with dementia by producing an up-to-date account of available treatments and interventions for all aspects of dementia, as well as outlining the nature of recent developments, which should lead to more effective therapies in the near future. Current and evolving therapeutic options, including anti-amyloid therapies, neuroprotective strategies, and symptomatic treatments (both pharmacological and non-pharmacological) all are discussed, and the pharmacoeconomics of treating dementia are addressed in detail.

We would like to thank Clinical Publishing, whose approach to us has resulted in what we think is a timely and comprehensive volume that addresses an area of enormous need. We have been very much impressed by the efficiency and enthusiasm of our publisher, which has led to an extremely short turnaround from the submission of edited manuscripts to final publication of this text. We also thank the individual contributors whose submission on schedule of the high quality chapters which follow has made our job as editors an easy and enjoyable task. Roz Seath processed a seemingly endless stream of edited manuscripts with cheerful enthusiasm; this book could not have been assembled without her efficient aid. We hope that readers will find *Therapeutic Strategies in Dementia* to be useful in their practice and research and that they will tell us how to make the second edition even better.

*Craig Ritchie, David Ames, Colin Masters, Jeffrey Cummings*
*London, Melbourne, Los Angeles*
*2006*

## REFERENCES

1. Ferri C, Prince M, Brayne C *et al*. Global prevalence of dementia: a Delphi consensus study. *Lancet* 2005; 366:2112–2117.
2. Burns A, O'Brien JT, Ames D. *Dementia*, 3rd edition, London, Hodder Arnold.

# Section I

## Current pharmacological approaches in dementia

# 1

# Cholinesterase inhibitors: synthesis of meta-analysis/randomized controlled trials

*C. W. Ritchie*

## INTRODUCTION

### *DO THE CURRENT TREATMENTS FOR ALZHEIMER'S DISEASE WORK?*

One approach to answering this question and perhaps the most conventional in an 'evidence-based medicine' medical culture is by conducting meta-analyses.

In terms of 'level of evidence', the meta-analysis is considered strongest [1]. However, whilst achieving much statistically by aggregating trials and synthesizing data to achieve greater precision of outcome estimates, the meta-analysis usually achieves only a very narrow conclusion. Also, by aggregating data from a variety of sources, meta-anlayses can miss out particular effects in subsample populations. Finally, because meta-analysis combines data from different sources, the meta-analysis is only as reliable as the data from which it is drawn.

If the condition being treated has a single (usually biological) outcome, then both trials and subsequent meta-analyses of trials will achieve the primary aim of meta-analyses, i.e. to answer 'does the drug work?'. For example, if the disease is due to an infection, then a meta-analysis of a new antimicrobial would combine trials looking at the efficacy of the drug in removing the underlying bacteria. This could be tested by the return of negative cultures after a certain duration of treatment. In this case, clear, relevant biological outcomes and a simple trial design are used, making interpretation of the meta-analysis straightforward.

How do we define a positive outcome in treating Alzheimer's disease (AD) though? Is it to be cognitive, functional, behavioural, quality of life, biological, mortality, avoidance of institutionalization, reduced carer stress, global clinical impression or neuropsychiatric? It is clear that in a complex illness such as AD, a positive outcome means different things to different parties. This efficacy vs. effectiveness [2] dilemma (Figure 1.1) has been underpinning the unenviable challenge that groups like the UK's National Institute for Health and Clinical Excellence (NICE) have been facing in describing whether AD treatments are 'effective' [3] and this is articulated in the chapter by Colin Green in this book. A further criticism of AD clinical trials has been levelled (usually without offering any sensible solution) which criticizes the design of the trials themselves and their analysis. The main thrust of the collective criticism is that analysis of data from conditions that are associated with inevitable decline would favour treatments that cause high dropout early in the trial if the standard 'last observation carried forward' method of imputing data is used. There are also criticisms of trials that last only several months in a condition that clinically usually lasts up to 10 years.

---

**Craig W. Ritchie**, MB ChB, MRCPsych, MSc, Director of Clinical Trials, Metabolic and Clinical Trials Unit, Department of Mental Health Sciences, Royal Free and University College Medical School, London, UK

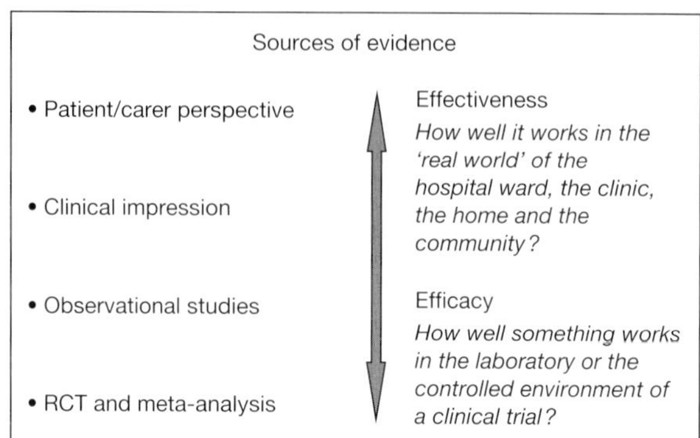


**Figure 1.1** Advantages and disadvantages of level of evidence in determining efficacy and effectiveness.

Whilst it is easy to identify problems, it is much harder to find solutions. Sensitivity analysis of data is often used whereby different methods of imputing missing data are compared with observed cases to determine if the type of analysis used affects the conclusions drawn from the trial. It is also clear that the longer the study the higher the dropout from double-blind randomized controlled trials (RCTs). To achieve a study of long duration (over 12 months) which is placebo-controlled could also be considered unethical. Finally, regulatory authorities have set guidelines for the necessary duration and outcome from clinical trials [4, 5], it is hard to criticize a sponsoring pharmaceutical company for designing trials to try and meet the criteria set down by others.

The ongoing debate about trial design, the modest efficacy of current treatments, the heterogeneity of the condition clinically and the vast array of relevant outcomes has meant that there is still much uncertainty regarding the answer to the question; 'do the drugs work?'

This chapter will present the findings from recent published meta-analysis and systematic reviews as well as summarizing and discussing their findings.

## *META-ANALYSES OF AD TRIALS*

### *Method of review*

There have been numerous meta-analyses conducted including the comprehensive and regularly updated meta-analyses of the Cochrane collaboration. They often focus on a particular question, e.g. neuropsychiatric symptoms or comparison of drugs. Table 1.1 lists the various publications and their main conclusions. To be included in this review, the publication has to be at least a systematic review (i.e. contains explicit and appropriate search criteria for papers), though some will include meta-analysis. The papers included will only be those that consider licensed, specific treatments for AD, i.e. donepezil (Aricept®), galantamine (Reminyl®), rivastigmine (Exelon®) and memantine (Ebixa®/Namenda®).

### *Findings from review*

Despite the distinct pharmacotherapy of the acetylcholinesterase inhibitors (AChEIs), they show remarkable similarity in terms of their cognitive efficacy. Differentiating between them based on tolerability would currently favour donepezil. However, as there is no observable dose effect with galantamine in terms of efficacy, it would appear that with dose titration to 16 mg a day, tolerability differences should not be clinically relevant. The suggestion that there may be a build-up of effect with galantamine over time noted in the Cochrane review, supports findings (unpublished) in the Ritchie meta-analysis (Figure 1.2). In the absence of any double-blind RCTs beyond 24 weeks with galantamine, it is impossible

**Table 1.1** A summary of the various publications looking at meta-analyses of AD

| *Drugs* | *Type* | *Aim* | *Conclusions* | *Authors' comments* | *Comments* |
|---|---|---|---|---|---|
| *Farlow et al.* [6] Rivastigmine | MA | Effect of Riva on cognitive 'rapid progression' of AD | Rapid progression over 26 weeks on placebo of ≥4 points on ADAS-Cog is associated with better response to Riva than less rapid progression | | Efficacy data was from open-label extension<br>Meta-analysis limited to ADAS-Cog as efficacy measure |
| *Kaduszkiewicz et al.* [7] Donepezil, Galantamine, Rivastigmine | SR | To examine 'efficacy' of AChEIs in AD | Showed efficacy for each drug in cognition and (where measured) global clinical change | Critical of methodology because of 'multiple testing' and 'exclusion of patients following randomization' | Authors' criticism of multiple testing is wrong when test of primary aim, do not need to correct $\alpha$<br>No meta-analysis conducted that would have helped and could have 'corrected' through weighting of trials<br>Imperfect trial design does not necessarily mean drugs lack efficacy |
| *Lingler et al.* [8] Donepezil, Galantamine, Rivastigmine | MA | Examine caregiver-specific outcomes | Four trials used in burden and six in time spent satisfied criteria. Don most frequently investigated. Small beneficial effects noted in both reducing caregiver burden and reducing time spent with patient | Small number of trials recording such 'important' outcomes<br>Included in analysis of unlicensed treatments | Improvement and consistent measurement of this outcome is becoming standard in newer licensing trials |

**Table 1.1** (Continued)

| | | | | | |
|---|---|---|---|---|---|
| *Gauthier et al.* [9] Memantine | MA | Effect specifically on NPI | Two trials included (one in combination with Don). Mem especially good for agitation/aggression and may reduce emergence of new symptoms over time | Aggression/agitation effect important due to impact of this symptom on carers. Mem may reduce the need for neuroleptic medication | Mechanism of action of Mem on this symptom merits further investigation and whether it is a specific effect of an NMDA antagonist |
| *Passmore et al.* [10] Donepezil | PA | Effect on cognition and global function in both AD and VaD | Clinical efficacy in both AD and VaD | AD benefit due to decline on placebo, whereas VaD benefit due to improvement in active treatment | Unclear from paper where the 'data' for this trial were sourced from though conclusions entirely consistent with other meta-analyses |
| *Harry and Zakzanis* [11] Donepezil, Galantamine | MA | Comparison between these 2 drugs on impact on cognition | Both drugs of modest though comparable efficacy with regard to cognition | Cohen D scores of $\sim$0.5 for both drugs suggest low to modest efficacy. Suggests functional outcomes (not reported) more relevant though | Several Don papers used in other published meta-analyses not included in this review, though this had no effect upon conclusions |
| *Livingston and Katona* [12] Memantine | PA/NNT | Derivation of NNT from rates of change in RCTs | Two trials used after data supplied by sponsor companies. NNT for global outcome were 3 and 6; cognitive outcome = 7; ADLs = 4 and 8. NNH comparable with placebo. Beneficial NNH for agitation | Mem of moderate efficacy by standard interpretation of NNTs. Trials only in severe AD. Advocate trials specifically on carer and BPSD outcomes | Strength of sourcing data from sponsor company to generate NNT/NNH. The effect on agitation consistent with Gauthier *et al.* is noteworthy |

| | | | | | |
|---|---|---|---|---|---|
| *Ritchie et al.* [13] Donepezil, Galantamine, Rivastigmine | RMA | Compare drugs on ADAS-Cog, CGI and dropout rate | All drugs equally efficacious. Low doses of Gal as effective as higher doses but better tolerated. Don across dose range had similar dropout rates to low dose Riva and Gal. Dose effect observed with Don | Improved tolerability of Gal and Riva through longer dose titration | Only concurrent meta-analysis of cognitive efficacy and global change, though no conclusion about other outcomes. Regression analyses regarding dose consistent with Cochrane review of Gal. Remarkable homogeneity of results of separate trials |
| *Whitehead et al.* [14] Donepezil | SR (PA) | To evaluate safety and efficacy of Don in AD | Don effective in both global change and cognition. Tolerability was good | Higher doses of donepezil associated with greater efficacy on cognition at 24 weeks. No effect on CGI by dose, nor at 12 weeks on ADAS | Same analysis set as Passmore *et al.* Greater efficacy at higher doses of Don on AD consistent with Ritchie *et al.* [13] through meta-regression analysis that combined 12-week and 24-week data |
| *Lanctot et al.* [15] Donepezil, Galantamine, Rivastigmine | MA/ NNT | Quantitative summary of efficacy and safety data | Results were initially polled and showed NNT~12. Tolerability with Don was best and Gal worst | Tolerability of Gal probably related to higher doses and more rapid titration in trials than used now clinically | Did not find a dose effect, but did not split analysis by dose and drug. However high dose effects were heterogeneous which may have been explained by the Don dose effect observed elsewhere |
| *Trinh et al.* [16] Donepezil, Galantamine, Rivastigmine | MA | To examine the effect of AChEIs on NPI and function | NPI and ADAS-Noncog used for measuring neuropsychiatric symptoms. AChEIs have a modest effect on both neuropsychiatric and functional outcomes | Author's advocate long-term studies to assess the benefit of improvement in these measures on function, quality of life, carer stress and institutionalization | MA included several AChEIs not licensed or not now used to treat AD |

**Table 1.1** (Continued)

| | | | | | |
|---|---|---|---|---|---|
| *Areosa et al.* [17]<br>Memantine | MA | Cochrane review to determine efficacy and safety of memantine for people with AD, VaD and mixed dementia. (Only AD results considered here) | *Cognition*<br>In moderate to severe disease, the SIB statistically improved and in mild to moderate disease the ADAS improved<br>*CGI*<br>In both mild to moderate and moderate to severe disease, CGI data supports efficacy | Two unpublished trials (where results are known) could negate positive findings in mild to moderate disease | Mem has shown benefit across a range of AD symptoms. The effect on agitation is again noteworthy |
| | | | *Other*<br>In moderate to severe disease ADLs and behaviour improved by Mem. NPI improved in mild to moderate disease, but no effect on ADLs in moderate patients | Beneficial effect of Mem on agitation both as part of NPI and as an emergent AE was confirmed in this analysis | |
| *Birks and Harvey* [18]<br>Donepezil | MA | Cochrane review to assess whether Don improves well-being | *Cognition*<br>Significant effect at both 5 mg and 10 mg – though no dose effect noted. Also effective up to 52 weeks<br>*CGI*<br>Significant effect at both 5 mg and 10 mg – though no dose effect noted | Combined with lower cost and better safety, authors consider that 5 mg may be optimal dose as consider that improved efficacy at 10 mg may be artefact of higher drop out at this dose | Non-significant effect of higher dose Don inconsistent with both Ritchie *et al.* and Whitehead *et al.* The greater drop out rate on 10 mg and its effect on cognitive outcome does not seem to have been tested statistically |
| | | | *Other*<br>Benefits noted in ADLs and behaviour though not on QOL. Safety was neutral with 5 mg though worse for 10 mg | The higher dropout with 10 mg may have explained the numercially better effect of Don at 10 mg | |

| | | | | | |
|---|---|---|---|---|---|
| *Loy and Schneider* [19]<br>Galantamine | MA | Cochrane review to assess whether Gal improves well-being | *Cognition*<br>No effect of 8 mg a day and 16 mg to 36 mg a day showed consistent effects<br>*CGI*<br>No effect of 8 mg a day and 16 mg to 36 mg a day showed consistent effects<br>*Other*<br>Other outcomes seldom tended to show benefit<br>Tolerability was dose-dependent | Suggestion that increased duration of treatment generated additional benefit | Findings consistent with Ritchie *et al.* that suggested no additional efficacy benefit with Gal over doses of 16 mg a day. As tolerability is dose dependent then optimal dose of Gal should be 16 mg. Interesting finding of increasing efficacy at 24 weeks compared to 12 weeks suggesting an accumulation of efficacy over time |
| *Birks et al.* [20]<br>Rivastigmine | MA | Cochrane review to determine the clinical efficacy and safety of Riva for patients with AD | *Cognition*<br>ADAS-Cog/MMSE improved by both low (1–4 mg) and higher dose (6–12 mg) Riva<br>*CGI*<br>Low dose Riva as effective as higher dose is<br>*Other*<br>Higher dose only improves ADLs. Higher doses associated with decreased tolerability | A small dose effect for ADAS may have been observed<br>No dose effect<br>Longer dose titrations associated with greater tolerability | Only higher doses, between 6 mg and 12 mg, are associated with efficacy across a range of outcomes that include CGI and ADLs. Cognitive efficacy similar at lower doses to higher doses. To achieve higher doses, titrations of up to 12 weeks may be necessary |

AChEIs = acetylcholinesterase inhibitors; ADAS-Cog = Alzheimer's Disease Assessment Scale – cognitive subscale; ADAS-Noncog = Alzheimer's Disease Assessment Scale – noncognitive subscale; ADLs = activities of daily living; AE = adverse event; BPSD = behavioural and psychological symptoms of dementia; CGI = clinical global impression; Don = donepezil; Gal = galantamine; MA = meta-analysis; Mem = memantine; NMDA = *N*-methyl-D-aspartate; NNT = number needed to treat analysis; NPI = Neuropsychiatric Inventory; PA = pooled analysis of individual patient data; QOL = cuality of life; Riva = rivastigmine; RMA = regression meta-analysis; SIB = severe impairment battery; SR = systematic review; VaD = vascular dementia.

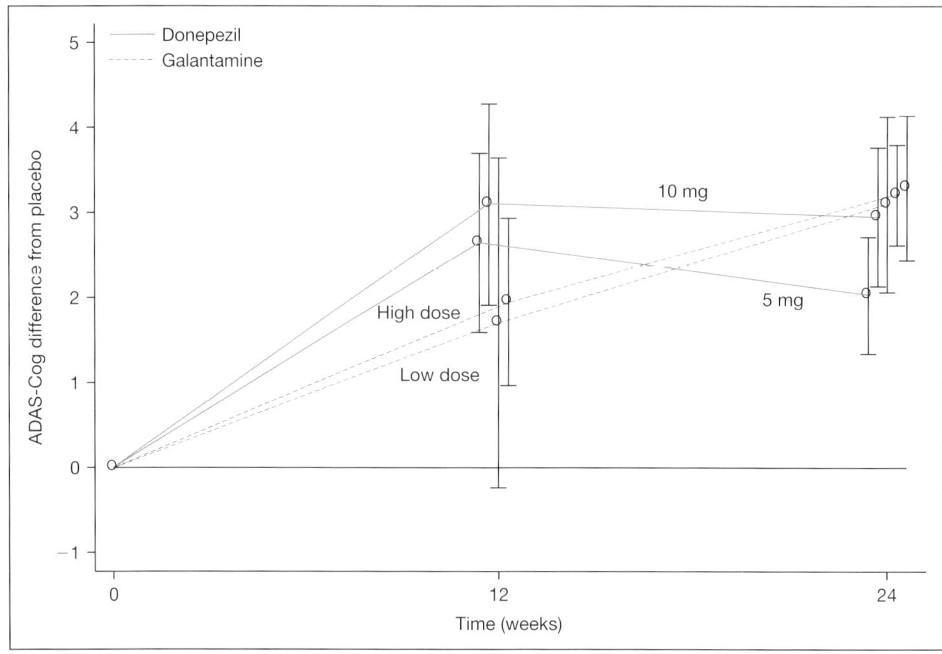


**Figure 1.2** Pooled effect estimates (95% CI) for donepezil and galantamine by dose and duration of study.

**Table 1.2** Summary of key findings from a review of the reviews

| | | |
|---|---|---|
| Donepezil | Effective at both 5 mg and 10 mg with some evidence of greater efficacy at 10 mg<br>Improved behaviour and ADLs though no effect on quality of life<br>May reduce caregiver burden<br>Well-tolerated with placebo rates of dropout at 5 mg | If dose effect and donepezil induces production of acetylcholinesterase (ref) then trials should investigate titrating doses above 10 mg |
| Galantamine | No dose effect on efficacy<br>Higher doses associated with reduced tolerability<br>Suggestion of build-up effect with longer treatment | Long-term double-blind RCTs necessary to confirm if galantamine has disease-modifying profile |
| Rivastigmine | Least well-tolerated and only higher doses effective<br>Dose titration and t.d.s. dosing may improve tolerability<br>May be of particular benefit in patients who are rapidly progressing | Head-to-head studies to determine if effect on rapid progression is specific to rivastigmine |
| Memantine | Effective only in moderate to severe disease<br>Very well-tolerated<br>Completely different class of drug suggests that may have role in combination with AChEIs<br>Very well-tolerated | Explanation of effect on agitation<br>Augmentation studies and specific studies (head-to-head) against neuroleptics for BPSD |

to be sure whether this accumulation of effect has maintained a characteristic that has been proposed as indicating an element of 'disease modification' [21].

Figure 1.2 also illustrates the similarity in effect estimation between doses of galantamine as well as the discrepancy between 5 mg and 10 mg doses of donepezil, most evident after 24 weeks of treatment.

The particular effect of memantine on agitation is also demonstrated consistently and merits further consideration through purposeful research of this clinical activity.

## SUMMARY

This review has limited itself to licensed drugs and has not considered meta-analysis of either unlicensed (selegiline [22], propentoffyline [23] and nicotine [24]) or experimental (clioquinol [25]) drugs (Table 1.2). A comprehensive review of ginkgo is included elsewhere in this book.

In general, while these drugs are only of modest efficacy in delaying clinical progression of disease, they are of benefit. AD is a fatal condition and delaying clinical progression even modestly may be of massive personal benefit to patients and carers as well as economic benefit to the wider community. Although not measurable in trials, an additional benefit of these licensed drugs has been to attract funding for and hope of finding a disease-modifying treatment for AD. The importance of the first step taken by AChEIs in the long journey towards finding a cure for AD cannot be measured scientifically, but should not be underestimated by society.

## REFERENCES


1. Centre for Evidence Based Medicine, Oxford. http://www.cebm.net/levels_of_evidence.asp#levels
2. Greenhalgh T. Papers that report drug trials. *Br Med J* 1997; 315:480–483.
3. National Institute of Clinical Excellence, UK. http://www.nice.org.uk/page.aspx?o=288826
4. Leber P. *Guidelines for Clinical Evaluation of Antidementia Drugs*. US Food and Drug Administration, Washington, DC.
5. European Agency for the Evaluation of Medicinal Products. Note for guidance on medicinal products in the treatment of Alzheimer's disease. http://www.emea.eu.int/pdfs/human/ewp/055395en.pdf; London, 1997.
6. Farlow MR, Small GW, Quarg P *et al*. Efficacy of rivastigmine in Alzheimer's disease patients with rapid disease progression: results of a meta-analysis. *Dement Geriatr Cogn Disord* 2005; 20:192–197.
7. Kaduszkiewicz H, Zimmerman T, Beck-Bornholdt HP *et al*. Cholinesterase inhibitors for patients with Alzheimer's disease: systematic review of randomized clinical trials. *BMJ* 2005; 331:321–327.
8. Lingler JH, Martire LM, Schulz R. Caregiver-specific outcomes in antidementia clinical drug trials: a systematic review and meta-anlaysis. *J Am Geriatr Soc* 2005; 53:983–990.
9. Gauthier S, Wirth Y, Mobius HJ. Effects of memantine on behavioural symptoms in Alzheimer's disease patients: analysis of the Neuropsychiatric Inventory (NPI) data of two randomized, controlled studies. *Int J Geriatr Psychiatry* 2005; 20:459–464.
10. Passmore AP, Bayer AJ, Steinhagen-Thiessen E. Cognitive, global, and functional benefits of donepezil in Alzheimer's disease and vascular dementia: results from large scale clinical trials. *J Neurol Sci* 2005; 229–230:141–146.
11. Harry RD, Zakzanis KK. A comparison of donepezil and galantamine in the treatment of cognitive symptoms of Alzheimer's disease: a meta-analysis. *Hum Psychopharmacol* 2005; 20:183–187.
12. Livingston G, Katona K. The place of memantine in the treatment of Alzheimer's disease: a number needed to treat analysis. *Int J Geriatr Psychiatry* 2004; 19:919–925.
13. Ritchie CW, Ames D, Clayton T *et al*. Metaanlaysis of randomized trials of the efficacy and safety of donepezil, galantamine, and rivastigmine for the treatment of Alzheimer's disease. *Am J Geriatr Psychiatry* 2004; 12:358–369.
14. Whitehead A, Perdomo C, Pratt RD *et al*. Donepezil for the symptomatic treatment of patients with mild to moderate Alzheimer's disease: a meta-analysis of individual patient data from randomized controlled trials. *Int J Geriatr Psychiatry* 2004; 19:624–633.

15. Lanctot KL, Herrmann N, Yau KK *et al.* Efficacy and safety of cholinesterase inhibitors in Alzheimer's disease: a meta-analysis. *Can Med Assoc J* 2003; 169:557–564.
16. Trinh NH, Hoblyn J, Mohanty S *et al.* Efficacy of cholinesterase inhibitors in the treatment of neuropsychiatric symptoms and functional impairment in Alzheimer's disease: a meta-analysis. *JAMA* 2003; 289:210–216.
17. Areosa SA, Sherriff F, McShane R. Memantine for dementia. *Cochrane Database Syst Rev* 2005; 3:CD003154.
18. Birks J, Harvey RJ. Donepezil for dementia due to Alzheimer's disease. *Cochrane Database Syst Rev* 2006; 1:CD001190.
19. Loy C, Schneider L. Galantamine for Alzheimer's disease and mild cognitive impairment. *Cochrane Database Syst Rev* 2006; 1:CD001747.
20. Birks J, Grimley Evans J, Iakovidou V *et al.* Rivastigmine for Alzheimer's disease. *Cochrane Database Syst Rev* 2006; 1:CD001191.
21. Maelicke A, Albuquerque EX. Allosteric modulation of nicotinic acetylcholine receptors as a treatment strategy for Alzheimer's disease. *Eur J Pharmacol* 2000; 393:165–170.
22. Birks J, Flicker L. Selegiline for Alzheimer's disease. *Cochrane Database Syst Rev* 2003; 1:CD000442.
23. Frampton M, Harvey RJ, Kirchner V. Propentofylline for dementia. *Cochrane Database Syst Rev* 2003; 2:CD002853.
24. Lopez-Arrieta JM, Rodriguez JL, Sanz F. Efficacy and safety of nicotine on Alzheimer's disease patients. *Cochrane Database Syst Rev* 2001; 2:CD001749.
25. Jenagaratnam L, McShane R. Clioquinol for the treatment of Alzheimer's disease. *Cochrane Database Syst Rev* 2006; 1:CD005380.

# 2

# Cholinesterase inhibitors: long-term studies

*R. Bullock*

## INTRODUCTION

Alzheimer's disease (AD) is characterized by a progressive loss of cognitive performance due to the degeneration of cortical neurones and the presence of amyloid plaques and tangles [1]. Memory impairment is the hallmark of AD, but other cognitive and language abilities are affected and functional ability also declines. The typical annual decline in untreated patients is reported to be 2–4 points on the Mini-mental State Examination (MMSE) [2], and 7 points on the Alzheimer's Disease Assessment Scale – cognitive subscale (ADAS-Cog) [3]. Initially, the more complex activities of daily living (ADL), such as handling finances, hobbies, and preparing meals, are increasingly impaired, but in the later stages there is a progressive loss of the more basic ADL, such as dressing and toileting [4]. Mood-related and psychiatric manifestations also become more notable as AD progresses [5]. Because of the progressive nature of the disease, an important aim is to stabilize and delay progression of these symptoms, ideally beyond the 6 months reported in randomized controlled trials.

The cholinesterase inhibitors (ChEIs) – donepezil, rivastigmine and galantamine – have demonstrated efficacy in large, 6-month, double-blind, placebo-controlled trials. This has been acknowledged by both the National Institute for Health and Clinical Excellence (NICE) in the UK and the American Academy of Neurology in their respective guidelines [6, 7] leading to widespread use for the symptomatic treatment of patients with mild-to-moderate AD. Over the past few years, data from extension studies to these original trials have emerged, suggesting that these agents may confer long-term benefits. This includes data on cognitive performance in patients remaining on rivastigmine for up to 5 years ($n = 83$), donepezil for up to 4.9 years ($n = 18$) and galantamine for up to 4 years ($n = 185$). The majority of these data come from open-label studies and so need to be interpreted with caution. However, the data appear to suggest that patients, caregivers and physicians will see some decline on ChEIs after a period of stabilization, but this appears to be slower and later than that expected in untreated patients. This appears to be true across all the recognized domains of AD (when measured) – not restricted solely to cognition. Importantly, in terms of the continuation of individual autonomy, function is often seen to be relatively preserved, even where cognitive scores are falling. So, in spite of the accepted limitations of these current data, the information summarized in this chapter may help practising clinicians assess

**Roger Bullock**, MBBS, Director and Principal Investigator, Kingshill Research Centre, Victoria Hospital, Swindon, UK

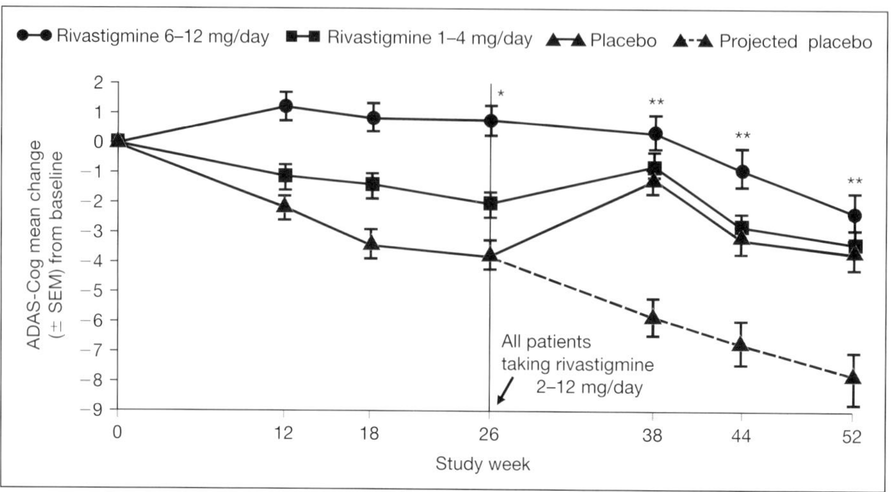


**Figure 2.1** Delayed start model to show 1-year effects of rivastigmine on cognition: ADAS-Cog. $*P \leq 0.001$ vs. placebo, $**P \leq 0.001$ vs. projected placebo. Adapted from Farlow *et al.* [21].

the relevance of the long-term value of using ChEIs in selected patients in this consistently progressive disease.

## THE DIFFICULTY IN PERFORMING LONG-TERM STUDIES WITH CHOLINESTERASE INHIBITORS

Randomized studies may offer the highest standard of data, but long-term placebo control in a degenerative condition does cause ethical dilemmas [8]. This means that most of the published evidence is non-controlled, open-label in nature and thus limited in its interpretation. Various methodological designs have attempted to add internal validity – the commonest being the 'delayed start' or the use of historical comparators.

The delayed start refers to 12-month studies where the first 6 months are randomized to placebo or treatment and the second 6 months sees everybody on treatment (Figure 2.1). This means that some participants receive 52 weeks of treatment, while others, after a 26-week delay then receive only 26 weeks of the same treatment. Comparisons of what happens after this delay, particularly whether this group fail to 'catch up' with those who have treatment throughout has posed questions about potential effects on disease progression. These are yet to be answered, but it does appear that while the individual benefits may be similar from wherever you start, any losses made while waiting to start are not made up over and above that effect. This suggests that acetyl ChEIs (AChEIs) do delay clinical decline *via* their symptomatic effects.

Historical and modelled data have also been used to predict placebo decline [9] (Figure 2.2). The difficulty here is matching the baseline demographics accurately. What the method achieves is a comparison of open–label findings to an expected outcome, based in part on a data driven model. The problem with this is when the line generated for the untreated group is taken too factually as it is not real or part of the same experiment. What is hoped for is that the treatment arm remains above the modelled line – supporting the notion of delay in decline. However, if the lines diverge, this may be an indication of slowing in disease progression, a desirable outcome, but not one that can be reliably demonstrated by this form of analysis.

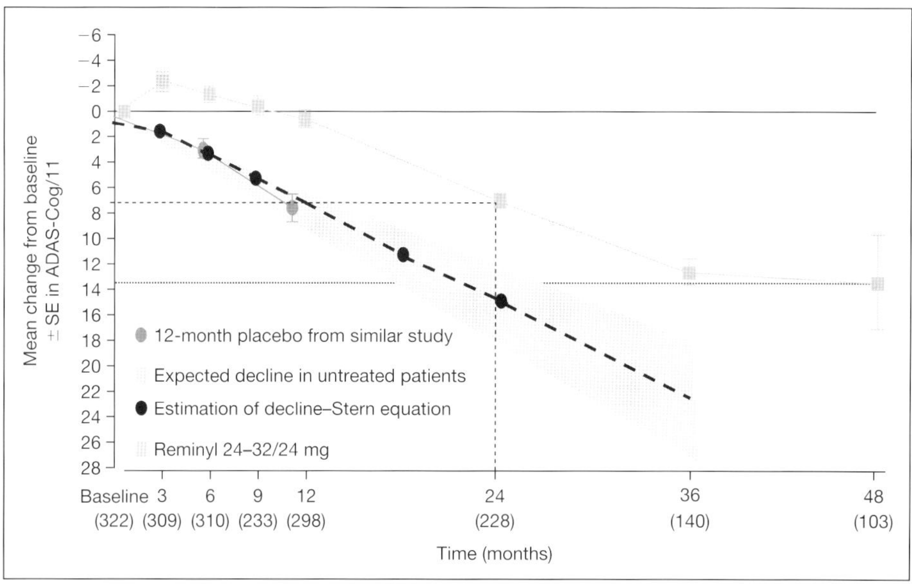


**Figure 2.2** The use of historical data and modelling in long-term studies of ChEIs.

Another factor to consider is the analysis type used on the study and in particular how dropouts were handled. Premature withdrawals may lead to incomplete drug efficacy and underestimation of drug effect. However, early dropout may also select out and leave in the study those who are doing best, thus overestimating the effect. The most conservative measure is the intention to treat (ITT) analysis where all randomized patients are included and their last observation is carried forward (LOCF). This does have some problems in degenerative disease though, because here early dropouts may still add to overestimation of effect, because they will show no change rather than any decline – irrespective of any treatment. The alternative analysis is to compare the completers alone with the 'control'. This is an observed case analysis. Some writers suggest this is preferable, though in general it should favour treatment, as only the best performers will be analysed. An ITT–LOCF analysis is still probably the more reliable report, provided sufficient numbers start the study.

In terms of withdrawals, the rates in published studies with ChEIs in AD are broadly similar, though difficult to compare as the number of studies reported for each drug varies considerably. A cautionary note is that the rates are all higher than audits of clinical practice published from the UK and USA and also are over shorter periods of treatment than most clinicians aim to achieve, which in many centres is further elongated by the practice of switching to a different ChEI should one fail due to efficacy or tolerability issues.

## LONG-TERM STUDIES OF CHOLINESTERASE INHIBITORS

### *DONEPEZIL*

Donepezil is an inhibitor of acetylcholinesterase (AChE) [10]. It is licensed for the treatment of mild-to-moderate AD. Two 52-week placebo-controlled studies of donepezil in mild-to-moderate AD have been carried out [11, 12]. In the first, 431 patients with moderate AD (mean baseline MMSE 17.1) underwent a survival design study (Figure 2.3). Most benefits of donepezil appeared early in the study, but then faded over time. Nevertheless, using LOCF analysis, the total mean scores on the MMSE, the functional outcome and the Clinical

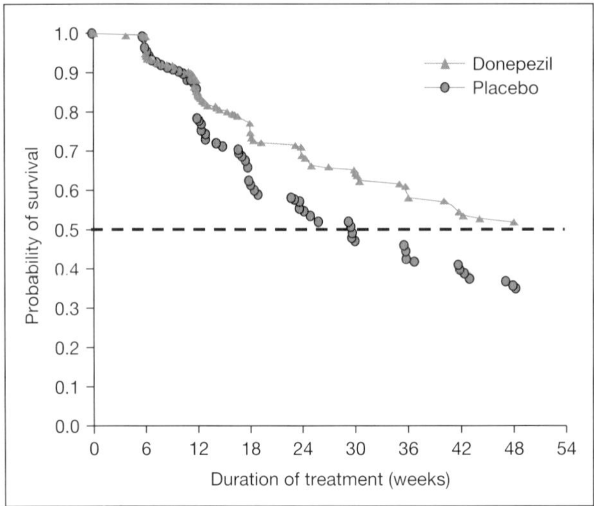


**Figure 2.3** Long-term effects of donepezil on preservation of function. Adapted from Mohs *et al.* [11].

Dementia Rating – Sum of Boxes (CDR–SB) were superior to placebo at endpoint [11]. The median time to clinically meaningful decline was delayed by 5 months on donepezil and this group were 38% less likely to deteriorate than those on placebo over the year of the study. In the second study of 286 patients with mild-to-moderate AD, donepezil provided initial symptomatic benefits that appeared to wane over time [12]. The primary outcome measure – the Gottfries–Bråne–Steen scale – did not reach statistical significance at the study end (LOCF population), even though at 24, 36 and 52 weeks it had a statistical advantage over placebo.

The results of a 144-week open-label extension of two US 6-month placebo-controlled studies were reported by Doody *et al.* [13]. Seven hundred and sixty-three patients with a mean baseline MMSE of 19.4 were recruited and scores for analysis were calculated from observed cases. Although 50% of the patients dropped out of the study over the first 108 weeks, continued donepezil treatment in the remaining patients resulted in improved ADAS-Cog scores relative to baseline for 24 weeks, after which the scores declined for the remainder of the study. By the end of the study, subgroups of patients who received placebo in the original two studies (followed by donepezil during the open-label extension) declined by 13–18 points on the ADAS-Cog, whereas scores of those who originally received donepezil (and then continued on with it) declined by 10–12 points. The rate of decline in both groups was within the range expected for untreated patients (4–6 points per annum). No modelling or historical comparison was made in this study.

A retrospective review of 130 patients receiving donepezil + vitamin E for up to 3 years compared clinical outcomes with historical untreated patients from an established AD database. The cognitive performance of patients remaining in the study at 3 years declined by 33% less than that reported in historical patients. MMSE scores fell by 6.3 points in the donepezil + vitamin E group, compared with 9.1 points in the historical patients [14]. These findings suggest that donepezil + vitamin E may slow cognitive decline in AD patients remaining on treatment over this period. No attempt to distinguish between the effects of the two individual agents was made.

The AD2000 Collaborative Group [15] published results of a planned 4-year study of donepezil – although only one patient was available for assessment at the end of those 4 years. A range of endpoints was considered, including institutionalization, progression of disability, cognitive performance, ADL, behavioural symptoms, caregiver burden and health economics. This study was placebo-controlled, and could have offered the opportunity to obtain robust data on the long-term benefits of cholinesterase inhibition. However, the study was underpowered for many of its endpoints [16, 17], suboptimal doses were used in the majority of patients (5 mg instead of 10 mg) and the (non-clinical practice) use of regular 4-week washout periods led to the study failing. Many patients did not recover from the 'crashes' experienced during these washout periods, and an insufficient number of participants were studied to enable detection of statistically significant differences. This led to reported findings that minimal benefits were seen in the donepezil group, compared with those in the placebo group, and that no delay was reported in reaching the severe cognitive disability milestone of MMSE <10. However, the cognitive and functional data at 2 years remained significantly better than placebo, very much in keeping with published open-label studies in donepezil and all the other AChEIs.

Rogers *et al.* [18] reported results of an open-label study that followed up patients involved in an initial 14-week randomized study of 161 participants for up to 4.9 years. In total, 133 patients enrolled in the open-label extension study, and the population fell to 18 patients by the time the study was terminated at week 254. Therefore, long-term data were based only on a small number of patients and should be interpreted with caution. Improvements on ADAS-Cog relative to baseline (at entry into the double-blind studies) were described for remaining patients until week 38, but a gradual decline relative to baseline was then observed in patients remaining in the study at week 50. Cognitive deterioration over the full study period was fairly consistent, with a mean annual decline of at least 6 points on ADAS-Cog. Because untreated patients may be expected to decline by 7 points each year on the ADAS-Cog, this suggests that, following initial symptomatic improvements, cognitive decline was largely unaffected. Similarly, MMSE and CDR-SB scores also remained close to baseline until week 26, before declining at expected rates.

### *RIVASTIGMINE*

Rivastigmine is an inhibitor of both AChE and butyrylcholinesterase (BuChE) [19], both enzymes responsible for regulating the neurotransmitter acetylcholine (ACh) in the human brain [20]. It is licensed for the treatment of mild-to-moderate AD. Farlow *et al.* [21] reported the results of a 52-week 'delayed start' rivastigmine study in 533 participants with mild-to-moderate AD (Figure 2.4). For the first 26 weeks, patients received either placebo or rivastigmine. Following this, patients were then eligible to receive open-label rivastigmine for a further 26 weeks. There was a significant treatment difference of 5.7 points with rivastigmine on ADAS-Cog for patients remaining on rivastigmine for 52 weeks ($P < 0.001$), as compared with the projected decline, using the Stern statistical model [9], as if they had been left 'untreated'. In addition, patients who received placebo for the first 26 weeks and were then commenced on rivastigmine for weeks 27–52 did not 'catch up' with those who were on rivastigmine from the beginning of the study (1.4-point difference on ADAS-Cog). These effects of rivastigmine on cognition were showed to persist for up to 2 years in a meta-analysis of 2010 AD patients entered in to four pivotal 26-week, placebo-controlled studies that were followed on by open-label extensions [22] (note: this includes the aforementioned study by Farlow). This demonstrated that the patients remaining on rivastigmine for up to 2 years showed 4–5 points less decline on the ADAS-Cog, compared with the Stern projected decline, than if they had received no treatment.

Recently, this meta-analysis was 'updated' by looking at the patients who had remained on treatment for up to 5 years [23] (Figure 2.4). These data represent the longest period of such efficacy data for any ChEI to date. Even though only 83 patients continued to remain under study conditions at this time, these data can be considered useful, because normally most patients would tend to have discontinued ChEI treatment over time [24, 25].

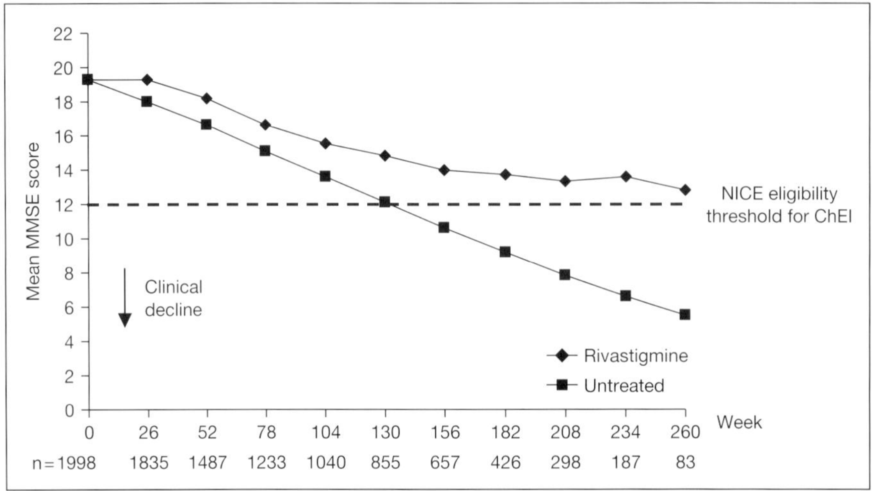


**Figure 2.4** Rivastigmine – efficacy (MMSE) data over 5 years.

However, what this 5-year study demonstrated was the continued relative preservation of cognition. Mean baseline MMSE and ADAS-Cog scores at entry into the placebo-controlled studies were 19.3 and 24.6, respectively. Mean MMSE and ADAS-Cog scores of patients remaining on rivastigmine for 5 years were 12.7 and 36.8 (both fitting into the 'moderate' AD range). Thus, patients remaining on rivastigmine for 5 years declined on average by 1.7 points each year on the MMSE and 3.9 points each year on ADAS-Cog. These cognitive declines were smaller than those predicted using baseline-dependent models of 'untreated' patients, and smaller than those reported for untreated patients in the literature [2, 3].

## GALANTAMINE

Galantamine is an inhibitor of AChE, but also has a reported allosteric action on the nicotinic receptor *in vitro* [26]. It is licensed for the treatment of mild-to-moderate AD. Raskind *et al.* [27] reported the results of an open-label extension study using galantamine in 636 patients who received placebo or galantamine 24 or 32 mg/day during the double-blind phase (weeks 1–26); after which 353 patients received galantamine 24 mg/day during the open-label phase (weeks 27–52). At 26 weeks both galantamine groups were superior to placebo, but by the study end, benefits in the 32 mg/day group were equivocal, whereas the group that had received galantamine 24 mg/day for the full study period maintained ADAS-Cog scores near baseline. A similar response was seen in ADL, as measured by the Disability Assessment for Dementia (DAD) scale. Raskind *et al.* [28] further showed that cognitive benefits of galantamine may be maintained for up to 3 years, as shown by an analysis of the completing 194 AD patients taking part in two 26-week placebo-controlled studies followed by open-label extension studies (including the original 52-week study by Raskind *et al.* [27]). This does mean that half of the patients were lost during this study due to dropouts, so results need to be interpreted with caution. However, 18% of those who finished the study still had maintained baseline cognitive function, though when considering the means, ADAS-Cog scores fell by 10.2 points in patients remaining on treatment for 3 years. A further analysis of these patients showed that over 4 years ($n$ = 185), the mean change on ADAS-Cog was 12.8 points in patients remaining on treatment [29] (Figure 2.5). These 3- and 4-year data suggested that cognitive decline in patients remaining on galantamine was 50% less than the predicted cognitive decline for untreated patients.

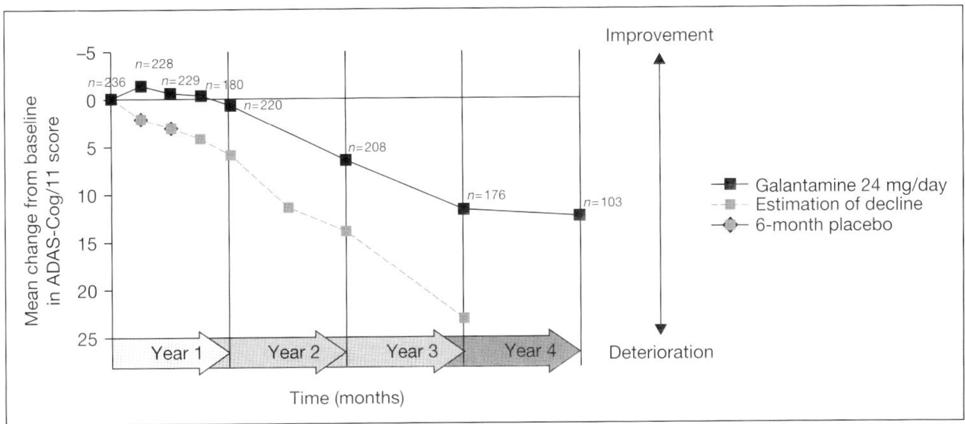


**Figure 2.5** Galantamine delays decline in cognitive function in 40% of treated participants for up to 4 years.

Another extension study was performed on the original Tariot *et al.* [30] 5-month pivotal study. Here 333 patients were followed up for 18 months after all commencing 24 mg at the end of the 5-month point. These patients started on placebo, 16 or 24 mg galantamine and by 4.5 months all had similar scores on the ADAS-Cog. They all then declined in parallel until the end of the study.

### *LONG-TERM COMPARATIVE STUDIES*

A 1-year rater blinded study comparing donepezil and galantamine using function as a primary endpoint showed the drugs to have similar efficacy, both crossing the baseline in this parameter at around 9 months [31]. In terms of cognition, galantamine had some statistical advantages, which appeared to reflect a superior effect on executive function – a measure that correlates with its additional nicotinic modulation.

A 2-year randomized head-to-head study of 998 patients given donepezil or rivastigmine, using the severe impairment battery as a primary endpoint also showed no difference between the two compounds at endpoint [32]. However, in subgroup analyses rivastigmine did appear of more benefit in patients younger than 75, those with potential Lewy body pathology and those with wild type BuChE genetics.

These two studies do confirm the clinical presumption that the drugs are very similar in effect, but also add to the impression that the differing pharmacology of the compounds may offer additional choice in certain circumstances.

## DISCUSSION

Data available to date are limited by the non-linear nature of AD and lack of long-term placebo-controlled studies. Withdrawal rates from long-term studies have tended to be high, leading to a considerable likelihood of positive selection bias, although data from galantamine studies shows that ADAS-Cog scores in both those who continue and the dropouts are not significantly different, suggesting that dropouts are not necessarily simply because of loss of effect [33] (Figure 2.6). Treatment withdrawal may also reflect unrealistic efficacy expectations and poor tolerability, as well as loss of efficacy or adverse effects emerging during the maintenance phase. Notwithstanding those points, results do need to be interpreted with caution, because they remain only applicable to relatively small subsets of patients who continued to remain in the studies for the duration. Nevertheless, data sug-

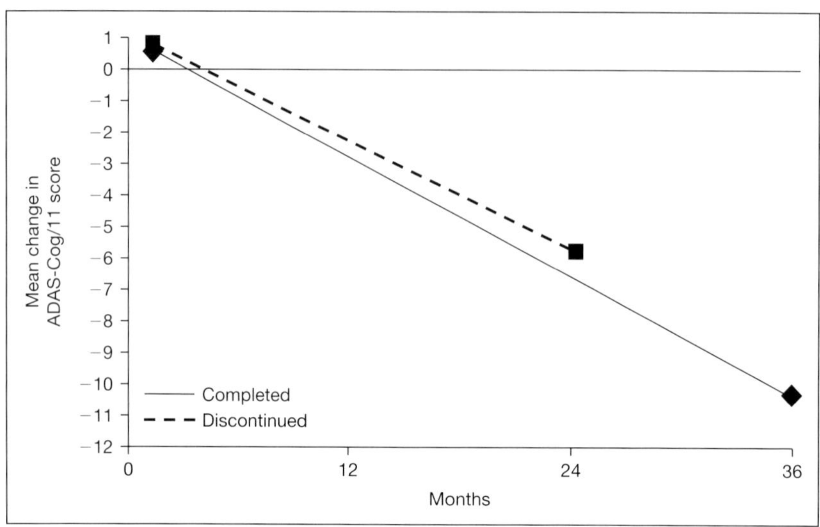


**Figure 2.6** Dropout analyses from galantamine study.

gest that cholinesterase inhibition may provide important benefits for patients remaining on treatment for up to 5 years.

This is useful for several reasons. Firstly, it does match clinical impression and experience. Secondly, at the individual level, any improvement is easily recognized, but the ongoing delay in symptomatology that these data imply persists, even in the presence of a continued decline, means that a person's autonomy continues to be relatively preserved. Finally, at a population level, this means that there is a net delay in reaching more advanced stages of AD, where much of the cost is incurred. It is postulated that a 2-year delay in progression of AD may reduce the prevalence of severe dementia by half [34] – clearly a desirable outcome. However, when the treatments are stopped, the person will then decline to the point where they would have been if left untreated. In effect then, symptomatic drugs may not have such a dramatic effect on reducing the prevalence of severe dementia – but they may shorten the length of time spent in this stage. Showing this is a key factor in cost-effectiveness arguments, as this stage is where admission to care homes is most likely. A retrospective analysis of patients participating in several of the galantamine studies which examined where they were residing after 7 years, showed that those who were exposed to galantamine for 3 years or more had half the chance of being in long-term care [35]. This effect was less in the UK than in the other seven countries studied (one reason why time to institutionalization is not a good outcome measure there). However, on an individual basis, what the symptomatic effect of these drugs undoubtedly achieves is an improvement in relevant symptoms and preservation of autonomy for a period of time in those people who respond favourably. What is now needed is a way of determining when the drug effect has diminished to the point that cessation does not produce any deterioration in the individual and further unnecessary prescribing of it does not continue. At this stage, other therapeutic strategies can be considered.

Evidence reviewed in this chapter from studies lasting up to 5 years suggests that patients receiving ChEIs all decline after a period of improvement or stability. With donepezil and galantamine, the rate of decline following the initial phase appears to be similar to the rate in untreated patients – though for an individual, this still means that the clinical symptoms are being kept above the expected untreated state. This was also demonstrated to be the case in the comparison study of these compounds [31]. The rate of decline with rivastigmine appears to be less than expected in the untreated state, which has led to suggestions of a slowing of disease as well as delay. This is yet to be proven – especially as in the 2-year comparison with donepezil, the total population outcomes on the cognitive scales were no different [32]. However, the subgroup analyses did suggest that the dual inhibition of both AChE and BuChE by rivastigmine may actually confer some additional effect, especially in younger patients with wild type BuChE genetics. If nothing else, at present this does imply that, through interpretation of randomized data, the compounds do behave differently in some clinical scenarios. It is not possible to make any other definitive comparisons across the other individual studies discussed in this chapter because of the variability in their methodology.

## SUMMARY

It is important for patients and caregivers to understand that they should not expect increasing improvements over the long term, but rather the aim is to maintain the patient's status at a manageable level, and for patients to 'continue to be as much as themselves as possible'. The studies all show that patients, caregivers and physicians will continue to see decline after a period of stabilization, but this will most likely be modified in some way from that which could have been expected if the patients were left untreated. For some this may last as long as five years. These findings appear to apply across several domains of AD – not simply cognition; with function especially sometimes continuing to be relatively preserved, even if cognitive scores are falling. Understanding the relevance and interactions of these complex measurements is the next task in determining what the best long term outcomes to measure will prove to be. Until then, ChEI treatment over the long term remains the necessary aim in the right patient.

## REFERENCES


1. Rosenstein LD. Differential diagnosis of the major progressive dementias and depression in middle and late adulthood: a summary of the literature of the early 1990s. *Neuropsychol Rev* 1998; 8:109–167.
2. Rainer M, Mucke HAM. Long-term cognitive benefits from galanthamine in Alzheimer's disease. *Int J Geriatr Psychopharmacol* 1998; 1:197–201.
3. Doraiswamy PM, Kaiser L, Bieber F, Garman RL. The Alzheimer's Disease Assessment Scale: evaluation of psychometric properties and patterns of cognitive decline in multicenter clinical trials of mild to moderate Alzheimer's disease. *Alzheimer Dis Assoc Disord* 2001; 15:174–183.
4. Gauthier S, Gelinas I, Gauthier L. Functional disability in Alzheimer's disease. *Int Psychogeriatr* 1997; 9(suppl 1):163–165.
5. Cummings JL, Kaufer D. Neuropsychiatric aspects of Alzheimer's disease: the cholinergic hypothesis revisited. *Neurology* 1996; 47:876–883.
6. Bryant J, Clegg A, Nicholson T *et al.* Clinical and cost-effectiveness of donepezil, rivastigmine and galantamine for Alzheimer's disease: a rapid and systematic review. *Health Technol Assess* 2001; 5:1–137.
7. Doody RS, Stevens JC, Beck C *et al.* Practice parameter: management of dementia (an evidence-based review). Report of the Quality Standards Subcommittee of the American Academy of Neurology. *Neurology* 2001; 56:1154–1166.
8. Kawas CH, Clark CM, Farlow MR *et al.* Clinical trials in Alzheimer's disease: debate on the use of placebo controls. *Alzheimer Dis Assoc Disord* 1999; 13:1124–1129.
9. Stern RG, Mohs RC, Davidson M *et al.* A longitudinal study of Alzheimer's disease: measurement, rate, and predictors of cognitive deterioration. *Am J Psychiatry* 1994; 151:390–396.
10. Weinstock M. Selectivity of cholinesterase inhibition. *CNS Drugs* 1999; 12:307–323.
11. Mohs RC, Doody RS, Morris JC *et al.* A 1-year, placebo-controlled preservation of function survival study of donepezil in AD patients. *Neurology* 2001; 57:481–488.
12. Winblad B, Engedal K, Soininen H *et al.* A 1-year, randomized, placebo-controlled, study of donepezil in patients with mild to moderate AD. *Neurology* 2001; 57:489–495.

13. Doody RS, Geldmacher DS, Gordon B *et al.* Open-label, multicenter, phase 3 extension study of the safety and efficacy of donepezil in patients with Alzheimer disease. *Arch Neurol* 2001; 58:427–433.
14. Klatte ET, Scharre DW, Nagaraja HN *et al.* Combination therapy of donepezil and vitamin E in Alzheimer disease. *Alzheimer Dis Assoc Disord* 2003; 17:113–116.
15. AD2000 Collaborative Group. Long-term donepezil treatment in 565 patients with Alzheimer's disease (AD) 2000: randomised double-blind trial. *Lancet* 2004; 363:2105–2115.
16. Bullock R, Passmore P, Wilkinson D *et al.* Participation in trials should be based on clinical uncertainty, not enforcement. *BMJ* 2000; 320:511.
17. Schneider L. AD2000: donepezil in Alzheimer's disease (Commentary). *Lancet* 2004; 363:2100–2101.
18. Rogers SL, Doody RS, Pratt RD, Leni JR. Long-term efficacy and safety of donepezil in the treatment of Alzheimer's disease: final analysis of a US multicentre open-label study. *Eur Neuropsychopharmacol* 2000; 10:195–203.
19. Darreh-Shori T, Almkvist O, Guan ZZ *et al.* Sustained cholinesterase inhibition in AD patients receiving rivastigmine for 12 months. *Neurology* 2002; 59:563–572.
20. Mesulam M, Guillozet A, Shaw P, Quinn B. Widely spread butyrylcholinesterase can hydrolyze acetylcholine in the normal and Alzheimer brain. *Neurobiol Dis* 2002; 9:88–93.
21. Farlow M, Anand R, Messina J Jr *et al.* A 52-week study of the efficacy of rivastigmine in patients with mild to moderately severe Alzheimer's disease. *Eur Neurol* 2000; 44:234–241.
22. Grossberg G, Irwin P, Satlin A *et al.* Rivastigmine in Alzheimer's disease: efficacy over two years. *Am J Geriatr Psychiatry* 2004; 12:420–431.
23. Small G, Kaufer K, Mendiondo MS, Quarg P, Spiegel R. Cognitive performance in Alzheimer's disease patients receiving rivastigmine for up to 5 years. *Int J Clin Pract* 2005; 59:473–477.
24. Tinklenberg J, Newkirk L, Thompson J. Donepezil treatment of Alzheimer's disease patients in California clinical practice: one-year follow-up. *14th Congress of the European College of Neuropsychopharmacology* (ECNP), 13–17 October 2001. Istanbul, Turkey (Abstract 444).
25. Cameron I, Curran S, Newton P *et al.* Use of donepezil for the treatment of mild–moderate Alzheimer's disease: an audit of the long-term cholinesterase inhibitor treatment of patients in routine clinical practice. *Int J Geriatr Psychiatry 2000*; 15:887–891.
26. Maelicke A. Allosteric sensitization of nicotinic receptors by galantamine, a new treatment strategy for Alzheimer's disease. *Biol Psychiatry* 2001; 49:279–288.
27. Raskind MA, Peskind ER, Wessel T *et al.* Galantamine in AD, a 6-month randomized placebo-controlled trial with a 6-month extension. *Neurology* 2000; 54:2261–2268.
28. Raskind MA, Peskind ER, Truyen L *et al.* The cognitive benefits of galantamine are sustained for at least 36 months: a long-term extension trial. *Arch Neurol* 2004; 61:252–256.
29. Burns A, Pirttila T, Gold M. 4-year safety and efficacy of galantamine in the treatment of Alzheimer's disease. *Poster presented at the 8th Congress of the European Federation of Neurological Societies (EFNS)*, Paris, France.
30. Morris JC, Kershaw P. Cognitive benefits of long term, continuous galantamine treatment in patients with Alzheimer's disease. *Poster presented at the 7th Geneva/Springfield symposium*, Geneva, Switzerland, 2002.
31. Wilcock G, Howe I, Coles H *et al.* A long-term comparison of galantamine and donepezil in the treatment of Alzheimer's disease. *Drugs Aging* 2003; 20:777–789.
32. Bullock R, Touchon J, Bergman H *et al.* Rivastigmine and donepezil treatment in moderate to moderately-severe Alzheimer's disease over a 2-year period. *Curr Med Res Opin* 2005; 21:1317–1328.
33. Raskind M. Cognition in AD: long-term treatment benefits. *Poster presented at the 8th International Montreal/Springfield Symposium on Advances in Alzheimer Therapy*, Montreal, Canada, 2004.
34. Brookmeyer R, Gray S, Kawas C. Predictions of Alzheimer's disease in the United States and public health impact of delaying onset. *Am J Public Health* 1998; 88:1377–1342.
35. Feldman H, Kavanagh S, Brashear R, van Baelen B. Effect of galantamine on time to residential or nursing home admission. *Poster presented at 8th EFNS*, Paris, France, 2004.

# 3

# Cholinesterase inhibitors: head-to-head studies

*R. W. Jones*

## INTRODUCTION

The cholinergic hypothesis, which states that one of the primary abnormalities in Alzheimer's disease (AD) is due to a deficiency in acetylcholine, has led to a number of therapeutic strategies. The most successful has been the development of cholinesterase inhibitors.

Four cholinesterase inhibitors – tacrine, donepezil, rivastigmine and galantamine – have been licensed for the treatment of mild to moderate AD. In 1993, tacrine became the first agent approved specifically for treating the cognitive symptoms of AD. Tacrine, an aminoacridine compound, became widely used in many countries including the USA, Sweden and France but was never marketed in the UK. It needed to be taken three or four times a day, was often poorly tolerated and caused a specific reversible hepatotoxicity. When donepezil became available in 1997 with its better tolerability and once daily dosing, not surprisingly it rapidly replaced tacrine as the drug of choice. Rivastigmine (since 1998) and galantamine (since 2000) are now also widely available, thus offering further options both to prescribers and to patients and carers.

A fifth drug, memantine, has been licensed since 2002 and is approved in Europe and the US for moderate to severe AD. In contrast to the cholinesterase inhibitors, memantine acts on another neurotransmitter glutamate and is a moderate affinity, uncompetitive antagonist at the *N*-methyl-D-aspartate receptor.

There have been no direct head-to-head comparisons either of tacrine with other cholinesterase inhibitors or of memantine with any of the cholinesterase inhibitors; neither tacrine nor memantine will therefore be discussed further in this chapter.

Donepezil is a piperidine-based reversible inhibitor of acetylcholinesterase that is highly selective for acetylcholinesterase with much less activity against butyrylcholinesterase. Red blood cell acetylcholinesterase inhibition at steady state was 64% with 5 mg/day and 77% with 10 mg/day. Inhibition up to 90% has been reported during long-term treatment with 10 mg/day [1]. Absorption is complete and neither food nor time of administration (morning or evening) influences the rate or extent of absorption. Peak plasma concentrations are reached after 3–4 h and steady state plasma levels after about 15 days. The effective dose range is 5–10 mg beginning with a single daily tablet of 5 mg and usually increasing after a minimum of 1 month to 10 mg according to efficacy and tolerability. Most patients are maintained on the maximum recommended daily dose of 10 mg [2, 3].

Rivastigmine is a centrally selective carbamate inhibitor of acetyl and butyrylcholinesterase. It forms a carbamylated complex with the enzyme and inactivates it for

**Roy W. Jones**, BSc (Hons), MBBS, Dip Pharm Med, FRCP, FFPM, Professor of Clinical Gerontology and Director, The Research Institute for the Care of the Elderly, St Martin's Hospital, Bath and School for Health, University of Bath, Bath, UK

about 10 h ('pseudo-irreversible' inhibition) despite a short plasma half-life of 1–2 h. A single 3 mg oral dose produces 30–40% inhibition of central acetylcholinesterase but minimal inhibition in the red cell or plasma. In contrast, it inhibits both acetyl and butyrylcholinesterase in the cerebrospinal fluid (CSF) to a similar extent [1]. Absorption is reported as rapid and complete, yet bioavailability increases with dose. Administration with food slows absorption and increases the area under the concentration–time curve by about 30%. Rivastigmine should be administered with food twice daily commencing at 1.5 mg b.d. (not a therapeutic dose) and increasing at a minimum of 2-weekly intervals to achieve the effective dose range of 3–6 mg b.d.

Galantamine is a phenanthrene alkaloid that is a reversible, competitive acetylcholinesterase inhibitor. Thirty–sixty percent inhibition of red blood acetylcholinesterase is obtained 30–45 min after oral galantamine [1]. Activity against acetylcholinesterase is more than 50-fold greater than inhibition of butyrylcholinesterase. In addition, galantamine is also an allosteric modulator of neuronal nicotinic receptors, a property that has been demonstrated in human nicotinic receptors expressed in cell lines [4]. The bioavailability of galantamine after oral administration is 85% with a plasma elimination half-life of about 6 h. One of the metabolites of galantamine is more active as an acetylcholinesterase inhibitor than the parent compound [1]. The relatively short half-life of galantamine requires twice-daily administration. Treatment should begin with 4 mg twice daily for 4 weeks following which the dose is increased to a clinically effective dose of 8 mg b.d.; the dose can be increased to 12 mg twice daily after a further 4 weeks. It is recommended that adequate fluid intake is ensured during treatment. More recently, a once-daily prolonged release capsule formulation of galantamine (8 mg, 16 mg and 24 mg) has been marketed.

There are numerous studies comparing each compound – donepezil, rivastigmine and galantamine – with placebo. Comparison of the relative efficacy and tolerability of the three compounds across clinical trials is inappropriate because of the different populations studied (with differing factors such as disease severity, comorbid conditions and concomitant medication use), differences in outcome measures, differences in safety evaluations and different dosing regimes [2, 5]. Randomized clinical trials that directly compare one agent with another are the best way of making appropriate comparisons [5]. Ideally these trials should also be conducted using standard double-blind methodology although this can be problematic when the drugs have different frequencies of dosing and different dosing regimes. This may necessitate the use of double-dummy techniques or reformulation (e.g. into capsules) that may increase both the frequency and the number of capsules/tablets to be taken. This may increase the artificiality of the clinical trial situation in contrast to the normal situation in clinical practice where a simpler dose titration or dose frequency may offer a potential practical advantage.

Nevertheless, four randomized clinical trials looking at head-to-head comparisons have now been published: two studies compare donepezil and rivastigmine (one sponsored by Eisai/Pfizer, makers of donepezil, and one by Novartis, makers of rivastigmine) and two studies compare donepezil and galantamine (again one sponsored by Eisai/Pfizer and one sponsored by Janssen/Shire, makers of galantamine). There are no published direct comparisons between rivastigmine and galantamine nor between donepezil and the recently marketed prolonged release galantamine.

## DONEPEZIL VS. RIVASTIGMINE: 12-WEEK STUDY [6]

The first published head-to-head study was a 12-week multinational comparison assessing the tolerability, compliance and cognitive effects of the recommended doses of donepezil (up to 10 mg once daily) and rivastigmine (up to 6 mg twice daily). Patients who had previously received either drug were excluded. Patients receiving donepezil commenced on 5 mg tablets once daily for 28 days and then 10 mg tablets once daily. Those receiving

**Table 3.1** Satisfaction/ease of use questionnaires

| |
|---|
| *Physician satisfaction/ease of use questionnaire** |
| 1. Ease of medication use by patient and caregiver |
| 2. Satisfaction with dosing frequency |
| 3. Satisfaction with titration schedule to achieve clinically effective dose |
| 4. Frequency of patient monitoring outside scheduled visits for side-effects or medication queries |
| 5. Overall convenience of medication |
| 6. Overall satisfaction with medication |
| *Caregiver satisfaction/ease of use questionnaire*** |
| 1. Ease of following directions of use |
| 2. Ease of ensuring correct dose given to patient each day |
| 3. Satisfaction with dosing frequency (number of times medication taken daily) |
| 4. Satisfaction with patient tolerability of medication |
| 5. Frequency of doctor contact regarding directions of use |
| 6. Frequency of doctor contact regarding side-effects |
| 7. Overall convenience of medication |
| 8. Overall satisfaction with medication |

*All questions scored 1–5 giving a total score range of 6–30. Lower scores indicate greater satisfaction/ease of use.
**All questions scored 1–5 giving a total score range of 8–40. Lower scores indicate greater satisfaction/ease of use.

rivastigmine initially received 1.5 mg capsules twice daily with food. At 14-day intervals, the patients were assessed and the dosages increased to 3 mg (day 14), 4.5 mg (day 28) and finally to a maximum of 6 mg (day 42) twice daily according to tolerability. In order to assess satisfaction and ease of use with two treatments that differ in terms of dosing frequency and dose escalation schedules, the medication was given open-label and dosage adjustments based on tolerability (down and up) were allowed throughout the study.

Nineteen sites in the UK, South Africa and Switzerland recruited patients with mild-to-moderate probable or possible AD (Mini-mental State Examination [MMSE], 10–26 inclusive). One hundred and twelve patients were randomized (1:1 ratio) using a stratified randomization scheme based on centre and disease severity split into mild (MMSE 21–26 inclusive) or moderate (MMSE 10–20 inclusive) categories. One subject received no study medication and the results were therefore presented for 111 patients (56 receiving donepezil, 55 receiving rivastigmine).

### *OUTCOME MEASURES*

Although not specifically stated as the primary outcome measure, the Alzheimer's Disease Assessment Scale – Cognitive subscale (ADAS-Cog) was the only measure administered by independent raters that were blinded to study treatment and outcome. The MMSE was a secondary outcome measure carried out at screening, baseline and at weeks 4 and 12 by clinicians who did have knowledge of the assigned medication.

Tolerability was assessed by comparing treatment groups with respect to adverse event (AE) monitoring together with other factors such as laboratory test abnormalities, electrocardiography (ECG) findings and compliance with study medication.

Physicians and caregivers rated the ease of use and their general satisfaction with the dosing frequency and titration of the assigned treatment by completing Likert-type questionnaires at weeks 4 and 12. These were developed by the Clinical and Outcomes Research

Group at Pfizer and Eisai in conjunction with an external consultant, Dr Jean Endicott of Columbia University, New York (Table 3.1) [6].

### *STATISTICAL ANALYSIS*

An analysis of covariance model was used for estimating and testing treatment effects. Both observed cases (OC) and last observation carried forward (LOCF) analyses were carried out for the intention-to-treat population (ITT). The publication only describes the OC analysis because of the potential for bias as a result of the large differences in discontinuation rates between the two drugs.

### *RESULTS*

Fifty (89.3%) patients in the donepezil group completed the study compared with 38 (69.1%; $P = 0.009$) in the rivastigmine group. In the donepezil group 10.7% and in the rivastigmine group 21.8% discontinued because of AEs. At the last study visit 87.5% of donepezil-treated patients and 47.3% of rivastigmine-treated patients remained on the maximum approved dose of each drug. In addition, 17.9% of donepezil- and 34.5% of rivastigmine-treated patients required a dose reduction or temporary discontinuation of study drug. Bradycardia was experienced by 2 donepezil- and 3 rivastigmine-treated patients respectively.

Both groups demonstrated similar improvements on the ADAS-Cog at both weeks 4 and 12. The mean change from baseline in MMSE total scores showed a similar result to the ADAS-Cog.

Physicians and caregivers both reported significantly better satisfaction/ease of use with donepezil in comparison to rivastigmine.

### *CONCLUSION AND COMMENT*

This study using the recommended dosing schedules demonstrated that donepezil was better tolerated than rivastigmine with fewer discontinuations due to AEs. Both agents appeared to improve cognition to a similar extent.

The data on physician and caregiver satisfaction/ease of use must be interpreted cautiously since it relied on a scale that appears to have been developed specifically for the study by Eisai/Pfizer working with an external consultant.

It is generally accepted, based on the pivotal double-blind placebo-controlled studies with the two drugs and on everyday clinical experience (e.g. data submitted in 2005–2006 to the National Institute for Health and Clinical Excellence [NICE] in the UK), that donepezil is better tolerated than rivastigmine and that more patients can tolerate the maximum recommended dose of donepezil than rivastigmine. In this study, the doses of the two drugs were increased using the minimum interval specified in the product labelling and it is possible that slower titration with either drug might have improved tolerability and reduced withdrawal.

## RIVASTIGMINE VS. DONEPEZIL: 2-YEAR STUDY [7]

This is the most recently published comparison reporting a large 2-year multinational double-blind randomized controlled study designed to evaluate the efficacy and tolerability of rivastigmine and donepezil. Ninety-four centres in Australia, Canada, France, Germany, Italy, Spain and the UK recruited patients with moderate to moderately-severe AD (MMSE 10–20 inclusive). Although the paper states that the study included probable AD only (NINCDS-ADRDA criteria) [8], subjects with symptoms suggestive of concomitant Lewy body disease were also allowed to enter. A diagnosis of probable AD requires the exclusion, as far as possible, of causes of dementia other than AD so there is some uncertainty about the nature of the subjects and the rigour with which the diagnosis of probable AD was applied. Nine hundred and ninety-eight patients were randomized in a 1:1 ratio; 994 actually received drug therapy (495 received rivastigmine and 499 received donepezil).

There was a 16-week dose titration period with increases in the rivastigmine dose every 4 weeks beginning at 3 mg/day, increasing in 3 mg steps to a maximum dose of 12 mg/day after 12 weeks (tolerability permitting). It is not stated how the dose was administered but presumably this was as capsules on a twice-daily basis with food as recommended in the product labelling. In order to maintain blinding, donepezil was also administered as capsules (together with placebo capsules) commencing at 5 mg/day for weeks 1–4 and weeks 5–8 increasing to 10 mg/day for weeks 9–16. It is not stated how donepezil, which is marketed as a tablet, was reformulated into the capsules.

### *OUTCOME MEASURES*

The primary efficacy measure was the Severe Impairment Battery (SIB), which assesses cognitive function in severely demented patients. This is an unusual choice for a study involving people with a starting MMSE score of up to 20, but was selected partly because of the intended duration of the study.

Secondary outcome measures included the Global Deterioration Scale (GDS), the Alzheimer's Disease Cooperative Study – Activities of Daily Living Scale (ADCS-ADL) although the version for more severely impaired subjects does not appear to have been used, the MMSE and the Neuropsychiatric Inventory (NPI) to assess behavioural problems.

Safety and tolerability assessments included monitoring and recording AEs and regular measurements of vital signs.

A single blood sample at screening was taken from a subpopulation who consented to pharmacogenetic evaluation. About one-third ($n = 340$) of subjects agreed to this, which allowed some secondary, exploratory analyses to be carried out. The objective was to identify genetic factors related to AD that might predict treatment response with rivastigmine or donepezil, or a subject's relative susceptibility to drug–drug interactions or serious side-effects.

### *STATISTICAL ANALYSIS*

The main efficacy analyses were based on mean change from baseline at 104 weeks in an ITT population, defined as all randomized patients who received study medication and from whom at least one efficacy measurement was obtained on treatment using the LOCF. An evaluable patient (EP) population was also assessed for those who received at least 16 weeks study medication with the LOCF. Finally an OC population was analysed. As for the previous study, an analysis of covariance model (ANCOVA) was used in the analyses.

Changes from baseline at 104 weeks were assessed for the primary outcome measure (the SIB) and all secondary efficacy variables (GDS, ADCS-ADL, MMSE and NPI). Additional secondary analyses on the SIB, NPI and ADCS-ADL were performed on patients with different baseline severities, gender, age and vascular risk factor profiles.

### *RESULTS*

Overall, 57.9% of patients completed the study, 52.7% (261/498) on rivastigmine but 63.5% (317/495) on donepezil. Premature discontinuations during the 16-week titration period were 18.8% for the rivastigmine group in comparison with 9.2% for the donepezil group. During the 88-week maintenance phase of the study, discontinuations on rivastigmine were 28.5% compared with 27.3% for donepezil. The most frequent reasons for premature discontinuation were AEs in 128 (25.9%) on rivastigmine (14.1% in the titration phase and 17.9% in the maintenance phase) and 80 (16.0%) on donepezil (7.0% in the titration phase and 14.1% in the maintenance phase). Consent was withdrawn in a further 34 (7.5%) on rivastigmine compared with 22 (4.6%) on donepezil whilst other reasons for discontinuation (abnormal laboratory values, unsatisfactory therapeutic effect, protocol violation, loss to follow-up, administrative problems and death) were similar for the two drugs.

More rivastigmine- than donepezil-treated patients reported 'any AE' during the titration phase (82.0% and 64.7%, respectively). The higher rate for rivastigmine appeared to be driven by an increased rate, relative to donepezil, of nausea (32.9% vs. 15.2%) and vomiting (27.9% vs. 5.8%). In the maintenance phase, AE rates were similar for the two groups when reported as totals for 'any AE reported' but there was still a much higher incidence with rivastigmine of those AEs that appeared in at least 5% of subjects within any treatment group (titration or maintenance phase). In particular, 12.9% of subjects on rivastigmine reported nausea and 15.3% vomiting in the maintenance phase, whereas the comparative figures for donepezil were 5.3% and 4.4%.

### *EFFICACY*

At the end of 2 years' treatment, the mean daily dose for each drug was 9.4 mg (indicating that more patients were on the maximum recommended dose of 10 mg for donepezil than the maximum recommended dose of 12 mg for rivastigmine). The main efficacy data presented in the publication is for the ITT-LOCF population which showed no statistically significant difference between the two drugs on measures of cognition (SIB, MMSE) or behaviour (NPI). Rivastigmine showed superior efficacy over donepezil on the ADCS-ADL and greater efficacy on the GDS. However, these differences were not maintained in the non-ITT-LOCF populations (EP and OC populations).

The published abstract within the paper suggests that in some of the secondary subgroup analyses, AD patients who had genotypes for full expression of the butyrylcholinesterase enzyme ($n = 226/340$), who were <75 years of age ($n = 362/994$) or who had symptoms suggestive of concomitant Lewy body disease ($n = 49/994$) showed significantly greater benefits from rivastigmine treatment. These data are not fully presented in the paper which again relies on the ITT-LOCF data; in addition, the data in the paper suggest that only 40 subjects were thought to have probable concomitant Lewy body dementia (DLB) in contrast to the 49 mentioned in the abstract but not elsewhere in the publication.

### *CONCLUSION AND COMMENT*

The abstract of the paper concludes that cholinesterase inhibitor treatment may offer continued therapeutic benefit for up to 2 years in patients with moderate AD. It goes on to state that although both drugs performed similarly on cognition and behaviour, rivastigmine may provide greater benefit in ADL and global functioning. It also reports the subanalyses that are mentioned above. These conclusions are misleading.

The major flaw in this study is the considerably greater number of dropouts on rivastigmine in comparison with those on donepezil (47.3% vs. 36.5%) such that only 261 subjects completed the study on rivastigmine in comparison with 317 on donepezil. Many of these withdrawals were due to AEs and occurred during the early (titration) phase of a study that lasted 2 years. Under these circumstances the ITT-LOCF analysis would favour rivastigmine because the natural course of AD is a steady decline. This is confirmed by the fact that the statistical significance of these findings disappears when the non-ITT-LOCF analysis is reported. Although the authors do discuss this point in their discussion they still concentrate on their erroneous conclusions in the abstract. It is noteworthy that the previous donepezil–rivastigmine comparison described above used an OC analysis rather than an ITT approach because of the same problem (a higher dropout rate on rivastigmine), even though the study was considerably shorter.

The abstract also glosses over the significantly different tolerability profile for the two compounds and only reports general comments about completion rates, AEs and serious AEs. For example, even in the maintenance phase of the study (i.e. excluding all subjects who withdrew in the titration phase), 15.3% of rivastigmine-treated patients report vomiting in comparison with 4.4% of donepezil-treated patients.

The conclusions of this Novartis sponsored study are therefore very similar to those of the shorter Eisai/Pfizer sponsored study. The two drugs appear fairly similar with regard to efficacy but, in general, donepezil is the better tolerated of the two drugs both in the titration phase and the maintenance phase.

## DONEPEZIL VS. GALANTAMINE: 12-WEEK STUDY [2]

This study used a similar randomized, open-label design to the 12-week donepezil–rivastigmine comparison. The primary objective of the study was to directly compare the ease of use, tolerability and compliance using the highest recommended doses of donepezil and galantamine in patients with mild to moderate probable or possible AD (MMSE 10–24 inclusive). Patients who had been treated previously with cholinesterase inhibitors were excluded. Fourteen centres in the UK, Finland, Germany and Norway recruited 120 patients randomized in a 1:1 ratio stratified for disease severity (into mild MMSE scores of 19–24 inclusive, or moderate MMSE scores of 10–18 inclusive). Sixty-four patients received donepezil and 56 galantamine.

The drugs were given orally and titrated to the maximum recommended dose according to the respective approved product labelling. Donepezil tablets were given once daily commencing with 5 mg for 4 weeks following which the dose was increased to 10 mg daily. Patients randomized to galantamine began on 4 mg tablets twice daily increasing to 8 mg tablets twice daily after 4 weeks and then, after a further 4 weeks, to 12 mg twice daily. The dose of either drug could be adjusted up and down for reasons of tolerability.

### *OUTCOME MEASURES*

The primary outcome measures were the Physician's and Caregiver's Satisfaction Questionnaires completed at weeks 4, 8 and 12 (Table 3.1).

Secondary efficacy assessments were two measures of cognition, the ADAS-Cog and the MMSE, and a measure of functional disability, the Disability Assessment for Dementia (DAD) scale. The cognitive assessments were both carried out by independent raters who were blinded to all other study information and used separate case report forms from the main study information.

Safety and tolerability were assessed by comparing treatment groups with respect to AE monitoring together with other factors such as laboratory test abnormalities, ECG findings and compliance with study medication.

### *STATISTICAL ANALYSIS*

The primary analyses were the total scores of the Physicians' and Caregivers' Satisfaction Questionnaire at endpoint (week 12 LOCF for the ITT population) and using an ANOVA model. Comparisons between study groups were performed for the secondary efficacy assessments using ANCOVA models. The safety data were summarized with no formal statistical analysis.

### *RESULTS*

Of the 120 patients who received study medication, 61 (95.3%) patients in the donepezil group and 51 (91.1%) in the galantamine completed the study. Three (4.7%) donepezil and

4 (7.1%) galantamine patients discontinued prematurely as a result of AEs. These AEs were considered to be related to study drug in one donepezil patient (depression) and three galantamine patients (depression, vomiting, nausea).

The maximum daily doses of donepezil (10 mg once daily) and galantamine (12 mg twice daily) were administered in 98.4% and 94.6% of patients respectively at some point in the study. However, more patients receiving donepezil remained at the maximum dose at the end of the study or at last study visit, compared with galantamine (92.2% vs. 71.4%, respectively).

Patients were permitted to return for unscheduled visits following clinic visits at weeks 4 and 8 in the event that a dose escalation was not tolerated. There were significantly less unscheduled visits overall for the patients in the donepezil group due to dose tolerability problems in comparison with the galantamine group (3 [4.7%] patients on donepezil and 13 [23.2%] patients on galantamine).

Both physicians and caregivers reported significantly greater overall satisfaction/ease of use for donepezil compared with galantamine at weeks 4, 12 and endpoint (week 12 LOCF). Significantly greater improvements in cognition were also observed for donepezil vs. galantamine on the ADAS-Cog at week 12 and endpoint. ADL also improved significantly in the donepezil group compared with the galantamine group at weeks 4, 12 and endpoint.

Treatment-emergent AEs (all causalities) were experienced by 43 (67.2%) donepezil patients and 41 (73.2%) galantamine patients. Most AEs were mild to moderate, however, 46% galantamine-treated patients reported gastrointestinal AEs vs. 25% donepezil patients. Seven patients (12.5%) on galantamine reported vomiting whereas no patients reported this with donepezil.

There were no clinically significant abnormal changes in heart rate and no patients on either drug discontinued as a result of laboratory abnormalities or physical findings.

### *CONCLUSION AND COMMENTS*

Physician and caregiver overall satisfaction and ease of use of treatment was significantly higher in the donepezil group compared with galantamine. This may partly reflect the reduced incidence of gastrointestinal AEs in the donepezil group and the reduced number of unscheduled visits in the donepezil group in comparison with those taking galantamine. These visits and the necessary reductions in dosage would have involved more physician, carer and patient time and the satisfaction/ease of use questionnaire would have reflected this. It is however relevant to mention that these questionnaires were developed by Eisai and Pfizer in discussion with an external consultant as previously mentioned in the donepezil vs. rivastigmine 12-week comparison. Nonetheless, the simpler dosing schedule for donepezil coupled with better tolerability during this period does potentially have both practical and cost implications.

Somewhat more surprising were the results on cognition carried out by blinded-rater assessments and assessments of ADL carried out by unblinded investigators. These showed a significantly greater improvement for donepezil vs. galantamine even though this was only a 12-week study. Although caution must be advised about these results, the results were consistent for all efficacy measures whether or not conducted by a blinded rater.

Both treatments were relatively well-tolerated, but there were more gastrointestinal AEs in the galantamine group in comparison with the donepezil group.

## GALANTAMINE VS. DONEPEZIL: 52-WEEK STUDY [3]

This study is presented as a pilot study that involved 182 patients randomized to galantamine ($n$ = 94) or donepezil ($n$ = 88) for 52 weeks. The study was a randomized, rater-blinded, parallel group multicentre study conducted at 18 outpatient clinics in the UK.

Patients with probable AD were included with a MMSE score between 9 and 18 at screening. It is not stated whether the patients were to have mild or moderate AD and usually MMSE scores of below 10 are used to indicate severe AD. This is an unusual choice for the MMSE range and would actually suggest that some of the patients recruited to the study would have had severe AD and the use of the drugs would therefore be technically outside the licensed indication. Patients who had previously received either galantamine or donepezil were excluded from the study. Randomization was stratified based on the baseline ADL scale score (the DAD). A cut-off point of 31 was chosen although no justification for this cut-off is included in the publication.

### *OUTCOME MEASURES*

The primary objective of this pilot study was to compare galantamine with donepezil on functional abilities as measured by the Bristol ADL Scale (BADL). This is a caregiver-rated instrument developed for brief community based assessment of ADL functioning and this was the first time this particular measure had been used as the primary endpoint in a therapeutic clinical trial setting. Secondary objectives were to compare the drugs on four further outcome measures, the MMSE, the ADAS-Cog, the NPI and a Screen for Caregiver Burden (SCGB).

Blinded evaluators were employed to make all clinical efficacy assessments because of the practical difficulties of achieving a full double-blind design for the two trial medications acknowledging the different dosing schedules and physical appearances.

Safety assessments performed throughout the study consisted of physical examinations, electrocardiography, standard laboratory tests, vital signs and monitoring for AEs which were then managed by the local investigator.

### *STATISTICAL ANALYSIS*

A one-way analysis of covariance was used to test treatment group differences for the change from baseline to last recorded assessment data on the BADL. All clinical efficacy results were reported on an intent-to-treat (OC) basis.

### *RESULTS*

There were no significant differences between the treatment groups in mean change from baseline to week 52 for the primary outcome, the BADL. In the total population, in terms of cognition, galantamine patients' scores on the MMSE at week 52 did not differ significantly from baseline, whereas donepezil patients' scores did. However, the between group differences in MMSE change did not reach statistical significance. There were also no between group differences for the total population with regard to the ADAS-Cog. However, a subgroup analysis looking at patients with MMSE scores of 12–18 demonstrated a significant between group difference in favour of galantamine. More caregivers of patients receiving galantamine reported reductions in burden compared with caregivers of patients receiving donepezil, whereas changes from baseline in the NPI were similar for both treatments.

Both treatments were reported as well-tolerated with most AEs being transient and of mild to moderate intensity and consistent with the findings of previous clinical trials. Although the paper comments that gastrointestinal effects, e.g. nausea and diarrhoea were the most commonly reported in both groups, no detailed figures are provided.

### *CONCLUSION AND COMMENTS*

ADL (measured using the BADL) was chosen as the primary outcome measure of this study because of 'the paramount importance of functional abilities for caregiver and patient quality of life in AD' but there were no differences between the drugs for this measure. The published abstract of the study concludes that significant advantages were found in the treatment response to galantamine (vs. donepezil) on cognition as measured by response rates on the MMSE and ADAS-Cog. This conclusion is mainly justified by the analysis of a subgroup with an MMSE score of between 12 and 18 (and not the whole population where the MMSE range was 9–18 although two subjects were reported with scores above this range. The paper comments that patients in this subgroup fulfil the criteria of the NICE Technology Appraisal Guidance report published in 2001 [3]. This Guidance states that acetylcholinesterase inhibitors should be made available as one component of the management of people with AD whose MMSE score is greater than 12 points although the Guidance comments that this score was selected for cost-effectiveness rather than clinical effectiveness reasons. Although the statistical section of this paper claims that all analyses were planned, it would not have been possible to plan this sub-analysis within the study protocol since the NICE Guidance was issued many months after this study had commenced. Some caution must therefore be observed with respect to the reasons for the additional analyses.

## SUMMARY: COMPARISON STUDIES OF CHOLINESTERASE INHIBITORS FOR ALZHEIMER'S DISEASE

In 2004, an article considering comparative studies of cholinesterase inhibitors for AD appeared in the personal view section of *Lancet Neurology* [5]. The authors did a MEDLINE search in May 2004 and only identified three randomized clinical trials where one cholinesterase was compared with another. These three studies are reported in this chapter together with the more recently published long-term rivastigmine–donepezil comparison. The authors of the personal view are critical of the three studies they reviewed and in particular draw attention to the fact that each study was sponsored by the manufacturers of one of the drugs and in general the results published appeared to favour that company's product. The additional study published since this review was also sponsored by one of the companies and again the publication appears to show benefit tending to favour the manufacturer's product.

There are a number of practical issues which have already been described earlier. These real life clinical trials are attempting to look at issues such as a simpler dosage schedule, which may offer a potential advantage to patients and their families, and this cannot easily be reflected in a double-blind, double-dummy study. It is worth noting that donepezil with its two-step, once-daily dosage regime was a comparator drug in all of the studies reported. However, there is inevitably a potential for bias in an unblinded study or a partially unblinded study and it is difficult to overcome this where different dosage regimes are involved. Manufacturers are likely to generate a protocol which they feel will identify positive factors in favour of their particular compound and this is a danger. There is no easy way to solve these problems in head-to-head studies unless funding is provided to independent groups that can then design a more independent protocol. A further factor is the analysis and writing up of the results which again would benefit from analysis and authorship completely independent from the manufacturers.

In conclusion, all three of the cholinesterase inhibitors reviewed here appear to demonstrate clinical efficacy as illustrated by the head-to-head studies but also by the many other studies that have now been carried out and published. There may be differences in favour of donepezil because of its simpler dosing schedule and it does appear that there are more gastrointestinal adverse effects with rivastigmine than with the other two compounds. In any therapeutic area it is important to have choice because not every drug or every dosage regimen will suit every patient and some patients may respond to or tolerate one drug better than another. Consideration should be given to trying to generate more independent head-to-head comparative studies with these and other drugs but this may not be easy particularly when the dosing regimes of the compounds are different.

## REFERENCES


1. Nordberg A, Svensson A-L. Cholinesterase inhibitors in the treatment of Alzheimer's disease: a comparison of tolerability and pharmacology. *Drug Safety* 1998; 19:465–480.
2. Jones RW, Soininen H, Hager K *et al.* A multinational, randomized, 12-week study comparing the effects of donepezil and galantamine in patients with mild to moderate Alzheimer's disease. *Int J Geriatr Psychiatry* 2004: 19:58–67.
3. Wilcock G, Howe I, Coles H *et al.* A long term comparison of galantamine and donepezil in the treatment of Alzheimer's disease. *Drugs Aging* 2003; 20:771–789.
4. Maelicke A, Albuquerque EX. Allosteric modulation of nicotine acetyl choline receptors as treatment strategy for Alzheimer's disease. *Eur J Pharmacol* 2000; 393:165–170.
5. Hogan DB, Goldlist B, Naglie G, Patterson C. Comparison studies of cholinesterase inhibitors for Alzheimer's disease. *Lancet Neurol* 2004; 3:622–626.
6. Wilkinson DG, Passmore AP, Bullock R *et al.* A multinational, randomized, 12-week comparative study of donepezil and rivastigmine in patients with mild to moderate Alzheimer's Disease. *Int J Clin Pract* 2002; 56:441–446.
7. Bullock R, Touchon J, Bergman H *et al.* Rivastigmine and donepezil treatment in moderate to moderately-severe Alzheimer's disease over a 2-year period. *Curr Med Res Opin* 2005; 21:1317–1327.
8. McKhann G, Drachman DA, Folstein M, Katzman R, Price DL, Stadlan EM. Clinical diagnosis of Alzheimer's disease – report of the NINCDS-ADRDA work group under the auspices of Department of Health and Human Services task force on Alzheimer's disease. *Neurology* 1984; 34:939–944.

# 4

# Ginkgo biloba

*R. W. McCarney, J. P. W. Warner*

## INTRODUCTION

Ginkgo is a herbal (or complementary or alternative) medicine classified as a dietary supplement in the UK and thus available for purchase without prescription. Its use amongst people with dementia is considerable, with surveys suggesting as many as 11% of individuals using Ginkgo. The therapeutic target for Ginkgo is the symptomatic improvement of cognitive functioning in dementia and a systematic review and meta-analysis of published trials has shown a modest but positive effect in achieving this. However, the more recent, better quality trials have been inconsistent in their conclusions and there is a need for more research.

## WHAT IS COMPLEMENTARY AND ALTERNATIVE MEDICINE?

Complementary and alternative medicine (CAM) is an umbrella term covering a large number of therapies from diverse origins, often with radically different theories and modes of delivery. It is dependent on the prevailing knowledge system within a culture and the availability of therapies within that culture: CAM use is essentially everything lying outside of the dominant health system within a given society and within the current epoch. As a result, definitions are relative. Ginkgo biloba is a 'biologically based practice', based on the definition of the National Centre for Complementary and Alternative Medicine (NCCAM).

The sheer number of available therapies means guidance as to what they are and what is effective is essential. The 'safe' image of CAM is often not justified as side-effects and interactions are widely reported [1–3] – so patients should be encouraged to keep their doctors informed of CAM use. One recent survey has reported just over half actively doing this. Furthermore, although a considerable number of healthcare professionals now offer many CAM treatments within the bounds of the National Health Service (NHS) [4, 5], a significant proportion are unregulated and sought privately; consequently advice on identifying reliable practitioners is important.

It is important that healthcare professionals are open to the notion of and actively enquire about CAM use. As Ginkgo is available over the counter it is imperative that this attitude is adopted, as concurrent use is possible.

## A HISTORY OF GINKGO BILOBA

The herbal medicine *Ginkgo biloba* is derived from the leaves of the tree *Ginkgo biloba* L. It is scientifically classified in its own division, the Ginkgophyta, within the genus *Ginkgo*. The

**Robert W. McCarney**, MPhil, Research Associate, Department of Psychological Medicine, Imperial College, London, UK

**James P. W. Warner**, MD, MRCPsych, Senior Lecturer/Honorary Consultant in Old Age Psychiatry, Department of Psychological Medicine, Imperial College, London, UK

German physician and botanist Englebert Kaempfer (1651–1716) gave the tree its common name after the Japanese word for it at the time, pronounced *'Ginkyo'* (meaning silver apricot: 'apricot' for the appearance of its seeds and 'silver' the bloom on the fruit). The Ginkgo is perhaps more commonly known in the UK as the maidenhair tree (its leaves similar in shape to *Adiantum monochlamys Eat.*, the maidenhair fern). Other popular names include the Kew tree (after the impressive example in Kew Gardens, London); the Fossil tree; and the Temple tree.

Fossilized remains of trees from the genus *Ginkgo* have been dated to the Jurassic period (206–144 million years ago) [6] and possibly earlier, and Ginkgo is probably what Charles Darwin (1809–1882) had in mind when he coined the phrase 'living fossil'! The tree was once present globally, as indicated by fossil finds up to the end of the Pilocene period (5.4–2.4 million years ago), subsequently surviving in China and Japan where its spiritual significance, as well as its ornamental, medicinal and culinary properties, ensured its cultivation. The current existence of wild specimens of Ginkgo is debated. Kaempfer re-introduced the tree to the West in the early 1700s.

The average, fully-grown Ginkgo is between 20 m and 35 m tall often with an angular crown and erratic branches. It is a deciduous tree and dioecious, with separate male and female trees. It is a gymnosperm, with seeds unprotected by fruit and with motive sperm. Its leaf has a very distinct fan shape (cf. 'maidenhair') and often has one single, deep groove in the middle that produces two distinct lobes (giving rise to the name 'biloba'). The leaf veins do not deliquesce; they are open-dichotomous, running in pairs from the base of the leaf to its edges.

Its good leaf cover, long life span and its high resistance to insects, infection and air pollution make it a common sight in cities. A good example can be seen on the Queen's Lawn of Imperial College London's South Kensington Campus. The male tree is most commonly used ornamentally as the female tree produces foul-smelling seeds. The tree has inspired artists over the centuries but of most interest to us here is its inspiration to scientists.

Exactly how long Ginkgo has been used in Traditional Chinese Medicine (TCM) is not known; some suggest more than 5000 years [7]. It is mentioned in the Chinese Materia Medica *Shen Nung Pen Tsao Ching*, although there does not seem to be a consensus on precisely when this book was written and considering the importance of the oral tradition in TCM [8], it is likely that Ginkgo use probably existed long before written records began. Ginkgo has many varied indications in TCM and Japanese Traditional Medicine (Kanpo), in which the seeds are more commonly but not exclusively used. In the West, its leaves are processed to produce the herbal supplement.

Christen sums up the scientific interest in Ginkgo with his term 'ginkgology' [9]. It has featured in publications on botany, evolution, ethnography, anthropology, mythology, chemistry, pharmacology and medicine; to name but a few. There has been an exponential rise in dedicated scientific publications from less than 50 a year up to and including 1984 to over 600 in 2001 [9]. This fascination with Ginkgo is fascinating in itself and shared by the general public (see Epidemiology): Ginkgo is one of the best selling herbal supplements in Europe and in the US [10]. But is the interest warranted?

## MECHANISM OF ACTION

It has not been firmly established how the purported cognitive enhancing effect of Ginkgo may work. It is thought to be a platelet-aggregation factor antagonist and a vasodilator, and so may improve the blood flow to the brain. It is also a powerful anti-oxidant which may counteract the effect of free radicals in the brain.

A more recent hypothesis [11] is that it is a combination of this purported effect on blood flow, as a vasodilator and through its influence on platelet activating factor; its anti-oxidant properties [12]; and also through a direct effect on the cholinergic system. This effect on the cholinergic system, neurotransmitters implicated in the dementias, is inferred from animal studies.

## EPIDEMIOLOGY OF GINKGO

Kelly's recent general population survey [13] of 8740 American adults found Ginkgo is one of the most widely used herbal medicines in the United States. In those aged 65 years or older, 4.0% of women and 2.2% of men reported weekly use, which made Ginkgo the 4th and 6th most commonly reported herbal medicine used by women and men respectively. Over a third of responders reported using Ginkgo specifically for 'memory', 'mental alertness' or 'their brain'.

Looking more specifically at use amongst people with dementia, Hogan [14] undertook a survey of CAM use in an outpatients clinic and found 10% were using CAM specifically for their cognitive problems: the most common form of CAM used was Ginkgo, although it does not state the exact number of users. This was a relatively small survey (115 individuals participated) and Ginkgo awareness, and so quite possibly use, has risen in the decade since it was conducted.

Dergal's survey [15] investigated the potential for interactions between herbal and conventional medication in memory clinic attendees. Although the interesting finding of this survey is how common reported concomitant use is: 22 of 195 patients sampled (11.3%) were using Gingko, of which over a third (eight of the 22) were also using aspirin. Their survey of 63 caregivers of attendees at an outpatient dementia clinic found six (9.5%) reported the use of Ginkgo for their care-recipient's dementia.

A much larger survey of 1222 participants of an Alzheimer's caregiver's health project [16] found 3.4% of the care-recipients used Ginkgo alone and a further 2.7% were using donepezil and Ginkgo concomitantly.

In conclusion amongst individuals with dementia, the evidence suggests the prevalence of Ginkgo use alone or in combination with other cognitive enhancement medication is currently somewhere between 6.1% and 11.3%.

## EVIDENCE FOR THE USE OF GINKGO IN TREATING DEMENTIA

A recent Cochrane review [17] reported 'promising' evidence for Ginkgo in treating 'cognitive impairment' (one criticism of the earlier studies is that they are imprecise in their use of diagnostic criteria) and dementia. The meta-analysis suggested a modest but positive effect of Ginkgo in improving cognition and general functioning. No data relating to other outcomes, e.g. quality of life or behavioural functioning were sufficiently and consistently used to be meta-analysed. It found that Ginkgo had a good safety profile with reporting of adverse events no greater in the Ginkgo than in the placebo groups. However, the review concludes that more research of this herbal treatment needs to be done and in particular there is a need for good quality, large-scale and valid trials undertaken with a sound methodological approach, that are representative of the populations most likely to use Ginkgo. For example, the data available (and which they report) are based on completer as opposed to intention-to-treat (ITT) analyses only. Other earlier systematic reviews exist [18, 19] and support the conclusions made by the Cochrane team.

Thirty-three trials were included in the Cochrane review [17], however there was significant heterogeneity with the majority of trials being either small or of short duration. The Cochrane reviewers stated they could not rule out publication bias. The three most recent, good quality, large-scale trials, published in English language journals and included in the review, are summarized and critically appraised below.

Le Bars *et al.* [20] designed a trial to assess the efficacy and safety of Ginkgo extract in Alzheimer's disease and multi-infarct dementia. It was a randomized, double-blind, placebo-controlled, parallel-group, multicentre trial with a long follow-up of 52 weeks. Participants received either 120 mg of the Ginkgo extract EGb761® per day or a similar placebo tablet. Of the 327 participants randomized to the trial, aged between 45 and 90 years, 251 had a diagnosis of Alzheimer's disease. The ITT analysis included 236 of the Alzheimer's participants. One hundred and thirty-seven (42% of those randomized) participants completed the 12-month follow-up. Reported outcome measures included an assessment of cognitive functioning, the Alzheimer's Disease Assessment Scale-Cognitive subscale (ADAS-Cog) [21] their carer's evaluation of daily living and social functioning, using the Geriatric Evaluation by Relative's Rating Instrument (GERRI) [22] and general clinical state using the Clinical Global Impression of Change (CGIC) [23]. A treatment response was described using two cut-offs previously employed in dementia trials; two-point and a four-point difference in means between the active treatment and placebo on the ADAS-Cog. The paper reports a statistically significant between-groups difference in favour of EGb761® at 52 weeks in the ITT analysis ($P < 0.04$), using the two-point mean difference cut-off on the ADAS-Cog. The safety of Ginkgo was reported as good, with a similar number of adverse events reported in both the Ginkgo and the placebo groups.

There are a number of potential shortcomings with this study. The ITT analysis was selected as the primary analysis *a posteriori* because of the large number of dropouts and their unequal distribution between the two arms. Perhaps the high rate of attrition led to the decision to use ITT and it is unusual that this was the initial choice. Although a large number dropped out, it is reasonable to assume that this would have been considered previously in a 52-week dementia trial; and the numbers finishing in each group were not considerably different (78 and 59 respectively in the Ginkgo and placebo groups). Also the ITT analysis was calculated using last observation carried forward (LOCF). This is a method of imputing missing data by using the last available value for that individual so the assumption is that the condition does not worsen after this point. The treatment effect could therefore be overestimated by using this method; however as more dropped out of the placebo group, this may still be conservative. The authors do comment that with a degenerative condition such as dementia this is not an ideal choice, however they still use this method.

Furthermore, the study employed a 'humanitarian' protocol. If there was a one-point change (worsening) as measured by the CGIC, the clinician could withdraw that individual from the study and treat them with Ginkgo. Although the ethics of this can be appreciated it could effectively remove progressive cases from the study and replace their missing data with their LOCF, which could further overestimate the treatment effect.

Statistical significance is defined as a two-point or four-point difference in mean ADAS-Cog score at 52 weeks. Whilst this is based on previous studies which use the ADAS-Cog, it could be argued that this does not indicate a *clinically* significant difference: this is less than a 6% change on a 70-point scale over a year.

No attempt was made to stratify the analyses by centre: this is important as there may be centre effects which were not controlled for. Finally, the manufacturers of the extract used in the trial (Schwabe) funded the study. There is evidence to suggest that the published results of commercially and non-commercially funded research differ [24], with commercially funded trials more likely to report positive findings. Research sponsored by non-independent bodies should therefore be viewed with some caution.

The Cochrane review [17] states that outpatients took part in this study, however this is not clear in the original article. Assuming that they are outpatients, this limits the applicability of the results as this is a select group of patients, whereas the potential for Ginkgo may be as an early, primary care intervention. It also highlights the difficulty of conducting trials in dementia with a follow-up period greater than 6 months: the high and unanticipated rate of attrition thus resulted in an analysis that was not ideal.

Van Dongen *et al.* [25] conducted a randomized, placebo-controlled, parallel-group, multicentre trial of EGb761® for treating dementia and age associated memory impairment

(AAMI). This was a 24-week study conducted in care homes for the elderly in The Netherlands and its three aims were: to determine the effectiveness of Ginkgo in treating cognitive decline by using randomized controlled trial (RCT) methodology; to address questions of dosage with Ginkgo by using 240 mg and 160 mg interventions; and to investigate whether there are persisting effects from Ginkgo by having a second randomization in the Ginkgo groups to either Ginkgo or placebo. The design was quite complex and featured two randomizations: one at baseline after a 3-week run-in period and another at 12 weeks. The first randomization was to 160 mg Ginkgo, 240 mg Ginkgo or placebo. The second (in the Ginkgo groups) was to either continue with that dosage of Ginkgo or to switch to a placebo for the remaining 12 weeks. Outcome assessment described in this paper included measures of: cognitive functioning (the ZN-G, testing short-term memory; the WL, a verbal learning test; and the ZVT-G, a trail-making test measuring cognitive speed); psychopathology (the Sandoz Clinical Assessment–Geriatric [SCAG], a geriatric symptom rating scale; the Global Deterioration Scale (GDS), measuring depressive mood; a measure of self-perceived health status and a measure of self-perceived memory status); and activities of daily living (the self-assessment version of the NAA). Most of the tests are German in origin. Pre-defined analysis were ITT conducted by replacing missing values with a pre-defined algorithm, based mainly on the LOCF principle: however, per-protocol analyses were also conducted. The paper reported no significant effects for any of the outcomes and no subgroup that benefited from Ginkgo. After 12 weeks of treatment, those taking Ginkgo seemed to perform slightly better with regard to self-reported activities of daily living (ADL) but slightly worse with regard to self-perceived health status compared with the placebo group. Gingko use was not associated with the occurrence of serious adverse events (SAEs).

This study, funded by a commercial company (Schwabe), appears on the whole well conducted and comprehensively reported. Of the 214 participants enrolled into the study, 63 (29%) were diagnosed as having dementia according to DSM-III-R criteria [26] and 151 (71%) were diagnosed with AAMI. This limits the applicability of the trial to dementia research. The number of Alzheimer's patients ($n = 63$) may mean analyses in this group are under-powered.

As with the Le Bars study [20] the LOCF principle of the ITT analysis is not ideal for degenerative conditions and the same criticism applies here as to that for Le Bar's trial [22].

Finally, there is a question with regard to blinding in the trial. It is not clear in the report but it is likely that the 160 mg and 240 mg tablets are different in size and, if so, which the placebo size matches. Although medication was administered by a member of the nursing staff and outcome assessment by another individual, it was possible that the assessor could have been aware of the medication and therefore treatment allocation could have been revealed to the assessor in one of the Ginkgo groups.

The study of Kanowski *et al.* [27] is a randomized, double-blind, placebo-controlled, multicentre trial of the Ginkgo extract EGb761® for Alzheimer's disease or multi-infarct dementia. After a 4-week run-in period, 216 participants were randomized to receive either 240 mg of Ginkgo daily or a placebo for 24 weeks. Outcomes were: Clinical Global Impressions (CGI) for psychopathology; Syndrom-Kurztest (SKT) (or Short Syndrome Test) for attention and memory; and the Nürnberger Alters-Beobachtungskala (NAB) for activities of daily living. Using a responder analysis (response in at least two of the three primary outcomes) to determine clinical efficacy, 156 participants were included in the per-protocol analysis and showed a statistically significant difference in favour of the Ginkgo extract. The ITT analysis also showed a statistically significant difference in favour of Ginkgo.

This study was conducted at 41 centres around three geographical locations in Germany, from a number of healthcare settings (primary and secondary care). The paper states that participants were only included if they could provide informed consent either written or orally in the presence of a witness. As the participants had mild to moderate dementia, it seems unlikely that they all would be able to provide informed consent so this could indicate a sampling bias against individuals without the capacity to provide informed consent. This may be a considerable number: a recent analysis of baseline data found that 75% of participants in a Ginkgo trial of mild to moderate dementia were unable to give informed consent. However, this study predates current guidelines [28] stating that in cases where potential participants in dementia research do not have the capacity to provide informed consent, their assent and the agreement of their legal representatives should be obtained. Again the ITT analysis used the LOCF principle.

The other 30 studies included in the Cochrane review [19] have in general small numbers of participants, short follow-up periods, and idiosyncratic outcomes or admissions criteria.

Since the publication of the Cochrane review, one further large-scale study has been published. Schneider *et al.* [29] compared two doses of Ginkgo (120 mg and 240 mg daily) against placebo in Alzheimer's patients. This study was conducted with 513 outpatients aged 60 and over with a 6-month follow-up. Recruitment was from 44 centres in the United States and the study was again funded by Schwabe. Diagnosis was made using DSM-IV [30] and NINCDS-ADRDA [31] criteria, with a scan from the year prior to enrolment consistent with the diagnosis. An MMSE [32] score between 10 and 24 inclusive and chronicity of at least 6 months formed part of the eligibility criteria, with a stipulation that each centre could not recruit more than a third of participants with an MMSE of 20 or above. Evidence of vascular comorbidity excluded potential participants. The use of anti-dementia drugs (cholinesterase inhibitors or 'cognitive-enhancing substances') 6 weeks prior or during the study period was not allowed. Evidence of behavioural or psychological symptoms or treatment were also grounds for exclusion (i.e. major or clinically significant depression as measured by the Hamilton rating scale for Depression (HAMD) [33] or any other current psychiatric disorder; psychotropic medication was 'prohibited' or allowed in the 3 months preceding randomization, apart from short-acting benzodiazepines).

The primary outcomes were change in ADAS-Cog score and Clinical Global Impression of Change with caregiver's input (CIBIC+) [34] from baseline to 6 months. The power calculation used a 2.5 point difference in ADAS-Cog score. Safety was assessed by an assessment of bleeding time in a subgroup of 280 of the participants (although it is not clear whether these were randomly selected from the three groups); and an analysis of adverse events and relevant laboratory tests on the whole sample.

No significant difference was found between the groups in the planned primary ITT analysis, which used LOCF to impute the missing data (although they do state other methods of imputation were be used in the sensitivity analysis, they were not reported). However, a subgroup analysis was conducted *ad hoc* using participants with behavioural and psychological symptoms of dementia (BPSD) and a significant difference between Ginkgo and placebo was reported. The conclusion made in this study is that the primary analysis is inconclusive as the participants are atypical, as evidenced by the lack of decline in ADAS-Cog score amongst the placebo group.

Four SAEs were reported, one in the 120 mg Ginkgo group and three in the 240 mg Ginkgo group. The SAE in the 120 mg group was retinal haemorrhage: although they report that this is probably due to vessel malformation, hypertension and aspirin intake, this is a safety concern of Ginkgo.

There appear to be a number of inconsistencies in the reporting of the study. Although a criterion for inclusion is age 60 years and over, the demographics report an age range of 56–98 years; but more significantly, psychotropics are prohibited but their use is reported during the trial (with 3.5% taking concomitant psychotropic medication at baseline and 13.6% using any during the study).

Of note is the robustness of the diagnostic process, as a counter to the heterogeneous samples (and 'looser' diagnoses) common in previous Ginkgo trials. Further, the elimination of the potential confounding effects from other psychoactive medication that may influence cognition is also of value. However, the *ad hoc* analysis uses a subgroup of participants with mild depression, based on their score on the HAMD at entry or behavioural problems, as defined by applying the categories from the Neuropsychological Inventory [35] to their medical histories recorded at baseline. It seems unconvincing to exclude BPSD and focus on uncomplicated AD only to conclude, with the support of evidence from the *ad hoc* analysis, that this is where Ginkgo is effective.

## SAFETY

Safety concerns over the use of Gingko have been raised [1–3, 36, 37]. In the main, these concerns arise from a number of reports of potential interactions with anti-coagulant proprietary medication and/or spontaneous haemorrhage associated with Ginkgo use [38–45]. These suggest that Ginkgo should not be used concomitantly with anti-coagulants (as it may produce a cumulative effect on blood clotting) or in individuals with bleeding problems [37].

This evidence however is in the form of case reports, which are essentially anecdotal and selective. Case reports are singular clinical events and possible confounders are not controlled for by this method: the reported event may be caused by a number of other factors such as a pre-existing medical condition or concurrent medication. The evidence from clinical trials, which are controlled with another treatment or a placebo arm and therefore a more reliable investigation of adverse events that can be attributed to the medication in question, suggests Ginkgo does have a good safety profile [17]. Adverse events reported in the clinical trial literature indicate possible mild gastrointestinal complaints, headaches and allergic skin reactions may occur from ingestion of Ginkgo with no evidence of serious (life-threatening) adverse events [17]. The occurrence of adverse events may be no greater than that seen with placebo [20], however, it is likely that randomized trials do not have sufficient power to detect small differences between groups for rarer (but potentially fatal) complications. A formal drug–drug interaction study [46] reported no findings suggestive of an enhancement of the anti-coagulant effect of aspirin by EGb761®. It should be noted that this is an internal report rather than a published one and therefore has not been peer-reviewed. There is also one (small) study that suggests Ginkgo does not alter the response to the oral anti-coagulant warfarin [47]. Further evidence from post-marketing surveillance surveys in Germany (where 3 billion daily doses of EGb761® were placed on the market of a 9-year period) found a very low rate of adverse events [16] but this study may be affected by reporting bias.

The use of aspirin as an anti-platelet agent is widespread in elderly populations, and it is reasonable to suggest that this may particularly be the case in patients with vascular dementia who have a history of vascular problems. Aspirin affects platelet-aggregation factor, thereby reducing the likelihood of clots forming, and so is commonly prescribed in such high-risk groups to prevent further cardio- or cerebrovascular incidents. Ginkgo is available over the counter and is widely marketed and used as a 'memory booster' among non-dementing individuals. By extension it is reasonable to assume usage would similarly be common amongst individuals with dementia because of its perceived efficacy for 'dysfunctional memory' in general (as the public understanding of efficacy tends to be more dichotomized than the complexities of precision inherent in scientific evidence). Concomitant use of the two medications is therefore likely to be widespread. There is some evidence to suggest this may be the case.

A number of potential interactions and contraindications have been noted [37], which also take the form of case reports. They include thiazide diuretics, trazodone, and drugs metabolized by CYP type enzymes. Kayne also discusses *theoretically* possible interactions: insulin and monoamine oxidase inhibitors, with theoretical contraindications including diabetes and epilepsy.

The need for caution in assessing case reports also applies to seizures. For example, a recent case report suggests a possible causal link between Ginkgo and seizures [48]. Haller's review of seizures reported with dietary supplement use [49] does acknowledge the possible association; however, it does not draw any conclusions.

To conclude, Ginkgo does seem quite safe in use but there is a need for improved reporting of adverse events with herbal medicines [50–52]. This relates to patient education about the need to tell their doctors about herbal medicine use. Patients appear reticent about reporting herbal medicine use because they do not believe that their doctors are knowledgeable about them, they are afraid of admitting such use and their perception is that herbs are not medicines [53].

## GINKGO AS A PHYTOMEDICINE

Phytomedicine is the term used to refer to the modern day, *scientific* use of herbal products in medicine. Current technology is employed in order to produce optimized extracts under rigorous pharmaceutical conditions. Optimization in phytomedicine generally entails producing a standardized, concentrated extract, where the main active constituents of the herb are isolated, removed and concentrated (i.e. formulated in a dose higher than would naturally occur in a comparative quantity of the herb) to yield a product of a standard (replicable and therefore reliable) strength. Other constituents of the whole-leaf are usually removed or ignored.

Schwabe (Schwabe Pharma, Willmar-Schwabe-Str. 4, 76227 Karlsruhe, Germany) was the first company to produce an extract of Ginkgo for the Western market and are currently the leading manufacturers worldwide. Their product is entitled EGb 761® and traded under the names Tebonin® and Tebonin forte®, Tanakan® and Rokan®. It is a high-purity, standardized, concentrated Ginkgo biloba extract. The active ingredients are 24% Ginkgo-flavone glycosides and 6% terpene lactones (3.1% ginkgolides A, B and C, 2.9% bilobalide). EGb 761® is the most widely researched Ginkgo extract on the market and most other manufacturers emulate the formulation.

There are a number of products marketed in the UK and all are available over the counter. EGb 761® is not currently available as an OTC product in the UK. As with all phytomedicines, variation in quality of manufacture and the purported content are problems. Phytomedicines are made from naturally occurring materials rather than being synthesized in a laboratory, and so are prone to natural variation. Successful attempts at synthesis of the ginkgolides have been made but at present this production is not commercially viable [54].

The bioequivalence of products has implications not just for the effectiveness and safety of the product but also for the generalizability of research [55]. For Ginkgo, comparisons have been made with products on general sale showing differences in pharmaceutical quality on specific markers [56] which may affect bioaviliability [57]. One study investigates only one other product [57] and neither study investigates consistency over batches from the same manufacturer. Two independent studies [58, 59] do show evidence that products do not always contain what their labelling claims they contain. What makes these studies difficult to compare is that the mechanism of action of Ginkgo has not been unequivocally proven and so they have looked at different aspects of the product. Mantle's study [62] investigates anti-oxidant activity, whereas the ConsumerLab [58] reports on the levels of constituent chemicals. Again neither study attempts to show a clinically relevant difference and ConsumerLab testing [58] is on products from the US market only.

To date studies have generally used standardized extracts doses of 120 mg or 240 mg, containing 24% flavenoids (Ginkgo-flavoneglycosides) and 6% terpenoids (3.1% ginkgolides A, B and C, 2.9% bilobalide) although it is unclear which is the optimum dose. Kayne [37] reports that the literature does not show evidence for other dosage forms or low concentration extracts made from the leaf.

A number of products are available, so care must be taken in selecting an appropriate one as there can be variation in their quality.

## SUMMARY: GINKGO OR CHOLINESTERASE INHIBITORS?

A comparison [60] of the long-term effects of cholinesterase inhibitors and Ginkgo suggests equivalence. However, this report should be viewed with caution as it compares data from a number of separate studies rather than trials with more than one treatment arm, which may lead to bias as the samples will be drawn from different populations. Furthermore, one of the two Gingko trials included [27] does not use the cognitive functioning assessment, the ADAS-Cog [21], which is the primary outcome measure in the review. The author argues that comparative studies indicate an improvement on the Short Syndrome Test is comparable to an improvement on the ADAS-Cog. The two Gingko trials also report milder impairment at baseline than in the cholinesterase inhibitor trials. There have been no randomized head-to-head trials of Ginkgo and cholinesterase inhibitors, which is the most reliable way of commenting on equivalence with any degree of confidence.

Kurz and van Baelen's review of Cochrane meta-analyses of Ginkgo and cholinesterase inhibitors [61] (reviewing the analyses separately) suggests that the evidence for cholinesterase inhibitors is more consistent and robust than that for Ginkgo, with a greater effect on cognition. Their conclusion is that cholinesterase inhibitors should remain the first-line treatment for mild to moderate dementia, with Ginkgo a 'last resort' in individuals who are unable to tolerate cholinesterase inhibitors.

## REFERENCES


1. Ernst E. Serious psychiatric and neurological adverse effects of herbal medicines – a systematic review. *Acta Psychiatr Scand* 2003; 108:83–91.
2. Ernst E. The risk-benefit profile of commonly used herbal therapies: Ginkgo, St. John's Wort, Ginseng, Echinacea, Saw Palmetto, and Kava. *Ann Intern Med* 2002; 136:42–53.
3. Izzo AA, Ernst E. Interactions between herbal medicines and prescribed drugs: a systematic review. *Drugs* 2001; 61:2163–2175.
4. Thomas KJ, Nicholl JP, Coleman P. Use and expenditure on complementary medicine in England: a population based survey. *Complement Ther Med* 2001; 9:2–11.
5. Thomas KJ, Nicholl JP, Fall M. Access to complementary medicine via general practice. *Br J Gen Pract* 2001; 51:25–30.
6. Zhao L, Ohana T, Kimaro T. A fossil population of *Ginkgo* leaves from the Xingyuan Formation, Inner Mongolia. *Transactions and Proceedings of the Palaeontological Society of Japan*. 1993, pp 73–96.
7. Foster S, Tyler VE. *Tyler's Honest Herbal: A Sensible Guide to the Use of Herbs and Related Remedies*, 4th edition. The Haworth Herbal Press, New York, 1999.
8. Hsu E. *The Transmission of Chinese Medicine*. Cambridge University Press, Cambridge, 1999.
9. Christen Y. The Ginkgo: past, present and future. In: Van Beek T (ed.). *Ginkgo Biloba*, 1st edition. Hartwood Academic, Amsterdam, 2000, pp 523–532.
10. Cooper R. Gin(kgo) and Tonic – With a Twist! *J Altern Complement Med* 2003; 9:599–601.
11. Nathan P. Can the cognitive enhancing effects of ginkgo biloba be explained by its pharmacology? *Med Hypotheses* 2000; 55:491–493.
12. Hoerr R. EGb 761® Investigator's Brochure: Dementia. Dr Willmar Schwabe GmbH & Co., Karlsruhe, 2000, Report No. 11.
13. Kelly JP, Kaufman DW, Kelley K, Rosenberg L, Anderson TE, Mitchell AA. Recent trends in use of herbal and other natural products. *Arch Intern Med* 2005; 165:281–286.
14. Hogan DB, Ebly EM. Complementary medicine use in a dementia clinic population. *Alzheimer Disease Assoc Disord* 1996; 10:63–67.
15. Dergal JM, Gold JL, Laxer DA *et al*. Potential interactions between herbal medicines and conventional drug therapies used by older adults attending a memory clinic. *Drugs Aging* 2002; 19:879–886.
16. Belle SH, Zhang S, Czaja SJ, Burns R, Schulz R. Use of cognitive enhancement medication in persons with Alzheimer disease who have a family caregiver: results from the Resources for Enhancing Alzheimer's Caregiver Health (REACH) project. *Am J Geriatr Psychiatry* 2004; 12:250–257.
17. Birks J, Grimley EV, Van Dongen M. Ginkgo biloba for cognitive impairment and dementia. *Cochrane Database Syst Rev* 2002; 4:CD003120.

18. Oken B, Storzbach D, Kaye J. The efficacy of Ginkgo biloba on cognitive function in Alzheimer's disease. *Arch Neurol* 1998; 55:1409–1415.
19. Ernst E, Pittler MH. Ginkgo biloba for dementia. A systematic review of double-blind, placebo-controlled trials. *Clin Drug Investig* 1999; 17:301–308.
20. Le Bars PL, Katz MM, Berman N, Itil TM, Freedman AM, Schatzberg AF. A placebo-controlled, double-blind, randomized trial of an extract of Ginkgo biloba for dementia. North American EGb Study Group. *JAMA* 1997; 278:1327–1332.
21. Rosen W, Mohs R, Davis K. A new rating scale for Alzheimer's disease. *Am J Psychiatry* 1984; 141:1356–1364.
22. Schwartz G. Development and validation of the Geriatric Evaluation by Relative's Rating Instrument (GERRI). *Psychol Rep* 1983; 53:479–488.
23. Guy W. ECDEU assessment manual for psychopharmacology. US National Institute of Health, Psychopharmacology Research Branch, Rockville, MD, 1976.
24. Yaphe J, Edman R, Knishkowy B, Herman J. The association between funding by commercial interests and study outcome in randomized controlled drug trials. *Fam Pract* 2001; 18:565–568.
25. van Dongen MC, van Rossum E, Kessels AG, Sielhorst HJ, Knipschild PG. The efficacy of ginkgo for elderly people with dementia and age-associated memory impairment: new results of a randomized clinical trial. *J Am Geriatr Soc* 2000; 48:1183–1194.
26. American Psychiatric Association. *Diagnostic and Statistical Manual of Mental Disorders DSM-IIIR*, 4th edition. American Psychiatric Press, Washington, 1987.
27. Kanowski S, Hermann W, Stephan K, Wierlich W, Horr R. Proof of efficacy of the Ginkgo biloba special extract EGb 761 in outpatients suffering from mild to moderate primary degenerative dementia of the Alzheimer type or multi-infarct dementia. *Pharmacopsychiatry* 1996; 29:47–56.
28. Brodaty H, Dresser R, Eisner M *et al.* Consensus statement of the Alzheimer's Disease International and International Working Group for Harmonization of Dementia Drug Guidelines for research involving human subjects with dementia. *Alzheimer Disease Assoc Disord* 1999; 13:71–79.
29. Schneider L, DeKosky S, Farlow MR, Tariot P, Hoerr R, Kieser M. A randomized, double-blind, placebo-controlled trial of two doses of ginkgo biloba extract in dementia of the Alzheimer's type. *Curr Alzheimer Res* 2005; 2:541–551.
30. American Psychiatric Association. *Diagnostic and Statistical Manual of Mental Disorders DSM-IV-TR (Text Revision)*, 4th edition. American Psychiatric Press, Washington, 2000.
31. McKhann G, Drachman D, Folstein M *et al.* Clinical diagnosis of Alzheimer's disease: report of the NINCDS-ADRDA Work Group under the auspices of Department of Health and Human Services Task Force on Alzheimer's Disease. *Neurology* 1984; 34:939–944.
32. Folstein M, Folstein S, McHugh P. 'Mini-mental state': a practical method for grading the cognitive state of patients for the clinician. *J Psychiatr Res* 1975; 12:189–198.
33. Hamilton M. A rating scale for depression. *J Neurol Neurosurg Psychiatry* 1980; 23:56–62.
34. Schneider L, Olin J, Doody R, Clark C, Morris J, Reisberg B. Validity and reliability of the Alzheimer's Disease Cooperative Study – Clinical Global Impression of Change. *Alzheimer Disease Assoc Disord* 1997; 11(suppl 2):S22–S32.
35. Cummings J, Mega M, Gray K *et al.* The Neuropsychiatric Inventory: comprehensive assessment of psychopathology in dementia. *Neurology* 1994; 44:2308–2314.
36. Fugh-Berman A. Herb-drug interactions. *Lancet* 2000; 355:134–138.
37. Kayne S. Ginkgo biloba: potential concern. *Good Clin Pract J* 2001; 8:8–10.
38. Benjamin J, Muir T, Briggs K, Pentland B. A case of cerebral haemorrhage – can Ginkgo biloba be implicated? *Postgrad Med J* 2001; 77:112–113.
39. Fessenden JM, Wittenborn W, Clarke L. Gingko biloba: a case report of herbal medicine and bleeding postoperatively from a laparoscopic cholecystectomy. *Am Surg* 2001; 67:33–35.
40. Fong KCK. Retrobulbar haemorrhage associated with chronic Gingko biloba ingestion. *Postgrad Med J* 2003; 79:531–532.
41. Hauser D, Gayowski T, Singh N. Bleeding complications precipitated by unrecognized Gingko biloba use after liver transplantation. *Transpl Int* 2002; 15:377–379.
42. Meisel C, Johne A, Roots I. Fatal intracerebral mass bleeding associated with Ginkgo biloba and ibuprofen. *Atherosclerosis* 2003; 167:367.
43. Rosenblatt M, Mindel J. Spontaneous hyphema associated with ingestion of Ginkgo biloba extract. *N Engl J Med* 1997; 336:1108.

44. Rowin J, Lewis SL. Spontaneous bilateral subdural hematomas associated with chronic Ginkgo biloba ingestion. *Neurology* 1996; 46:1775–1776.
45. Vale S. Subarachnoid haemorrhage associated with Ginkgo biloba. *Lancet* 1998; 352:36.
46. Köhler S. *Examination of the Effect of Ginkgo Biloba Special Extract EGb761® and of the Interaction Between ASA and Ginkgo Biloba Special Extract EGb761® Regarding Coagulation*. Dr Willmar Schwabe GmbH&Co, Karlsruhe, 1999.
47. Engelsen J, Nielsen JD, Winther K. Effect of coenzyme Q10 and Ginkgo biloba on warfarin dosage in stable, long-term warfarin treated outpatients. A randomized, double blind, placebo-crossover trial. *Thromb Haemost* 2002; 87:1075–1076.
48. Kupiec T, Raj V. Fatal seizures due to potential herb – drug interactions with ginkgo biloba. *J Anal Toxicol* 2005; 29:755–758.
49. Haller CA, Meier K, Olson K. Seizures reported in association with use of dietary supplements. *Clin Toxicol* 2005; 1:23–30.
50. Barnes J, Mills SY, Abbot NC, Willoughby M, Ernst E. Different standards for reporting ADRs to herbal remedies and conventional OTC medicines: face-to-face interviews with 515 users of herbal remedies. *Br J Clin Pharmacol* 1998; 45:496–500.
51. Fugh-Berman A, Ernst E. Herb – drug interactions: review and assessment of report reliability. *Br J Clin Pharmacol* 2001; 52:587–595.
52. Haller CA, Anderson IB, Kim SY, Blanc PD. An evaluation of selected herbal reference texts and comparison to published reports of adverse herbal events. *Adverse Drug React Toxicol Rev* 2002; 21:143–150.
53. Kaye AD, Clarke RC, Sabar R *et al*. Herbal medicines: current trends in anesthesiology practice – a hospital survey. *J Clin Anesth* 2000; 12:468–471.
54. Van Beek T, Bombardelli E, Morazzoni P, Peterlongo F. Ginkgo biloba L. *Fitoterapia* 1998; LXIX:195–244.
55. Loew D, Kaszkin M. Approaching the problem of bioequivalence of herbal medicinal products. *Phytother Res* 2002; 16:705–711.
56. Kressmann S, Muller WE, Blume HH. Pharmaceutical quality of different Ginkgo biloba brands. *J Pharm Pharmacol* 2002; 54:661–669.
57. Kressmann S, Biber A, Wonnemann M, Schug B, Blume HH, Muller WE. Influence of pharmaceutical quality on the bioavailability of active components from Ginkgo biloba preparations. *J Pharm Pharmacol* 2002; 54:1507–1514.
58. ConsumerLab. Product Review: Ginkgo Biloba and Huperzine A – Memory Enhancers. www.ConsumerLab.com 2003.
59. Mantle DWR, Gok M. Comparison of antioxidant activity in commercial Ginkgo biloba preparations. *J Altern Complement Med* 2003; 9:625–629.
60. Wettstein A. Cholinesterase inhibitors and Gingko extracts – are they comparable in the treatment of dementia? Comparison of published placebo-controlled efficacy studies of at least six months' duration. *Phytomedicine* 2000; 6:393–401.
61. Kurz A, Van Baelen B. Ginkgo biloba compared with cholinesterase inhibitors in the treatment of dementia: a review based on meta-analyses by the Cochrane Collaboration. *Dement Geriatr Cogn Disord* 2004; 18:217–226.

# 5

# Memantine

*D. Wilkinson*

## INTRODUCTION

Glutamate is an excitatory amino acid neurotransmitter found in cortical and hippocampal neurones. Evidence is accumulating to suggest that the sustained presence of synaptic glutamate due to poor reuptake by glial cells may lead to loss of calcium homeostasis within the neurone [1]. During normal synaptic transmission full depolarization of the membrane occurs when glutamate binds with the *N*-methyl-D-aspartate (NMDA) receptor after partial depolarization by other ionotropic glutamate receptors, e.g. alpha-amino-3-hydroxy-5-methyl-4-isoxazolepropionic acid (AMPA) and kainate. This opens the cation channel which, at rest, is closed by a magnesium ion, allowing calcium ions into the neurone. Memantine, which is an uncompetitive NMDA receptor antagonist, like magnesium, blocks the cation channel in the resting state, however, the binding of magnesium and memantine to the receptor are voltage dependent. It is postulated that during the chronic partial depolarization of the membrane, caused by the abnormal persistence of glutamate in the synapse and its effects on AMPA receptors the voltage change causes magnesium to leave the channel, allowing calcium through. However, memantine which requires a greater potential difference to dislodge it remains in place blocking the channel until full depolarization from a physiological stimulus occurs thus allowing normal synaptic transmission (Figure 5.1). Chronic excessive calcium influx impairs neuronal homeostasis causing eventual neurodegeneration and may result in synaptic or dendritic damage, necrosis or apoptosis [2, 3] resulting in cell death [4–6]. The excessive stimulation of the NMDA receptor, under conditions of energy deprivation such as ischaemia and the resulting excitotoxicity will impair long-term potentiation, a process necessary for memory and learning.

Memantine has been available in Germany for many years for use in neurodegenerative disorders and a number of clinical studies have shown memantine to improve cognition in various stages of dementia. These data have been sufficient to achieve a licence in the USA and Europe for moderate to severe Alzheimer's disease (AD) and more recently for mild to moderate AD in Turkey and Mexico. However, in its early development its mode of action and potential neuroprotective effect was seen as being relevant to the treatment of the ischaemia related to vascular dementia (VaD).

## MEMANTINE IN VASCULAR DEMENTIA

Two studies have been published in VaD which had very similar designs. The MMM 300 study was a 28-week multicentre double-blind study conducted in France, which enrolled

**David Wilkinson**, MB, ChB, MRCGP, FRCPsych, Consultant in Old Age Psychiatry, Memory Assessment and Research Centre, Moorgreen Hospital, University of Southampton Division of Neuroscience, Southampton, UK

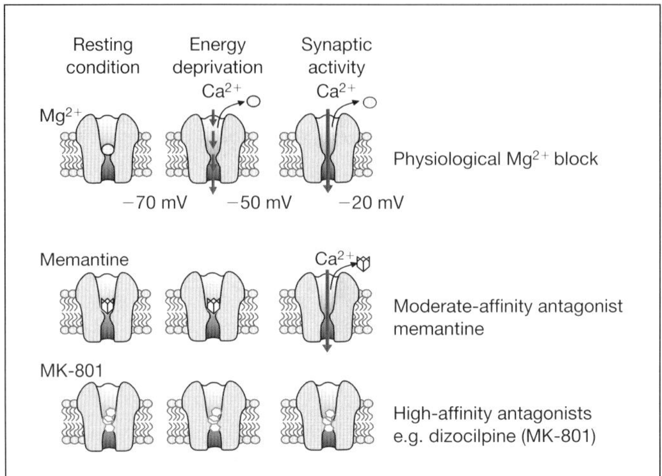


**Figure 5.1** Differentiation from other NMDA antagonists (with permission from [23]).

321 patients with mild to moderate dementia (using DSM-III and MMSE 12–20) satisfying the criteria for probable VaD according to NINDS-AIREN criteria [7]. Patients with AD were excluded according to the protocol.

Overall, the results were rather equivocal finding statistically significant improvements only on cognition using the Alzheimer's Disease Assessment Scale cognitive portion (ADAS-Cog) and Mini-mental State Examination (MMSE) although with some numerical advantage for memantine in all parameters. As has become familiar in subsequent VaD studies, the placebo group showed a lack of the deterioration normally seen in AD trials. Although there was a significant advantage for memantine in the cognitive subscale of the Gottfries–Bråne–Steen (GBS) scale, a composite measure of cognition and function, overall the GBS, the Clinical Global Impression of Change (CGIC) and Nurses Geriatric Observation scale (NOSGER) all failed to show a significant advantage for memantine.

The authors argue that the demonstration of a cognitive advantage in a VaD population was a proof of concept and that the lack of decline in the placebo group may have meant that the study was underpowered leading to the equivocal results. This is something of a recurring theme in the memantine data set.

Recruitment for the second study which was already underway was extended as a result (MMM 500), perhaps giving the chance to test the assumption that the initial study was underpowered. In this study, 548 patients were randomized to either 20 mg memantine daily or placebo in a 28 week multicentre study in the UK [8]. The same entry criteria were used for probable VaD but the mean MMSE at entry was slightly higher (range 10–22). The results were similar showing that, whilst there was some slight advantage for memantine in a number of sub-analyses, the only significant outcome was in cognition as determined by the ADAS-Cog. In the placebo population, the MMSE did not change over the 28 weeks in common with many VaD studies but unfortunately neither did the memantine group.

Again subgroup analysis showed that there were greater benefits for the memantine by grouping the patients with more severe dementia as defined by entry MMSE and with small vessel disease on imaging [9] (Figure 5.2). This latter finding was confirmed in a combined analysis of the two studies when the baseline computed tomography/magnetic resonance imaging (CT/MRI) findings were separated into those with larger cortical infarctions, or large vessel disease, and those with white matter lesions and lacunes, or small vessel disease [9]. Those with small vessel disease showed progressive decline in cognitive function

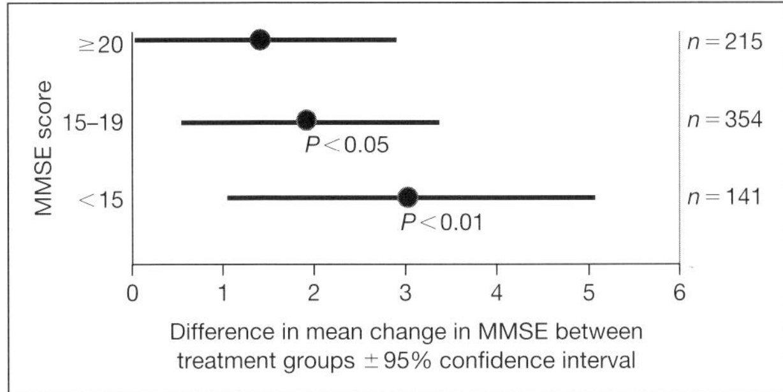


**Figure 5.2** Cognitive benefit increases with severity of VaD. MMM 300 + 500: Pooled subgroup analysis by severity at baseline, difference in mean change from baseline in ADAS-Cog total scores. (With permission from [35]).

compared with the large vessel group who showed no change after 28 weeks and as a result the symptomatic improvements were much greater in the small vessel group. This may suggest that whilst stoke and multiple infarctions are a risk factor for dementia they represent brain damage rather than dementia and the cognitive decline we see in VaD patients is caused by small vessel disease. It was then felt that there could be a rationale for treating more severe AD and the most influential memantine study was undertaken in a group of moderately severe AD patient.

## MEMANTINE IN AD

Memantine has demonstrated neuroprotective qualities in a number of model systems, both *in vivo* and *in vitro*. Prevention of NMDA- and glutamate-induced cell death has been shown in a number of culture systems, including rat retinal ganglion, cerebellar, cortical, mesencephalic and hippocampal neurones. Interestingly, in other tissue culture experiments, memantine reduced tau hyperphosphorylation [10] and promoted non-amyloidogenic amyloid precursor protein (APP) processing [3]. These effects may contribute to the observed efficacy of memantine in patients with AD. Other studies have shown reduced cell loss in rat models with administration of memantine [3, 11, 12].

## CLINICAL TRIALS

### *MODERATELY SEVERE AD*

Seven randomized controlled trials of memantine in AD have been completed to date, six of which have been of 6 months' duration (Table 5.1). The first controlled trial to report positive findings in AD was unlike the others in that it was of 12 weeks' duration, undertaken in a severe nursing home population (mean baseline MMSE 6.3) and only tested 10 mg daily rather than the currently licensed dose of 10 mg twice daily used in the others [13]. This study undertaken in Latvian nursing homes included 166 patients of whom 51% had AD and 49% VaD. The primary outcome measures were the CGIC as rated by a physician and the Behavioural rating scale for Geriatric Patients (BGP) subscore 'care dependence' as rated by a nurse. The overall outcomes of the study demonstrated a statistically significant advantage for memantine over placebo for both primary outcomes with 73% of the memantine-treated patients improving on CGIC compared with only 43% of the placebo group. After a responder analysis the functional improvements were judged to be clinically relevant. A separate

**Table 5.1** Completed phase III, placebo-controlled clinical studies with Memantine in AD

| *Study no.*<br>*Author* | *AD severity*<br>*MMSE inclusion range (Mean)* | *Duration/design* | *Number of randomized patients* | *Key efficacy parameters* |
|---|---|---|---|---|
| **M-Best**<br>Winblad and Poritis [13] | Severe NH patients<br><10 (6.3) | 12 weeks DB, PBO-controlled mixed AD/VaD patients<br>10 mg/day | *n* = 166 | CGI-C<br>BGP<br>D-scale |
| **MRZ-9605**<br>Reisberg *et al.* [14] | Moderate to severe<br>3–14 (7.7) | 28-week/DB, PBO-controlled | 252<br>PBO: 126<br>MEM: 126 | SIB<br>CIBIC+<br>ADCS-ADL<br>NPI |
| **MD-02**<br>Tariot *et al.* [15] | Moderate to severe<br>5–14 (10.0) | 24-week/DB, PBO-controlled in combination with donepezil | 403<br>PBO: 201<br>MEM: 202 | SIB<br>CIBIC+<br>ADCS-ADL<br>NPI |
| **99679**<br>Backchine *et al.* [17] | Mild to moderate<br>11–23 (18.7) | 24-week/DB, PBO–controlled | 470<br>PBO: 152<br>MEM: 318 | ADAS-Cog<br>CIBIC+<br>ADCS-ADL<br>NPI |
| **MD-10**<br>Peskind *et al.* [16] | Mild to moderate<br>10–22 (17.3) | 24-week/DB, PBO-controlled | 403<br>PBO: 202<br>MEM: 201 | ADAS-Cog<br>CIBIC+<br>ADCS-ADL<br>NPI |
| **MD-12**<br>Forest data on file [18, 24] | Mild to moderate<br>10–22 (16.9) | 24-week/DB, PBO-controlled in combination with donepezil, rivastigmine, or galantamine | 433<br>PBO: 216<br>MEM: 217 | ADAS-Cog<br>CIBIC+<br>ADCS-ADL<br>NPI |
| **MD-01**<br>[18, 24] | Moderate to severe<br>5–14 (10.1) | 24-week/DB, PBO-controlled | 350<br>PBO: 172<br>MEM: 178 | SIB<br>CIBIC+<br>ADCS-ADL<br>NPI |

DB = double-blind; MEM = memantine; PBO = placebo.

analysis of the AD patients which in fact only amounted to about 20 patients in each group showed an advantage for memantine which was used to support the licensing applications for moderate to severe AD along with the data published by Reisberg on the most important trial to date [14].

This study was a 28-week double-blind placebo-controlled trial of 252 moderately severe outpatients (mean baseline MMSE 7.9) undertaken in the US. The main outcome measures were the severe impairment battery (SIB) a cognitive scale validated to demonstrate change in severe AD patients, the Clinicians Interview Based Impression of Change plus caregiver information (CIBIC+), the 19 item Alzheimer's Disease Cooperative Study severe activities of daily living scale (ADCS-ADL) and the functional assessment staging tool (FAST). Other measures including the MMSE, Neuropsychiatric Inventory (NPI) and a resource utilization scale were also used. There were significant advantages for the treated group on the SIB, ADCS-ADL and FAST. Sub analysis of the NPI showed a significant advantage for memantine in the domains of delusions and agitation/aggression. This study was important in

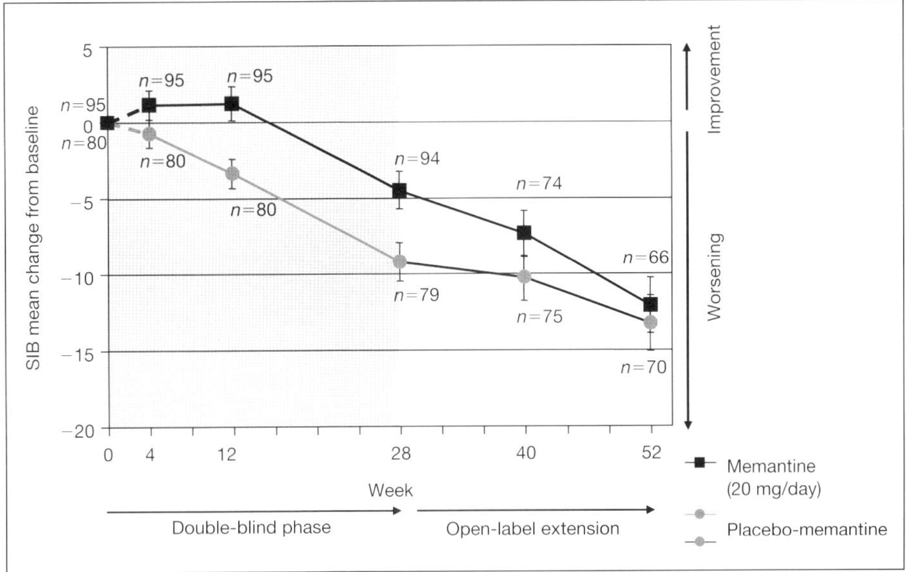


**Figure 5.3** Memantine in moderate to severe AD: SIB mean change (±SEM) observed case analysis (with permission from [14]).

showing that a new therapeutic agent different from the cholinergic drugs had a clinically significant effect and that these benefits could be achieved in the more severe stages of the disease. Also crucial when generalizing the trial data to clinical practice was the fact that, whilst there was a clear advantage for the treated patients, nevertheless at this advanced stage all patients were deteriorating (Figure 5.3). This is important when treating patients clinically when one has no placebo group for reference, as one has to consider that despite continued decline the patient may be getting the benefit of a slowed rate of deterioration.

The other published trial of memantine a 26-week double-blind placebo-controlled study in moderately severe dementia was in 404 patients who were already stabilized on donepezil [15]. The patients had to have been on donepezil for at least 6 months and a stable dose for 3 months but in fact the mean length of treatment was 2.5 years with nearly 90% on treatment for over 1 year prior to entry. The outcome measures were SIB, $\text{ADCS-ADL}_{\text{sev}}$, CIBIC+, NPI and the BGP care dependency subscore. In this study, the patients who were slightly less severe than in the two previous studies (mean baseline MMSE 10) who had memantine added to their donepezil showed significant improvements over those patients who continued donepezil with placebo on all measures. Patients on memantine and donepezil treatment compared with donepezil monotherapy also sustained improved cognitive performance relative to baseline compared with a progressive decline in the latter group over the same duration of treatment (Figure 5.4).

The last study in moderately severe AD, similar in design to the study published by Reisberg [14], was also conducted in the US and according to press releases this did not reach significance although the data have not yet been published for comment in this review.

### *MILD TO MODERATE AD*

Two studies have studied memantine monotherapy against placebo in mild to moderate AD and although as yet neither study has been published in a peer-reviewed journal, data have been presented showing benefits in cognition.

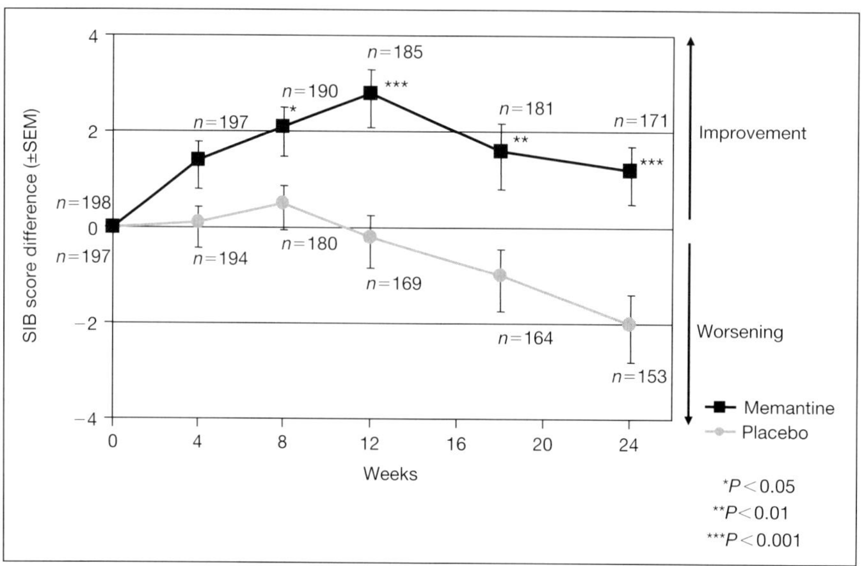


**Figure 5.4** Cognitive outcome in the Memantine 'Add on Study' in moderate to severe AD (MMSE 5–14) using SIB (with permission from [15]).

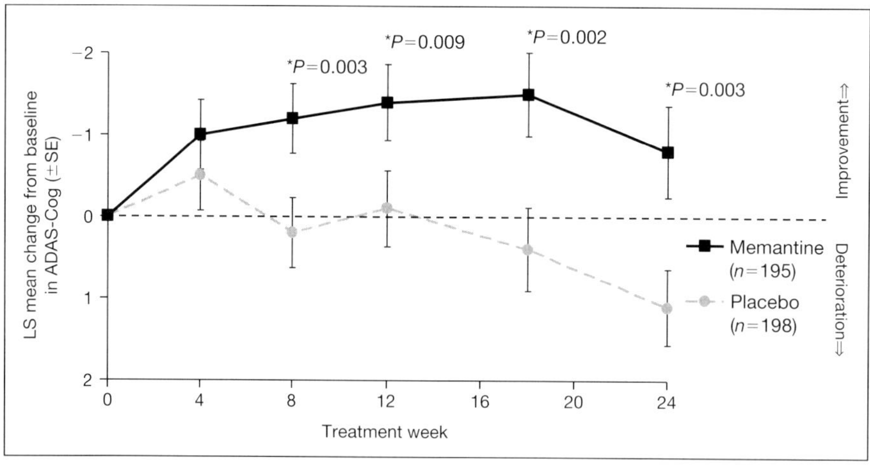


**Figure 5.5** MD-10 mild to moderate Alzheimer's disease ADAS-Cog (ITT-LOCF) (with permission from [16]).

The first a, 24-week randomized double-blind parallel group study, of memantine 20 mg/day (10 mg b.d.) or placebo, in 403 US outpatients (MMSE scores of 10–22, mean 17.3), used the ADAS-Cog and the CIBIC+ as primary outcomes and also measured the ADCS-ADL and NPI [16]. Although this was a monotherapy study 62% had been on acetylcholinesterase inhibitors (AChEIs) prior to study. There was no difference in completer rates between groups and those that stopped did so twice as often for poor response than for tolerability. The study showed significant improvements in the primary outcomes ADAS-Cog, CIBIC+ and in behaviour (NPI) but not in function (ADCS-ADL) (Figure 5.5).

The second study in mild to moderate AD was conducted in 470 patients with probable AD in 65 sites in 12 countries in Europe and was an identical design but for ethical reasons used a

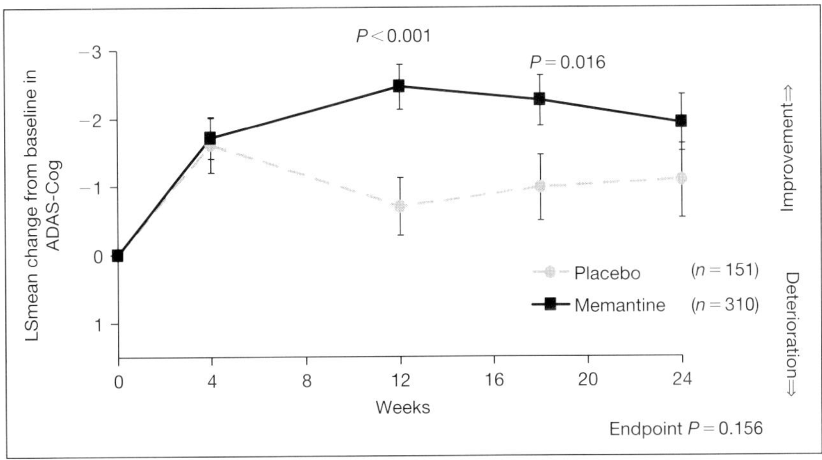


**Figure 5.6** Study 99679 mild to moderate AD ADAS-Cog (observed cases) (with permission from [17]).

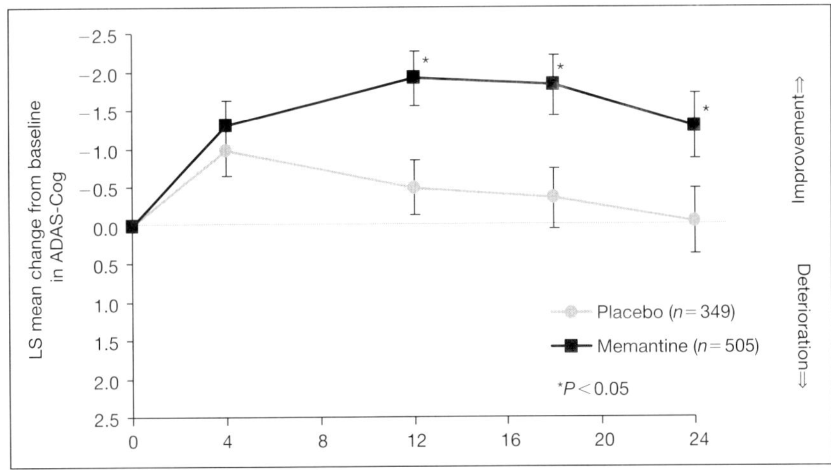


**Figure 5.7** Mild to moderate AD: studies MD-10 and 99679 integrated analysis (ADAS-Cog) (with permission from [17]).

2:1 randomization of memantine to placebo. This may have influenced the power of the study as in this case the placebo group showed very little decline in cognition over 6 months and so although there was a trend in favour of memantine on the ADAS-Cog which was significant at 12 and 18 weeks this did not reach significance at endpoint [17] (Figure 5.6).

In this study, as in the other mild to moderate study, many patients had prior treatment with AChEIs and an integrated analysis of both these mild to moderate studies in view of the similarity of study designs and the smaller placebo group in the European study did suggest that the second study may have been underpowered. (Figure 5.7).

The third mild to moderate study was a placebo-controlled 'add on' study, this time adding memantine or placebo to patients already stable on donepezil, rivastigmine or galantamine. This did not achieve statistically significant endpoints in favour of the memantine group (Table 5.1).

A combined analysis of all 6-month studies has been presented separately [18]. In this analysis, the three mild to moderate studies which used the ADAS-Cog were combined separately from the three moderately severe studies which used the SIB. Consistent with the results of the published studies, memantine-treated patients with AD showed statistically significant benefits compared to placebo-treated patients on the SIB total score and on the ADAS-Cog total score, suggesting a benefit of memantine on cognition throughout the course of AD. Single item and subscale analyses of the ADAS-Cog and SIB showed statistically significant differences between memantine and placebo on: Commands, Orientation, Comprehension and Test Instructions (ADAS-Cog), and Language, Memory, Orientation, Praxis, Construction, and Visuospatial Ability (SIB). Memantine significantly improved orientation and language abilities in AD patients. The findings support the efficacy of memantine in improving the patients' ability to communicate and interact with their environment, as well as their comprehension of spoken language which has been reported anecdotally from naturalistic treatment.

### *SAFETY AND TOLERABILITY*

Overall the tolerability of memantine has been very good in all the trials so far reported and a meta-analysis of all the 6-month studies showed all-cause discontinuations of memantine treatment similar to placebo [24]. Hypertension, constipation, abnormal gait, vomiting, and somnolence were significantly more frequent in memantine-treated patients, but none of these occurred in more than 5% of patients and no more than 2.2% more than in placebo-treated patients. The fact that glutamate is an excitotoxic neurotransmitter and that in the Reisberg trial there was a slight increase in hallucinations ($n$ = 11; 8.7%) in the memantine group as against $n$ = 4;3.2 % in the placebo group, and insomnia ($n$ = 13; 10.3% vs. $n$ = 10 7.9%) in the placebo group raised some concern. However, the numbers were very small and any concerns that use of memantine may increase neuropsychiatric symptoms have not been borne out in the subsequent studies. What was of considerable interest, however, was that agitation seemed to be much less frequent in the memantine group ($n$ = 23; 18%) than in the placebo group ($n$ = 40; 32%) and subsequent *post hoc* analyses of the combined trial data seem to indicate that memantine may exert a protective effect against the emergence of psychosis and agitation in AD. An interesting finding in view of the Reisberg [14] data is that in this combined analysis agitation was significantly less frequent in memantine-treated patients, occurring at a rate of 4% less than in placebo-treated patients.

Another important finding was that there appear to be very few cholinergic side-effects overall and that in the Tariot [15] study where all the patients were taking donepezil there was a reduction in diarrhoea and faecal incontinence suggesting that it may have effect on reducing the gastrointestinal side-effects of the AChEIs.

## EFFECTS OF MEMANTINE ON NEURODEGENERATION

Preclinical studies have shown an extensive array of effects that demonstrate a neuroprotective effect for memantine *in vitro* and in animal models. In various studies memantine has been shown to protect neuronal cells against toxicity due to mitochondrial dysfunction and chronic neuroinflammatory effects on cholinergic neurones; protects cholinergic neurones after NMDA-induced lesions. In animal models memantine can prevent neuronal damage, preserve acetylcholine terminals, reduce Aβ-induced learning deficits, protect against Aβ-induced apoptosis and neurotoxicity in rat brains and reduce tau phosphorylation in AD-like models possibly by its effects on stimulating protein phosphatase 2a which is known to prevent tau phosphorylation. Whether any of these effects remain hypothetical in man is unknown and its neuroprotective potential remains to be confirmed in clinical studies. One such study using serial MRI measures is underway [19–22].

## SUMMARY

Memantine is an important and interesting addition to the available treatments for AD. There is now a growing body of evidence particularly in moderate to severe AD, with some supporting evidence for an effect on patients with small vessel disease VaD that confirm a symptomatic effect [9]. The neuroprotective effects remain to be proved but further analysis and studies may elucidate this in time. There is no doubt that memantine at licenced doses of 10 mg twice daily is particularly well-tolerated, but more extensive use in clinical practice will show if that continues to be the case.

At present there is not enough evidence to decide whether memantine should be started prior to cholinesterase inhibitors as findings from the studies in mild to moderate AD have not been as robust as the AChEIs. Equally there are no data to indicate whether the two treatments should be started together or whether the two treatments have an additive or synergistic effect when combined. It also offers a clear treatment option in patients who cannot tolerate AChEIs or in whom their efficacy is in doubt. Practical considerations related to the pharmacokinetics of memantine are that, as it is 100% bioavailable, absorption is unaffected by food; it rapidly diffuses across the blood–brain barrier; and has an elimination half-life of 60–80 h, which is why it continues to be prescribed twice daily, particularly in patients with moderately severe AD where once daily dosing would be an advantage. A study has been undertaken to assess once daily dosing and one hopes this can soon be recommended. The other concern is that, whilst there are a number of notably positive studies, an equal number seem to have just failed to reach significance in the sum of the measure used. Whether this suggests a modest effect of the drug or in fact, in view of the very good safety profile supported by many years' use in Germany prior to licensing for AD, it suggests that the dose of 20 mg daily is at the borderlines of efficacy is not clear. One hopes studies with higher doses will be undertaken to see if there is a dose response which would consolidate the positive findings seen so far, without compromising the impressive tolerability profile.

## REFERENCES


1. Parsons CG, Danysz W, Quack G. Memantine is a clinically well tolerated *N-methyl-D-aspartate* (NMDA) receptor antagonist – a review of preclinical data. *Neuropharmacology* 1999; 38:735–767.
2. Lipton SA, Chen HS. Paradigm shift in neuroprotective drug development: clinically tolerated NMDA receptor inhibition by memantine. *Cell Death Differ* 2004; 11:18–20.
3. Rogawski MA, Wenk GL. The neuropharmacological basis for the use of memantine in the treatment of Alzheimer's disease. *CNS Drug Rev* 2003; 9:275–308.
4. Cacabelos R, Takeda M, Winblad B. The glutamatergic system and neurodegeneration in dementia: preventive strategies in Alzheimer's disease. *Int J Geriatr Psychiatry* 1999; 14:3–47.
5. Greenamyre J, Young A. Excitatory amino acids and Alzheimer's disease. *Neurobiol Aging* 1988; 10:593–602.
6. Greenamyre JT, Maragos WF, Albin RL *et al.* Glutamate transmission and toxicity in Alzheimer's disease. *Prog Neuropsychopharmacol Biol Psychiatry* 1988; 12:421–430.
7. Orgogozo JM, Rigaud AS, Stoffler A *et al.* Efficacy and safety of memantine in patients with mild to moderate vascular dementia: a randomized, placebo-controlled trial (MMM 300). *Stroke* 2002; 33:1834–1839.
8. Wilcock G, Mobius HJ, Stoffler A. A double-blind, placebo-controlled multicentre study of memantine in mild to moderate vascular dementia (MMM500). *Int Clin Psychopharmacol* 2002; 17:297–305.
9. Mobius HJ, Stoffler A. New approaches to clinical trials in dementia: memantine in small vessel disease. *Cerebrovasc Dis* 2002; 13(suppl 2):61–66.
10. Li L, Sengupta A, Haque N *et al.* Memantine inhibits and reverses the Alzheimer type abnormal hyperphosphorylation of tau and associated neurodegeneration. *FEBS Lett* 2004; 566:261–269.
11. Seif EL, Nasr M, Peruche B *et al.* Neuroprotective effect of memantine demonstrated in vivo and in vitro. *Eur J Pharmacol* 1990; 185:19–24.
12. Wenk GL, Zajaczkowski W, Danysz W. Neuroprotection of acetylcholinergic basal forebrain neurones by memantine and neurokinin-b. *Behav Brain Res* 1997; 83:129–133.

13. Winblad B, Poritis N. Memantine in severe dementia: results of the 9 M-best study (benefit and efficacy in severely demented patients during treatment with memantine). *Int J Geriatr Psychiatry* 1999; 14:135–146.
14. Reisberg B, Doody R, Stöffler A *et al.* Memantine in moderate-to-severe Alzheimer's Disease. *N Engl J Med* 2003; 348:1333–1341.
15. Tariot PN, Farlow MR, Grossberg GT *et al.* Memantine treatment in patients with moderate to severe Alzheimer's disease already receiving donepezil. A randomized controlled trial. *JAMA* 2004; 291:317–324.
16. Peskind ER, Potkin SG, Pomara N *et al.* Memantine monotherapy is effective and safe for the treatment of mild to moderate Alzheimer's disease: a randomized, controlled trial (abstract). *Eur J Neurol* 2004; 11(suppl 2):186.
17. Backchine S, Pascual-Gangnant L, Loft H. Results of a randomized, placebo-controlled 6-month study of memantine in the treatment of mild to moderate Alzheimer's disease in Europe. Poster presented at the European Federation of the Neurological Societies, (EFNS), Athens, Greece, 2005 Lundbeck data on file.
18. Mecocci P, Hefting N, Loft H. Memantine benefit on cognition in mild to severe Alzheimer's disease. Poster presented at the 9th Congress of the European Federation of the Neurological Societies, (EFNS), Athens, Greece, 2005 Lundbeck data on file.
19. Jain KK. Evaluation of memantine for neuroprotection in dementia. *Expert Opin Investig Drugs* 2000; 9:1397–1406.
20. Li L, Sengupta A, Haque N *et al.* Memantine inhibits and reverses the Alzheimer type abnormal hyperphosphorylation of tau and associated neuro degeneration. *FEBS Lett* 2004; 566:261–269.
21. Willard LB, Hauss-Wegrzyniak B, Danysz W *et al.* The cytotoxicity of chronic neuroinflammation upon basal forebrain cholinergic neurones of rats can be attenuated by glutamatergic antagonism or cyclooxygenase-2 inhibition. *Exp Brain Res* 2000; 134:58–65.
22. Miguel-Hidalgo JJ, Alvarez XA, Cacabelos R *et al.* Neuroprotection by memantine against neurodegeneration induced by beta-amyloid (1–40). *Brain Res* 2002; 958:210–221.
23. Danysz W, Parsons CG, Quack G *et al.* NMDA channel blockers: memantine and amino-aklyclohexanes-in vivo characterization. *Amino Acids* 2000; 19:167–172.
24. Doody RS, Tariot PN, Pfeiffer E *et al.* Meta-Analysis of 6-month memantine Clinical Trials in Alzheimer's disease. Poster presented at NCDEU, Boca Raton, US, 2005.

# 6

# Anti-oxidant drugs

*D. M. Stein, M. Sano*

## INTRODUCTION

Alzheimer's disease (AD) represents one of the most challenging healthcare problems world-wide. While the incidence and prevalence grows with life expectancy there are few treatment options and little knowledge of effective prevention strategies. Oxidative damage in the brain has been implicated in the pathophysiology of AD, suggesting a possible role for anti-oxidant interventions in treatment and prevention. Current clinical practice involves the use of anti-oxidant treatment in AD, and a number of clinical trials and observational studies have in the past and are currently exploring the efficacy and safety of the use of anti-oxidants in preventing and/or delaying progression of neurodegenerative processes. The scientific basis of this approach is grounded in *in vitro* and *in vivo* studies, which have demonstrated that oxidative stress is at least a significant player in what is likely a multi-factorial pathogenesis of neurodegenerative disorders such as AD. Epidemiological and clinical studies provide some support for a beneficial effect in AD. Recently meta-analyses and *post hoc* examination of large clinical trials using vitamin E suggest possible risks particularly within clinically relevant subgroups. We will review the information regarding our current understanding of anti-oxidants as an intervention for AD.

## BIOLOGICAL BASIS FOR ANTI-OXIDANT USE IN AD

The idea that oxidative injury plays a role in AD likely originated from the free radical hypothesis of ageing, proposed formally in the 1950s [1]. This theory states that a 'single common process, modifiable by genetic and environmental factors... [is] responsible for the ageing and death of all living things' [2]. The process implicated is that of the initiation of free radical reactions, which are innate to biological systems and produce random, and deleterious changes to cellular structures and chemical composition. That AD is significantly correlated with ageing led to a natural question of whether oxidative stress is a contributing factor to the disease. The fact that brain tissue is a particularly susceptible target of reactive oxygen species (ROS), due to its relatively low content of anti-oxidants, its high content of polyunsatureated fatty acids, and its high metabolic activity, underscores this possibility [3].

A number of studies show evidence of the role of oxidative stress in the pathogenesis of AD. Early studies showed evidence of a relative increase of ROS release. This was thought

**Daniel M. Stein**, MD, Research Associate, Department of Psychiatry, The Mount Sinai Medical Center, New York, Research and Development Program, James J. Peters VA Medical Center, Bronx, New York, USA

**Mary Sano**, PhD, Director of the Alzheimer's Disease Research Center, Professor of Psychiatry, Department of Psychiatry, The Mount Sinai Medical Center, New York, Research and Development Program, James J. Peters VA Medical Center, Bronx, New York, USA

to be secondary to one or more of the following: a deficiency of cytochrome oxidase activity (involved in mitochondrial electron transfer), an alteration of iron homeostasis, a reduced potency of normal anti-oxidative systems, and an unbalanced activity of physiological anti-oxidants such as superoxide dismutase and monamine oxidase isoenzyme B [4].

'Surrogate markers' of free radical injury include lipid peroxidation, protein oxidation, glyco-oxidation, and oxidation of nucleic acids [5, 6]. The past several years of study in this area have shown that patients with AD have increased levels of oxidation of all of these biological macromolecules, and have led researchers to conclude that 'oxidative imbalance is a prominent feature of AD' [7]. One of the most commonly studied of these markers in AD is brain lipid peroxidation. Patients with a clinical diagnosis of AD have been shown to have increased levels of isoprostanes (IPs), markers of *in vivo* lipid peroxidation, in blood, urine and cerebrospinal fluid (CSF) [8, 9]. Evidence of increased oxidative stress in AD patients has been found in peripheral cells and tissues. Lymphocytes were used to detect increased oxidation peripheral cells of AD patients [10, 11]. Levels of the end processes of lipid peroxidation were measured in skin fibroblasts and lymphoblasts in patients with AD and in healthy controls. This study demonstrated an increase in lipid peroxides in AD patients, suggesting an attack by free radicals on cell membrane phospholipids [12]. Animal studies involving transgenic/knockout mice that model AD support this theory, as these models have been shown to display signs of increased oxidative stress [13–15].

While it is apparent that increased oxidative stress is present in AD, it is not as clear whether it is a cause or an effect of the pathology that leads to the disease. There are several findings, however, that hint that it may play a causal role rather than a secondary one.

Signs of oxidative damage have been shown to be present in the regions of vulnerable neurones associated with amyloid-β plaques and neurofibrillary tangles [16, 17]. These findings suggest a link in the pathophysiology of AD between plaques and tangles, and the aforementioned oxidative imbalance. Several other studies have suggested amyloid-β itself can lead to increased levels of ROS, and vice versa [18–21].

Patients with mild cognitive impairment (MCI), a precursor or early stage of AD, have been shown to have signs of increased oxidative stress. As with AD patients, MCI patients were shown to have increased levels of IPs [22]. A recent study showed increased DNA damage secondary to oxidized purines and pyrimidines in peripheral leukocytes of both patients with AD and those with MCI [23]. Another recent study showed a pattern of increased homocysteine (another risk factor for AD, and one that contributes to oxidative stress) and decreased total anti-oxidant capacity in both AD and MCI patients [24]. These findings of high levels of oxidation in MCI patients as compared to normal controls stress the role of oxidative damage in neurodegenerative disease even in its very early stages. Such early involvement suggests that oxidative stress could play a primary role in the neurodegenerative process of AD.

Another interesting source of evidence stems from studies in Down's syndrome (DS), in which nearly all individuals develop a pathology that is akin to AD. Oxidative damage plays a significant role in the pathology and DS patients demonstrate similar amyloid-β pathology. One study suggested the causal role of oxidative injury in DS by actually linking apoptotic neuronal death to lipid peroxidation and showing that this could be inhibited by the use of free radical scavengers [25]. Another group showed that increased oxidative stress in DS temporally precedes amyloid-β deposition, suggesting it is not merely secondary to this process [26]. This group subsequently showed that in AD itself, oxidative damage to RNA and amino acids is perhaps the earliest pathological sign even in AD, and that it occurs more in the early stages of the disease than in the later stages [27].

The abundance of evidence that oxidative stress plays a role in AD, coupled with the evidence suggesting that the role is causative or primary in nature and not merely a side-effect of other pathological mechanisms, leads one to seek out ways to determine whether interventions to reduce oxidative damage in the brains of patients with AD is a viable therapeutic or even preventive strategy. While there are a number of laboratory/experimental studies that suggest this [28–36], the clinical evidence is taken from both epidemiological studies and clinical trials which are reviewed below.

## CLINICAL EVIDENCE OF ANTI-OXIDANT EFFECT IN AD

Many observational studies support the notion that anti-oxidants may have a beneficial effect in AD either by reducing the risk or by modifying disease severity. Table 6.1 summarizes several of the observational studies supporting this notion.

Six of these are reports from ageing, population-based studies which have longitudinally followed subjects measuring anti-oxidant use with food frequency questionnaires and various forms of self-reported vitamin and supplement intake [37–42]. The most commonly studied agents are vitamins E and C, both from food and from vitamin supplementation. The results of these studies range from mild beneficial effect to no effect. For example, high intake of vitamins C and E from foods has been associated with a decreased risk of dementia in three studies [40–42] with one of these only finding a benefit among those who took both vitamins C and E. These samples had relatively long follow-up time permitting sufficient cases to convert to dementia thereby ensuring sufficient power to see an effect if it was there. Two other studies were unable to observe a benefit using similar methodologies [38–39]. In one the observation period was briefer, although the conversion rate was relatively high suggesting that the risk of low power may not have interfered with the results [39]. In the Honolulu Asia Aging Study cohort, a beneficial effect was seen for supplements of vitamins E and C on vascular dementia [38], the more common diagnosis in this cohort, but not on AD. Since this cohort depends on clinical diagnosis and there is little autopsy, it is not possible to determine in this data set if AD pathology may be affected by the use of these anti-oxidants.

Other studies have used clinical convenience samples such as the report of Fillenbaum *et al.* [43], which describes a secondary analysis of a sub-sample of cases from a 10-year prospective cohort study of community-dwelling elderly. The presence or absence of vitamin supplement use was recorded, although dose and frequency were not available. This sample, in which only 10% used any vitamin supplement, was unable to identify any benefit to vitamins E or C. Klatte *et al.* [44] reported on a chart review which identified 130 patients from memory disorders clinic, with a diagnosis of probable AD by NINCDS-ADRDA criteria who were taking donepezil (at least 5mg daily) and vitamin E (at least 1000 U daily). He examined the change in Mini-mental State Examination Score among those who were followed for at least 1 year and found a slower rate of decline than among historical controls not exposed to these treatments.

Overall the strongest observational data for a beneficial effect of vitamin E use comes from studies of dietary intake, which in general yields lower amounts than reported in studies of supplement use. It is also important to consider that dietary vitamin E is not in isolation and may reflect other aspects of dietary habits that contribute to positive outcomes. While studies have controlled for some of these, such as caloric intake there may be other aspects of food and lifestyle associated with these intake patterns that could be considered in multifactorial models.

Few clinical trials have been conducted examining the effect of vitamin E use as a treatment for dementia. Table 6.2 summarizes those trials in which dementia or cognitive loss was a primary or secondary outcome. One multicentre randomized trial examined vitamin E use (2000 IU/day) among community-residing patients with AD of moderate severity [45]. The trial examined vitamin E, selegiline and the combination compared to placebo. The primary outcome was the time to reach any of several clinical endpoints (nursing home placement, loss of basic activities of daily living, advancement to severe dementia or death). After adjustment for baseline imbalances in cognition, a beneficial effect was observed with

**Table 6.1** Observational studies of anti-oxidant use

| *References* | *Population, Study Design and Outcome Measures* | *Results and Comments* |
|---|---|---|
| Morris *et al.* [37] | **Population and Design:** 633 random sample of healthy, aged ≥65 years. Vitamin supplements taken in 'last 2 weeks' determined by direct inspection. Prospective follow-up<br>**Outcome:** Clinical diagnosis of AD | **Results:** 91 cases of AD in 4.3 years. Lower rate of AD in those taking vitamin E (both unadjusted and adjusted) and lower adjusted rate of AD in those taking vitamin C<br>**Comment:** No effect of multi-vitamin on rate of AD |
| Masaki *et al.* [38] | **Population and Design:** 3385 community-based males aged 71–93 from the Honolulu-Asia Aging Study, prospectively followed. Vitamins E and C supplements were ascertained by interview<br>**Outcomes:** Presence of dementia and type (Vascular, AD, Mixed) bases on CASI | **Results:** Reduced risk of vascular dementia in those taking both vitamins E and C supplements. No protective effect for AD. Vitamin E or C alone had better cognitive test performance at follow-up<br>**Comment:** Vitamin use reported at one time-point only. No measures of cognitive function at baseline |
| Commenges *et al.* [53] | **Population and Design:** 1367 subjects randomly selected from 5554 of the Paquid Study, SW France, age 65 years followed prospectively, for cognitive loss and dementia<br>**Outcome:** DSM-IIIR Diagnosis of dementia assessed with psychometric testing confirmed by neurologist | **Results:** Reduced risk of incident dementia with increased flavenoid intake<br>**Comment:** Small number of incident cases ($n = 65$) and large dropout (16% before 5 years, 20% before 8 years) |
| Luchsinger *et al.* [39] | **Population and Design:** 980 subjects >65 years old, random sample of healthy Medicare beneficiaries from North Manhattan (WHICAP) with at least 1 year follow-up. Observational prospective cohort. Food frequency questionnaire used to assess vitamin intake<br>**Outcome:** Incident AD by NINCDS-ADRDA | **Results:** 242 incident cases of AD. No effect of intake of carotenes and vitamin C, or vitamin E in supplemental or dietary form or in both forms, on risk of AD<br>**Comment:** Relatively high intake of dietary anti-oxidants, high conversion rate and short observation period |
| Engelhart *et al.* [40] | **Population and Design:** 5395 subjects age >55 years, non-demented from population based prospective, cohort Rotterdam Study. Evaluated with dietary assessment mean follow-up period 6 years<br>**Outcome:** Incident AD (DSM-IIIR; NINCDS-ADRDA) | **Results:** High dietary intake of vitamins C and E from food was associated with lower risk of AD<br>**Comment:** Positive effect of diet may require long observation period which is difficult to achieve in a randomized clinical trial |

| | | |
|---|---|---|
| Morris *et al.* [41] | **Population and Design:** 815 subjects ≥65 years old, non-demented random sample from biracial community in Chicago (CHAPS). Observational prospective cohort with mean follow-up of 3.9 years. Dietary assessment with food frequency and reported supplement use<br>**Outcome:** Incident AD based on NINCDS-ADRDA | **Results:** Increased dietary vitamin E associated with decreased risk of AD. The effect of vitamin E was reduced when dietary differences were controlled (fats, other anti-oxidants. Supplement use (vitamins C and E, β-carotene) had no effect<br>**Comment:** No dietary vitamin E effect in ApoE-ε4 subjects. Increased vitamin E supplement use during study, with possibility of inadequate exposure to see an effect |
| Klatte *et al.* [44] | **Population and Design:** 130 subjects from memory disorders clinic, probable AD by NINCDS-ADRDA criteria, taking donepezil (at least 5 mg daily) and vitamin E (at least 1000 U daily) with at least 1 year follow-up on these meds<br>**Outcome:** Mini-mental State Examination average cumulative score change compared to those of historical control (CERAD) before these treatments were available | **Results:** Subjects taking vitamin E declined at significantly lower rate than those in CERAD cohort<br>**Comment:** Many limitations of CERAD cohort (dropouts not included and vitamin E use not available and age differences) |
| Zandi *et al.* [42] | **Population and Design:** 4740 subjects, ≥65 years old, from Cache County Study, a population-based study of prevalence and incidence of AD and other dementias. Observational cross-sectional and prospective data review. In-home direct observation of current supplement use<br>**Outcome:** Diagnosis of AD by means of multistage assessment procedures | **Results:** Vitamins C and E combination supplement use was associated with reduced prevalence and risk of incidence of AD. No evidence of a protective effect when vitamin C or E used alone or with other vitamin complexes<br>**Comment:** Vitamin users were younger, more educated, and in better general health |
| Fillenbaum *et al.* [43] | **Population and Design:** 616 subjects from a secondary analysis of subsample of cases from Duke EPSE project, aged 65–105. Prospective cohort study of community-dwelling elderly. Vitamin use by subject report<br>**Outcome:** Time to dementia/AD on consensus conference using NINCDS-ADRDA criteria | **Results:** 8% subjects used vitamins; 141 subjects had dementia (93 AD). Use of low- or high-dose vitamin supplement of C and/or E did not delay incidence of dementia or AD<br>**Comment:** Did not record dose or duration of vitamin use. Few used vitamin but high conversion rate |

**Table 6.2** Randomized clinical trials of anti-oxidants

| *References* | *Subjects, Study Design and Outcome Measures* | *Results and Comments* |
|---|---|---|
| Sano *et al.* [45] | **Subjects and Study Design:** 342 subjects with moderate probable AD aged 55–90. Randomized, double-blind, placebo-controlled 2-year, multi-centre (23 sites) study of 4 treatment groups: selegiline (10 mg), $\alpha$-tocopherol (2000 IU)l, both, placebo<br>**Primary Outcome:** Time to any endpoint (death, institutionalization, loss of activities of daily living or severe dementia)<br>**Secondary Outcome:** Cognition, function, behaviour, extrapyramidal signs | **Results:** Delay in the time to the primary outcome for patients treated with selegiline, $\alpha$-tocopherol, or both, as compared to placebo<br>**Secondary Outcome:** Slower decline in functional outcomes. No improvement on cognitive, behavioural or extra-pyramidal measures<br>**Safety:** More falls in combined treatment group, unclear aetiology<br>**Comment:** Adjusted analysis due to imbalance in baseline MMSE scores |
| Le Bars *et al.* [54] | **Subjects and Study Design:** 309 subjects, with mild to severe dementia (AD or multi-infarct). Randomized, double-blind, placebo-controlled multicentre study of two groups: EGb 761 (extract of ginkgo) 120 mg/day or placebo for l52 weeks<br>**Primary Outcome:** Cognitve (ADAS-Cog), and two Clinical Global (GERRI) and CGIC | **Results:** EGb group did significantly better on the ADAS-Cog (1.4 points) and better in GERRI (0.14) than placebo. CGIC not significantly different<br>**Comment:** Significant dropout rate |
| Adair *et al.* [59] | **Subjects and Study Design:** 43 mild to moderate probable AD (MMSE of 12–26). Randomized, double-blind, placebo-controlled trial of NAC (50 mg/kg/day) with assessments at 3 and 6 months<br>**Primary Outcome:** Change in MMSE and ADL scale<br>**Secondary Outcome:** Performance on cognitive battery components | **Results:** No significant effect of treatment with NAC on primary outcome. Significant benefit on some subtests of the cognitive battery<br>**Safety:** Fatigue, headache and appetite loss were the most common side-effects<br>**Comment:** Trend toward a positive result in some other outcomes |
| Gutzmann *et al.* [60] | **Subjects and Study Design:** 203 subjects aged 40–90 with mild to moderate primary dementia (DSM-IIIR) and probable AD (NINCDS-ADRDA). Double-blind, parallel-group, multicentre study randomized to either idebenone (360 mg/day) or tacrine (up to 160 mg/day) and treated for 60 weeks | **Results:** Higher benefit from treatment in patients randomized to idebenone, very high dropout rates in both groups<br>**Comment:** Did not focus on drug vs. placebo, but on improvement after set 60-week time period |

| | | |
|---|---|---|
| | **Primary Outcome:** The efficacy index score (EIS), a 'multi-dimensional evaluation' including physician, psychologist, patient's relative<br>**Secondary Outcome:** ADAS-Cog, NOSGER-IADL, CGIC | |
| HPSCG [47] | **Subjects and Study Design:** 20 536 UK adults, aged 40–80 with coronary/occlusive artery disease, or diabetes. Randomized placebo-controlled factorial design 5-year study of anti-oxidant supplementation (600 mg vitamin E, 250 mg vitamin C, 20 mg β-carotene/day) and simvastatin (40 mg/day)<br>**Primary Outcome (non-cognitive):** Major coronary or vascular events<br>**Secondary Outcome (cognitive):** Cognitive impairment measured by a telephone interview at study end and incident dementia by record review of report | **Results:** No benefit of anti-oxidant supplements on cognitive performance or incident dementia<br>**Comment:** Cognition was an 'add-on' to the cardiovascular study and no baseline evaluation of cognition or incident dementia was conducted |
| Thal *et al.* [58] | **Subjects and Study Design:** 536 subjects, age >50 years with mild to moderate (MMSE 12–25) probable AD (NINCDS-ADRDA), randomized, placebo-controlled trial for 1 year with 3 treatment groups: idebenone 120, 240, or 360 mg t.i.d., each of which was compared with placebo<br>**Primary Outcome:** ADAS-Cog,ADCS-CGIC<br>**Secondary Outcome:** ADCS-ADL (activities of daily living scale), MMSE, BEHAVE-AD (behavioural rating scale) | **Results:** There were no significant differences between any dose group and placebo for the primary or secondary outcomes<br>**Comment:** In an exploratory two-group analysis comparing all three treated groups combined to placebo, drug-treated patients performed better on the ADAS-Cog but not the CGIC |
| Petersen *et al.* [46] | **Subjects and Study Design:** 769 subjects with amnestic MCI, aged 55–90. Multicentre (69 sites), randomized, double-blind placebo-controlled, 3-year study of vitamin E (200 IU/day), donepezil (10 mg/day) each compared to placebo<br>**Primary Outcome:** Incident AD<br>**Secondary Outcome:** Cognitive battery and IADL | **Results:** No effect of vitamin E on primary outcome. A few significant differences in secondary outcomes (executive, language, overall cog scores) for first 18 months only<br>**Comment:** Incident dementia occurred primarily in the ApoE-ε4 group |

**Table 6.2** (continued)

| *References* | *Subjects, Study Design and Outcome Measures* | *Results and Comments* |
|---|---|---|
| Schneider *et al.* [56] | **Subjects and Study Design:** 513 subjects with mild to moderate (MMSE of 24–10) AD<br>Multicentre randomized placebo-controlled study for 26-week treatment with GbE at 120 mg or 240 mg/day or placebo<br>**Primary Outcome:** Alzheimer's Disease Assessment Scale (ADAS-Cog), Clinical Global Impression of Change (ADCS-CGIC) | **Results:** There were no significant between-group differences for the whole sample. In a subgroup with behavioural disturbance there was significantly better cognitive and global assessment scores for the patients on GbE<br>**Comment:** There was little cognitive and functional decline of the placebo-treated patients |
| van Donegan *et al.* [63] | **Subjects and Study Design:** 214 institutionalized subjects AD, VAD or MCI. Randomized, double-blind, placebo-controlled, parallel-group, multicentre 24-week trial of Ginkgo (either 240 mg/day or 160 mg/day) or placebo<br>**Primary Outcome:** Syndrome Kurz Test (SKT) a cognitive measure. CGIC, psychopathology assessed by nursing staff, and ADL scale | **Results:** No differences in SKT or ADL found between Ginkgo and placebo were found on any measure<br>**Comment:** No trend of benefit based on dose or diagnosis |
| Kanowski *et al.* [61] | **Subjects and Study Design:** 216 subjects with AD or MID *via* DSM-IIIR. Alzheimer disease and multi-infarct dementia randomized, double-blind, placebo-controlled, multicentre study of 24 weeks with a 4 week run-in, Ginkgo (240 mg/day) or placebo<br>**Primary Outcome:** CGIC, SKT, the NAB for behavioural assessment of activities of daily life. Responders defined as response in at least two of the three primary variables.<br>ADAS-Cog and CGIC reported later [62] | **Results:** 156 of 216 completed the study. Frequency of therapy responders was greater with Ginkgo ($P < 0.005$). Later report demonstrated benefit in ADAS-Cog and CGIC [62]<br>**Comment:** Drug was well-tolerated |
| Nathan *et al.* [64] | **Subjects and Study Design:** 11 healthy volunteers received *Ginkgo biloba* (120 mg) or placebo in double-blind placebo-controlled crossover design trial. Testing was conducted pre- and 90 min post-drug administration for each treatment condition. Treatment conditions were separated by 7 days | **Results:** No acute effects of *Ginkgo biloba* were found for any of the memory tests examined. The findings suggest that 120 mg of *Ginkgo biloba* has no acute nootropic effects in healthy older humans<br>**Comment:** Crossover design may have carryover effects for measures of learning and memory |

| | | |
|---|---|---|
| | **Primary Outcomes:** Memory functioning using the computer battery of memory tests, Rey auditory verbal learning task | |
| Mix and Crews [65] | **Subjects and Study Design:** 262 cognitively healthy individuals 60 years of age and older enrolled in a randomized, double-blind, placebo-controlled, parallel-group, clinical trial, Ginkgo (180 mg/day) or placebo for 6 weeks<br>**Primary Outcome:** Cognitive measures: Selective Reminding Test (SRT), block design and digit symbol-coding face memory (WMS-III FI) and self-reported memory | **Results:** Ginkgo group had more improvement on SRT and on face memory and self-report of memory function<br>**Comment:** Baseline differences in cognitive measures may be responsible for the effect |
| Stough *et al.* [66] | **Subjects and Study Design:** 61 young healthy volunteers enrolled in a randomized, double-blind, placebo-controlled clinical trial for 30 days receiving 120 mg of Ginkgo or placebo<br>**Primary Outcome:** A battery of validated neuropsychological tests | **Results:** Benefit in the Ginkgo group for memory consolidation and working memory.<br>Also significant improvements in speed of information processing, executive processing |
| van Donegan [67] | **Subjects and Study Design:** 214 persons with dementia (either Alzheimer's dementia or vascular dementia; mild to moderate degree) or age-associated memory impairment (AAMI) enrolled for 24 weeks in a randomized, double-blind, placebo-controlled, parallel-group, multicentre trial. Treated with EGb 761 (240 or 160 mg/day) or placebo for 24 weeks<br>**Primary Outcome:** Cognitive tests and geriatric symptoms(SCAG), depressive mood (GDS), self-perceived health and memory status, self-reported level of instrumental daily life activities | **Results:** No effect on these outcomes, secondary analyses found slight improvement in combined Ginkgo doses than placebo on activities of daily and slightly worse on self-perceived health status. No beneficial effects of a higher dose or a prolonged duration of Ginkgo treatment were found<br>**Comment** No subgroup benefited from Ginkgo though no occurrence of (serious) adverse events |
| Maurer *et al.* [68] | **Subjects and Study Design:** 20 subjects with AD. Randomized to 240 mg/day of *Ginkgo biloba* special extract EGb 761, a double-blind, randomized, placebo-controlled, parallel-group design of 3 months<br>**Primary Outcome:** SKT, other tests (trailmaking test, ADAS, CGI) and EEG topography was evaluated descriptively | **Results:** Gingko-treated group performed better than placebo, trend of benefit on CGI and EEG<br>**Comment:** No effect on all other measures |

**Table 6.2** (continued)

| *References* | *Subjects, Study Design and Outcome Measures* | *Results and Comments* |
|---|---|---|
| Weyer *et al.* [69] | **Subjects and Study Design:** 300 subjects with AD randomized to either placebo, idebenone 30 mg or 90 mg t.i.d. and treated for 6 months<br>**Primary Outcome:** ADAS-Total<br>**Secondary Outcome:** ADAS-Cog and ADAS-Noncog, CGIC, MMSE, the Digit Symbol Substitution test (DSS) and scales of daily activities | **Results:** 90 mg t.i.d. significantly better on ADAS-Total and in ADAS-Cog. A responders' analysis for CGICC, ADAS-Cog, and ADAS-Noncog showed significant benefit over placebo (idebenone 90 mg)<br>**Comment:** Safety results were inconspicuous for all assessments |

all treatment groups on these outcomes and vitamin E also demonstrated a benefit on a measure of activities of daily living. However no benefit was observed on other secondary outcomes which included measures of cognitive benefit and behavioural disturbance.

An attempt to replicate this finding in individuals with Mild Cognitive Impairment (MCI), a prodrome to AD, was reported in 2005 [46]. This 3-year study compared vitamin E (2000 IU/day) and donepezil (10 mg/day) to placebo for the rate of conversion from MCI to AD. There was no benefit to either drug at the end of the 3-year period. There were also very few benefits noted on secondary measures in the vitamin E group.

Other studies have examined vitamin E in randomized trials designed to test other outcomes and have added on a secondary outcome to assess cognition. One such trial used a $2 \times 2$ factorial design to assess an anti-oxidant combination that included 600 IU of vitamin E and simvastatin for the prevention of cardiac disease outcomes in trial participants who were at risk for cardiovascular disease [47]. At the end of the study of over 20 000 participants, a telephone cognitive assessment was conducted on the part of the cohort who were age 65 and older. No benefit on the cognitive outcome was seen among those treated with anti-oxidants.

Other ongoing studies are designed to determine if vitamin E may have a beneficial effect on dementia and cognitive loss. The PREADVISE study is designed to add a cognitive assessment to a trial to assess the benefit of low dose vitamin E (65 IU) and selenium on prevention of prostate cancer [48]. The benefit of this add-on design is to gain information about a secondary outcome such as dementia without the expense of a separate trial. The disadvantage of this approach is that the population is selected for the primary trial and may not be the most ideal cohort for the secondary outcomes. For example the age of the cohort recruited for the prevention of prostate cancer may be younger than the cohort selected for dementia. Nevertheless, it provides an opportunity to ask an important question.

Another study examining the effect of vitamin E (2000 IU/day) on cognitive decline is a multicentre, randomized placebo-controlled trial of older individuals with DS [49]. This ongoing study by Aisen and colleagues is using the brief praxis test as the primary outcome to measure cognition and will provide information on the use of vitamin E in a cohort that has a very high risk of developing AD.

## VITAMIN E SAFETY CONCERNS AND IMPLICATIONS FOR TREATMENT OF AD

Recently, the safety of high-dose vitamin E therapy has been questioned. A meta-analysis of randomized studies of vitamin E therapy for various indications indicated that high-dose vitamin E increases the risk of all-cause mortality; the authors of this article and the editors of the journal in which it was published concluded that high-dose vitamin E should be avoided [50, 51]. Several aspects of the report are noteworthy including the exclusion of all studies with follow-up less than or equal to one year or with fewer than 10 deaths in the trial. The initial analysis examined all published trials regardless of dose and found no effect on mortality. Secondary analyses divided the trial using an arbitrary dose of 400 IU as a cut-off and found reduced mortality in studies using up to 400 IU and an increased mortality in studies exceeding this dose.

The safety of the chronic use of vitamin E has also been questioned by analysis of the results of a follow-up study to the Heart Outcomes Prevention Evaluation (HOPE) trial, one of the studies included in the above described meta-analysis [52]. The HOPE trial evaluated the impact of natural vitamin E, 400 IU daily, as well as ramipril, on cardiovascular events and cancer in over 9000 individuals with vascular disease or diabetes at least 55 years of age; mean follow-up was 4.5 years. For HOPE-The Ongoing Outcomes (HOPE-TOO), the trial was then extended, with about 4000 subjects continuing study medication (vitamin E or placebo) for a mean total duration of 7 years. The primary analyses of both HOPE and HOPE-TOO were negative, showing no impact of vitamin E on cancer or the composite of myocardial infarction, stroke and death from cardiovascular causes. But a planned secondary analysis revealed an excess of all heart failure events (relative risk [RR] 1.19; 95% confidence interval [CI] 1.05–1.35), and heart failure requiring hospital admission (RR 1.40; 95% CI 1.13–1.73), in subjects taking vitamin E. This increased risk has not been confirmed in other trials [52].

It is difficult to know how to integrate this information into clinical practice and future research. It appears that high-dose vitamin E supplements may be associated with poor outcomes specifically among those with cardiovascular risk factors. At present the only efficacy of high-dose vitamin E has been observed in moderately severe AD. Thus the use in that population in those without cardiac disease may have value clinically. However, no other clinical indication is supported. Yet the promise of vitamins as an anti-oxidant strategy seems reasonable and only continued evaluation through controlled clinical trials of dementia and perhaps of dementia prevention will provide viable answers. Given that so little is available as interventions for this disease, the potential risk in a subgroup must be weighed against the larger potential public health benefit. It is this risk ratio that should perhaps be used to determine the fate of ongoing clinical trials with vitamin E, rather than the results of any single study or meta-analysis.

## OTHER ANTI-OXIDANT AGENTS

Many agents appear to have some anti-oxidant activity as well as other potential mechanisms of action. Other agents with anti-oxidant properties have been studied including flavenoids. In 2000, Commenges *et al.* [53] described flavenoid intake in a cohort of 1367 subjects who were taken from a larger group of participants in a longitudinal study in the south of France [53]. The population was over age 65 and living in their homes. The primary outcome was the diagnosis of dementia, made according to DSM-IIIR criteria established by a clinician and psychometric testing. Flavenoid intake, estimated from food frequency questionnaires, was associated with a reduced risk of dementia. These findings, though hopeful, have several limitations including limited standardization of identifying flavenoid intake by food history and limited knowledge about the bioavailability of different sources of dietary flavenoids.

Clinical trials have examined agents which purport to have their anti-oxidant effect because they contain flavenoids. Most notable is *Ginkgo biloba*, which has been tested in Alzheimer's disease and is reviewed in detail elsewhere in this book. A multicentre study of 202 subjects, with mild to severe AD or multi-infarct dementia were enrolled in this year long study, which used EGb 761, an extract of ginkgo [54]. Results showed a small benefit on a cognitive measure and on a global scale in the treated group compared to placebo group and this difference was significant. An unusual trend was noted which indicated that there were more dropouts in the placebo group than in the treatment group. A meta-analysis by the Cochrane review (2003) summarized all reported trials with individuals with any cognitive complaint including dementia and found benefit for low (<200 mg/day) and high doses (>200 mg/day) of Ginkgo on clinical global measures, cognition and activities of daily living [55]. The authors caution, however that much of the data comes from early trials, which were subject to significant publication bias in favour of positive results, and which have inferior methodology (e.g. mixed patient populations, absence of intent-to-treat analysis, and atypical approach to statistical design). When the review is confined to those trials with modern trial designs the results are inconsistent with several clearly negative studies. Since that time an additional study of relatively good methodology reported no benefit on any cognitive global or functional measure [56].

In general, the overview of clinical trials indicates somewhat better response in subjects without dementia, particularly on outcomes of cognitive status and well-being. These findings raise the possibility Ginkgo may prevent cognitive loss and dementia. An ongoing placebo-controlled trial of Ginkgo is assessing the ability to prevent AD and all-cause dementia in healthy elderly people, aged 75 and above. Results of this study are projected to be available in 2009 [57].

Idebenone, a benzoquinone derivative, is structurally similar to coenzyme Q, which is an intermediate in the oxidative phosphorylation pathway. While anti-oxidant activity has been touted as a likely mechanism of action for therapeutic benefit, there are several others. Idebenone inhibits lipid peroxidation through free radical scavenger activity and appears to act as an anti-oxidant. Idebenone has also been studied in patients with dementia with mixed results. Most recently, a well-controlled multicentre trial of three doses of idebenone (120, 240 and 360 mg tid) in patients with mild to moderate AD was unable to demonstrate any benefit over placebo on cognitive, functional or behavioural measures [58]. Secondary analysis with all treated groups combined vs. placebo did show difference in a cognitive measure (ADAS-Cog), but no other measures were significant. Overall, the limited positive finding across the controlled clinical trials provides little support for clinical relevance of this agent in the treatment of AD.

## SUMMARY

While evidence from the basic science literature supports the potential benefit of anti-oxidants as treatments for cognitive loss and dementia, epidemiological and clinical studies are less clear. Some observational studies of supplement use have provided evidence of benefit while others do not. The same can be said for dietary studies, but it is unclear how well the beneficial effects of vitamin levels achieved by diet reflect supplement intervention. Perhaps the most convincing data are basic science studies that identify multiple mechanisms by which anti-oxidants could slow ageing changes and reduce the burden of amyloid in the AD brain.

Recent results with a range of agents tested in AD suggest that our current animal and cellular models have significant limitations. First it is not clear that the pathology being modelled reflects the mechanism of disease or symptoms. Second, these isolated models do not permit the simultaneous assessment of safety, which though relevant in any populations is of particular note in an ageing population with a significant amount of frailty. Safety concerns particularly when biological models provide so little confidence about dose selection are exacerbated as agents are proposed in conditions that will require long-term use. Furthermore, in developing agents for disease prevention, recruitment of healthy volunteers is required and the potential of increased risk to a population which is healthy at the study start significantly raises the risk–benefit ratio.

Perhaps most striking about the anti-oxidant story is how the use of the agents has proceeded beyond the data both in the AD population and in the general public. This is particularly true of vitamin E supplementation which appears to be >10% in the population over 65. It is important to remember that safety with any agent is too often presumed rather than tested and efficacy as suggested by epidemiological data is seldom as prominent in clinical trials as in observational studies. These observations should lead the practitioner to caution when prescribing treatments with little clinical evidence-based support. On the other hand, this lack of knowledge should be the specific impetus for the clinician to encourage participation in research and in particular clinical trials where the robustness of efficacy can be demonstrated. This approach will permit the most efficient and rapid means to create reasonable recommendations.

At present, clinical recommendation for the use of vitamin E may continue among those who are moderately impaired possibly with a reduction in dose from the 2000 IU/day used in the only trial demonstrating benefit. Caution is indicated among those with cardiac disease. Currently, there are insufficient data to recommend this agent for any other clinical population with cognitive disorders or complaints. In particular, there are no data to support its use to prevent cognitive loss or dementia. Ongoing trials may provide support for additional indications and the potential benefit must be weighed against known risks for individual agents.

## ACKNOWLEDGEMENTS

The authors' work is supported by P50AG05138 and U01 AG10483.

## REFERENCES

1. Harman D. Aging: a theory based on free radical and radiation chemistry. *J Gerontol* 1956; 11:298–300.
2. Harman D. The free radical theory of aging. *Antioxid Redox Signal* 2003; 5:557–561.
3. Christen Y. Oxidative stress and Alzheimer disease. *Am J Clin Nutr* 2000; 71:621S–629S.
4. Benzi G, Moretti A. Are reactive oxygen species involved in Alzheimer's disease? *Neurobiol Aging* 1995; 16:661–674.
5. Pratico D, Delanty N. Oxidative injury in diseases of the central nervous system: focus on Alzheimer's disease. *Am J Med* 2000; 109:577–585.
6. Levine RL, Williams JA, Stadman ER, Sharter E. Carbonyl assays for determination of oxidatively modified proteins. *Methods Enzymol* 1994; 233:346–357.
7. Zhu X, Lee HG, Casadesus G *et al.* Oxidative imbalance in Alzheimer's disease. *Mol Neurobiol* 2005; 31:205–217.
8. Montine TJ, Markesbery WR, Morrow JD, Roberts LJ 2nd. Cerebrospinal fluid F2-isoprostane levels are increased in Alzheimer's disease. *Ann Neurol* 1998; 44:410–413.
9. Pratico D, Clark CM, Lee VM, Trojanowski JQ, Rokach J, FitzGerald GA. Increased 8,12-iso-iPF2alpha-VI in Alzheimer's disease: correlation of a noninvasive index of lipid peroxidation with disease severity. *Ann Neurol* 2000; 48:809–812.
10. Mecocci P, Polidori MC, Cherubini A *et al.* Lymphocyte oxidative DNA damage and plasma antioxidants in Alzheimer disease. *Arch Neurol* 2002; 59:794–798.
11. Mecocci P, Polidori MC, Ingegni T *et al.* Oxidative damage to DNA in lymphocytes from AD patients. *Neurology* 1998; 51:1014–1017.
12. Cecchi C, Fiorillo C, Sorbi S *et al.* Oxidative stress and reduced antioxidant defenses in peripheral cells from familial Alzheimer's patients. *Free Radic Biol Med* 2002; 33:1372–1379.
13. Poppolla MA, Chyan YJ, Omar RA *et al.* Evidence of oxidative stress and in vivo neurotoxicity of beta-amyloid in a transgenic mouse model of Alzheimer's disease: a chronic oxidative paradigm for testing antioxidant therapies in vivo. *Am J Pathol* 1998; 152:871–877.
14. Smith MA, Hirai K, Hsiao K *et al.* Amyloid-beta deposition in Alzheimer transgenic mice is associated with oxidative stress. *J Neurochem* 1998; 70:2212–2215.
15. Li F, Calingasan NY, Yu F *et al.* Increased plaque burden in brains of APP mutant MnSOD heterozygous knockout mice. *J Neurochem* 2004; 89:1308–1312.
16. Smith MA, Perry G, Richey PL *et al.* Oxidative damage in Alzheimer's. *Nature* 1996; 382:120–121.
17. Pappolla MA, Omar RA, Kim KS, Robakis NK. Immunohistochemical evidence of oxidative [corrected] stress in Alzheimer's disease. *Am J Pathol* 1992; 140:621–628.
18. Behl C, Davis J, Cole GM, Schubert D. Vitamin E protects nerve cells from amyloid beta protein toxicity. *Biochem Biophys Res Commun* 1992; 186:944–950.
19. Sagara Y, Dargusch R, Klier FG, Schubert D, Behl C. Increased antioxidant enzyme activity in amyloid beta protein-resistant cells. *J Neurosci* 1996; 16:497–505.
20. Misonou H, Morishima-Kawashima M, Ihora Y. Oxidative stress induces intracellular accumulation of amyloid beta-protein (Abeta) in human neuroblastoma cells. *Biochemistry* 2000; 39:6951–6959.
21. Butterfield DA, Griffin S, Munch G, Pasinetti GM. Amyloid beta-peptide and amyloid pathology are central to the oxidative stress and inflammatory cascades under which Alzheimer's disease brain exists. *J Alzheimers Dis* 2002; 4:193–201.
22. Pratico D, Clark CM, Liun F, Rokach J, Lee VY, Trojanowski JQ. Increase of brain oxidative stress in mild cognitive impairment: a possible predictor of Alzheimer disease. *Arch Neurol* 2002; 59:972–976.
23. Migliore L, Fontana I, Trippi F *et al.* Oxidative DNA damage in peripheral leukocytes of mild cognitive impairment and AD patients. *Neurobiol Aging* 2005; 26:567–573.
24. Guidi I, Galimberti D, Lonati S *et al.* Oxidative imbalance in patients with mild cognitive impairment and Alzheimer's disease. *Neurobiol Aging* 2006; 27:262–269.

25. Busciglio J, Yankner BA. Apoptosis and increased generation of reactive oxygen species in Down's syndrome neurons in vitro. *Nature* 1995; 378:776–779.
26. Nunomura A, Perry G, Pappolla MA *et al.* Neuronal oxidative stress precedes amyloid-beta deposition in Down syndrome. *J Neuropathol Exp Neurol* 2000; 59:1011–1017.
27. Nunomura A, Perry G, Aliev G *et al.* Oxidative damage is the earliest event in Alzheimer disease. *J Neuropathol Exp Neurol* 2001; 60:759–767.
28. Bruce AJ, Malfroy B, Baudry M. Beta-Amyloid toxicity in organotypic hippocampal cultures: protection by EUK-8, a synthetic catalytic free radical scavenger. *Proc Natl Acad Sci USA* 1996; 93:2312–2316.
29. Escames G, Guerrero JM, Reiter RJ *et al.* Melatonin and vitamin E limit nitric oxide-induced lipid peroxidation in rat brain homogenates. *Neurosci Lett* 1997; 230:147–150.
30. Pappolla MA, Sos M, Omar RA *et al.* Melatonin prevents death of neuroblastoma cells exposed to the Alzheimer amyloid peptide. *J Neurosci* 1997; 17:1683–1690.
31. Urano S, Asai Y, Makabe S *et al.* Oxidative injury of synapse and alteration of antioxidative defense systems in rats, and its prevention by vitamin E. *Eur J Biochem* 1997; 245:64–70.
32. Subramaniam R, Koppal T, Green M *et al.* The free radical antioxidant vitamin E protects cortical synaptosomal membranes from amyloid beta-peptide(25–35) toxicity but not from hydroxynonenal toxicity: relevance to the free radical hypothesis of Alzheimer's disease. *Neurochem Res* 1998; 23:1403–1410.
33. Tagami M, Yamagata K, Ikeda K *et al.* Vitamin E prevents apoptosis in cortical neurons during hypoxia and oxygen reperfusion. *Lab Invest* 1998; 78:1415–1429.
34. Bastianetto S, Ramassamy C, Dore S, Christen Y, Poirier J, Quirion R. The Ginkgo biloba extract (EGb 761) protects hippocampal neurons against cell death induced by beta-amyloid. *Eur J Neurosci* 2000; 12:1882–1890.
35. Gibson GE, Huang HM. Oxidative stress in Alzheimer's disease. *Neurobiol Aging* 2005; 26:575–578.
36. Tucker S, Ahl M, Bush A, Westaway D, Huang X, Rogers JT. Pilot study of the reducing effect on amyloidosis in vivo by three FDA pre-approved drugs via the Alzheimer's APP 5′ untranslated region. *Curr Alzheimer Res* 2005; 2:249–254.
37. Morris MC, Beckett LA, Scherr PA. Vitamin E and vitamin C supplement use and risk of incident Alzheimer disease. *Alzheimer Dis Assoc Disord* 1998; 12:121–126.
38. Masaki KH, Losonczy KG, Izmirlian G *et al.* Association of vitamin E and C supplement use with cognitive function and dementia in elderly men. *Neurology* 2000; 54:1265–1272.
39. Luchsinger JA, Tang MX, Shea S, Mayeux R. Antioxidant vitamin intake and risk of Alzheimer disease *Arch Neurol* 2003; 60:203–208.
40. Engelhart MJ, Geerlings MI, Ruitenberg A *et al.* Dietary intake of antioxidants and risk of Alzheimer disease. *JAMA* 2002; 287:3223–3229.
41. Morris MC, Evans DA, Bienias JL *et al.* Dietary intake of antioxidant nutrients and the risk of incident Alzheimer disease in a biracial community study. *JAMA* 2002; 287:3230–3237.
42. Zaondi PP, Anthony JC, Khachaturian AS *et al.* Reduced risk of Alzheimer disease in users of antioxidant vitamin supplements: the Cache County Study. *Arch Neurol* 2004; 61:82–88.
43. Fillenbaum GG, Kuchibhatla MN, Hanlon JT *et al.* Dementia and Alzheimer's disease in community-dwelling elders taking vitamin C and/or vitamin E. *Ann Pharmacother* 2005; 39:2009–2014.
44. Klatte ET, Scharre DW, Nagaraja HN, Davis RA, Beversdorf DQ. Combination therapy of donepezil and vitamin E in Alzheimer disease. *Alzheimer Dis Assoc Disord* 2003; 17:113–116.
45. Sano M, Ernesto C, Thomas RG *et al.* A controlled trial of selegiline, alpha-tocopherol, or both as treatment for Alzheimer's disease. The Alzheimer's Disease Cooperative Study. *N Engl J Med* 1997; 336:1216–1222.
46. Petersen RC, Thomas RG, Grundman M *et al.* Vitamin E and donepezil for the treatment of mild cognitive impairment. *N Engl J Med* 2005; 352:2379–2388.
47. Heart Protection Study Collaborative Group. MRC/BHF Heart Protection Study of antioxidant vitamin supplementation in 20,536 high-risk individuals: a randomized placebo-controlled trial. *Lancet* 2002; 360:23–33.
48. Kryscio RJ, Mendiondo MS, Schmitt FA, Markesbery WR. Designing a large prevention trial: statistical issues. *Stat Med* 2004; 23:285–296.
49. Aisen PS, Dalton AJ, Sano M, Lott IT, Andrews HF, Tsai W-Y and the IDSADC. Design and implementation of a multicenter trial of Vitamin E in aging individuals with Down syndrome. *J Policy Pract Intellect Disabil* 2005; 2:86–93.

50. Miller ER 3rd, Pastor-Barriuso R, Dalal D, Riemersma RA, Appel LJ, Guallar E. Meta-analysis: high-dosage vitamin E supplementation may increase all-cause mortality. *Ann Intern Med* 2005; 142:37–46.
51. Greenberg ER. Vitamin E supplements: good in theory, but is the theory good? *Ann Intern Med* 2005; 142:75–76.
52. Lonn E, Bosch J, Yusuf S *et al*. Effects of long-term vitamin E supplementation on cardiovascular events and cancer: a randomized controlled trial. *JAMA* 2005; 293:1338–1347.
53. Commenges D, Scotet V, Renaud S *et al*. Intake of flavonoids and risk of dementia. *Eur J Epidemiol* 2000; 16:357–363.
54. Le Bars PL, Katz MM, Berman N *et al*. A placebo-controlled, double-blind, randomized trial of an extract of Ginkgo biloba for dementia. North American EGb Study Group. *JAMA* 1997; 278:1327–1332.
55. Birks J, Grimley EV, Van Dongen M. Ginkgo biloba for cognitive impairment and dementia. *Cochrane Database Syst Rev* 2002;CD003120.
56. Schneider LS, DeKosky ST, Farlow MR, Tariot PN, Hoerr R, Kieser M. A randomized, double-blind, placebo-controlled trial of two doses of Ginkgo biloba extract in dementia of the Alzheimer's type. *Curr Alzheimer Res* 2005; 2:541–551.
57. DeKosky ST, Fitzpatrick A, Ives DG *et al*. The Ginkgo Evaluation of Memory (GEM) study: design and baseline data of a randomized trial of Ginkgo biloba extract in prevention of dementia. *Contemp Clin Trials* 2006; 27:238–253. Epub 2006; 19.
58. Thal LJ, Grundman M, Berg J *et al*. Idebenone treatment fails to slow cognitive decline in Alzheimer's disease. *Neurology* 2003; 61:1498–1502.
59. Adair JC, Knoefel JE, Morgan N. Controlled trial of N-acetylcysteine for patients with probable Alzheimer's disease. *Neurology* 2001; 57:1515–1517.
60. Gutzmann H, Kuhl KP, Hadler D *et al*. Safety and efficacy of idebenone versus tacrine inpatients with Alzheimer's disease: results of a randomized, double-blind, parallel-group multicenter study. *Pharmacopsychiatry* 2002; 35:12–18.
61. Kanowski S, Herrmann WM, Stephan K, Wierich W, Horr R. Proof of efficacy of the ginkgo biloba special extract EGb 761 in outpatients suffering from mild to moderate primary degenerative dementia of the Alzheimer type or multi-infarct dementia. *Pharmacopsychiatry* 1996; 29:47–56.
62. Kanowski S, Hoerr R. Ginkgo biloba extract EGb 761 in dementia: intent-to-treat analyses of a 24-week, multi-center, double-blind, placebo-controlled, randomized trial. *Pharmacopsychiatry* 2003; 36:297–303.
63. van Donegan M, van Rossum E, Kessels A, Sielhorst H, Knipschild P. Ginkgo for elderly people with dementia and age-associated memory impairment: a randomized clinical trial. *J Clin Epidemiol* 2003; 56:367–376.
64. Nathan PJ, Ricketts E, Wesnes K, Mrazek L, Greville W, Stough C. The acute nootropic effects of Ginkgo biloba in healthy older human subjects: a preliminary investigation. *Hum Psychopharmacol* 2002; 17:45–49.
65. Mix JA, Crews WD Jr. A double-blind, placebo-controlled, randomized trial of Ginkgo biloba extract EGb 761 in a sample of cognitively intact older adults: neuropsychological findings. *Hum Psychopharmacol* 2002; 17:267–277.
66. Stough C, Clarke J, Lloyd J, Nathan PJ. Neuropsychological changes after 30-day Ginkgo biloba administration in healthy participants. *Int J Neuropsychopharmacol* 2001; 4:131–134.
67. van Donegan MC, van Rossum E, Kessels AG, Sielhorst HJ, Knipschild PG. The efficacy of ginkgo for elderly people with dementia and age-associated memory impairment: new results of a randomized clinical trial. *J Am Geriatr Soc* 2000; 48:1183–1194.
68. Maurer K, Ihl R, Dierks T, Frolich L. Clinical efficacy of Ginkgo biloba special extract EGb 761 in dementia of the Alzheimer type. *J Psychiatr Res* 1997; 31:645–655.
69. Weyer G, Babej-Dolle RM, Hadler D, Hofmann S, Herrmann WM. A controlled study of 2 doses of idebenone in the treatment of Alzheimer's disease. *Neuropsychobiology* 1997; 36:73–82.

# 7

# Pharmacoeconomic studies

*C. Green*

## INTRODUCTION

In healthcare systems around the world there are limits on the funding available for healthcare and there is a growing demand for a broadening range of health services. These factors create an environment where healthcare systems are unable to provide all healthcare interventions that are known to be clinically effective and potentially beneficial to respective patient groups. This gives rise to an increasing number of difficult decisions, and increasing pressure is placed on those involved in decision-making within healthcare. Nevertheless, decisions have to be made. The focus of pharmacoeconomics is on making the most of available healthcare resources, and on the provision of information to help with difficult health policy decisions (e.g. which health services should be available, and to whom).

Pharmacoeconomics considers the relative value of specific health interventions using the framework of economic evaluation. Economic evaluation is the comparative analysis of alternative courses of action in terms of both their costs and consequences [1]. It aims to promote efficiency, or to use more familiar terminology, it considers the issue of 'value for money'.

There are a number of forms of economic evaluation (*cost minimization analysis, cost-effectiveness analysis, cost utility analysis*), but they have the common feature that some combination of inputs to a healthcare service or programme are compared with some combination of outputs. Economic evaluation presents information on the cost-effectiveness of alternative strategies – with efficiency often one of a number of considerations relevant to decision makers. This form of information is now prominent in the world of health policy. In the UK, the explicit use of economic evaluation and cost-effectiveness analysis to guide health policy decisions is highlighted in the health technology appraisal process of the National Institute for Health and Clinical Excellence (NICE) [2], and the guidance published by NICE. However, there are a great number of other decision-making bodies that take account of cost-effectiveness when making health policy decisions at what may be a local, regional, national or international level.

In order to offer some understanding of pharmacoeconomics in the area of dementia, I offer a commentary on the economic evaluation of drugs for Alzheimer's disease (AD). I present a broad review of the literature on the cost-effectiveness of (i) acetylcholinesterase inhibitors for the treatment of mild to moderately-severe AD, and (ii) memantine for the treatment of moderately-severe to severe disease. The chapter begins with an outline summary of the literature to inform on the cost-effectiveness of these drugs for AD, followed by a critical summary of the published studies. This summary draws out some important issues and concerns when interpreting the literature.

**Colin Green**, BA (Hons), MSc, Principal Research Fellow, Southampton Health Technology Assessments Centre (SHTAC), Wessex Institute for Health Research and Development, University of Southampton, Southampton, UK

## PHARMACOECONOMIC STUDIES *(COST-EFFECTIVENESS ANALYSES)* IN ALZHEIMER'S DISEASE

This summary review is based on a detailed systematic review of the literature undertaken to inform decision makers in the UK National Health Service (NHS). The methods for the literature review have been reported in detail elsewhere [3]. The search strategy considered literature available from inception of databases (e.g. MEDLINE, EMBase) up to mid-2004. It identified a growing literature (with the majority of studies published since 2000), with 18 published economic evaluations, six published abstracts, and two published UK NHS regional reports. There were also a number of review papers, either on individual drugs [4–7] or providing a broader review on one or more of these drugs [8, 9]. The current discussion is on the published studies, and review papers have not been covered. Interested readers will find these review papers accessible and helpful in combination with this chapter if they have a keen interest in the cost-effectiveness literature.

Table 7.1 provides a summary of the scope of the literature, the headline messages and the basic characteristics of the published literature. The majority of studies are on the assessment of donepezil, and this reflects the fact that donepezil was the first of these products to be available for the treatment of AD. Of some concern, is that at least 16 of these cost-effectiveness studies are directly or indirectly supported by the pharmaceutical industry (manufacturers), and may therefore, but not necessarily, have biases due to competing interests. All studies are drug-specific, with single drug comparisons to placebo (usual care), and they all present country-specific analysis. All except two of the cost-effectiveness studies have used a model as the analytical framework for analysis. Models, using clinical, economic and epidemiological data, are used to consider AD progression over time. Studies have relied on modelling due to the absence of longer-term effectiveness data, with clinical trials rarely extending beyond 48 weeks. Given that available effectiveness data is on specific intermediate markers of disease progression (e.g. scores on cognitive function) and that there is an absence of longer-term data on patient related outcomes (e.g. reduced rates of institutionalization, reduced need for full-time care, and quality of life gains), some form of modelling has been unavoidable. Studies have extrapolated from short-term trial data to longer-term outcomes, using a number of different modelling approaches, and these are discussed below.

Perspective (viewpoint) of the analysis is an important issue for those wishing to draw some conclusions from the literature. In at least 10 studies the perspective is that of a societal decision maker, and in much of the remainder the perspective is often unclear.

Almost all studies report that drugs offer health benefits and cost savings over time, indicating that their use is cost-effective. Yet, this may not be the case when considering treatment under certain conditions, for example when using a third party payer perspective (e.g. UK NHS). One study [10] reports that treatment incurs added costs, but indicates that it is a cost-effective use of resources, whilst one study [11] indicates cost savings when not including the cost for the drug used. A recent UK study [12] reports that donepezil vs. placebo results in a reduction in cognitive decline, but that donepezil is not a cost-effective use of UK NHS resources.

## CRITICAL APPRAISAL OF ECONOMIC EVALUATIONS

The basic tasks of any economic evaluation are to identify, measure, value and compare the costs and consequences of the alternatives being considered. There are always challenges in the conduct of economic evaluation and studies can vary greatly in the methods they use and in their quality. Therefore, it is important to critically appraise the cost-effectiveness literature available when it is being used to inform a particular policy question. Any user of cost-effectiveness data should take note of the methods used and the generalizability of the data, as well as their results. A decision maker should have in their mind the important

**Table 7.1** Economic evaluations of drugs for AD – study characteristics

| *References* | *Drug* | *Country/ setting* | *Perspective* | *Base year costs/prices* | *Modelling studies* | *Results presented* | | *Competing interests** |
|---|---|---|---|---|---|---|---|---|
| | | | | | | *Cost saving or cost neutral* | *Benefits: delays to disease progression* | |
| Stewart *et al.* [21] | Donepezil | UK | NS/societal | 1996/1997 | ✓ | ✓ | ✓ | ✓ |
| Jonsson *et al.* [22] | | Sweden | NS/societal | 1995? | ✓ | ✓ | ✓ | ✓ |
| O'Brien *et al.* [23] | | Canada | Societal | 1997 | ✓ | ✓ | ✓ | ✓ |
| Neumann *et al.* [16] | | USA | Societal | 1997 | ✓ | ✓ | ✓ | ✓ |
| Ikeda *et al.* [24] | | Japan | TPP | 2000 | ✓ | ✓ | ✓ | ✓ |
| Fagnani *et al.* [25] | | France | Societal | 2003 | ✓ | ✓ | ✓ | ✓ |
| Wimo *et al.* [17] | | Sweden | Societal | 1999 | X Trial based | ✓ | ✓ | ✓ |
| AD Collaborative Group [12] | | UK | Societal | 2002/3 | X Trial based | Added costs | ✓ | None |
| Fenn and Gray [11] | Rivastigmine | UK | UK NHS and PSS | 1997 | ✓ | ✓ | ✓ | ✓ |
| Hauber *et al.* [43] | | USA | NS/unclear | 1997 | ✓ | ✓ | ✓ | ✓ |
| Hauber *et al.* [38] | | Canada | Societal | 1997 | ✓ | ✓ | ✓ | ✓ |
| Getsios *et al.* [58] | Galantamine | Canada | NS/TPP | 1999 | ✓ | ✓ | ✓ | ✓ |
| Garfield *et al.* [44] | | Sweden | NS/TPP | 1998 | ✓ | ✓ | ✓ | ✓ |
| Caro *et al.* [45] | | Netherlands | Part societal | 1998 | ✓ | ✓ | ✓ | ✓ |
| Migliaccio-Walle *et al.* [46] | | USA | Third party payer | 2000 | ✓ | ✓ | ✓ | ✓ |
| Ward *et al.* [10] | | UK | UK NHS | 2001 | ✓ | Added costs | ✓ | ✓ |
| François *et al.* [30] | Memantine | Finland | Societal | 2001 | ✓ | ✓ | ✓ | ✓ |
| Jones *et al.* [19] | | UK | NS/TPP | 2003 | ✓ | ✓ | ✓ | ✓ |

TPP = third party payer; NS = not stated; NS/societal = not stated but appears societal; NS/TPP = not stated but appears third party payer.

*Manufacturer involvement.

**Table 7.2** Checklist for assessing economic evaluations (adapted with permission from Drummond *et al.* [1])

1. Was a well-defined question posed in answerable form?
2. Was a comprehensive description of the competing alternatives given?
3. Was the effectiveness of the programmes or services established?
4. Were all the important and relevant costs and consequences for each alternative identified?
5. Were costs and consequences measured accurately in appropriate physical units?
6. Were costs and consequences valued credibly?
7. Were costs and consequences adjusted for differential timing?
8. Was an incremental analysis of costs and consequences of alternatives performed?
9. Was allowance made for uncertainty in the estimates of costs and consequences?
10. Did the presentation and discussion of study results include all issues of concern to users?

elements of a sound economic evaluation when taking account of whether the cost-effectiveness analyses available are useful in their particular setting. There are a number of published sources of methodological standards for economic evaluation [1, 13], and there is useful guidance on the elements of good practice in cost-effectiveness modelling studies [14]. Detail on these methodological standards will not be offered here; that job has been done well by others elsewhere [1, 14, 15]. But one of the objectives of this paper is to outline the basic methods underlying economic evaluation, therefore Table 7.2 presents a summary of the important elements of an economic evaluation, which are often summarized in the form of a checklist of questions to ask about a published study [1, 13].

Table 7.3 reports basic data from a critical appraisal of the published economic evaluations. The framework for critical appraisal used is adapted from that presented by Drummond *et al.* [1], and in this instance – for presentational purposes only – some simple and crude symbols have been used to draw attention to those areas of the literature that are deserving of particular attention. Ticks are used to indicate a favourable (acceptable) response to a review area, crosses to indicate a non-favourable response, and question marks to indicate issues which are unknown or uncertain. I would not advocate this simple approach generally, and would recommend that when undertaking a critical review of this nature it is advisable to use the checklist as a prompt, and to note in a descriptive manner the findings from studies. A more detailed account of the review can be found elsewhere [3]. However, Table 7.3 is useful in drawing attention to the areas of particular concern within the published cost-effectiveness studies. Whilst there may be some concerns with the style of reporting and presentation of analysis (e.g. stated study question, use of incremental analysis, reporting of sensitivity analysis) these areas are not a major concern in the context of the current discussion. Those areas that are of greater concern, and form the basis of our discussion of the literature, are (a) analytical perspective, (b) the reporting and use of effectiveness data, (c) the methods used to model progression of disease, and (d) the related issues of identification, measurement and valuation of relevant costs and consequences.

### THE IMPORTANCE OF PERSPECTIVE/VIEWPOINT

The perspective, or viewpoint, of an economic evaluation determines the scope of the analysis, i.e. which combination of inputs and outputs are relevant. The analytical perspective of a study can be that of the individual patient, a specific institution, a target group for specific services, the national health budget, the overall public sector budget, or a broad societal perspective. Indeed a study can address any or all of these perspectives. With perspective, it is not a simple question of which perspective an economic evaluation should take, as an economic evaluation can aim to inform against a number of different objectives and perspectives. Any analysis should be clear about the perspective taken, or the multiple perspectives

**Table 7.3** Critical appraisal of economic evaluations (outline summary review)

| *Study* | *Question? Alternatives?* | *Effectiveness established?* | *Effect related to population of interest?* | *Relevant costs and consequences* | | | *Differential timing considered?* | *Incremental analysis undertaken?* | *Sensitivity analysis undertaken?* | *Modelling conducted reasonably?* |
|---|---|---|---|---|---|---|---|---|---|---|
| | | | | *Identified?* | *Measured accurately?* | *Valued credibly?* | | | | |
| *Donepezil* | | | | | | | | | | |
| Stewart *et al.* [21] | ✓ | X | X/? | ? | ? | ? | ✓ | ✓ | ✓ | ? |
| Jonsson *et al.* [22] | ✓ | ✓/? | X/? | ✓/? | ? | ? | ✓ | ✓ | ✓ | ? |
| O'Brien *et al.* [23] | ✓ | ✓ | ✓/? | ✓ | ? | ✓ | ✓ | ✓ | ✓ | ? |
| Neumann *et al.* [16] | ✓ | X | ✓ | ✓ | ? | ? | ✓ | ✓ | ✓ | ? |
| Ikeda *et al.* [24] | ✓ | X | ?/X | ✓ | ? | ✓/X | ✓ | ✓ | ✓ | ? |
| Fagnani *et al.* [25] | ✓ | X | ✓/? | ✓ | ? | ✓/? | ✓ | ? | ✓ | ? |
| Wimo *et al.* [17] | ✓ | ✓ | ✓ | ✓ | ✓ | ✓ | N/A | X | ✓ | N/A |
| AD Collaborative Group [12] | ✓ | ✓ | ✓ | ✓ | ✓ | ✓ | ✓ | X | ✓ | N/A |
| *Rivastigmine* | | | | | | | | | | |
| Fenn and Gray [11] | ✓ | ?/✓ | ? | ✓/? | ? | ? | X | ✓ | X | ? |
| Hauber *et al.* [43] | ✓/? | X | ✓/? | ? | ? | ? | ✓ | ✓ | X | ? |
| Hauber *et al.* [38] | ✓ | X | ✓/? | ✓/? | ? | ? | ✓ | ✓ | X | ? |

**Table 7.3** (Continued)

| | | | | | | | | | | |
|---|---|---|---|---|---|---|---|---|---|---|
| *Galantamine* | | | | | | | | | | |
| Getsios *et al.* [58] | ✓ | ✓ | ? | ✓/? | ? | ? | ✓ | ✓ | ✓ | ?/✓ |
| Garfield *et al.* [44] | ✓ | X | X | ✓/? | ? | ? | ✓/? | ✓ | ✓ | ?/✓ |
| Caro *et al.* [45] | ✓ | X | X | ✓/? | ? | ? | ✓ | ✓ | ✓ | ?/✓ |
| Migliaccio-Walle *et al.* [46] | ✓ | X | ? | ✓/? | ? | ? | ✓ | ✓ | ✓ | ?/✓ |
| Ward *et al.* [10] | ✓ | X | X | ✓/? | ✓/? | ✓/? | ✓ | ✓ | ✓ | ?/✓ |
| *Memantine* | | | | | | | | | | |
| François *et al.* [30] | ✓ | X | X | ? | ✓/? | ✓/? | ✓ | ✓ | ✓ | ?/✓ |
| Jones *et al.* [19] | ✓ | X | X | ? | ?/X | ?/X | ✓ | ✓ | ✓ | ?/✓ |

Reviewer (CG) opinion: ✓ = judged OK; X = judged not OK or insufficient information reported; ? = unknown/uncertain; ✓/? = judged potentially OK but uncertain; X/? = judged to be not OK, but uncertain.

presented, and the component parts of the cost-effectiveness calculation, i.e. which costs and consequences have been taken into account. A health intervention which looks attractive from one perspective may look much less attractive when other perspectives are considered. This can be the case for AD. AD is not a simple condition for evaluation. Treatment for AD involves a number of different provider and funding sectors, and patients and carers often contribute to the cost of care. Informal care (often family members, but also volunteers) is one of the most important resources in AD care, but different perspectives will dictate whether informal care forms part of the economic analysis. Drug treatments are relatively low cost interventions, in the context of broader care costs, but still remain a significant budgetary concern for healthcare providers, and will be very important from a third party payer perspective. A societal perspective will include all relevant costs and benefits regardless of where they occur and regardless of who pays. A specific payer perspective will limit the economic analysis to take into account only the costs that fall on the budget of that payer (i.e. exclude patient and carer costs). However, even where a decision is taken to include societal costs (e.g. informal care costs) there are a great number of difficulties estimating and valuing resource inputs and benefits from a societal perspective, and these remain methodological issues that have yet to be resolved.

When reviewing the literature, in a number of cases the perspective is not clearly stated, and often when it is stated there remain uncertainties over the actual scope of the input data used. Table 7.1 reports summary detail on perspective in published studies, with six of the 18 studies not stating the perspective of their analysis. Where possible the perspective that is apparently taken has been indicated (e.g. societal or third party payer), but this is not always possible. Even where a perspective is clearly stated it is important to consider if that perspective has been pursued correctly in the analysis undertaken. It is clear from the review undertaken that there are some ambiguities and/or uncertainties when interpreting the literature in the context of stated perspective. For example, where societal perspective is stated by a number of studies [16, 17], all of the consequences of treatment may not have been investigated (e.g. the effect of treatment on carers is not included, other than in the estimation of longer-term cost consequences). While six studies state, or indicate, that their perspective is that of a third party payer (e.g. NHS and personal social services in the UK), we can easily conclude that certain costs are included in the analysis which are not met by the third party payer. For example, in UK studies [10, 11], costs that are not met by the payer (e.g. UK NHS) are included in the analysis. In the UK the costs for longer-term care (i.e. institutional costs) are not met by the UK or public sector budget for all patients. Support for such costs is dependent on the financial status of the patient (means tested) and around 30% of those patients with AD in a UK long-term institutional setting are responsible for their own care costs [18]. The UK cost-effectiveness analysis for memantine, presented by Jones *et al.* [19] as a reflection of a third party payer perspective (although this is not directly stated) includes estimates of longer-term care costs that far exceed the usual (or typical) level of funding provided by the UK NHS and personal social services.

### METHODS USED TO MODEL DISEASE PROGRESSION AND TREATMENT EFFECT

It is now well accepted that in economic evaluation we often require a model of the disease and its management. It is rare that a single clinical trial will provide all the necessary information on costs and outcomes, and even if this were to be the case it would still be necessary to model the available data in the setting and population of interest (outside of clinical trial protocol). Indeed there has been an acceptance that models and trials are not alternative analytical frameworks, and that they are both necessary components of the evaluation process. AD is a good example of the necessity to use a model to synthesize available clinical trial data with data on costs, epidemiology and other data on disease management, in order to predict longer-term outcomes and costs. In the studies identified to inform on the cost-effectiveness of drugs for AD, we see a variety of methods used to model disease progression and the impact of treatment. In each of the four drugs of interest, we see a different approach to the modelling of cost-effectiveness data. For the three cholinesterase inhibitors this makes the comparison of the drugs more difficult, and does not allow the reader to consider how each of the drugs would compare when using a common analytical framework and similar model parameter inputs. Memantine is available for the treatment of more severe disease, therefore it is understandable that a different modelling approach is adopted. In all studies using cost-effectiveness models there are concerns related to structure and/or data used. I offer a brief summary of the methods applied for each of the four drugs, and highlight those areas of greatest concern.

Economic models have typically been structured and analysed using decision trees or Markov models. Markov models represent the course of a disease in terms of mutually exclusive 'health states' and the transitions among them [20]. Markov models are particularly useful when a decision problem involves clinical changes that are ongoing over time. The progression of AD with time is a good clinical example.

The cost-effectiveness studies for donepezil are almost entirely based on the use of Markov type models of disease progression. Health states defined according to categories of cognitive function have been used to estimate disease progression across different levels of disease severity, with treatment effects based on trial-specific data. Three studies have used Mini-mental State Examination (MMSE) scores to define either four or five levels of AD severity [21–23], two studies used Clinical Dementia Rating (CDR) scale scores to define three levels of disease severity [16, 24], and one study [25] used MMSE in a continuous manner. Progression of disease is modelled using transition probabilities between health states at each model cycle (e.g. 6-month cycle), with an ongoing risk of death over time included in the models. There are variations between studies in the methods used to determine appropriate transition probabilities for the disease progression models. Three studies obtained transition probabilities for donepezil-treated and untreated groups from clinical trial data [22, 23, 25]. One study [21] used epidemiological data for the untreated control group and trial data for the donepezil-treated group, while the others used epidemiological data to calculate transition probabilities for the untreated group and then applied a risk reduction factor derived from clinical trial data to generate transition probabilities for the treatment group [16, 22, 24]. In some studies [21, 23, 25] the effect of donepezil on disease progression was assumed to last for only part of the overall time horizon, but other studies [16, 22, 24] assumed that the treatment effect persisted for the entire time horizon. Generally models incorporated an ongoing mortality risk that was the same for both treated and untreated patients; this mortality risk was dependent on disease severity in three studies [16, 22, 24]. Cycle length, time horizon, and the characteristics of the baseline patient cohorts varied across studies. All the studies assumed that donepezil treatment would stop when patients reached a state of severe AD.

The studies informing on the cost-effectiveness of rivastigmine have all used the same modelling framework. They have used the hazard model of disease progression presented by Fenn and Gray [11]. This model uses individual patient data from clinical trials on rivastigmine [26, 27] to estimate the time taken for each patient to move from one level of AD severity to another. The model estimates the likelihood that a patient will remain at a particular MMSE score at any given time. Statistical techniques are used to model disease progression. The model is used to generate survival curves for both placebo and rivastigmine treatment groups, with these extrapolated beyond the end of the trial period. The impact of treatment on disease progression is measured as days saved by preventing patients from entering the next, more severe, stage of AD. This delay in disease progression is represented by the area between the placebo and treatment survival curves. The hazard model does not incorporate a mortality risk directly in the disease progression process. The proportional difference in cognitive decline between the placebo and treatment groups estimated by the model is assumed to persist until patients reach the most severe stage of disease at which point the treatment effect declines to zero.

All published economic evaluations for galantamine use the same methodology for modelling disease progression – the Assessment of Health Economics in Alzheimer's Disease (AHEAD) model developed by Caro *et al.* [28]. The AHEAD model rests on the concept of need for full-time-care (FTC), and simulates the experience of a cohort of patients across three possible health states: pre-FTC, FTC and death. The model uses patient characteristics at a given point in time to estimate the likelihood of disease progression over time to a level at which FTC is required. When in the pre-FTC health state patients are assumed to live at home or in a residence that does not provide extensive care. When in FTC patients have a requirement for a significant amount (for the greater part of the day) of paid care and supervision each day, regardless of the location of care (institution or community setting), or who provides the care, incorporating paid care received at home or elsewhere in the community as well as care in an institutional setting. Regardless of disease progression to FTC patients are subject to the simultaneous risk of death.

The AHEAD model determines the proportion of the patient cohort in each state over time using predictive risk (hazard) equations. A similar risk equation is used to predict time of death. The predictive risk equations are based on longitudinal epidemiological data reported by Stern *et al.* [29] and derive the time-dependent hazards of requiring FTC, and of death, according to patient characteristics present at a given point in time. The data underpinning the risk equations, from Stern *et al.* [29] are from a prospective cohort study of 236 patients (USA), followed up semi-annually, for up to 7 years. The predictive equation for 'requiring FTC' used data on age, the presence of extrapyramidal symptoms (EPS), the presence of psychotic symptoms (e.g. delusions, hallucinations), age at onset, duration of illness, and cognitive score as measured by the modified MMSE. Predictions for mortality are based on presence of EPS, duration of illness, gender and MMSE.

The AHEAD model simulates the experiences of a cohort of patients over 10 years, following an initial treatment period of 6 months, for patients treated with galantamine, and for those same patients if they did not receive galantamine. Galantamine effectiveness is reflected in the model using trial data on difference (treatment vs. controls) in cognitive function (e.g. ADAS-Cog values) and the presence of psychotic symptoms (two studies) following an initial 6-month treatment period (effectiveness data taken from galantamine randomized controlled trials [RCTs]). Patients treated with galantamine are assumed to remain on treatment until they require FTC.

The two cost-effectiveness studies for memantine both use the same modelling approach, with different data inputs and time horizons. Memantine is modelled for the treatment of a more severely affected patient group and there is less reliance on cognitive function, to define health states and model treatment effect. The time period (horizon) used for the models is shorter than in the mild to moderately-severe group, with studies from François *et al.* [30] (Finland) and Jones *et al.* [19] (UK) reporting analysis over 5-year and 2-year periods, respectively. The model categorizes patients by severity level (using MMSE), by dependency level, and care setting. The model uses a multiplicative probability to move patients between health states defined according to a combination of severity, dependency and location. Where patients are defined as institutionalized (either at the start of the model, or on entering an institutionalized health state) they remain in that state, with transit probabilities only applied to patients in a community setting (either remain in community or enter institutional care setting). The primary outcome of the model is 'time to dependency', with 'time to institutionalizaton' considered as an additional outcome. The UK study also estimates small health gains in terms of quality-adjusted life-years (QALYs). Epidemiological data (country-specific) are used in each of the studies to define the initial distribution of patients.

Transit probabilities covering severity, dependency and institutionalization, for the no treatment cohort were based on clinical trial data (Reisberg *et al.* [31]) and data from the

LASER-AD Study (UK observational study [32]). Transit probabilities for dependency and location were based on a transformation of the rates from the no pharmacological treatment group using an estimated odds ratio for memantine vs. placebo, using clinical trial data. Treatment effect was applied to the first 12 months (2 × 6-month cycles), using data from the RCT by Reisberg *et al.* [31] (6-month RCT), and an open-label follow-up study (6 months post trial) (Reisberg *et al.* 2000, unpublished). Dropouts from treatment were not considered within the model.

The critical review of published studies discussed here has highlighted concerns over the methods used in studies to model disease progression, and to estimate the cost-effectiveness of each of the drugs. A brief summary of the modelling method used in the studies reported has been given above. As well as considering the checklist for economic evaluations presented in Table 7.2, modelling studies have also been considered in the context of the good practice methodology for cost-effectiveness models presented by Philips *et al.* [14]. The framework from Philips *et al.* does overlap with that of Drummond *et al.*, but importantly it addresses key aspects of the modelling process. In summary these good practice guidelines for modelling consider four main areas, essential for the delivery of a good quality model, which are model structure, data, consideration of uncertainty, and consistency.

In most of the cost-effectiveness studies on drugs for AD, model structure is not discussed in any detail (if at all). There is no (or limited) rationale provided for the model structure used, and structural assumptions are not always transparent. The main concern with all of the models used is their reliance on the use of cognition (scores for cognitive function) to model disease progression over time. There is a growing literature that indicates cognitive function is an unreliable approach to predicting AD progression [33–35] and outcomes such as time to institutionalization [12, 36, 37]. A number of the donepezil studies [16, 21–23] have used transition probabilities from clinical trials to model AD using MMSE (cognitive function) to define health states and progression to endpoints (e.g. severe disease). The rivastigmine studies [11, 38, 39] have used a similar structure and similar trial data to determine disease progression over time. The galantamine cost-effectiveness studies have used a model and a disease structure that is less dependent upon cognition for baseline progression of disease, but they do apply effectiveness data on differences in cognitive scores to model treatment effect over time. However, this is the basis for reported efficacy and effectiveness of galantamine in RCTs.

As part of the detailed review undertaken on the cost-effectiveness of drugs for AD a systematic search of the literature has been undertaken to identify the methods available to model disease progression over time. As well as those methods reported above, in the context of published cost-effectiveness studies, we also identified a number of other general approaches [40, 41]. Neumann *et al.* [40] used the Consortium to Establish a Registry in Alzheimer's Disease (CERAD) database [42] to examine the progression of disease to mild, moderate and severe stages. The transition probabilities estimated by Neumann and colleagues underscore the rapid and progressive nature of AD. The CERAD data showed a varied course of disease progression in AD, with age, gender and behavioural symptoms shown to have an impact on transition probabilities, supporting a view (in my opinion) that modelling disease progression around cognitive function is a suboptimal approach. The CERAD stage transition matrix (in various presentations) may be a helpful tool to model baseline disease progression in a cohort of patients with AD (used in part in the study by Neumann *et al.* [16]), but issues over generalizability of the patient group, and adjustment to transit probabilities when patients are subject to drug therapy (e.g. donepezil, rivastigmine, or galantamine) are issues that would require attention in any further application of the data.

Mendiondo and colleagues present an approach for the modelling of AD progression over time [41]. They use data from CERAD to model change in MMSE as a function of time in the CERAD population. The model uses MMSE alone to predict disease progression over time, with the authors arguing that the different symptoms of AD, including daily function, cognitive impairment, or global impression of severity or change, all reflect the same underlying pathological process. Mendiondo and colleagues present a mathematical representation of decline in MMSE over time, with decline dependent on average MMSE score between time intervals examined. They also present findings to show that age is a significant factor in AD progression and education was seen to be a marginally significant factor. Data suggested that disease progression is more rapid when it affects younger individuals, and given the effect of education on disease progression, the authors speculate that it may be a result of a better initial performance on MMSE by those regarded as better educated (delaying diagnosis, and making the course of disease apparently more rapid). Mendiondo and colleagues warn that there was considerable heterogeneity in the raw observational data used in the modelling of disease progression, with data showing variability in measurement of MMSE unrelated to disease progression, with environmental and patient factors also offering a potential to influence estimates of disease progression. As above, I believe that there is a strengthening view that cognitive function (especially alone) is a poor predictor of disease progression for AD, therefore the application of the method presented by Mendiondo *et al.* may be of limited use when considering the cost-effectiveness of drugs for treatment of AD.

The cost-effectiveness studies on drugs for AD have limitations due to the methods used to model disease progression, yet, this may be reflective of the general literature available to inform on the area of AD. Unfortunately, despite the growing literature on the epidemiology of AD, and on the cost-effectiveness of treatments, it is still not possible at the present time to identify a methodology which appears to capture the nature of the disease (i.e. functioning, cognition, and activities of daily living) and which is able to reliably estimate disease progression to important and meaningful patient outcomes.

However, there are also concerns over the form of the data used in many of the models as well as the problems with the structure of the models used to model disease progression. It is difficult in the current summary review to provide detail on all of these studies and concerns. Some concerns with the reporting and use of effectiveness data are outlined here, but interested readers are also urged to give some consideration to the data inputs for costs, healthstate utilities, mortality, etc., when using the results from cost-effectiveness studies in a decision-making context. Where cost-effectiveness studies report methods and data used, they should provide adequate information on the data used on the effectiveness of treatments. This should give the reader an outline of the data used, its source, and the methods used to derive the data (e.g. some detail on trial design, patient characteristics), and not merely be a citation to clinical trials. As can be seen from Table 7.3, a number of studies have failed to establish the appropriateness of the effectiveness data used. At least four of the donepezil studies [16, 21, 24, 25] have not reported sufficient information to establish the appropriateness of the effectiveness data used; they cite clinical trials but do not offer any summary information. For rivastigmine, we see that two of the three studies fail to establish the appropriateness of effectiveness data [38, 43], and this is the case in four of the five galantamine studies [10, 44–46], and in both of the memantine studies [19, 30]. In the studies using transition probabilities (e.g. many of the donepezil studies, and the memantine studies), where the reader does go back to the cited studies to assess the effectiveness data, there is no way of reconciling the effectiveness data presented in clinical trials with the transition probabilities used in the cost-effectiveness studies. RCTs do not present data on transitions between health states defined by category of cognitive function. The data presented in RCTs on cognition is against a mean difference on scores such as the MMSE or ADAS-Cog, with only modest differences reported against these cognitve scores. However, when considering the transition probabilities used in the economic models we see a large difference in the numbers of patients expected to have a delay in reaching severe AD as a consequence of treatment. This issue should be discussed further by the authors of the studies and, in the absence of such discussion, those using the cost-effectiveness literature should treat it with some caution.

**Table 7.4** Data on AD health state values reported by Neumann *et al.* [49]

| *AD stage/setting* | *Patients* | *Caregivers* |
|---|---|---|
| *Mild AD* | | |
| Community | 0.68 | 0.86 |
| Nursing home | 0.71 | 0.86 |
| *Moderate AD* | | |
| Community | 0.54 | 0.86 |
| Nursing home | 0.48 | 0.86 |
| *Severe AD* | | |
| Community | 0.37 | 0.86 |
| Nursing home | 0.31 | 0.86 |

## HEALTH STATE VALUES FOR HEALTH STATES USED TO MODEL ALZHEIMER'S DISEASE

Health state values, usually on a scale of 0 (equivalent to death) and 1 (equivalent to full health), are used to calculate QALYs, in order to combine morbidity and mortality in a single index of health-related quality of life. The data available to inform on the health state values associated with stages of AD are very sparse. Where cost-effectiveness studies have used QALYs in their analysis, readers are urged to consider the source of the information used in the cost-effectiveness analysis, to consider how the health state values have been derived (e.g. techniques such as standard gamble, time trade-off, visual analogue scales), and from whom the values have been elicited (e.g. patients or carers, general public, clinicians). I have undertaken a systematic literature search to identify data on the health-related quality of life associated with AD, in terms of health state values [3], but find little to help the analyst or decision maker in their assessment of health state values for the health states used to model disease. A scarcity of data to inform on this issue was identified, which is of great importance in cost-effectiveness analysis when decision makers are seeking summary cost-effectiveness estimates presented as cost per QALY. The focus of the quality of life (QOL) literature for AD is on cognitive function and not QOL *per se* [47].

The most commonly used health state valuation estimates are those from Neumann *et al.* [48], who obtained health state utility weights for AD from a US cross-sectional study of 679 caregivers of AD patients, stratified by disease severity/stage using the CDR scale stages of disease. This study used the combined Mark II and Mark III Health Utility Index (HUI-II/HUI-III) to obtain utility weights, with respondents also completing a number of other health-related quality of life (HRQL) instruments. Neumann *et al.* [49], in an earlier presentation of their findings, report health state values for AD by severity and location (community or nursing home), see Table 7.4. There are a number of concerns with the health state valuation methods generally, be it with individual techniques such as the standard gamble, or with multi-attribute instruments such as the HUI, and I am not able to go into detail at present. However, the interested reader may find earlier work on the use of health status measures, and health state valuation techniques in economic evaluations helpful [50, 51]. The values presented by Neumann *et al.* do offer a basis for considering the notion of HRQL in AD, but given the general methodological concerns, and the sparse literature upon which we are able to compare or validate any findings, users of these data are urged to be cautious.

For information, other studies offering estimates of health state values for AD, are Kerner *et al.* [52] and Sano *et al.* [53], but the literature is generally sparse and undeveloped, and not too helpful in the area of cost-effectiveness analysis, where a summary measure of health (i.e. QALY) is often preferred.

### *ESTIMATING LONGER-TERM CARE COST FOR ALZHEIMER'S DISEASE*

As highlighted above, when discussing perspective, treatment for AD involves a number of different agencies, and therefore different areas of service provision and often multiple funding sources (often including the patient and carer in payment for services). The main areas for resource use are treatment costs (e.g. drugs), monitoring costs (e.g. ongoing outpatient and office visits, regular tests), and longer-term costs of care (e.g. support services in a community setting, costs for care in an institutional setting, informal care). When reviewing the cost-effectiveness literature, it is important to ask whether the relevant costs have been identified, measured, and valued appropriately. Table 7.3 highlights that the appropriate identification of resource use, or cost items, is more common than the subsequent appropriate measurement and valuation of those resources. Essentially, this is indicative of the information that is available to inform on the costs of care for AD. As with the literature on modelling methods and health state values, we find that the literature on the costs associated with AD is also sparse, and often unhelpful to the analyst. There is a very sparse literature on the costs associated with treatment. Costing studies are often a combination of burden of illness studies, using aggregate data on costs and prevalence [11, 39] and survey studies often related to dementia rather than AD [18, 36]. Cost estimates tend to be based on data analysis (involving assumptions) and modelling, to determine estimates of care (based on various inputs to packages of care) over time, i.e. annual average cost estimates. A number of cost-effectiveness studies have used data from trial patients, or observational studies, to inform their analyses [12, 17, 23] but the majority of studies cite sources for cost items that have modelled cost data for health states, defined according to cognitive function (e.g. MMSE). Often these studies have failed to provide sufficient information to allow the reader to draw conclusions on the adequacy of the data used [19, 21, 39, 44].

## SUMMARY

Whilst the conduct of economic evaluation has obvious challenges, one question for the current reader is whether there are particular challenges for economic evaluation in the area of dementia. When reviewing the literature on AD we find that there are specific challenges, and that we must pay particular attention to the nature of the effectiveness data used, and subsequent methods used to model disease progression and outcomes of interest (i.e. the use of intermediate outcomes such as MMSE or ADAS-Cog scores). We must also consider the problems encountered when estimating longer-term costs of care, and to the importance of the decision-making perspective applied in analyses (e.g. third party payer, NHS, or societal perspective). I have spent some time above on these core elements of economic evaluation for AD. I believe all of these are key areas of concern in the current literature, and that future studies should give these areas greater attention when estimating the cost-effectiveness of interventions for AD. I hope that those reading this chapter feel better armed to critically appraise the literature on the cost-effectiveness of treatments for AD, and to advise those responsible for the design of trials and cost-effectiveness studies on the areas that require specific attention.

A priority area for future research must be the more comprehensive modelling of disease progression over time, using data and methods that capture the broad spectrum of AD, and not merely using cognition as a proxy for disease progression. Where trials are undertaken, it is important to capture both costs and consequences of treatment (and control groups) more effectively. The use of instruments in the trials to measure resource use, and to address the data requirements for consequences (i.e. measures of health-related quality of life, QALYs), must be encouraged.

The review reported here has included studies published up to mid-2004. A number of other studies [54–56] have been published more recently, but the general messages from the literature, and the methodological concerns in analyses, remain the same in my opinion. The current cost-effectiveness literature is unhelpful to policy makers such as the UK NHS who generally take a third party payer perspective (in the first instance). The feel from the current literature that cholinesterase inhibitors are a cost-effective use of NHS resources has not been supported by a recent economic analysis for these treatments in the UK. Colleagues and I have estimated the cost-effectiveness of cholinesterase inhibitors for the treatment of mild to moderately severe AD in the UK, and we find that the NHS could expect cost per QALY estimates in the region of £50–£70,000 [57]. These analyses are recently published and are therefore not included in the more detailed review above. In summary, our analysis adapts modelling methods and data inputs from the sparse literature, in a UK context-specific manner, and the findings are a function of the modest clinical effects from treatment (differences in cognitive scores) and the expected mean costs per patient from an NHS and personal social services perspective. Interested readers are encouraged to consider the methods and results of our analysis in further detail. Importantly, decision makers, at whatever level (local, regional, or national) are encouraged to interpret the cost-effectiveness literature in the context of their specific policy environment. Furthermore, clinical trial teams and decision analysts are encouraged to give greater thought to the challenges present when attempting to estimate the cost-effectiveness of treatments for AD.

## ACKNOWLEDGEMENTS

The basis for this chapter is a detailed review on the clinical and cost-effectiveness of drugs for AD undertaken by The Southampton Health Technology Assessments Centre (SHTAC), University of Southampton, on behalf of the UK NHS R&D Health Technology Assessment Programme, and commissioned on behalf of the UKs' NICE. However, the views expressed here are my own and do not necessarily reflect those of the Department of Health. I would like to thank my colleagues within SHTAC for there assistance, especially Dr Joanna Picot for comments on the cost-effectiveness literature.

## REFERENCES

1. Drummond MF, O'Brien B, Stoddart GL, Torrance GW. *Methods for the Economic Evaluation of Health Care Programmes*, 2nd edition. Oxford University Press, New York, 1997.
2. National Institute for Clinical Excellence. *Guide to the Methods of Technology Appraisal*. National Institute for Clinical Excellence, London, 2004.
3. Loveman E, Green C, Kirby J *et al*. The clinical and cost effectiveness of donepezil, rivastigmine, galantamine, and memantine for Alzheimer's disease. *Health Technol Assess* 2006; 10:1–160. www.ncchta.org
4. Foster RH, Plosker GL. Donepezil. Pharmacoeconomic implications of therapy. *Pharmacoeconomics* 1999; 16:99–114.
5. Lyseng-Williamson K, Plosker GL. Galantamine: a pharmacoeconomic review of its use in Alzheimer's disease. *Pharmacoeconomics* 2002; 20:919–942.
6. Lamb HM, Goa KL. Rivastigmine – a pharmacoeconomic review of its use in Alzheimer's disease. *Pharmacoeconomics* 2001; 19:303–318.
7. Plosker GL, Lyseng-Williamson KA. Memantine. A pharmacoeconomic review of its use in moderate-to-severe Alzheimer's disease. *Pharmacoeconomics* 2005; 23:193–206.
8. Clegg A, Bryant J, Nicholson T *et al*. Clinical and cost-effectiveness of donepezil, rivastigmine and galantamine for Alzheimer's disease: a rapid and systematic review. *Health Technol Assess* 2001; 5:1–137.
9. Wolfson C, Oremus M, Shukla V *et al*. Donepezil and rivastigmine in the treatment of Alzheimer's disease: a best-evidence synthesis of the published data on their efficacy and cost-effectiveness. *Clin Ther* 2002; 24:862–886.
10. Ward A, Caro JJ, Getsios D *et al*. Assessment of health economics in Alzheimer's disease (AHEAD): treatment with galantamine in the UK. *Int J Geriatr Psychiatry* 2003; 18:740–747.

11. Fenn P, Gray A. Estimating long term cost savings from treatment of Alzheimer's disease: a modelling approach. *Pharmacoeconomics* 1999; 16:165–174.
12. AD2000 Collaborative Group. Long term donepezil treatment in 565 patients with Alzheimer's disease (AD2000): randomized double-blind trial. *Lancet* 2004; 363:2105–2115.
13. Drummond M, Jefferson TO. Guidelines for authors and peer reviewers of economic submissions to the BMJ. The BMJ Economic Evaluation Working Party. *BMJ* 1996; 313:275–283.
14. Philips Z, Ginnelly L, Sculpher M *et al.* A review of guidelines for good practice in decision-analytic modelling in health technology assessment. *Health Technol Assess* 2004; 8:1–158.
15. Gold MR, Siegel JE, Russell LB, Weinstein MC. *Cost-effectiveness in Health and Medicine.* Oxford University Press, New York, 1996.
16. Neumann PJ, Hermann RC, Kuntz KM *et al.* Cost-effectiveness of donepezil in the treatment of mild or moderate Alzheimer's disease. *Neurology* 1999; 52:1138–1145.
17. Wimo A, Winblad B, Engedal K *et al.* An economic evaluation of donepezil in mild to moderate Alzheimer's disease: results of a 1-year, double-blind, randomized trial. *Dement Geriatr Cogn Disord* 2003; 15:44–54.
18. Netten A, Darton R, Bebbington A *et al.* Residential and nursing home care of elderly people with cognitive impairment: prevalence, mortality and costs. *Aging Ment Health* 2001; 5:14–22.
19. Jones RW, Soininen H, Hager K *et al.* A multinational, randomized, 12-week study comparing the effects of donepezil and galantamine in patients with mild to moderate Alzheimer's disease. *Int J Geriatr Psychiatry* 2004; 19:58–67.
20. Beck JR, Pauker SG. The Markov process in medical prognosis. *Med Decis Making* 1983; 3:419–458.
21. Stewart A, Phillips R, Dempsey G. Pharmacotherapy for people with Alzheimer's disease: a Markov-cycle evaluation of five years' therapy using donepezil. *Int J Geriatr Psychiatry* 1998; 13:445–453.
22. Jonsson L, Lindgren P, Wimo A, Jonsson B, Winblad B. The cost-effectiveness of donepezil therapy in Swedish patients with Alzheimer's disease: A Markov model. *Clin Ther* 1999; 21:1230–1240.
23. O'Brien BJ, Goeree R, Hux M *et al.* Economic evaluation of donepezil for the treatment of Alzheimer's disease in Canada. *J Am Geriatr Soc* 1999; 47:570–578.
24. Ikeda S, Yamada Y, Ikegami N. Economic evaluation of donepezil treatment for Alzheimer's disease in Japan. *Dement Geriatr Cogn Disord* 2002; 13:33–39.
25. Fagnani F, Lafuma A, Pechevis M *et al.* Donepezil for the treatment of mild to moderate Alzheimer's disease in France: the economic implications. *Dement Geriatr Cogn Disord* 2003; 17:5–13.
26. Rosler M, Anand R, Cicin SA *et al.* Efficacy and safety of rivastigmine in patients with Alzheimer's disease: International randomized controlled trial. *BMJ* 1999; 318:633–640.
27. Corey-Bloom J, Anand R, Veach J. A randomized trial evaluating the efficacy and safety of ENA 713 (rivastigmine tartrate), a new acetylcholinesterase inhibitor, in patients with mild to moderately severe Alzheimer's disease. *Int J Geriatr Psychopharmacol* 1998; 1:55–65.
28. Caro JJ, Getsios D, Migliaccio-Walle K, Raggio G, Ward A. Assessment of health economics in Alzheimer's disease (AHEAD) based on need for full-time care. *Neurology* 2001; 57:964–971.
29. Stern Y, Tang MX, Albert MS *et al.* Predicting time to nursing home care and death in individuals with Alzheimer disease. *JAMA* 1997; 277:806–812.
30. François C, Sintonen H, Sulkava R. The cost-effectiveness of memantine in moderately severe to severe Alzheimer's disease. A Markov model in Finland. *Clin Drug Investig* 2004; 27:373–384.
31. Reisberg B, Doody R, Stoffler A *et al.* Memantine in moderate-to-severe Alzheimer's disease. *N Engl J Med* 2003; 348:1333–1341.
32. Livingston G, Katona C, Roch B *et al.* A dependency model for patients with Alzheimer's disease: its validation and relationship to the costs of care – the LASER-AD Study. *Curr Med Res Opin* 2004; S7:1007–1016.
33. Bowie P, Branton T, Holmes J. Should the mini mental state examination be used to monitor dementia treatments? *Lancet* 1999; 354:1527–1528.
34. Davey RJ, Jamieson S. The validity of using the mini mental state examination in NICE dementia guidelines. *J Neurol, Neurosurg Psychiatry* 2004; 75:343–344.
35. Tombaugh TN, Mcintyre NJ. The mini-mental-state-examination – a comprehensive review. *J Am Geriatr Soc* 1992; 40:922–935.
36. Wolstenholme J, Fenn P, Gray A, Keene J, Jacoby R, Hope T. Estimating the relationship between disease progression and cost of care in dementia. *Br J Psychiatry* 2002; 181:36–42.
37. Clark CM, Sheppard L, Fillenbaum G *et al.* Variability in annual mini-mental state examination score in patients with probably Alzheimer's disease. *Arch Neurol* 1999; 56:857–862.

38. Hauber AB, Gnanasakthy A, Mauskopf JA. Savings in the cost of caring for patients with Alzheimer's disease in Canada: an analysis of treatment with rivastigmine. *Clin Ther* 2000; 22:439–451.
39. O'Shea E, O'Reilly S. The economic and social cost of dementia in Ireland. *Int J Geriatr Psychiatry* 2000; 15:208–218.
40. Neumann PJ, Araki SS, Arcelus A *et al.* Measuring Alzheimer's disease progression with transition probabilities: estimates from CERAD. *Neurology* 2001; 57:957–964.
41. Mendiondo MS, Ashford JW, Kryscio RJ, Schmitt FA. Modelling mini mental state examination changes in Alzheimer's disease. *Stat Med* 2000; 19:1607–1616.
42. Morris JC, Heyman A, Mohs RC *et al.* The Consortium to Establish a Registry for Alzheimer's Disease (CERAD). Part I. Clinical and neuropsychological assessment of Alzheimer's disease. *Neurology* 1989; 39:1159–1165.
43. Hauber AB, Gnanasakthy A, Snyder EH, Bala MV, Richter A, Mauskopf JA. Potential savings in the cost of caring for Alzheimer's disease – treatment with rivastigmine. *Pharmacoeconomics* 2000; 17:351–360.
44. Garfield FB, Getsios D, Caro JJ, Wimo A, Winblad B. Assessment of Health Economics in Alzheimer's Disease (AHEAD): treatment with galantamine in Sweden. *Pharmacoeconomics* 2002; 20:629–637.
45. Caro JJ, Salas M, Ward A, Getsios D, Mehnert A. Economic analysis of galantamine, a cholinesterase inhibitor, in the treatment of patients with mild to moderate Alzheimer's disease in the Netherlands. *Dement Geriatr Cogn Disord* 2002; 14:84–89.
46. Migliaccio-Walle K, Getsios D, Caro JJ *et al.* Economic evaluation of galantamine in the treatment of mild to moderate Alzheimer's disease in the United States. *Clin Ther* 2003; 25:1806–1825.
47. Whitehouse P. Measurements of quality of life in dementia. In: Wimo A, Jonsson B, Karlsson G, Winblad B (eds). *Health Economics of Dementia.* John Wiley & Sons, Chichester, 1998.
48. Neumann PJ, Kuntz KM, Leon J *et al.* Health utilities in Alzheimer's disease: a cross-sectional study of patients and caregivers. *Med Care* 1999; 37:27–32.
49. Neumann PJ. Measuring QALYS in dementia. In: Wimo A, Jonsson B, Karlsson G, Winblad B (eds). *Health Economics of Dementia.* John Wiley & Sons, Chichester, 1998.
50. Brazier J, Deverill M, Green C, Harper R, Booth A. A review of the use of health status measures in economic evaluation. *Health Technol Assess* 1999; 3:1–164.
51. Green C, Brazier J, Deverill M. Valuing health-related quality of life. A review of health state valuation techniques. *Pharmacoeconomics* 2000; 17:151–165.
52. Kerner DN, Patterson TL, Grant I, Kaplan RM. Validity of the quality of well-being scale for patients with Alzheimer's disease. *J Aging Health* 1998; 10:44–61.
53. Sano M, Albert SM, Tractenberg R, Schittini M. Developing utilities: quantifying quality of life for stages of Alzheimer's disease as measured by the clinical dementia rating. *J Ment Health Aging* 1999; 5:59–68.
54. Jonsson L. Cost-effectiveness of memantine for moderate to severe Alzheimer's disease in Sweden. *Am J Geriatr Pharmacother* 2005; 3:77–86.
55. Caro J, Salas M, Ward A, Getsios D, Migliaccio-Walle K, Garfield F. Assessing the health and economic impact of galantamine treatment in patients with Alzheimer's disease in the healthcare systems of different countries. *Drugs Aging* 2004; 21:677–686.
56. Feldman H, Gauthier S, Hecker J *et al.* Economic evaluation of donepezil in moderate to severe Alzheimer disease. *Neurology* 2004; 63:644–650.
57. Green C, Picot J, Loveman E, Takeda A, Kirby J, Clegg A. Modelling the cost effectiveness of cholinesterase inhibitors in the management of mild to moderately severe Alzheimer's disease. *Pharmacoeconomics* 2005; 23:1271–1282.
58. Getsios D, Caro JJ, Caro G, Ishak K, AHEAD Study Group. Assessment of health economics in Alzheimer's disease (AHEAD): galantamine treatment in Canada. *Neurology* 2001; 57:972–978.

# Section II

## Biological developments and future therapies

# 8

# Disease-modifying therapeutic strategies for Alzheimer's disease: targeting the APP/Aβ pathway

*C. L. Masters, K. Beyreuther*

## INTRODUCTION

The ultimate goal of current research into Alzheimer's disease (AD) and related disorders of the ageing nervous system is to develop a disease-modifying therapeutic strategy. In numerical terms, the current emphasis is on the biochemical and molecular genetic pathways surrounding the amyloid β (Aβ) and the amyloid precursor protein (APP). In 2005 alone, more than 780 papers appeared on APP/Aβ, many of which deal with pre-clinical and clinical therapeutic strategies directed at the APP/Aβ pathway (Figure 8.1). In this chapter, we survey the 2005/2006 literature, which includes several useful reviews [1–8]. We have also reviewed the two public databases of clinical trials which enumerate the current status of clinical activity in this area (Novatis International, maintained by Kwon and Herrling [9] and the clinical trials registry sponsored by the National Institutes of Health (NIH) [www.clinicaltrials.gov]).

Why is there so much interest in the APP/Aβ pathway? The theory which underlies this pathway as the principal and proximal causal mechanism in AD is pinned to two critical series of observations: first, mutations in the gene encoding APP (and the presenilin [PS] genes as components of the γ-secretase machinery) are causally linked to early onset familial AD; second, genetically engineered mice with these mutations recapitulate the human disease. More recently, a very tight association between the mean age at onset of pedigrees with PS mutation-related familial AD and the ratio of secreted $A\beta_{40}$ to $A\beta_{42}$ has emerged [10]. This, together with the development of a robust Aβ-neuroimaging ligand (a thioflovin T analogue) which as a biomarker clearly differentiates AD and mild cognitive impairment (MCI) from normal controls and other neurologic diseases [11, 12], adds much more strength to the Aβ theory. But the single most important challenge to test the theory remains the demonstration that a drug targeting the APP/Aβ pathway actually modifies the natural history of the disease. To this end, the criteria set out by Cummings [13], and listed in Table 8.1, have clarified the standards to be met when we come to assess this test of the Aβ theory of AD. The first criterion (a plausible mechanism of action in a validated model) has been achieved by many of the therapeutic strategies reviewed below. But no drug has yet met any of the other four criteria, although we remain optimistic that the current pace of activity will deliver a result in the not too distant future.

**Colin L. Masters**, MD, Department of Pathology, The University of Melbourne and The Mental Health Research Institute of Victoria, Australia

**Konrad Beyreuther**, PhD, Centre for Molecular Biology Heidelberg, Zentrum für Molekulare Biologie Heidelberg, Heidelberg, Germany

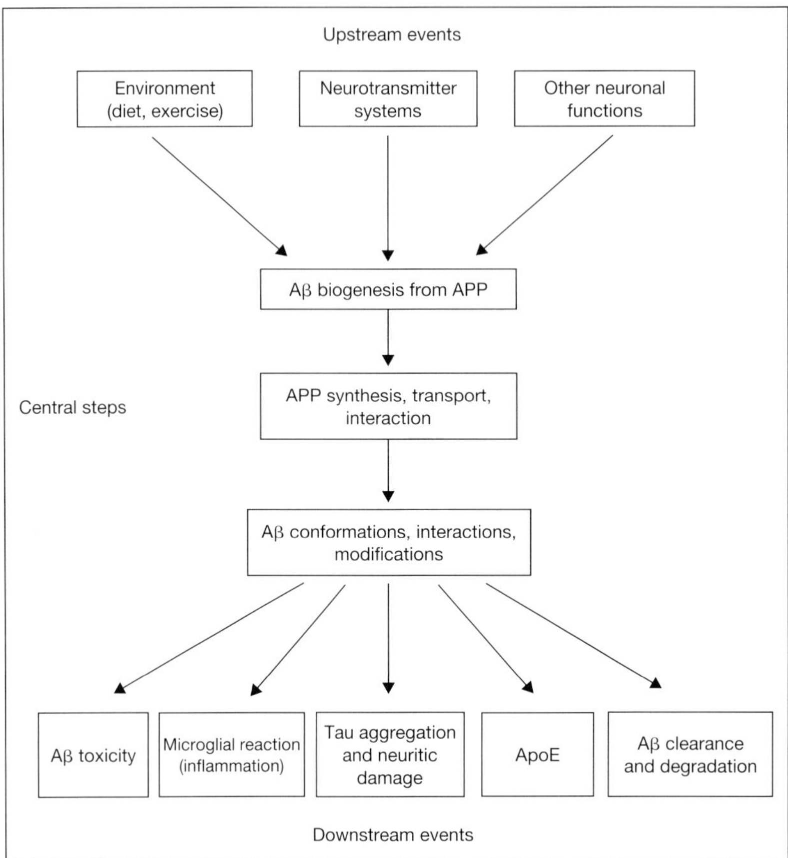


**Figure 8.1** Schematic outline of the upstream and downstream events which surround the central APP/Aβ pathway.

**Table 8.1** Alzheimer's disease modification by drug intervention: criteria (modified with permission from Cummings [13]).

1. Plausible mechanism of action in a validated model.
2. Clinical trial evidence based on the Lerber staggered start design.
3. Difference in survival to a meaningful clinical outcome.
4. Change in rate (slope) of decline.
5. Demonstrable drug–placebo difference on an accepted biomarker of disease progression.

## UPSTREAM EVENTS IN THE APP/Aβ PATHWAY

The targets derived from the APP/Aβ pathway outlined in Figure 8.1 are listed in more detail in Table 8.2. While it is not a comprehensive or exhaustive listing, it does present a novel and logical way of classifying the wide range of current research activity being undertaken in this area.

### *AGE AND ENVIRONMENTAL FACTORS*

Of all the external variables which determine risk of getting AD, age and the environment stand out as factors which demand explanations. Yet for all their obviousness, no reasonable

**Table 8.2** Alzheimer's disease therapeutic targets derived from the APP/Aβ pathway

| *Pathway step/event* | *Target/drug* |
|---|---|
| **Upstream events** | |
| *Ageing* | |
| Environment | Exercise, diet |
| Neurotransmitter systems modulation | Cholinergic: AChE/BuChE inhibition<br>Glutamatergic: NMDA antagonism<br>Serotonergic: Anti-depressants |
| Other cerebral or general systemic factors | |
| **Central steps: Aβ biogenesis from APP** | |
| *APP gene target* | |
| APP interactions, transport | X11 gene target, growth factors, metal homeostasis, ZnT3, oestrogen, cholesterol |
| APP proteolytic processing | |
| γ-secretase (PS, Aph1, PEN2, Nct) | Inhibitor, modulator (NSAID), gene target and associated ε- and ζ-cleavages |
| β-secretase (BACE 1) | Inhibitor, modulator/interaction (PAR 4), immunomodulations of β-cleavage site, gene target |
| α-secretase | Stimulation (PKC activation) |
| *Aβ and its varied conformations* | |
| Monomers/dimer/trimer ($A_4$, $A_8$, $A_{12}$) | |
| Metal binding sites | Metal–protein attenuating compounds (MPAC) |
| GAG binding sites | |
| Oxidative modifications | Di-tyrosine, methionine oxidation |
| Aβ–lipid interactions | Lipid–protein attenuating compounds (LPAC) |
| Aβ–protein interactions | Protein–protein attenuating compounds (PPAC) |
| β-oligomers/protofibrils | Anti-aggregants/dis-aggregants |
| Polymers/fibrils | Anti-fibrillogenics/de-fibrillants |
| **Downstream events** | |
| Aβ-induced 'toxicity' through oxidative damage (protein, mitochondria, lipid, sterols, nucleic acid, etc.) | Anti-oxidants, natural product screens, oestrogen |
| Anti-inflammatory (anti-microglia) | Sigma 1 receptor, PPAR-γ, $PGE_2$, NSAID, iNOS inhibition |
| Aβ–tau direct/indirect interactions | Microtubule stabilizers, kinase, inhibitors, anti-aggregants, etc. |
| Aβ–ApoE interactions | Statins/cholesterol |
| Aβ–clearance/neutralization | Immunization, immunomodulation |
| Aβ–degradation | IDE, NPE, ACE |

explanations have been forthcoming. While many of the biochemical events listed in the APP/Aβ pathway are known to be developmentally regulated, very little information is yet available on what happens under normal ageing conditions. Partial loss of function of a critical biochemical reaction would seem to be a good starting point for investigation, either as an upstream or downstream event; or a 'double hit' phenomenon could be invoked, as seen in the early development of ideas on oncogenesis. Whichever, the incontrovertible link between ageing and AD remains obscure in mechanistic terms.

Similarly, the interactions between the environment and the risk for AD have attracted many epidemiological studies. Diet and exercise remain as the two most interesting variables. General caloric restriction has often been associated with longevity in rodent models of ageing, and recent studies in transgenic AD models [14, 15] and normal rodents [16] suggest an effect on Aβ plaque load or α-secretase processing of APP. The effects of exercise [17] and environmental enrichment [18, 19] have also been examined in transgenic AD models with encouraging results. One group [19] found a change in a downstream event, an increase in the enzymatic activity of neprilysin, an Aβ-degrading protease, in response to environmental enrichment. These downstream events are discussed in the section 'Modulating the Aβ Degradation Pathway'.

Specific dietary intakes, especially naturally occurring anti-oxidants (see section: 'Ameliorating the toxic gain-of-function of Aβ: anti-oxidants, neuroprotectants, and other products of natural origin') or metal ions (see section: 'Monomers ($A_4$), dimers ($A_8$) and trimers ($A_{12}$)') remain largely under-investigated as AD risk factors. As methods for diagnosis and population-based screening improve (using plasma biomarkers or specific ligands of Aβ for neuroimaging), it will become more feasible to examine analytically the dietary risk profiles of discrete populations, overcoming current limitations on sensitivity and specificity of case-ascertainment. A surprising study has already pre-empted dietary modulation of AD through the consumption of transgenic Aβ-expressing potatoes [20]! The proposed mechanism involves low-level immune-mediated clearance of Aβ deposits (see section: 'Using immunization and immunomodulation of Aβ to promote clearance and inhibit toxicity (neutralization)'). One wonders where this approach might lead – perhaps the production of transgenic Aβ-over expressing beef or lamb stock will appear on future menus?

## *THE EFFECT OF MODULATION OF NEUROTRANSMITTER SYSTEMS ON APP PROCESSING*

Acetylcholinesterase (AChE) was discovered to be present in AD amyloid plaques 40 years ago, and the activity of choline acetyl transferase (CAT) was found to be decreased in the AD brain 30 years ago. From these observations the cholinergic hypothesis/theory of AD arose, which led to the development of AChE inhibitors (AChEI) as a therapeutic strategy, with apparent success, despite the lack of any plausible explanation for the presence of AChE in plaques and the underlying loss of CAT. A paradox then emerged: subjects treated with AChEI responded with a compensatory increase in AChE levels. This might have been expected to negate the intended effect of the AChEI on the availability of ACh for cholinergic transmission. At the same time, clinical trials of AChEIs and their meta-analyses continued to show favourable, albeit mild, effects on cognitive parameters, at least during the first 6–12 months of treatment. Against this background, basic and clinical investigators have recently turned their attention towards other possible mechanisms of action of the AChEIs, especially on the APP/Aβ pathway, and have begun to ask whether these drugs might have any disease-modifying effects [21].

Various aspects of AChEI actions on the upstream and downstream APP/Aβ pathway have been reported: attenuating the effects of Aβ-induced neuronal cytoxicity [22], promoting α-secretase or decreasing β-secretase activity [21, 23], inhibiting Aβ aggregation [24, 25] or inhibiting GSK 3β activity and tau phosphorylation [21]. One group found no effect on Aβ amyloid plaque load while still improving behavioural deficits in a transgenic mouse model [26], while another group found that inhibitors of butyrylcholinesterase had a lowering effect on cellular APP and Aβ and brain Aβ in transgenic mice [27].

The modulation of glutamatergic transmission in AD has also received increasing attention with the results of the memantine clinical trials aimed at blocking (non-competitively) the action of *N*-methyl-D-aspartase (NMDA) receptors. With the growing awareness that the toxic soluble oligomers of Aβ may inhibit long-term potentiation (LTP) at the pre-synaptic level and that Aβ promotes the endocytosis of the NMDA receptor (mediated in part through α7 nicotinic receptor, protein phosphatase PP2B, and tyrosine phosphase STEP [28]), the finding that memantine has beneficial behavioural effects in both Aβ toxicity models [29] and APP transgenic mouse models [30] requires further work which might tie all these observations together.

Finally, behavioural intervention with antidepressants has also been explored in relation to *in vitro* APP processing [31]. It would seem less likely that the tricyclics or serotonin reuptake inhibitors will ever be subjected to AD-modification trials, but if further pre-clinical studies emerge showing effects on APP processing, then an argument could be made for additional clinical studies in the early phases of AD.

### *OTHER CEREBRAL OR GENERAL SYSTEMIC FACTORS*

One suspects that there will be many other upstream factors which play into the APP/Aβ pathway, but few have been identified to date. A particularly contentious area has been the role of the vascular supply to the brain and the effects of ischaemia (atherosclerosis) and hypertension. Historically, this has deep roots, going back to the days when 'arteriosclerosis' was thought to cause all forms of dementia. Similarly, head trauma has been considered as a risk factor for AD, and APP has been identified as a sensitive marker of axonal damage following traumatic brain injury. But neither hypoxia nor trauma has yet been shown to be major risk factors for AD, and neither has been shown to promote the long-term amyloidogenic processing of APP.

## CENTRAL STEPS IN THE APP/Aβ PATHWAY

### *TARGETING THE APP GENE OR GENES WITH PRODUCTS INTERACTING DIRECTLY WITH APP*

With the advent of RNA interference (RNAi) silencing, it is to be expected that attempts at direct APP gene regulation will emerge. As a forerunner to this, models in which the over-expressed human APP transgene in mice can be downregulated with doxycline provide a proof-of-principle that rapid control over Aβ expression and deposition can be obtained without gross adverse side-effects [32]. Unexpectedly, Aβ deposits formed before the onset of downregulation seemed to be remarkably stable, indicating that any treatment of this type in isolation might have to be administered early in the natural history of AD. Using RNAi techniques in transfected cell lines [33], targeting the X11 gene (APAB) successfully increased APP C-terminal fragments and lowered Aβ levels; X11 is a known interactor with the cytoplasmic domain of APP, and presents a novel method of possibly modulating γ-secretase cleavage.

### *APP-INTERACTING SYSTEMS*

As a presumptive cell surface receptor, APP probably has ligands and effector mechanisms for signal transduction. Nearly 200 proteins have been reported as having direct interactions with APP. Suspected ligands in the extracellular domain include growth factors (nerve growth factor [NGF] in particular), heparin-containing extracellular matrix, metals (through the extracellular Cu/Zn binding domain) and APP itself through hetero- and homo-dimerization. Small compounds such as propentofyline [34] can affect NGF release, and through this modulate the amyloidogenic pathway. Other small compounds may bind directly to APP [35] and affect its processing.

A controversial area involves the effects of hormones (oestrogens and testosterone especially) and how they may affect APP metabolism. Conflicting results in experimental models have appeared, in which oestrogen deficiency exacerbates Aβ in the APP23 transgenic model [36] and neither oestrogen deprivation nor replacement affected Aβ deposition in the PDAPP transgenic model [37]. Further studies are clearly required to unravel this important area where there is an epidemiological impression that females have a higher incidence of AD than males (this impression does not appear to have ever been subjected to a prospective analytical epidemiological study). The mechanisms through which oestrogen/testosterone might act remain obscure, but include oestrogen-dependent regulation of metal homeostasis in the brain through the expression of the neuronal zinc-transporter, ZnT3 (see also chapter 12).

Cholesterol and inhibitors of cholesterol synthesis (statins) have been shown to significantly alter APP processing *in vitro*, with a reduction in β-secretase cleavage and lessened Aβ production. While some early phase clinical trials with stains have shown encouraging results [38], others have not [39, 40]. Cholesterol-independent effects have also been noted for statins acting on isoprenyl intermediates in the cholesterol biosynthetic pathways, with a putative anti-inflammatory effect induced by reactive microglia [41, 42]. This might conflict with the current theory that microglia are involved in the beneficial process of clearing Aβ deposits (see sections: 'Suppressing Brain "inflammation"' and 'Using Immunization and Immunomodulation of Aβ to Promote Clearance and Inhibit Toxicity (Neutralization)'). Statins also have been implicated in the toxic gain-of-function of Aβ interacting with $\alpha_7$-nicotinic AChR [43], although the mechanism for this remains unclear.

If eventually cholesterol does prove to be a risk factor for AD, then the observations [44] of an association between AD and the expression levels and haplotypes of the 5′ region of the cholesterol 25-hydroxylase (CH25H) gene on chromosome 10 may provide a plausible explanation: one in which cerebral cholesterol metabolism (as distinct from systemic cholesterol and its association with atherosclerosis) directly plays into the APP processing and transport pathways.

## *APP PROTEOLYTIC PROCESSING*

The biogenesis of Aβ has been the prime validated drug target for AD since the discovery of the proteolytic processing of APP in 1987 (providing the fertile ground for nearly 20 years of intensive research). Molecular details of the C-terminal cleavage (γ-secretase) were the first to emerge, followed by the α- and β-cleavage mechanisms. Subsequent elucidation of δ-, ε-, and ζ-cleavages has added another layer of complexity. Drug discovery programs reflect this sequence of events: many large pharmaceutical companies have γ-secretase inhibitors or modulators in clinical development, while the β-secretase inhibitors are several years behind, largely in pre-clinical discovery.

### *γ-secretase inhibitors and modulators*

During 2005, the first publications of *in vivo* γ-secretase inhibition/modulation of $A\beta_{42}$ biogenesis appeared. One of the first known inhibitors (DAPT) was shown to be effective in acute experiments in behavioural tests (contextual fear conditioning) in the Tg 2576 AD mouse model [45]. Modifications to the chemical structure of DAPT has now improved its delivery to the brain [46], as with other compounds [47], in the hope of achieving lower effective dosages minimizing the risk of adverse peripheral effects. Many diverse classes of inhibitors and modulators are showing very favourable acute pharmacokinetics, with rapid lowering of plasma and CSF Aβ levels [48–53]. Importantly, there is now strong evidence linking plasma and cerebrospinal fluid (CSF) Aβ levels, indicating that the brain/CSF pool of Aβ is at least in part a significant proportion of the plasma Aβ pool. There are still methodological issues in measuring Aβ, using either enzyme-linked immunosorbent assay (ELISA) or Western blotting techniques (which soluble oligomeric species are being measured, and what forms of Aβ: total, $A\beta_{40}$, $A\beta_{42}$?). Nevertheless, these preliminary data offer some hope that plasma Aβ species may eventually prove to be a reliable marker of cerebral Aβ turnover. Further explorations of the properties of γ-secretase inhibitors are revealing unanticipated effects on synaptic function [54]. New classes of γ-secretase inhibitors/modulators continue to be disclosed [55–57], as part of the effect to develop compounds devoid of side-effects. The major concern is the inhibition of signalling in the Notch pathway, which affects cellular differentiation [58, 59]. Ironically, γ-secretase inhibitor compounds originally developed for AD are now being trialled in phase II studies of acute lymphoblastic leukaemia (NCT00100152-Clinical Trials.gov [60]) and advanced breast cancer (NCT00106145-Clinical Trials.gov [61]).

The first in-human phase I results to be published [62, 63] have shown that the Lilly compound LY450139 achieved a significant lowering of plasma Aβ, but not CSF Aβ, in normal volunteers (up to 50 mg/day for 14 days) or subjects with AD (up to 40 mg/day for 6 weeks). The drug was well-tolerated. Higher dosages may be required to achieve a reduction in CSF levels. The results of phase II studies with readouts on cognitive variables are eagerly awaited. In the meantime, further research on the mechanistic operations of the γ-secretase complex [64] may lead to new paths of drug discovery, as might gene targeting of PS, PEN-2, APH-1, and nicastrin lead to selective regulation of γ-secretase activity [65, 66].

#### *β-secretase (BACE) inhibitors*

Although approximately 5 years behind the development of the γ-secretase inhibitors, much progress has been made in the discovery and design of compounds which target the active site of BACE-1. Improved assays [67] and structural-based *in silico* designs [68–72] have added to the existing pipe-line of drugs in early pre-clinical development [73–76] or early discovery programs [77, 78]. Other proteins interacting with BACE-1 may become drug targets [79], and gene targeting of BACE-1 mRNA using siRNA is also producing encouraging preliminary results [80]. As with γ-secretase, unanticipated side-effects on other BACE-1 substrates or downstream consequences of BACE-1 inhibition may prove difficult to circumvent. As a consolation, inhibitors of BACE-1 may also turn out to have anti-angiogenic and anti-neoplastic activities [81].

## *DRUGS TARGETING Aβ AND ITS VARIED CONFORMATIONS*

#### *Monomers ($A_4$), dimers ($A_8$) and trimers ($A_{12}$)*

In contrast to the inhibition of Aβ biogenesis, therapeutic strategies which directly target Aβ itself should inherently have a lower risk of throwing up unanticipated side-effects, as the accumulated Aβ molecule is restricted to AD. If the Aβ fragment (or its domain within APP) does, however, subserve some critical normal function, then targeting Aβ itself might interfere with this function and thereby lead to adverse side-effects, but to date, a normal function for Aβ has not been identified. APP knockout mice are viable and healthy, providing some support for this idea.

Current models of the physical state of Aβ are evolving. Whilst resident in the membrane, Aβ is assumed to be in an α-helical conformation. Following sequential β- and γ-cleavages, Aβ as a monomer ($A_4$), dimer ($A_8$) [or perhaps even as a trimer ($A_{12}$)] is translocated into the extra-cytosolic space, and may transition there into a β-strand enriched structure. These structures may then progress towards β-oligomers/protofibrils through to polymers/fibrils of amyloid filaments.

The mechanisms through which Aβ causes damage to neurones ('the toxic gain of function') are slowly emerging. There are many theories: the two most favoured include the ability of Aβ to generate oxidative stress and the hydrophobic interaction of Aβ with lipid membranes, particularly the synaptic plasma membrane. Our current working model incorporates both theories: we have defined a metal binding domain near the N-terminus of Aβ which is capable of binding $Zn^{2+}$ (which causes Aβ to precipitate) or redox-active $Cu^{2+}$. When $Cu^{2+}$ binds Aβ, it not only causes a significant increase in insolubility, but induces a series of electron transfers which result in histidine bridge formation, tyrosine 10 radicalization, di-tyrosine cross-linking and oxidation of methionine 35. Ultimately, in the presence of reductants, this results in the production of $H_2O_2$ and hydroxyl radicals, capable of inflicting short-range oxidative damage to proteins, lipids, sterols, nucleic acids, etc. Our studies show that toxicity to neurones in culture is associated with the ability of Aβ to associate with the lipid head-group on the outer surface of the plasma membrane.

If this schema is only partially correct, then it is clear that any therapeutic strategy targeting Aβ directly might have multiple routes, many intersecting and overlapping. Thus, targeting the metal binding site of Aβ might relate to Aβ in one or more of its varied conformations (α-helix, β-strand, β-sheet; $A_4$, $A_8$, $A_{16}$ vs. higher order oligomers vs. polymerized fibril) or whilst interacting with other proteins or lipids.

In consideration of targeting the metal binding site on Aβ, we have developed the concept of an MPAC – a metal–protein attenuating compound – in distinction to the more widely known term of metal chelator. The MPAC has relatively weak binding constants for metals, and is able to compete with the target site for the metal ion. As a consequence, an MPAC should not alter the general homeostasis of metal ions in the whole animal. In contrast, a metal chelator has high, effectively irreversible, binding constants for metal ions. A chelator might affect the metal binding to Aβ through deletion of the total pool of bioavailable metal, but is not expected necessarily to interact with the Aβ metal binding site itself.

The utility of MPACs in AD has been initiated with studies of clioquinol, an 8-OH quinoline, with encouraging pre-clinical [82, 83] and early phase II clinical [84, 85] results. Other groups have considered chelators [86, 87] or other novel compounds [88–92]. Our own studies have progressed with a new chemical entity based around the 8-OH quinoline structure. This compound (PBT2-Prana Biotechnology) has passed phase I and will soon commence phase II clinical development.

Additional binding sites on Aβ, such as the glycosaminoglycan (GAG) site, (HHQK [13–16]), have been targeted with compounds such as 3-amino-1-propanesulfonic acid [3-APS (Alzhemed) – Neurochem Inc.]. The results of early clinical trials have been released by the company, with some effects seen on CSF $A\beta_{42}$, but none on the Alzheimer's Disease Assessment Scale Cognitive subscale (ADAS-Cog) or Mini-mental State Examination (MMSE). A large phase III study is under way, coupled to an open-label extension study. The double-blind study results are expected in January 2007.

We have identified other structural changes or mechanisms of toxicity for Aβ which include the oxidative modifications of Tyr10 and Met35, the interaction of Aβ with the polar head groups of the lipid bilayer, or the interaction of Aβ with other proteins. These areas remain very much in the early discovery phase and may deliver LPACs – lipid–protein attenuating compounds, or PPACs (protein–protein attenuating compounds) [93, 94].

#### *β-oligomers/protofibrils/and polymers/fibrils of Aβ*

The pharmaceutical industry has for a long time interrogated their libraries for compounds that are anti-aggregants and/or anti-fibrillogenic. Many hits with compounds that look similar to Congo Red have never been developed. Similarly, compounds capable of disaggregating or defibrillating Aβ have been sought, but not with the intensity of the search for anti-aggregants. While many peptidyl/protein-like designs have been examined [95–99], other small molecules have been discovered which hold some promise [100–107]. However, most interesting, is the development of assays specifically designed to examine the effects of soluble β-oligomers of Aβ (possibly the trimeric form $A_{12}$) and to use these assays in a discovery process of small compounds capable of inhibiting β-oligomer formation [108].

## TARGETING THE DOWNSTREAM EFFECTS OF Aβ

There are many productive lines of enquiry being applied to the downstream effects of Aβ, beginning with the direct consequences of Aβ toxicity and oxidative damage through to the promotion of Aβ clearance/degradation. Big questions remain on the role of the innate immune system and the value of targeting neurofibrillary tangle formation.

### AMELIORATING THE TOXIC GAIN-OF-FUNCTION OF Aβ: ANTI-OXIDANTS, NEUROPROTECTANTS, AND OTHER PRODUCTS OF NATURAL ORIGIN

Existing knowledge and screens of natural product libraries have thrown up a wide variety of anti-oxidants and 'neuroprotectants' which have an effect on the actions of Aβ in experimental assays of its toxicity. Many of these assays are difficult to control, and there is little agreement in the field as to their validity. Nevertheless, an increasing number of papers are appearing reporting efficacy of compounds derived from plants (ferulic acid [109–114], green tea extracts [115–117], curcumin [118–119], resveratol [120], fucoidan [121] and various other plant materials [122–125]), other natural products (docosahexaenoic acid [126, 127], vitamin E [128, 129], oestrogens [129, 130], glutathione [131, 132], melatonin [133], coenzyme Q10 [134], gelsolin [135] and insulin-like growth factor 1 [136]) or a variety of small compounds [137–139]). From these investigations, a common theme emerges: that a wide variety of anti-oxidants can ameliorate the toxic gain-of-function of Aβ. This is consistent with our argument that Aβ itself is the principal pro-oxidant in AD. Other lines of evidence are emerging which contribute to an understanding of the oxidative stress [140] or form a feed-forward mechanism [141] to account for the progressive nature of AD.

### SUPPRESSING BRAIN 'INFLAMMATION'

"*Inflammation* [L. *inflammare* to set on fire] a localized protective response elicited by injury or destruction of tissues... Histologically, it involves a complex series of events, including dilation of arterioles, capillaries, and venules, with increased permeability and blood flow; exudation of fluids...; and leukocyte migration..."

*Dorland's Illustrated Medical Dictionary*

There is considerable controversy around the concept that the AD brain is undergoing inflammation. As usually understood, inflammatory changes are not visible. What Alzheimer, Cajal and their contemporaries recognized was that microglia were increased in number, activated and together with astrocytes were reacting to some underlying factor, possibly the amyloid within the plaque. They also recognized that the dystrophic neurites and "drusige Entartung" associated with the perivascular amyloid deposits could represent the reactive and regenerative response of neurones to the same injurious process. Therefore, it is surprising that the idea of 'inflammation' in AD has gained such ground in recent times. In this scenario, the microglia are seen as inflammatory invaders causing damage through their release of cytokines and other powerful destructive molecules designed to respond to injury. This innate immune reaction would therefore exacerbate the clinical expression of AD and lead to its progression towards neuronal dysfunction and death. From this, trials of anti-inflammatories in AD have been conducted, and considerable research efforts undertaken to examine the effects of anti-inflammatories in a variety of experimental models. These include the non-steroidal anti-inflammatories (NSAIDs) [142, 143], peroxisome proliferator-activated receptor-γ (PPAR-γ) agonists [144–148], cannabinoids [149], glucocorticoids [150] and zingansikpoongtang – a Korean herbal medicine [151]! To date, no prospective clinical trial with an anti-inflammatory has shown a convincing beneficial outcome. Perhaps the underlying theory is wrong? In the light of the data emerging around the immunization/immunomodulation strategies against Aβ, the counter-hypothesis that microglia are actually beneficial could prove to be correct.

### TARGETING TAU AGGREGATION IN THE Aβ PATHWAY

While Aβ has captured the imagination of most AD researchers, studies of the neurofibrillary tangle and its constituent, the tau microtubule-associated protein, have progressed to a point where clear therapeutic strategies are emerging. The exact form of tau which causes neuronal degeneration is now being re-examined [152], with data emerging that the soluble aggregated species, akin to soluble β-oligomers of Aβ, might represent the best target. The binding sites on tau [153] for a variety of interactors are potential targets. Downregulation of expression of the tau gene [154] or altering the alternative splicing [155] also offer some new strategies.

As the molecular basis for the accumulation of tau in the AD brain becomes clearer, so will the precise therapeutic target. If tau accumulation is closely linked to Aβ toxicity, then oxidative modifications of tau become understandable [156–160] and subject to anti-oxidative classes of drugs. Metal ions might also affect this pathway [161–162]. Looking at the normal function and processing of tau has raised the possibility of using microtubule-stabilizing agents such as paclitaxel (Taxol) [163]. Great controversy still persists on the role of normal and abnormal phosphorylation of tau in its passage from a highly soluble cytoskeletal-associated protein into an aggregated neurofibrillary tangle. If phosphorylation of specific amino acids by specific kinases such as c-Abl [164], Cdk5 [165], GSK-3 [166] or MAPK [167] proves to be pathogenic, then specific kinase inhibitors (including lithium [166]) might be developed for AD – indeed, a trial with lithium is currently in progress in the UK. However, if phosphorylation proves to be a secondary event, following aggregation and accumulation of intracellular tau, then this approach would not be expected to be useful. Other post-translational modifications including proteolytic cleavages have been proposed [168] – all amenable to therapeutic drug discoveries. As with Aβ, small compounds capable of inhibiting aggregation and fibrillization of tau are now being examined *in vitro* [169, 170], but require much more work in animal models.

### HOW DOES APOE FIT WITHIN THE Aβ PATHWAY?

As the major (if not the sole) genetic risk factor for determining the age at onset of AD, it is surprising that we still do not have a definitive explanation of the mechanism of action of ApoE. Targeting the ApoE gene directly, or aiming for the delivery of the protective ApoE isoform [171], offer some prospect of therapeutic intervention. However, understanding the precise interaction between ApoE and the processing of APP/Aβ is likely to yield more amenable therapeutic strategies.

### USING IMMUNIZATION AND IMMUNOMODULATION OF Aβ TO PROMOTE CLEARANCE AND INHIBIT TOXICITY (NEUTRALIZATION)

Since 1999, increasing evidence has accumulated to make a compelling antibody-mediated Aβ clearance/neutralization strategy. Experiments in mouse models continue to demonstrate efficacy [172–177]. The aborted clinical trial with the Elan $A\beta_{42}$ antigen (AN1792) has provided a wealth of clinical information [178–181] which will assist further development of strategies designed to avoid the auto-immune adverse events [182, 183]. Chief among these will be avoidance of T-cell mediated responses [184] and the development of passive immunization protocols [185–190]. The results of the current clinical trials by Elan using passive immunization are awaited with great interest. In the meantime, novel methods of antigen presentation [20, 191–195] and the use of neo-epitopes [196–198] are under investigation. Neo-epitopes generated post-transationally by modification of Aβ (through oxidative mechanisms, as discussed above) should have inherently less potential to generate an auto-immune adverse reaction.

A startling process of lateral thinking has emerged with the report [199] of the use of Cerebrolysin in a successful phase II study of AD in Spain and Romania. The product is a proteolytic extract of pig brain, and is administered by multiple intravenous infusions over an 8-week period. Putting aside the possibility of transmitting a porcine form of prion

**Table 8.3** Drugs in clinical development directly targeting the Aβ pathway

| *Target* | *Drug* | *Company* | *Status* | *Clinical Trials.gov Identifier* |
|---|---|---|---|---|
| *γ-secretase inhibition* | | | | |
| | R-flurbiprofen (Flurizan) MCP-7869 | Myriad Genetics | Phase 3 (in progress) | NCT00105547 |
| | LY-450139 | Eli Lilly & Co | Phase 2 | NCT00244322 |
| | Merck compound | Merck Inc. | Phase 2 | |
| *Aβ monomer/oligomer* | | | | |
| Metal binding site | PBT2(PBT1) | Prana Biotechnology | Phase 2 | |
| GAG binding site | 3APS (Alzhemed) | Neurochem Inc. | Phase 3 | NCT00217769 |
| *Aβ clearance/neutralization* | | | | |
| | AN-1792 (acute immunization synthetic $A\beta_{42}$) | Elan/Wyeth | Phase 3 (discontinued) | |
| | AAB-001 (passive immunotherapy) | Elan/Wyeth | Phase 2 | NCT00112073 |
| | ACC-001 (immunization) | Elan/Wyeth | Phase 1 | |
| *APP/Aβ processing* | | | | |
| Cholesterol synthesis | Statins | Merck/Pfizer | Phase 2 | |
| *Antioxidants* | | | | |
| | Curcumin | French Foundation | Phase 2 | NCT00099710 |
| | VitE/VitC/ α-lipoic acid. Coenzyme Q | NIH | Phase 1 | NCT00117403 |

disease, the method raises interesting regulatory and religious issues. Should someone look at the sera of these subjects to see what forms of reactivity to Aβ have been generated?

### *MODULATING THE Aβ DEGRADATION PATHWAY*

The re-uptake, clearance and degradation of Aβ is still subject to considerable uncertainties. If sporadic AD is the result of a low level shift (e.g. $<10\%$) in the efficiency in any of these mechanisms, then a therapeutic strategy aimed at restoring or bypassing this faulty mechanism could be very useful. Each of the different pools of Aβ probably have slightly different mechanisms of elimination, varying with the cellular compartment in which Aβ resides over the course of its catabolic cycle. Several pieces of evidence point towards the enzymes neprilysin (NPE) and insulin degrading enzyme (IDE) as key players [200, 201], but the highly sought evidence from gene linkage studies remains elusive [202]. A new candidate, angiotensin-converting enzyme (ACE), has emerged [203], and it will be of great interest to learn whether the ACE inhibitors could be having an adverse influence over the natural history of AD.

## SUMMARY

The clinical development of drugs directly targeting the Aβ pathway is at an early stage of evolution. In Table 8.3 we list the publically disclosed trials that are in progress or which have completed/discontinued with drugs which have been developed specifically to target the Aβ pathway. The γ-secretase inhibitor trials are of immense theoretical interest, as they are likely to provide the most compelling support for the Aβ theory of AD. The trials around the Aβ metal binding site or the GAG binding sites also have the potential to address this aspect. Immunization/immunomodulation of Aβ holds great promise for elucidating the Aβ clearance/neutralization strategies in which there is currently a dearth of information. A variety of prospective statin-mediated approaches will also test the hypothesis that cholesterol has an important role in the biogenesis of AD. The anti-oxidant trials have the disadvantage of lacking specificity for Aβ, but nonetheless will continue to provide much needed guidance for the general theory of the AD brain being under oxidative stress.

It is extremely unlikely that a single class of compound or targeting a single mechanism of action will be sufficient to treat AD. For this complex disease, it is far more likely that a combination of drugs targeting various aspects of the greater APP/Aβ pathway will evolve into some form of rational therapy. Trials now in progress should represent the very beginning of the enlightenment required to find the right combinations... all predicated on the assumption that the APP/Aβ pathway underlies the cause of AD.

## ACKNOWLEDGEMENTS AND DISCLOSURES

Some of the work described in this chapter is supported by research grants from the National Health and Medical Research Council of Australia (to CLM) and the Deutsche Forschungsgemeinschaft and the Bundesministerium fur Forschung und Technologie (to KB).

Colin L Masters discloses interests in Prana Biotechnology.

## REFERENCES

1. Benson A. Alzheimer's disease: a tangled issue. *Drug Discov Today* 2005; 10:749–751.
2. Bloom FE, Reilly JF, Redwine JM *et al.* Mouse models of human neurodegenerative disorders. Requirements for medication development. *Arch Neurol* 2005; 62:185–187.
3. Golde TE. The Aβ hypothesis: leading us to rationally-designed therapeutic strategies for the treatment or prevention of Alzheimer disease. *Brain Pathol* 2005; 15:84–87.
4. Higuchi M, Iwata N, Saido TC. Understanding molecular mechanisms of proteolysis in Alzheimer's disease: Progress toward therapeutic interventions. *Biochim Biophys Acta* 2005; 1751:60–67.
5. Pangalos MN, Jacobsen SJ, Reinhart PH. Disease modifying strategies for the treatment of Alzheimer's disease targeted at modulating levels of the β-amyloid peptide. *Biochem Soc Trans* 2005; 33:553–558.
6. Selkoe DJ. Defining molecular targets to prevent Alzheimer disease. *Arch Neurol* 2005; 62:192–195.
7. Hilbush BS, Morrison JH, Young WG *et al.* New prospects and strategies for drug target discovery in neruodegenerative disorders. *NeuroRx: J Am Soc Exp Neurother* 2005; 2:627–697.
8. Wisniewski T, Frangione B. Immunological and anti-chaperone therapeutic approaches for Alzheimer disease. *Brain Pathol* 2005; 15:72–77.
9. Kwon MO, Herrling P. List of drugs in development for neurodegenerative diseases. *Neurodegenerative Dis* 2005; 2:61–108.
10. Duering M, Grimm M, Grimm HS *et al.* Mean age of onset in familial Alzheimer's disease is determined by amyloid beta 42. *Neurobiol Ageing* 2005; 26:785–788.
11. Mathis CA, Klunk WE, Price JC *et al.* Imaging technology for neurodegenerative diseases. *Arch Neurol* 2005; 62:196–200.
12. Rowe CC, Ackermann U, Gong SJ *et al.* In vivo Aβ imaging in Alzheimer's disease and dementia with Lewy bodies (submitted).
13. Cummings JL. What we can learn from open-label extensions of randomized clinical trials. *Arch Neurol* 2006; 63:18–19.
14. Patel NV, Gordon MN, Connor KE *et al.* Caloric restriction attenuates Aβ-deposition in Alzheimer transgenic models. *Neurobiol Aging* 2005; 26:995–1000.
15. Wang J, Ho L, Qin W *et al.* Caloric restriction attenuates β-amyloid neuropathology in a mouse model of Alzheimer's disease. *FASEB J* 2005; 19:659–661.
16. Tang BL. Alzheimer's disease: channeling APP to non-amyloidogenic processing. *Biochem Biophys Res Commun* 2005; 331:375–378.

17. Adlard PA, Perreau VM, Pop V *et al.* Voluntary exercise decreases amyloid load in a transgenic model of Alzheimer's disease. *J Neurosci* 2005; 25:4217–4221.
18. Jankowsky JL, Melnikova T, Fadale DJ *et al.* Environmental enrichment mitigates cognitive deficits in a mouse model of Alzheimer's disease. *J Neurosci* 2005; 25:5217–5224.
19. Lazarov O, Robinson J, Tang YP *et al.* Environmental enrichment reduces Aβ levels and amyloid deposition in transgenic mice. *Cell* 2005; 120:701–713.
20. Youm JW, Kim H, Han JH *et al.* Transgenic potato expressing Aβ reduce Aβ burden in Alzheimer's disease mouse model. *FEBS Lett* 2005; 579:6737–6744.
21. Caccamo A, Oddo S, Billings LM *et al.* M1 receptors play a central role in modulating AD-like pathology in transgenic mice. *Neuron* 2006; 49:671–682.
22. Kimura M, Akasofu S, Ogura H *et al.* Protective effect of donepezil against Aβ(1–40) neurotoxicity in rat septal neurons. *Brain Res* 2005; 1047:72–84.
23. Zimmermann M, Borroni B, Cattabeni F *et al.* Cholinesterase inhibitors influence APP metabolism in Alzheimer disease patients. *Neurobiol Dis* 2005; 19:237–242.
24. Belluti F, Rampa A, Piazzi L *et al.* Cholinesterase inhibitors: xanthostigmine derivatives blocking the acetylcholinesterase-induced β-amyloid aggregation. *J Med Chem* 2005; 48:4444–4456.
25. Bolognesi ML, Andrisano V, Bartolini M *et al.* Propidium-based polyamine ligands as potent inhibitors of acetylcholinesterase and acetylcholinesterase-induced amyloid-β aggregation. *J Med Chem* 2005; 48:24–27.
26. Dong H, Csernansky CA, Martin MV *et al.* Acetylcholinesterase inhibitors ameliorate behavioral deficits in the Tg2576 mouse model of Alzheimer's disease. *Psychopharmacology (Berl)* 2005; 181:145–152.
27. Greig NH, Utsuki T, Ingram DK *et al.* Selective butyrylcholinesterase inhibition elevates brain acetylcholine, augments learning and lowers Alzheimer β-amyloid peptide in rodent. *Proc Nat Acad Sci USA* 2005; 102:17213–17218.
28. Snyder EM, Nong Y, Almeida CG *et al.* Regulation of NMDA receptor trafficking by amyloid-β. *Nat Neurosci* 2005; 8:1051–1058.
29. Yamada K, Takayanagi M, Kamei H *et al.* Effects of memantine and donepezil on amyloid β-induced memory impairment in a delayed-matching to position task in rats. *Behav Brain Res* 2005; 162:191–199.
30. Van Dam D, Abramowski D, Staufenbiel M *et al.* Symptomatic effect of donepezil, rivastigmine, galantamine and memantine on cognitive deficits in the APP23 model. *Psychopharmacology (Berl)* 2005; 180:177–190.
31. Pákáski M, Bjelik A, Hugyecz M *et al.* Imipramine and citalopram facilitate amyloid precursor protein secretion in vitro. *Neurochem Int* 2005; 47:190–195.
32. Jankowsky JL, Slunt HH, Gonzales V *et al.* Persistent amyloidosis following suppression of Aβ production in a transgenic model of Alzheimer disease. *PLoS Med* 2005; 2:e355.
33. Xie Z, Romano DM, Tanzi RE. RNA interference-mediated silencing of X11α and X11β attenuates amyloid β-protein levels via differential effects on β-amyloid precursor protein processing. *J Biol Psychiatry* 2005; 280:15413–15421.
34. Chauhan NB, Siegel GJ, Feinstein DL. Propentofylline attenuates tau hyperphosphorylation in Alzheimer's Swedish mutant model Tg2576. *Neuropharmacology* 2005; 48:93–104.
35. Espeseth AS, Xu M, Huang Q *et al.* Compounds that bind APP and inhibit Aβ processing *in vitro* suggest a novel approach to Alzheimer's disease therapeutics. *J Biol Chem* 2005; 280:17792–17797.
36. Yue X, Lu M, Lancaster T *et al.* Brain estrogen deficiency accelerates Aβ plaque formation in an Alzheimer's disease animal model. *Proc Nat Acad Sci USA* 2005; 102:19198–19203.
37. Green PS, Bales K, Paul S *et al.* Estrogen therapy fails to alter amyloid deposition in the PDAPP model of Alzheimer's disease. *Endocrinology* 2005; 146:2774–2781.
38. Masse I, Bordet R, Deplanque D *et al.* Lipid lowering agents are associated with a slower cognitive decline in Alzheimer's disease. *J Neurol Neurosurg Psychiatry* 2005; 76:1624–1629.
39. Höglund K, Thelen KM, Syversen S *et al.* The effect of simvastatin treatment on the amyloid precursor protein and brain cholesterol metabolism in patients with Alzheimer's disease. *Dement Geriatr Cogn Disord* 2005; 19:256–265.
40. Höglund K, Syversen S, Lewczuk P *et al.* Statin treatment and a disease-specific pattern of β-amyloid peptides in Alzheimer's disease. *Exp Brain Res* 2005; 164:205–214.
41. Cordle A, Landreth G. 3-hydroxy-3-methylglutaryl-coenzyme a reductase inhibitors attenuate β-amyloid-induced microglial inflammatory responses. *J Neurosci* 2005; 25:299–307.
42. Cole SL, Grudzien A, Manhart IO *et al.* Statins cause intracellular accumulation of amyloid precursor protein, β-secretase-cleaved fragments, and amyloid β-peptide via an isoprenoid-dependent mechanism. *J Biol Chem* 2005; 280:18755–18770.

43. Si ML, Long C, Yang DI *et al.* Statins prevent β-amyloid inhibition of sympathetic α7-nAChR-mediated nitrergic neurogenic dilation in porcine basilar arteries. *J Cereb Blood Flow Metab* 2005; 25:1573–1585.
44. Papassotiropoulos A, Lambert JC, Wavrant-De Vrièze F *et al.* Cholesterol 25-hydroxylase on chromosome 10q is a susceptibility gene for sporadic Alzheimer's disease. *Neurodegenerative Dis* 2005; 2:233–241.
45. Comery TA, Martone RL, Aschmies S *et al.* Acute γ-secretase inhibition improves contextual fear conditioning in the Tg2576 mouse model of Alzheimer's disease. *J Neurosci* 2005; 25:8898–8902.
46. Quéléver G, Kachidian P, Melon C *et al.* Enhanced delivery of γ-secretase inhibitor DAPT into the brain *via* an ascorbic acid mediated strategy. *Org Biomol Chem* 2005; 3:2450–2457.
47. Laras Y, Quéléver G, Garino C *et al.* Substituted thiazolamide coupled to a redox delivery system: a new γ-secretase inhibitor with enhanced pharmacokinetic profile. *Org Biomol Chem* 2005; 3:612–618.
48. Best JD, Jay MT, Otu F *et al. In vivo* characterization of Aβ[40] changes in brain and CSF using the novel γ-secretase inhibitor MRK-560 (N-[cis-4-[(4-chlorophenyl)sulfonyl]-4- (2,5-difluorophenyl) cyclohexyl]-1,1,1-trifluoromethanesulfonamide) in the rat. *J Pharmacol Exp Ther* 2006; 317:786–790.
49. Anderson JJ, Holtz G, Baskin PP *et al.* Reductions in β-amyloid concentrations in vivo by the γ-secretase inhibitors BMS-289948 and BMS-299897. *Biochem Pharmacol* 2005; 69:689–698.
50. Barten DM, Guss VL, Corsa JA *et al.* Dynamics of β-amyloid reductions in brain, cerebrospinal fluid, and plasma of β-amyloid precursor protein transgenic mice treated with a γ-secretase inhibitor. *J Pharmacol Exp Ther* 2005; 312:635–643.
51. Lanz TA, Fici GJ, Merchant KM. Lack of specific amyloid-β(1–42) suppression by nonsteroidal anti-inflammatory drugs in young, plaque-free Tg2576 mice and in guinea pig neuronal cultures. *J Pharmacol Exp Ther* 2005; 312:399–406.
52. Peretto I, Radaelli S, Parini C *et al.* Synthesis and biological activity of flurbiprofen analogues as selective inhibitors of β-amyloid$_{1-42}$ secretion. *J Med Chem* 2005; 48:5705–5720.
53. Grimwood S, Hogg J, Jay MT *et al.* Determination of guinea-pig cortical γ-secretase activity ex vivo following the systemic administration of a γ secretase inhibitor. *Neuropharmacology* 2005; 48:1002–1011.
54. Dash PK, Moore AN, Orsi SA. Blockade of γ-secretase activity within the hippocampus enhances long-term memory. *Biochem Biophys Res Commun* 2005; 338:777–782.
55. Ravi Keerti A, Ashok Kumar B, Parthasarathy T *et al.* QSAR studies – potent benzodiazepine γ-secretase inhibitors. *Bioorg Med Chem* 2005; 13:1873–1878.
56. Gundersen E, Fan K, Haas K *et al.* Molecular-modeling based design, synthesis, and activity of substituted piperidines as γ-secretase inhibitors. *Bioorg Med Chem Lett* 2005; 15:1891–1894.
57. Lewis SJ, Smith AL, Neduvelil JG *et al.* A novel series of potent γ-secretase inhibitors based on a benzobicyclo[4.2.1]nonane core. *Bioorg Med Chem Lett* 2005; 15:373–378.
58. Curry CL, Reed LL, Golde TE *et al.* Gamma secretase inhibitor blocks Notch activation and induces apoptosis in Kaposi's sarcoma tumor cells. *Oncogene* 2005; 24:6333–6344.
59. van Es JH, van Gijn ME, Riccio O *et al.* Notch/γ-secretase inhibition turns proliferative cells in intestinal crypts and adenomas into goblet cells. *Nature* 2005; 435:959–963.
60. ClinicalTrials.gov. A notch signalling pathway inhibitor for patients with T-cell acute lymphoblastic leukaemia/lymphoma (ALL). *ClinialTrials.gov Identifier:* NCT00100152. http://www.clinicaltrials.gov/ct/show/NCT00100152?order=2
61. ClinicalTrials.gov. A Notch signalling pathway inhibitor for patients with advanced breast cancer. *ClinialTrials.gov Identifier:* NCT00106145. http://www.clinicaltrials.gov/ct/show/NCT00106145?order=1
62. Siemers E, Skinner M, Dean RA *et al.* Safety, tolerability, and changes in amyloid β concentrations after administration of a γ-secretase inhibitor in volunteers. *Clin Neuropharmacol* 2005; 28:126–132.
63. Siemers ER, Quinn JF, Kaye J *et al.* Effects of a γ-secretase inhibitor in a randomized study of patients with Alzheimer disease. *Neurology* 2006; 66:602–604.
64. Sato T, Tanimura Y, Hirotani N *et al.* Blocking the cleavage at midportion between γ- and ε-sites remarkably suppresses the generation of amyloid β-protein. *FEBS Lett* 2005; 579:2907–2912.
65. Saura CA, Chen G, Malkani S *et al.* Conditional inactivation of presenilin 1 prevents amyloid accumulation and temporarily rescues contextual and spatial working memory impairments in amyloid precursor protein transgenic mice. *J Neurosci* 2005; 25:6755–6764.
66. Xie Z, Romano DM, Tanzi RE. Effects of RNAi-mediated silencing of PEN-2, APH-1a, and Nicas wild-type vs FAD mutant forms of presenilin 1. *J Mol Neurosci* 2005; 25:67–77.
67. Pietrak BL, Crouthamel MC, Tugusheva K *et al.* Biochemical and cell-based assays for characterization of BACE-1 inhibitors. *Ana Biochem* 2005; 342:144–151.

68. Turner RT 3rd, Hong L, Koelsch G *et al.* Structural locations and functional roles of new subsites $S_5$, $S_6$, and $S_7$ in memapsin 2 (β-secretase). *Biochemistry* 2005; 44:105–112.
69. Polgár T, Keserü GM. Virtual screening for β-secretase (BACE1) inhibitors reveals the importance of protonation states at Asp32 and Asp228. *J Med Chem* 2005; 48:3749–3755.
70. Huang D, Lüthi U, Kolb P *et al.* Discovery of cell-permeable non-peptide inhibitors of β-secretase by high-throughput docking and continuum electrostatics calculations. *J Med Chem* 2005; 48:5108–5111.
71. Hanessian S, Yun H, Hou Y *et al.* Structure-based design, synthesis, and memapsin 2 (BACE) inhibitory activity of carbocyclic and heterocyclic peptidomimetics. *J Med Chem* 2005; 48:5175–5190.
72. Ghosh AK, Devasamudram T, Hong L *et al.* Structure-based design of cycloamide-urethane-derived novel inhibitors of human brain memapsin 2 (β-secretase). *Bioorg Med Chem Lett* 2005; 15:15–20.
73. Kimura T, Shuto D, Hamada Y *et al.* Design and synthesis of highly active Alzheimer's β-secretase (BACE1) inhibitors, KMI-420 and KMI-429, with enhanced chemical stability. *Bioorg Med Chem Lett* 2005; 15:211–215.
74. Kornacker MG, Lai Z, Witmer M *et al.* An inhibitor binding pocket distinct from the catalytic active site on human β-APP cleaving enzyme. *Biochemistry* 2005; 44:11567–11573.
75. Lefranc-Jullien S, Lisowski V, Hernandez JF *et al.* Design and characterization of a new cell-permeant inhibitor of the β-secretase BACE1. *Br J Pharmacol* 2005; 145:228–235.
76. Pietrancosta N, Quéléver G, Laras Y *et al.* Design of β-secretase inhibitors by introduction of a mandelyl moiety in DAPT analogues. *Aust J Chem* 2005; 58:585–594.
77. Byun H-G, Kim Y-T, Park P-J *et al.* Chitooligosaccharides as a novel β-secretase inhibitor. *Carbohydr Polym* 2005; 61:198–202.
78. Lee HJ, Seong YH, Bae KH *et al.* β-secretase (BACE1) inhibitors from Sanguisorbae radix. *Arch Pharm Res* 2005; 28:799–803.
79. Xie J, Guo Q. Par-4 is involved in regulation of β-secretase cleavage of the Alzheimer amyloid precursor protein. *J Biol Chem* 2005; 280:13824–13832.
80. Singer O, Marr RA, Rockenstein E *et al.* Targeting BACE1 with siRNAs ameliorates Alzheimer disease neuropathology in a transgenic model. *Nat Neurosci* 2005; 8:1343–1349.
81. Paris D, Quadros A, Patel N *et al.* Inhibition of angiogenesis and tumor growth by β and γ-secretase inhibitors. *Eur J Pharmacol* 2005; 514:1–15.
82. Cherny RA, Atwood CS, Xilinas ME *et al.* Treatment with a copper-zinc chelator markedly and rapidly inhibits β-amyloid accumulation in Alzheimer's disease transgenic mice. *Neuron* 2001; 30:665–676.
83. Raman B, Ban T, Yamaguchi K *et al.* Metal ion-dependent effects of clioquinol on the fibril growth of an amyloid β peptide. *J Biol Chem* 2005; 280:16157–16162.
84. Ritchie CW, Bush AI, Mackinnon A *et al.* Metal-protein attenuation with iodochlorydroxyquin (clioquinol) targeting Aβ amyloid deposition and toxicity in Alzheimer disease: a pilot Phase 2 clinical trial. *Arch Neurol* 2003; 60:1685–1691.
85. Ibach B, Haen E, Marienhagen J *et al.* Clioquinol treatment in familiar early onset of Alzheimer's disease. A case report. *Pharmacopsychiatry* 2005; 38:178–179.
86. Liu G, Garrett MR, Men P *et al.* Nanoparticle and other metal chelation therapeutics in Alzheimer disease. *Biochim Biophys Acta* 2005; 1741:246–252.
87. Gaeta A, Hider RC. The crucial role of metal ions in neurodegeneration: the basis for a promising therapeutic strategy. *Br J Pharmacol* 2005; 146:1041–1059.
88. Zheng H, Youdim MB, Weiner LM *et al.* Synthesis and evaluation of peptidic metal chelators for neuroprotection in neurodegenerative diseases. *J Pept Res* 2005; 66:190–203.
89. Zheng H, Youdim MB, Weiner LM *et al.* Novel potential neuroprotective agents with both iron chelating and amino acid-based derivatives targeting central nervous system neurons. *Biochem Pharmacol* 2005; 70:1642–1652.
90. Sutoh Y, Nishino S, Nishida Y. Metal chelates to prevent or clear the deposits of amyloid β-peptide (1–40) induced by Zinc(II) Chloride. *Chem Lett* 2005; 34:140.
91. Ji HF, Zhang HY. A new strategy to combat Alzheimer's disease. Combining radical-scavenging potential with metal-protein-attenuating ability in one molecule. *Bioorg Med Chem Lett* 2005; 15:21–24.
92. Cui Z, Lockman PR, Atwood CS *et al.* Novel D-penicillamine carrying nanoparticles for metal chelation therapy in Alzheimer's and other CNS diseases. *Eur J Pharm Biopharm* 2005; 59:263–272.
93. Yang SP, Kwon BO, Gho YS *et al.* Specific interaction of $VEGF_{165}$ with β-amyloid, and its protective effect on β-amyloid-induced neurotoxicity. *J Neurochem* 2005; 93:118–127.
94. Mettenburg JM, Arandjelovic S, Gonias SL. A chemically modified preparation of α2-macroglobulin binds β-amyloid peptide with increased affinity and inhibits Aβ cytotoxicity. *J Neurochem* 2005; 93:53–62.

95. Gibson TJ, Murphy RM. Design of peptidyl compounds that affect β-amyloid aggregation: importance of surface tension and context. *Biochem* 2005; 44:8898–8907.
96. Lee S, Carson K, Rice-Ficht A *et al.* Hsp20, a novel α-crystallin, prevents Aβ fibril formation and toxicity. *Protein Sci* 2005; 14:593–601.
97. Schmuck C, Frey P, Heil M. Inhibition of fibril formation of Aβ by guanidiniocarbonyl pyrrole receptors. *Chembiochem* 2005; 6:628–631.
98. Schuster D, Rajendran A, Hui SW *et al.* Protective effect of colostrinin on neuroblastoma cell survival is due to reduced aggregation of β-amyloid. *Neuropeptides* 2005; 39:419–426.
99. Szegedi V, Fülöp L, Farkas T *et al.* Pentapeptides derived from Aβ1–42 protect neurons from the modulatory effect of Aβ fibrils – an in vitro and in vivo electrophysiological study. *Neurobiol Dis* 2005; 18:499–508.
100. Liu R, Barkhordarian H, Emadi S *et al.* Trehalose differentially inhibits aggregation and neurotoxicity of beta-amyloid 40 and 42. *Neurobiol Dis* 2005; 20:74–81.
101. Hennessy EJ, Buchwald SL. Synthesis of 4,5-dianilinophthalimide and related analogues for potential treatment of Alzheimer's disease via palladium-catalyzed amination. *J Org Chem* 2005; 70:7371–7375.
102. Kanapathipillai M, Lentzen G, Sierks M *et al.* Ectoine and hydroxyectoine inhibit aggregation and neurotoxicity of Alzheimer's β-amyloid. *FEBS Lett* 2005; 579:4775–4780.
103. Sabaté R, Estelrich J. Stimulatory and inhibitory effects of alkyl bromide surfactants on β-amyloid fibrillogenesis. *Langmuir* 2005; 21:6944–6949.
104. Wang SS, Chen YT, Chou SW. Inhibition of amyloid fibril formation of β-amyloid peptides via the amphiphilic surfactants. *Biochim Biophys Acta* 2005; 1741:307–313.
105. Lee KH, Shin BH, Shin KJ *et al.* A hybrid molecule that prohibits amyloid fibrils and alleviates neuronal toxicity induced by β-amyloid (1–42). *Biochem Biophys Res Commun* 2005; 328:816–823.
106. Török M, Abid M, Mhadgut SC *et al.* Organofluorine inhibitors of amyloid fibrillogenesis. *Biochemistry* http://pubs.acs.org.ezproxy.lib.unimelb.edu.au/cgi-bin/asap.cgi/bichaw/asap/pdf/bi0601104.pdf.
107. Cohen T, Frydman-Marom A, Rechter M *et al.* Inhibition of amyloid fibril formation and cytotoxicity by hydroxyindole derivatives. *Biochemistry* http://pubs.acs.org.ezproxy.lib.unimelb.edu.au/cgi-bin/asap.cgi/bichaw/asap/pdf/bi051525c.pdf
108. Walsh DM, Townsend M, Podlisny MB *et al.* Certain inhibitors of synthetic amyloid β-peptide (Aβ) fibrillogenesis block oligomerization of natural Aβ and thereby rescue long-term potentiation. *J Neurosci* 2005; 25:2455–2462.
109. Sultana R, Ravagna A, Mohmmad-Abdul H *et al.* Ferulic acid ethyl ester protects neurons against amyloid β- peptide(1–42)-induced oxidative stress and neurotoxicity: Relationship to antioxidant activity. *J Neurochem* 2005; 92:749–758.
110. Ono K, Hirohata M, Yamada M. Ferulic acid destabilizes preformed β-amyloid fibrils in vitro. *Biochem Biophys Res Commun* 2005; 336:444–449.
111. Mohmmad Abdul H, Butterfield DA. Protection against amyloid β-peptide (1–42)-induced loss of phospholipid asymmetry in synaptosomal membranes by tricyclodecan-9-xanthogenate (D609) and ferulic acid ethyl ester: implications for Alzheimer's disease. *Biochem Biophys Acta* 2005; 1741:140–148.
112. Jin Y, Yan EZ, Fan Y *et al.* Sodium ferulate prevents amyloid-beta-induced neurotoxicity through suppression of p38 MAPK and upregulation of ERK-1/2 and Akt/protein kinase B in rat hippocampus. *Acta Pharmacol Sin* 2005; 26:943–951.
113. Cho JY, Kim HS, Kim DH *et al.* Inhibitory effects of long-term administration of ferulic acid on astrocyte activation induced by intracerebroventricular injection of β-amyloid peptide (1–42) in mice. *Prog Neuropsychopharmacol Biol Psychiatry* 2005; 29:901–907.
114. Ono K, Hirohata M, Yamada M. Ferulic acid destabilizes preformed β-amyloid fibrils in vitro. *Biochem Biophys Res Commun* 2005; 336:444–449.
115. Rezai-Zadeh K, Shytle D, Sun N *et al.* Green tea epigallocatechin-3-gallate (EGCG) modulates amyloid precursor protein cleavage and reduces cerebral amyloidosis in Alzheimer transgenic mice. *J Neurosci* 2005; 25:8807–8814.
116. Lee SY, Lee JW, Lee H *et al.* Inhibitory effect of green tea extract on β-amyloid-induced PC12 cell death by inhibition of the activation of NF-κB and ERK/p38 MAP kinase pathway through antioxidant mechanisms. *Brain Res Mol Brain Res* 2005; 140:45–54.
117. Mandel S, Amit T, Reznichenko L *et al.* Green tea catechins as brain-permeable, natural iron chelators-antioxidants for the treatment of neurodegenerative disorders. *Mol Nutr Food Res* 2006; 50:229–234.
118. Ono K, Hasegawa K, Naiki H *et al.* Curcumin has potent anti-amyoidogenic effects for Alzheimer's β-amyloid fibrils in vitro. *J Neurosci Res* 2004; 75:742–750.

119. Yang F, Lim GP, Begum AN *et al.* Curcumin inhibits formation of amyloid β oligomers and fibrils, binds plaques, and reduces amyloid *in vivo*. *J Biol Chem* 2005; 280:5892–5901.
120. Marambaud P, Zhao H, Davies P. Resveratrol promotes clearance of Alzheimer's disease amyloid-β peptides. *J Biol Chem* 2005; 280:37377–37382.
121. Jhamandas JH, Wie MB, Harris K *et al.* Fucoidan inhibits cellular and neurotoxic effects of β-amyloid (Aβ) in rat cholinergic basal forebrain neurons. *Eur J Neurosci* 2005; 21:2649–2659.
122. Yu MS, Leung SK, Lai SW *et al.* Neuroprotective effects of anti-ageing oriental medicine *Lycium barbarum* against β-amyloid peptide neurotoxicity. *Exp Gerontol* 2005; 40:716–727.
123. Jeong JC, Yoon CH, Lee WH *et al.* Effects of *Bambusae concretio* Salicea (Chunchukhwang) on amyloid β-induced cell toxicity and antioxidative enzymes in cultured rat neuronal astrocytes. *J Ethnopharmacol* 2005; 98:259–266.
124. Kim H, Park BS, Lee KG *et al.* Effects of naturally occurring compounds on fibril formation and oxidative stress of β-amyloid. *J Agric Food Chem* 2005; 53:8537–8541.
125. Lecanu L, Yao W, Piechot A *et al.* Identification, design, synthesis, and pharmacological activity of (4-ethyl-piperazin-1-yl)-phenylmethanone derivatives with neuroprotective properties against β-amyloid-induced toxicity. *Neuropharmacology* 2005; 49:86–96.
126. Hashimoto M, Tanabe Y, Fujii Y *et al.* Chronic administration of docosahexaenoic acid ameliorates the impairment of spatial cognition learning ability in amyloid β-infused rats. *J Nutr* 2005; 135:549–555.
127. Lim GP, Calon F, Morihara T *et al.* A diet enriched with the omega-3 fatty acid docosahexaenoic acid reduces amyloid burden in an aged Alzheimer mouse model. *J Neurosci* 2005; 25:3032–3040.
128. McDaid DG, Kim EM, Reid RE *et al.* Parenteral antioxidant treatment preserves temporal discrimination following intrahippocampal aggregated Aβ(1–42) injections. *Behav Pharmacol* 2005; 16:237–242.
129. Quintanilla RA, Muñoz FJ, Metcalfe MJ *et al.* Trolox and 17β-estradiol protect against amyloid β-peptide neurotoxicity by a mechanism that involves modulation of the Wnt signalling pathway. *J Biol Chem* 2005; 280:11615–11625.
130. Coma M, Guix FX, Uribesalgo I *et al.* Lack of oestrogen protection in amyloid-mediated endothelial damage due to protein nitrotyrosination. *Brain* 2005; 128:1613–1621.
131. Ju TC, Chen SD, Liu CC *et al.* Protective effects of *S*-nitrosoglutathione against amyloid β-peptide neurotoxicity. *Free Radic Biol Med* 2005; 38:938–949.
132. Woltjer RL, Nghiem W, Maezawa I *et al.* Role of glutathione in intracellular amyloid-α precursor protein/carboxy-terminal fragment aggregation and associated cytotoxicity. *J Neurochem* 2005; 93:1047–1056.
133. Quinn J, Kulhanek D, Nowlin J *et al.* Chronic melatonin therapy fails to alter amyloid burden or oxidative damage in old tg2576 mice: implications for clinical trials. *Brain Res* 2005; 1037:209–213.
134. Moreira PI, Santos MS, Sena C *et al.* CoQ10 therapy attenuates amyloid β-peptide toxicity in brain mitochondria isolated from aged diabetic rats. *Exp Neurol* 2005; 196:112–119.
135. Qiao H, Koya RC, Nakagawa K *et al.* Inhibition of Alzheimer's amyloid-β peptide-induced reduction of mitochondrial membrane potential and neurotoxicity by gelsolin. *Neurobiol Ageing* 2005; 26:849–855.
136. Aguado-Llera D, Arilla-Ferreiro E, Campos-Barros A *et al.* Protective effects of insulin-like growth factor-I on the somatostatinergic system in the temporal cortex of β-amyloid-treated rats. *J Neurochem* 2005; 92:607–615.
137. Youdim MB, Maruyama W, Naoi M. Neuropharmacological, neuroprotective and amyloid precursor processing properties of selective MAO-B inhibitor antiparkinsonian drug, rasagiline. *Drugs Today (Barc)* 2005; 41:369–391.
138. Caraci F, Chisari M, Frasca G *et al.* Nicergoline, a drug used for age-dependent cognitive impairment, protects cultured neurons against β-amyloid toxicity. *Brain Res* 2005; 1047:30–37.
139. Marrazzo A, Caraci F, Salinaro ET *et al.* Neuroprotective effects of sigma-1 receptor agonists against β-amyloid-induced toxicity. *Neuroreport* 2005; 16:1223–1226.
140. Nathan C, Calingasan N, Nezezon J *et al.* Protection from Alzheimer's- like disease in the mouse by genetic ablation of inducible nitric oxide synthase. *J Exp Med* 2005; 202:1163–1169.
141. Tong Y, Zhou W, Fung V *et al.* Oxidative stress potentiates BACE1 gene expression and Aβ generation. *J Neural Transm* 2005; 112:455–469.
142. Morihara T, Teter B, Yang F *et al.* Ibuprofen suppresses interleukin-1β induction of pro-amyloidogenic $\alpha_1$-antichymotrypsin to ameliorate β-amyloid (Aβ) pathology in Alzheimer's models. *Neuropsychopharmacology* 2005; 30:1111–1120.

143. Farías GG, Godoy JA, Vázquez MC *et al.* The anti-inflammatory and cholinesterase inhibitor bifunctional compound IBU-PO protects from β-amyloid neurotoxicity by acting on Wnt signalling components. *Neurobiol Dis* 2005; 18:176–183.
144. Sastre M, Dewachter I, Rossner S *et al.* Nonsteroidal anti-inflammatory drugs repress β-secretase gene promoter activity by the activation of PPARγ. *Proc Nat Acad Sci USA* 2006; 103:443–448.
145. Heneka MT, Sastre M, Dumitrescu-Ozimek L *et al.* Acute treatment with the PPARγ agonist pioglitazone and ibuprofen reduces glial inflammation and Aβ1–42 levels in APPV717I transgenic mice. *Brain* 2005; 128:1442–1453.
146. Costello DA, O'Leary DM, Herron CE. Agonists of peroxisome proliferator-activated receptor-γ attenuate the Aβ-mediated impairment of LTP in the hippocampus in vitro. *Neuropharmacology* 2005; 49:359–366.
147. Echeverria V, Clerman A, Doré S. Stimulation of $PGE_2$ receptors EP2 and EP4 protects cultured neurons against oxidative stress and cell death following β-amyloid exposure. *Eur J Neurosci* 2005; 22:2199–2206.
148. Shie FS, Montine KS, Breyer RM *et al.* Microglial eEP2 as a new target to increase amyloid β phagocytosis and decrease amyloid β-induced damage to neurons. *Brain Pathol* 2005; 15:134–138.
149. Ramírez BG, Blázquez C, Gómez del Pulgar T *et al.* Prevention of Alzheimer's disease pathology by cannabinoids: neuroprotection mediated by blockade of microglial activation. *J Neurosci* 2005; 25:1904–1913.
150. Boedker M, Boetkjaer A, Bazan NG *et al.* Budesonide epimer R, LAU-8080 and phenyl butyl nitrone synergistically repress cyclooxygenase-2 induction in [IL-1β + Aβ42]-stressed human neural cells. *Neurosci Lett* 2005; 380:176–180.
151. Kim SJ, Jeong HJ, Lee KM *et al.* Zingansikpoongtang modulates β-amyloid and IL-1β-induced cytokine production and cyclooxygenase-2 expression in human astrocytoma cells U373MG. *J Ethnopharmacol* 2005; 96:279–285.
152. Duff K, Planel E. Untangling memory deficits. *Nat Med* 2005; 11:826–827.
153. Mukrasch MD, Biernat J, von Bergen M *et al.* Sites of tau important for aggregation populate β-structure and bind to microtubules and polyanions. *J Biol Chem* 2005; 280:24978–24986.
154. Santacruz K, Lewis J, Spires T *et al.* Tau suppression in a neurodegenerative mouse model improves memory function. *Science* 2005; 309:476–481.
155. Rodriguez-Martin T, Garcia-Blanco MA, Mansfield SG *et al.* Reprogramming of tau alternative splicing by spliceosome-mediated RNA trans-splicing: Implications for tauopathies. *Proc Nat Acad Sci USA* 2005; 102:15659–15664.
156. Santa-Maria I, Hernandez F, Smith MA *et al.* Neurotoxic dopamine quinone facilitates the assembly of tau into fibrillar polymers. *Mol Cell Biochem* 2005; 278:203–212.
157. Zhang YJ, Xu YF, Chen XQ *et al.* Nitration and oligomerization of tau induced by peroxynitrite inhibit its microtubule-binding activity. *FEBS Lett* 2005; 579:2421–2427.
158. Reynolds MR, Berry RW, Binder LI. Site-specific nitration and oxidative dityrosine bridging of the τ protein by peroxynitrite: implications for Alzheimer's disease. *Biochemistry* 2005; 44:1690–1700.
159. Reynolds MR, Berry RW, Binder LI. Site-specific nitration differentially influences τ assembly in vitro. *Biochemistry* 2005; 44:13997–14009.
160. Reynolds MR, Lukas TJ, Berry RW *et al.* Peroxynitrite-mediated τ modifications stabilize preformed filaments and destabilize microtubules through distinct mechanisms. *Biochemistry* 2006; 45:4314–4326.
161. Ma QF, Li YM, Du JT *et al.* Binding of copper (II) ion to an Alzheimer's tau peptide as revealed by MALDI-TOF MS, CD, and NMR. *Biopolymers* 2005; 79:74–85.
162. Ma Q, Li Y, Du J *et al.* Copper binding properties of a tau peptide associated with Alzheimer's disease studied by CD, NMR, and MALDI-TOF MS. *Peptides* 2006; 27:841–849.
163. Michaelis ML, Ansar S, Chen Y *et al.* β-amyloid-induced neurodegeneration and protection by structurally diverse microtubule-stabilizing agents. *J Pharmacol Exp Ther* 2005; 312:659–668.
164. Derkinderen P, Scales TM, Hanger DP *et al.* Tyrosine 394 is phosphorylated in Alzheimer's paired helical filament tau and in fetal tau with c-Abl as the candidate tyrosine kinase. *J Neurosci* 2005; 25:6584–6593.
165. Sakaue F, Saito T, Sato Y *et al.* Phosphorylation of FTDP-17 mutant tau by cyclin-dependent kinase 5 complexed with p35, p25, or p39. *J Biol Chem* 2005; 280:31522–31529.
166. Noble W, Planel E, Zehr C *et al.* Inhibition of glycogen synthase kinase-3 by lithium correlates with reduced tauopathy and degeneration *in vivo*. *Proc Nat Acad Sci USA* 2005; 102:6990–6995.
167. Lambourne SL, Sellers LA, Bush TG *et al.* Increased tau phosphorylation on mitogen-activated protein kinase consensus sites and cognitive decline in transgenic models for Alzheimer's disease and

FTDP-17: evidence for distinct molecular processes underlying tau abnormalities. *Mol Cell Biol* 2005; 25:278–293.
168. Cotman CW, Poon WW, Rissman RA *et al.* The role of caspase cleavage of tau in Alzheimer disease neuropathology. *J Neuropathol Exp Neurol* 2005; 64:104–112.
169. Taniguchi S, Suzuki N, Masuda M *et al.* Inhibition of heparin-induced tau filament formation by phenothiazines, polyphenols, and porphyrins. *J Biol Chem* 2005; 280:7614–7623.
170. Necula M, Chirita CN, Kuret J. Cyanine dye N744 inhibits tau fibrillization by blocking filament extension: implications for the treatment of tauopathic neurodegenerative diseases. *Biochemistry* 2005; 44:10227–10237.
171. Dodart JC, Marr RA, Koistinaho M *et al.* Gene delivery of human apolipoprotein E alters brain Aβ burden in a mouse model of Alzheimer's disease. *Proc Nat Aca Sci USA* 2005; 102:1211–1216.
172. Bales KR, Tzavara ET, Wu S *et al.* Cholinergic dysfunction in a mouse model of Alzheimer disease is reversed by an anti-Aβ antibody. *J Clin Invest* 2006; 116:825–832.
173. Klyubin I, Walsh DM, Lemere CA *et al.* Amyloid β protein immunotherapy neutralizes Aβ oligomers that disrupt synaptic plasticity *in vivo*. *Nat Med* 2005; 11:556–561.
174. Buttini M, Masliah E, Barbour R *et al.* β-amyloid immunotherapy prevents synaptic degeneration in a mouse model of Alzheimer's disease. *J Neurosci* 2005; 25:9096–9101.
175. Brendza RP, Bacskai BJ, Cirrito JR *et al.* Anti-Aβ antibody treatment promotes the rapid recovery of amyloid-associated neuritic dystrophy in *PDAPP* transgenic mice. *J Clin Invest* 2005; 115:428–433.
176. Banks WA, Pagliari P, Nakaoke R *et al.* Effects of a behaviourally active antibody on the brain uptake and clearance of amyloid beta proteins. *Peptides* 2005; 26:287–294.
177. Rowan MJ, Klyubin I, Wang Q *et al.* Synaptic plasticity disruption by amyloid β protein: modulation by potential Alzheimer's disease modifying therapies. *Biochem Soc Trans* 2005; 33:563–567.
178. Bayer AJ, Bullock R, Jones RW *et al.* Evaluation of the safety and immunogenicity of synthetic Aβ42 (AN1792) in patients with AD. *Neurology* 2005; 64:94–101.
179. Gilman S, Koller M, Black RS *et al.* Clinical effects of Aβ immunization (AN1792) in patients with AD in an interrupted trial. *Neurology* 2005; 64:1553–1562.
180. Lee M, Bard F, Johnson-Wood K *et al.* Aβ42 immunization in Alzheimer's disease generates Aβ N-terminal antibodies. *Ann Neurol* 2005; 58:430–435.
181. Masliah E, Hansen L, Adame A *et al.* Aβ vaccination effects on plaque pathology in the absence of encephalitis in Alzheimer disease. *Neurology* 2005; 64:129–131.
182. Racke MM, Boone LI, Hepburn DL *et al.* Exacerbation of cerebral amyloid angiopathy-associated microhemorrhage in amyloid precursor protein transgenic mice by immunotherapy is dependent on antibody recognition of deposited forms of amyloid β. *J Neurosci* 2005; 25:629–636.
183. Lee EB, Leng LZ, Lee VM *et al.* Meningoencephalitis associated with passive immunization of a transgenic murine model of Alzheimer's amyloidosis. *FEBS Lett* 2005; 579:2564–2568.
184. Agadjanyan MG, Ghochikyan A, Petrushina I *et al.* Prototype Alzheimer's disease vaccine using the immunodominant b cell epitope from β-amyloid and promiscuous T cell epitope pan HLA DR-binding peptide. *J Immunol* 2005; 174:1580–1586.
185. Hartman RE, Izumi Y, Bales KR *et al.* Treatment with an Amyloid-β antibody ameliorates plaque load, learning deficits, and hippocampal long-term potentiation in a mouse model of Alzheimer's disease. *J Neurosci* 2005; 25:6213–6220.
186. Gaugler MN, Tracy J, Kuhnle K *et al.* Modulation of Alzheimer's pathology by cerebro-ventricular grafting of hybridoma cells expressing antibodies against Aβ in vivo. *FEBS Lett* 2005; 579:753–756.
187. Chauhan NB, Siegel GJ. Efficacy of anti-Aβ antibody isotypes used for intracerebroventricular immunization in TgCRND8. *Neurosci Lett* 2005; 375:143–147.
188. Asami-Odaka A, Obayashi-Adachi Y, Matsumoto Y *et al.* Passive immunization of the Aβ42(43) C-terminal-specific antibody BC05 in a mouse model of Alzheimer's disease. *Neurodegenerative Dis* 2005; 2:36–43.
189. Maier M, Seabrook TJ, Lemere CA. Modulation of the humoral and cellular immune response in Aβ immunotherapy by the adjuvants monophosphoryl lipid A (MPL), cholera toxin B subunit (CTB) and *E. coli* enterotoxin LT(R192G). *Vaccine* 2005; 23:5149–5159.
190. Li SB, Wang HQ, Lin X *et al.* Specific humoral immune responses in rhesus monkeys vaccinated with the Alzheimer's disease-associated β-amyloid 1–15 peptide vaccine. *Chin Med J (Engl)* 2005; 118:660–664.
191. Zurbriggen R, Amacker M, Kammer AR *et al.* Virosome-based active immunization targets soluble amyloid species rather than plaques in a transgenic mouse model of Alzheimer's disease. *J Mol Neurosci* 2005; 27:157–166.

192. Solomon B. Generation of anti-β-amyloid antibodies via phage display technology towards Alzheimer's disease vaccination. *Vaccine* 2005; 23:2327–2330.
193. Qu B, Boyer PJ, Johnston SA *et al.* A$\beta_{42}$ gene vaccination reduces brain amyloid plaque burden in transgenic mice. *J Neurol Sci* 2006; 244:151–158.
194. Bowers WJ, Mastrangelo MA, Stanley HA *et al.* HSV amplicon-mediated Aβ vaccination in Tg2576 mice: differential antigen-specific immune responses. *Neurobiol Ageing* 2005; 26:393–407.
195. Frenkel D, Maron R, Burt DS *et al.* Nasal vaccination with a proteosome-based adjuvant and glatiramer acetate clears β-amyloid in a mouse model of Alzheimer disease. *J Clin Invest* 2005; 115:2423–2433.
196. Yamamoto N, Yokoseki T, Shibata M *et al.* Suppression of Aβ deposition in brain by peripheral administration of Fab fragments of anti-seed antibody. *Biochem Biophys Res Commun* 2005; 335:45–47.
197. Paganetti P, Calanca V, Galli C *et al.* β-site specific intrabodies to decrease and prevent generation of Alzheimer's Aβ peptide. *J Cell Biol* 2005; 168:863–868.
198. Arbel M, Yacoby I, Solomon B. Inhibition of amyloid precursor protein processing by β-secretase through site-directed antibodies. *Proc Nat Acad Sci USA* 2005; 102:7718–7723.
199. Alvarez XA, Cacabelos R, Laredo M *et al.* A 24-week, double-blind, placebo-controlled study of three dosages of Cerebrolysin in patients with mild to moderate Alzheimer's disease. *Eur J Neurol* 2006; 13:43–54.
200. Saido TC, Iwata N. Metabolism of amyloid β peptide and pathogenesis of Alzheimer's disease: towards presymptomatic diagnosis, prevention and therapy. *Neurosci Res* 2006; 54:235–253.
201. Saito T, Iwata N, Tsubuki S *et al.* Somatostatin regulates brain amyloid β peptide A$\beta_{42}$ through modulation of proteolytic degradation. *Nat Med* 2005; 11:434–439.
202. Eckman EA, Eckman CB. Aβ-degrading enzymes: modulators of Alzheimer's disease pathogenesis and targets for therapeutic intervention. *Biochem Soc Trans* 2005; 33:1101–1105.
203. Hemming ML, Selkoe DJ. Amyloid β-protein is degraded by cellular angiotensin-converting enzyme (ACE) and elevated by an ACE inhibitor. *J Biol Chem* 2005; 280:37644–37650.

# 9

# Anti-inflammatory drugs

*M. Woodward*

## INTRODUCTION

While Alzheimer's disease (AD) is pathologically best recognized for the presence of amyloid plaques and neurofibrillary tangles, there is also considerable evidence for active inflammation. Alzheimer himself recognized the presence of activated microglial cells around the plaques and tangles and subsequently other markers of inflammation have been identified. This has led to the neuroinflammatory hypothesis for the neurodegeneration of AD. This hypothesis has gained additional support from large epidemiological studies, which have demonstrated that use of anti-inflammatory agents, particularly the non-steroidal anti-inflammatory drugs (NSAIDs), is associated with a reduced risk of developing AD. There have now been several trials of NSAIDs and other anti-inflammatory agents for the treatment of AD and one trial commenced to assess whether NSAIDs may play a role in preventing AD.

To date no trial has demonstrated a role for anti-inflammatory therapy in AD, but the strong evidence for inflammation in the pathogenesis of AD and the results from population studies will lead to further research in this area.

## INFLAMMATION IN AD

AD is characterized by the presence of activated microglial cells – enlarged, rod-like cells with long tortuous processes that are quite different from the thin, straight processes of resting microglia [1]. These cells belong to the mononuclear phagocyte system and are the main cell line that initiates and controls inflammatory reactions in the central nervous system. It is unclear what leads to activation of microglial cells in AD. Upon activation, these cells generate a number of neurotrophic substances, which are important in the development, homeostasis and repair of the central nervous system [2]. Activated microglia are also the source and target for various cytokines that are used for communication between themselves and other cells. Foremost among these is interleukin-1 (IL-1) that amplifies the inflammatory response and, it is hypothesized, may induce damage, including death, in surrounding nerve cells. Many markers of inflammation have been identified in AD brain tissue [3]. The complement cascade is also activated in AD [4]. Indeed, the whole neuropathological cascade of AD, including the development of plaques and tangles, may be generated by this inflammatory response [5]. IL-1 drives a number of cellular and molecular responses that are central to Alzheimer pathogenesis, as shown in Table 9.1.

**Michael Woodward**, MBBS, FRACP, Associate Professor, Consultant Geriatrician and Medical Director, Aged and Residential Care, Heidelberg Repatriation Hospital, Austin Health, Heidelberg, Victoria, Australia

**Table 9.1** IL-1 driven responses central to AD pathology (with permission from reference [6])

| |
|---|
| Excessive synthesis, translation and processing of neuronal APP |
| Activation of astrocytes |
| Excessive synthesis of acetylcholinesterase |
| Phosphorylation of tau |
| Decreased expression of synaptic proteins |

It may be that inflammation converts diffuse amyloid plaques into mature senile plaques [3], although it is now recognized that these senile plaques may not be the pathogenic element in AD.

There are also peripheral markers of inflammation in AD. In a case cohort study within a large epidemiological study, the Rotterdam study, high plasma levels of the inflammatory markers $\alpha_1$-anti-chymotrypsin, IL-6 and, to a lesser extent, C-reactive protein were associated with an increased risk of dementia [7]. Prospectively, increased levels of C-reactive protein have been associated with an increased risk of dementia 25 years later [8]. Higher plasma levels of $\alpha_1$-anti-chymotrypsin have also been associated with an increased risk of cognitive decline [9].

## ANTI-INFLAMMATORY DRUGS AND NEUROINFLAMMATION

Non-steroidal anti-inflammatory drugs may modify the neuroinflammation seen in AD. There is *in vivo* evidence that NSAIDs diminish microglial activation [10, 11]. There are also *in vitro* studies showing that NSAIDs inhibit not only production of prostaglandins, which are central to inflammation, but also a number of other inflammatory functions of microglia including production of inflammatory cytokines and directly neurotoxic agents [12–16].

The effects of NSAIDs may be more related to their cyclo-oxygenase -1 (COX-1) inhibitory effects than COX-2 inhibition. This is supported by findings that the anti-neurotoxic actions of various NSAIDs are independent of their selectivity towards the two COX isoforms [12] and that COX-1 appears to be the predominant COX isoform expressed by human microglial cells [17–19]. Therapeutic trials of NSAIDs need to consider this, and results with COX-2 selective inhibitors may not automatically translate to similar results with COX-1 or non-selective inhibitors.

NSAIDs may interfere with the formation of senile plaques or suppress the microglial-mediated inflammation associated with these plaques. In post-mortem brain tissue there was no difference between NSAID-treated and untreated groups in the mean number of plaques or in the type of plaques, but NSAID use was associated with less microglial activation. These results suggest that if NSAID use is effective in treating AD, the mechanism is more likely to be through suppression of microglial activity than through directly inhibiting the formation of senile plaques [3].

## ANTI-INFLAMMATORY DRUGS AND THE RISK OF AD

In support of the possibly central role that inflammation plays in the pathogenesis of AD, many observational studies have demonstrated a link between longer-term anti-inflammatory drug use and a reduced risk of AD [20–42]. These individual studies have, however, not all shown such an association. This variability of results may be explained by varying designs, sample sizes and populations. In most of these studies information about NSAID use was obtained retrospectively from patients or relatives, or from medical records. These approaches may lead to inaccurate conclusions as they can misclassify drug exposure.

A more accurate approach is a prospective population-base cohort study design. Such a study was carried out using the Rotterdam study cohort and examined 6,989 subjects

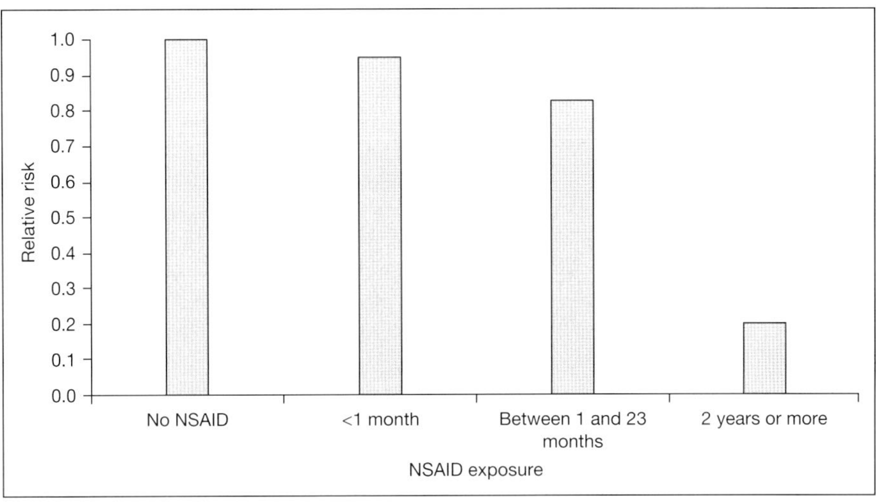


**Figure 9.1** Relative risk of Alzheimer's disease (with permission from reference [43]).

**Table 9.2** Risk of Alzheimer's disease in NSAID users [44]

| *Relative risk (95% CIs)* | *Length of use of NSAID* |
|---|---|
| 0.95 (0.70–1.29) | <1 month |
| 0.83 (0.65–1.06) | <24 months |
| 0.27 (0.13–0.58) | >24 months |
| 0.72 (0.56–0.94) | Any use |
| 0.97 (0.70–1.07) | Aspirin use |

initially 55 years of age or older and who were free of dementia at baseline [43]. The risk of AD was estimated in relation to the use of NSAIDs as documented in pharmacy records. Four mutually exclusive categories of use were defined: non-use, short-term use (1 month or less of cumulative use), intermediate-term use (more than 1 but less than 24 months of cumulative use) and long-term use (24 months or more of cumulative use). During an average follow-up period of 6.8 years, dementia developed in 394 subjects, of which most (293) had AD; 56 developed vascular dementia and 45 other types of dementia. Cox regression analysis adjustments were made for age, sex, education, smoking status and the use or non-use of salicylates (aspirin was not classified as an NSAID), histamine $H_2$-receptor antagonists, antihypertensive agents and hypoglycaemic agents. The relative risk of AD was 0.95 (95% confidence interval [CI] 0.70–1.29) in subjects with short-term use compared to non-use of NSAIDs, 0.20 (95% CI 0.05–0.83) in those with long-term use (Figure 9.1).

The risk did not vary according to age. The use of NSAIDs was not associated with a reduction in the risk of vascular dementia. This study provides powerful evidence for an association between NSAID use and a reduced risk of developing AD, and supports a central role of neuroinflammation in AD pathogenesis. More recently a systematic review and meta-analysis of observational studies between 1966 and October 2002 has also supported this possible protective effect [44]. The analysis included nine studies of NSAID use in adults over age 55. Six were cohort studies, with a total population of 13,211 participants, and three were case–control studies with a total of 1,443 participants. The results are shown in Table 9.2.

These results do need to be seen simply as hypothesis-generating rather than evidence of a protective effect of NSAIDs. Epidemiological evidence is subject to a range of potential biases including recall bias, prescription bias and publication bias. An analysis of 25 case–control and cohort studies used relative risks weighted by the inverse of their variances to obtain pooled relative risks and 95% confidence intervals [45]. These pooled relative risks were 50% in studies with prevalent dementia cases but declined to 20% in studies with incident dementia cases and there was no protective effect where cognitive decline was used as the endpoint. These differences suggested that biases were indeed influencing this proposed protective effect of NSAID use.

Individual studies have suggested a protective effect of NSAID use on cognitive decline, which can be seen as further supporting a potential protection against AD. In a prospective study of 16,128 Nurses' Health Study participants, six tests of cognitive function were administered by telephone over 6 years [46]. Compared to never users, the relative risk of a low baseline cognitive score was 0.75 (95% CI 0.59–0.96) for current users of aspirin with at least 15 years' use, and 0.79 (95% CI 0.62–1.02) for current NSAID users of at least 8 years' use. The relative risk for substantial subsequent cognitive decline was 0.93 (95% CI, 0.68–1.26) for long-term aspirin users and 0.77 (95% CI 0.57–1.05) for long-term NSAID users. Those results suggest an association between aspirin use and a baseline better cognitive score, but the follow-up showed no definite association between NSAID use and a lack of cognitive decline.

In an analysis of 2,651 participants in the UK Medical Research Council (MRC) treatment trial of hypertension in older adults, there was a significant but modest association between NSAID use and less decline over 54 months in one measure of cognition, the Paired Associate Learning Test [47]. A population-based sample of 7,671 subjects in three communities showed that those who had used NSAIDs for at least 3 years had better cognitive function than non-users, as assessed by the Short Portable Mental Status Questionnaire [48]. After controlling for potential confounders, the relative risk of cognitive decline in NSAID users was 0.82 (95% CI 0.69–0.98) compared to non-users.

## THERAPEUTIC TRIALS OF NSAIDs IN DEMENTIA

The finding that NSAIDs may attenuate or reverse the neuropathological changes of AD has led to several trials of NSAIDs in the treatment of established AD. Initially (1993) there was a small promising pilot trial of indomethacin [49]. This was followed by a small trial of diclofenac with misoprostol conducted in Melbourne, Australia [50]. This 25-week trial with 41 participants fell well short of statistical significance on all primary endpoints (ADAS-Cog, Global Deterioration Scale [GDS] and Clinical Global Impression of Change [CGIC]), largely as the placebo group failed to decline as expected. Another small trial with 40 participants found nimesulide to be ineffective over 24 weeks [51]. Larger trials have assessed the therapeutic effects of several other agents and are summarized in Table 9.3. To date, there has been no statistically significant evidence of a benefit of any anti-inflammatory agent on AD.

These negative results probably indicate that anti-inflammatory agents will not in the future have a role in the treatment of AD and other dementias. However, it is possible that these results could be explained by other factors [57]. The doses used may have been inadequate, but higher doses would almost certainly have increased the risk of adverse effects. The dose of prednisone used, for instance, at 10 mg in the maintenance phase, was quite low [55]. However, the 25 mg daily dose of rofecoxib used in both trials was at the upper limit of the usual dose used for inflammatory conditions [53, 54].

It may be that anti-inflammatory agents are more effective if initiated early in the disease process. In the therapeutic trials to date, baseline Mini-mental State Examination (MMSE) score has been around 20, and the disease duration at trial entry has averaged over a year but is often considerably longer. The ultimate test of the benefits of early use of NSAIDs

**Table 9.3** Large trials of anti-inflammatory agents in AD

| *Agent* | *Reference* | *Duration (months)* | *Trial design* | *No of participants* | *Primary endpoint* | *Results* |
|---|---|---|---|---|---|---|
| Hydroxy-chloroquine | [52] | 18 | Double-blind placebo-controlled | 168 | ADL (function) Cognition Behaviour | No significant differences in any outcome, compared to placebo |
| Rofecoxib | [53] | 12 | Double-blind placebo-controlled | 692 | ADAS-Cog CIBIC+ | No significant differences compared to placebo |
| Rofecoxib or Naproxen | [54] | 12 | Double-blind placebo-controlled | 351 | ADAS-Cog | No significant differences with either agent compared to placebo |
| Prednisolone | [55] | 12 | Double-blind placebo-controlled | 138 | ADAS-Cog | No significant difference compared to placebo |
| Celecoxib | [56] | 12 | Double-blind placebo-controlled | 425 | ADAS-Cog CIBIC+ | No significant difference compared to placebo |

would be primary prevention trials, and at least one has commenced. It is also possible that the endpoints chosen in the trials to date are inappropriate. The ones chosen reflect a symptomatic response and are the standard endpoints in AD therapeutic trials. These endpoints, however, may miss an underlying disease–modifying effect of therapy. The separation of disease-modifying and symptomatic effects is however problematic [58] and any purported disease-modifying effect would be difficult to support if not accompanied by a symptomatic effect. Disease modification could generally be expected to take longer to demonstrate and all but one trial to date was only of a relatively short 12 months' duration.

It is also possible that only specific anti-inflammatory agents are effective in AD. The majority of trials have selected cyclo-oxygenase-2 (COX-2) inhibitors, due to concerns about gastrointestinal toxicity with the non-selective inhibitors. However, this COX-2 selectivity may not be as useful in the reduction of brain inflammation. For instance, in the brain COX-2 is preferentially expressed by neurones but not by the microglial cells that are key to inflammation [17, 59]. It is possible that some beneficial effects of NSAIDs in AD could be mediated in part by their action on neuronal COX. There is upregulation of neuronal COX-2 in early AD [17, 59, 60]. Alternatively, COX-2 may play a compensatory, beneficial effect in AD pathology, and inhibition of COX-2 would have adverse effects. It is known that COX-1 is the predominant COX isoform expressed by microglia in the human brain [17–19] and this suggests that it will be the non-selective COX inhibitors, that are relatively more active towards COX-1, that may be a better choice for AD treatment [61]. Thus, it may be that we need trials of other, non-selective NSAIDs in the treatment of AD before we completely close the door on their possible beneficial effects. At this stage, NSAIDs and other anti-inflammatory agents cannot be recommended for the treatment of AD.

## NSAIDs IN THE PREVENTION OF AD

While NSAIDs appear ineffective in the treatment of established AD, they may have a role in the prevention of AD. Both the epidemiological and neuropathological evidence could be interpreted as demonstrating that NSAIDs will be most effective if used early and long-term. The main trial to test this hypothesis has been the Alzheimer's Disease Anti-inflammatory Prevention Trial (ADAPT). This trial, sponsored by the USA National Institute of Aging (NIA) randomized 2,400 cognitively normal people over age 70 and at increased risk of developing AD to either celecoxib, naproxen or placebo. The trial planned for treatment for 3 years but due to concerns about the possible safety of celecoxib was terminated prematurely, in December 2004. All patients continue to be followed up and it may be that treatment effects will become apparent despite the early termination. At the time of termination, no significant safety concerns of celecoxib were apparent. There was, however, an apparent increase in cardiovascular and cerebrovascular events compared to placebo among patients taking 220 mg of naproxen twice-daily. No other primary prevention trials with anti-inflammatory agents are in progress or completed and at this time NSAIDs and other anti-inflammatories cannot be recommended for the primary prevention of AD.

A logical target group for primary prevention trails is those with mild cognitive impairment (MCI). This group of people have an increased risk of progression to AD – around 15% 'convert' to AD [62] each year. There have been trials of several agents for MCI, including cholinesterase inhibitors but no agent to date has demonstrated efficacy in preventing progression to AD or other dementias. No trial of NSAIDs in MCI has yet been reported.

An alternative approach to preventing or treating AD is to utilize an NSAID that has additional effects apart from attenuating inflammation. One such potential agent is flurbiprofen, an anti-inflammatory drug that also appears to reduce $A\beta_{1-42}$ production [63]. Trials of this agent have commenced but results are not expected until around 2007. There are other COX-independent activities of NSAIDs that may lead to further trials. These include activation of peroxisome proliferators-activated receptor-$\gamma$ (PPAR-$\gamma$), which may modify amyloid production [64]. The concentration of drug required for these COX-independent actions are higher than those currently used and risk considerable toxicity so such trials have as yet not proceeded [2].

## SUMMARY

While there is strong evidence for inflammation as a pivotal event in the pathogenesis of AD, at this stage there is no proven role for anti-inflammatory agents in the treatment of AD. These agents may have a role in AD prevention, but this has yet to be proven. Newer agents with additional actions, such as flurbiprofen, may have a role but evidence is awaited.

So what is the clinician to do? If an anti-inflammatory agent is required longer term for the treatment of an inflammatory condition such as rheumatoid or other arthritis, it may be reasonable to tell the patient that such treatment may also have beneficial effects on the risk of AD. However, such agents should not be primarily prescribed to prevent, or treat, AD. It would appear that selective COX-2 inhibition offers no advantage in AD prevention or treatment, and indeed non-selective NSAIDs may be more effective than COX-2 selective inhibitors.

More research is needed, especially with newer agents and in AD prevention. Anti-inflammatory agents may also have a role in the prevention or treatment of non-AD dementias, but this has yet to be proven.

## REFERENCES

1. McGeer PL , McGeer EG. Inflammation of the brain in Alzheimer's disease: implications for therapy. *J Leukoc Biol* 1999; 65:409–415.

2. Klegeris A , McGeer PL. Non-steroidal anti-inflammatory drugs (NSAIDs) and other anti-inflammatory agents in the treatment of neurodegenerative disease. *Curr Alzheimer Res* 2005; 2:355–365.
3. Mackenzie IRA, Munoz DG. Nonsteroidal anti-inflammatory drug use and Alzheimer-type pathology in aging. *Neurology* 1998; 50:986–990.
4. Aisen PS. Inflammation and Alzheimer's disease: mechanisms and therapeutic strategies. *Gerontology* 1997; 43:143–149.
5. Griffin WS, Stanley LC, Ling C *et al.* Brain interleukin 1 and S-100 immunoreactivity are elevated in Down syndrome and Alzheimer disease. *Proc Natl Acad Sci USA* 1989; 86:7611–7615.
6. Griffin WST, Mrak RE. The role of microglial activation, interleukin-1, and neuroinflammation in Alzheimer pathogenisis. In: Iqbal K, Winblad B (eds). *Alzheimer's Disease and Related Disorders: Research Advances*. Ana Aslan Intl. Acad. of Aging, Bucharest, Romania, 2003, p 484.
7. Engelhart MJ, Geerlings MI, Meijer J *et al.* Inflammatory proteins in plasma and the risk of dementia. *Arch Neurol* 2004; 61:668–672.
8. Schmidt R, Schmidt H, Curb D, Maraki K, White LR, Launer LJ. Early inflammation and dementia: a 25-year follow-up of the Honolulu-Asia Aging Study. *Ann Neurol* 2002; 52:168–174.
9. Dik MG, Jonker C, Hack CE, Smit JH, Comijs HC, Eikelenboom P. Serum inflammatory proteins and cognitive decline in older persons. *Neurology* 2005; 64:1371–1377.
10. Netland EE, Newton JL, Majocha RE, Tate BA. Indomethacin reverses the microglial response to amyloid β-protein. *Neurobiol Aging* 1998; 19:201–204.
11. Scali C, Prosperi C, Vannucchi MG, Pepeu G, Casamenti F. Brain inflammation reaction in an animal model of neuronal degeneration and its modulation by an anti-inflammatory drug; implication in Alzheimer's disease. *Eur J Neurosci* 2000; 12:1900–1912.
12. Klegeris A, Walker DG, McGeer PL. Toxicity of human THP-1 monocytic cells towards neuron-like cells is reduced by non-steroidal anti-inflammatory drugs (NSAIDs). *Neuropharmacology* 1999; 38:1017–1025.
13. Klegeris A, Maguire J, McGeer PL. S- but not R-enantiomers of flurbiprofen and ibuprofen reduce human microglial and THP-1 cell neurotoxicity. *J Neuroimmunol* 2004; 152:73–77.
14. Dzenko KA, Weltzien RB, Pachter JS. Suppression of Aβ-induced monocyte neurotoxicity by antiinflammatory compounds. *J Neuroimmunol* 1997; 80:6–12.
15. Combs CK, Johnson DE, Cannady SB, Lehman TM, Landreth GE. Inflammatory mechanisms in Alzheimer's disease: inhibition of β-amyloid-stimulated proinflammatory responses and neurotoxicity by PPARγ agonists. *J Neurosci* 2000; 20:558–567.
16. Morihara T, Chu T, Ubeda O, Beech W, Cole GM. Selective inhibition of Aβ42 production by NSAID R-enantiomers. *J Neurochem* 2002; 83:1009–1012.
17. Hoozemans JJ, Rozemuller AJ, Janssen I, De Groot CJ, Veerhuis R, Eikelenboom P. Cyclooxygenase expression in microglia and neurons in Alzheimer's disease and control brain. *Acta Neuropathol* 2001; 101:2–8.
18. Hoozemans JJ, Veerhuis R, Janssen I, van Elk EJ, Rozemuller AJ, Eikelenboom P. The role of cyclo-oxygenase 1 and 2 activity in prostaglandin $E_2$ secretion by cultured human adult microglia: implications for Alzheimers disease. *Brain Res* 2002; 951:218–226.
19. Yermakova AV, Rollins J, Callahan LM, Rogers J, O'Banion MK. Cyclooxygenase-1 in human Alzheimer and control brain: quantitive analysis of expression by microglia and CA3 hippocampal neurons. *J Neuopath Exp Neurol* 1999; 58:1135–1146.
20. Andersen K, Launer LJ, Ott A, Hoes AW, Breteler MM, Hofman A. Do nonsteriodal anti-inflammatory drugs decrease the risk for Alzheimer's disease? The Rotterdam Study. *Neurology* 1995; 45:1441–1445.
21. Broe GA, Henderson AS, Creasey H *et al.* A case-control study of Alzheimer's disease in Australia. *Neorology* 1990; 40:1698–1707.
22. Heyman A, Wilkinson WE, Stafford JA, Helms MJ, Sigmon AH, Weinberg T. Alzheimer's disease: a study of epidemiological aspects. *Ann Neurol* 1984; 15:335–341.
23. Graves AB, White E, Koepsell TD *et al.* A case-control study of Alzheimer's disease. *Ann Neurol* 1990; 28:766–774.
24. Li G, Shen YC, Li YT, Chen CH, Zhau YW, Silverman JM. A case-control study of Alzheimer's disease in China. *Neurology* 1992; 42:1481–1488.
25. French LR, Schuman LM, Mortimer JA, Hutton JT, Boatman RA, Christians B. A case-control study of dementia of the Alzheimer type. *Am J Epidemiol* 1985; 121:414–421.
26. Jenkinson ML, Bliss MR, Brain AT, Scott DL. Rheumatoid arthritis and senile dementia of the Alzheimer's type. *Br J Rheumatol* 1989; 28:86–88.

27. Beard CM, Kokman E, Kurland LT. Rheumatoid arthritis and susceptibility to Alzheimer's disease. *Lancet* 1991; 337:1426.
28. McGeer PL, McGeer E, Rogers J, Sibley J. Anti-Inflammatory drugs and Alzheimer disease. *Lancet* 1990; 335:1037.
29. Amaducci LA, Fratiglioni L, Rocca WA *et al.* Risk factors for clinically diagnosed Alzheimer's disease: a case-control study of an Italian population. *Neurology* 1986; 36:922–931.
30. Henderson AS, Jorm AF, Korten AE *et al.* Environmental risk factors for Alzheimer's disease: their relationship to age of onset and to familial or sporadic types. *Psychol Med* 1992; 22:429–436.
31. Breitner JC, Gau BA, Welsh KA *et al.* Inverse association of anti-inflammatory treatments and Alzheimer's disease: initial results of a co-twin control study. *Neurology* 1994; 44:227–232.
32. Breitner JC, Welsh KA, Helms MJ *et al.* Delayed onset of Alzheimer's disease with nonsteroidal anti-inflammatory and histamine H2 blocking drugs. *Neurobiol Aging* 1995; 16:523–530.
33. The Canadian Study of Health and Aging. Risk factors for Alzheimer's disease in Canada. *Neurology* 1994; 44:2073–2080.
34. Brooks W, Grayson D, Nicholson G *et al.* APOE-ε4 predicts, but anti-inflammatory drugs do not prevent, incident Alzheimer's disease in an elderly community sample. *Neurobiol Aging* 1998; 19(suppl 4):S140.
35. Anthony JC, Breitner JC, Zandi PP *et al.* Reduced prevalence of AD in users of NSAIDs and H2 receptor antagonists: the Cache County study. *Neurology* 2000; 54:2066–2071.
36. Kukull WA, Larson EB, Stergachis A *et al.* Non-steroidal anti-inflammatory drug use and risk of Alzheimer's disease. *Neurology* 1994; 44(suppl 2):A37.
37. Fourrier A, Letenneur L, Begaud B, Dartigues JF. Nonsteroidal anti-inflammatory drug use and cognitive function in the elderly: inconclusive results from a population-based cohort study. *J Clin Epidemiol* 1996; 49:1201.
38. Stewart WF, Kawas C, Corrada M, Metter EJ. Risk of Alzheimer's disease and duration of NSAID use. *Neurology* 1997; 48:626–632.
39. Henderson AS, Jorm AF, Christensen H, Jacomb PA, Korten AE. Aspirin, anti-inflammatory drugs and risk of dementia. *Int Geriatr Psychiatry* 1997; 12:926–930.
40. Beard CM, Waring SC, O'Brien PC, Kurland LT, Kokmen E. Nonsteroidal anti-inflammatory drug use and Alzheimer's disease: a case-control study in Rochester, Minnesota, 1980 through 1984. *Mayo Clin Proc* 1998; 73:951–955.
41. In't Veld BA, Launer LJ, Hoes AW *et al.* NSAIDs and incidence of Alzheimer's disease: the Rotterdam Study. *Neurobiol Aging* 1998; 19:607–611.
42. Cornelius C, Fratiglioni L, Fastbom J, Guo Z, Vitanen M, Winblad B. No support for a protective effect of NSAIDs against Alzheimer's disease from a follow-up population-based study. *Neurobiol Aging* 1998; 19(suppl 4):S28.
43. In't Veld BA, Ruitenburg A, Hofman A *et al.* Nonsteriodal antiinflammatory drugs and the risk of Alzheimer's Disease. *N Engl J Med* 2001; 345:1515–1521.
44. Etminan M, Gill S, Samii A *et al.* Effect of non-steroidal anti-inflammatory drugs on risk of Alzheimer's disease: systematic review and meta-analysis of observational studies. *BMJ* 2003; 327:128–131.
45. De Craen AJM, Gussekloo J, Vrijsen B, Westendorp RC. Meta-analysis of nonsteroidal antiinflammatory drug use and risk of dementia. *Am J Epidemiol* 2005; 161:114–120.
46. Kang JH, Grodstein F. Regular use of nonsteroidal anti-inflammatory drugs and cognitive function in aging women. *Neurology* 2003; 60:1591–1597.
47. Prince M, Rabe-Hesketh S, Brennan P. Do antiarthritic drugs decrease the risk for cognitive decline? An analysis based on data from the MRC Treatment Trial of Hypertension in Older Adults. *Neurology* 1998; 50:374–379.
48. Rozzini R, Ferruci L, Losonczy K, Havlik R and Guralnik JM. Protective effect of chronic NSAID use on cognitive decline in older persons. *J Am Geriatr Soc* 1996; 44:1025–1029.
49. Rogers J, Kirby LC, Hempelmen SR *et al.* Clinical trial of indomethacin in Alzheimer's disease. *Neurology* 1993; 43:1609–1611.
50. Scharf S, Mander A, Ugoni A, Vajda F, Christophidis N. A double-blind, placebo-controlled trial of diclofenac/misoprostol in Alzheimer's disease. *Neurology* 1999; 53:197–201.
51. Aisen PS, Schmeidler J, Pasinetti GM. Randomised pilot study of nimesulide treatment in Alzheimer's disease. *Neurology* 2002; 58:1050–1054.
52. Van Gool WA, Weinstein HC, Scheltens PK, Walstra GJ. Effect of hydroxychloroquine on progression of dementia in early Alzheimer's disease: an 18 month randomised, double blind, placebo-controlled study. *Lancet* 2001; 358:455–460.

53. Reines SA, Block GA, Morris JC *et al*. Rofecoxib. No effect on Alzheimer's disease in a 1-year, randomised, blinded, controlled study. *Neurology* 2004; 62:66–71.
54. Aisen PS, Schafer KA, Grundman M *et al*. Effects of rofecoxib or naproxen vs placebo on Alzheimer disease progression. *JAMA* 2003; 289:2819–2826.
55. Aisen PS, Davies KL, Berg JD *et al*. A randomised controlled trial of prednisone in Alzheimer's disease. *Neurology* 2000; 54:588–593.
56. Sainati SM, Ingram DM, Talwalker S, Geis GS. Results of a double-blind, randomised, placebo-controlled study of celecoxib in the treatment of progression of Alzheimer's disease. Sixth International Stockholm/Springfield Symposium on Advances in Alzheimer Therapy. Abstract book 2000, p 180.
57. Breitner JC. NSAIDs and Alzheimer's disease: how far to generalise from trials? *Lancet Neurol* 2003; 2:527.
58. Leber P. Slowing the progression of Alzheimer disease: methodological issues. *Alzheimer Dis Assoc Disord* 1997; 11(suppl 5):S10–S21.
59. Yasojima K, Schwab S, McGeer EG, McGeer PL. Distribution of cyclooxygenase-1 and cyclooxygenase-2 mRNAs and proteins in human brain and peripheral organs. *Brain Res* 1999; 830:226–236.
60. Ho L, Purohit D, Haroutunian V *et al*. Neuronal cyclooxygenase 2 expression in the hippocampal formation as a function of the clinical progression of Alzheimer disease. *Arch Neurol* 2001; 58:487–492.
61. McGeer PL. Cyclo-oxygenase-2 inhibitors rationale and therapeutic potential in Alzheimer's disease. *Drugs Aging* 2000; 17:1–11.
62. Petersen RC, Thomas RG, Grundman M *et al*. Vitamin E and donepezil for the treatment of mild cognitive impairment. *N Engl J Med* 2005; 352:2379–2388.
63. Eriksen JL, Sagi SA, Smith TE *et al*. NSAIDs and enantiomers of flurbiprofen target gamma-secretase and lower Aβ42 in vivo. *J Clin Invest* 2003; 112:440–449.
64. Lehmann JM, Lenhard JM, Oliver BB, Ringold GM, Kliewer SA. Peroxisome proliferators-activated receptors α and γ are activated by indomethacin and other non-steroidal anti-inflammatory drugs. *J Biol Chem* 1997; 272:3406–3410.

# 10

# Nicotine and amyloid-β

*M. Svedberg, C. Unger, A. Nordberg*

## INTRODUCTION

Alzheimer's disease (AD) is a progressive neurodegenerative disease characterized by memory impairments and increasingly severe dementia. Alois Alzheimer described the two major pathological hallmarks present in the AD brain: amyloid plaques, which are mainly composed of amyloid β (Aβ), and neurofibrillary tangles, consisting of hyperphosphorylated tau protein. Although genetic and biochemical studies have suggested a cardinal role for Aβ in AD, the underlying mechanism(s) of how Aβ induces degeneration in the central nervous system is still unclear [1]. The aggregated form of Aβ (i.e. insoluble), soluble as well as intra/extracellular deposition, seems to be an important factor. The exact identity of the active species is still unclear. Fibrils, smaller peptide oligomers, water-soluble non-filamentous forms of Aβ, dimeric and trimeric species have all been suggested to be the toxic form [2–6]. During the last 10–15 years there has been intensive ongoing research with the aim of finding the underlying pathophysiological mechanisms of AD and how these abnormal processes could be influenced in order to prevent or slow down the progression of the disease [7]. Figure 10.1 shows several pathological processes that might be involved in the ongoing neurodegenerative processes in AD, including inflammatory processes, oxidative stress mechanisms, growth factor activation, microglial activation and synaptic impairments. The final cognitive disturbances are strongly related to impairment of the cholinergic system.

## NEURONAL NICOTINIC RECEPTORS

The cholinergic system in the brain is involved in higher cognitive functions and mediates its effect via the muscarinic and nicotinic acetylcholine receptors (nAChRs): the nAChRs seem to play an important role in AD. The nAChRs are ion channel receptors present in neuronal and non-neuronal cells. They belong to the same receptor family as glutamate, γ-aminobutyric acid (GABA) and serotonin 3 (5-$HT_3$) receptors that transduce cations, $Na^+$ and $Ca^{2+}$ [8, 9]. The nAChRs are transmembrane allosteric proteins formed by five subunits arranged around a central core that is perpendicular to the membrane [10].

The neuronal nAChRs are composed of α and β subunits. To date, six different α subunits (α2–α7), and three β subunits (β2–β4) have been cloned and sequenced from human brain tissue. The neuronal nAChRs can be homo-oligomers composed of α7, or hetero-oligomers,

**Marie Svedberg**, PhD, Researcher, Karolinska Institutet, Department of Neurobiology, Care Sciences and Society, Division of Molecular Neuropharmacology, Karolinska University, Hospital Huddinge, Stockholm, Sweden

**Christina Unger**, PhD, Researcher, Karolinska Institutet, Department of Neurobiology, Care Sciences and Society, Division of Molecular Neuropharmacology, Karolinska University, Hospital Huddinge, Stockholm, Sweden

**Agneta Nordberg**, MD, PhD, Professor, Karolinska Institutet, Department of Neurobiology, Care Sciences and Society, Division of Molecular Neuropharmacology, Karolinska University, Hospital Huddinge, Stockholm, Sweden

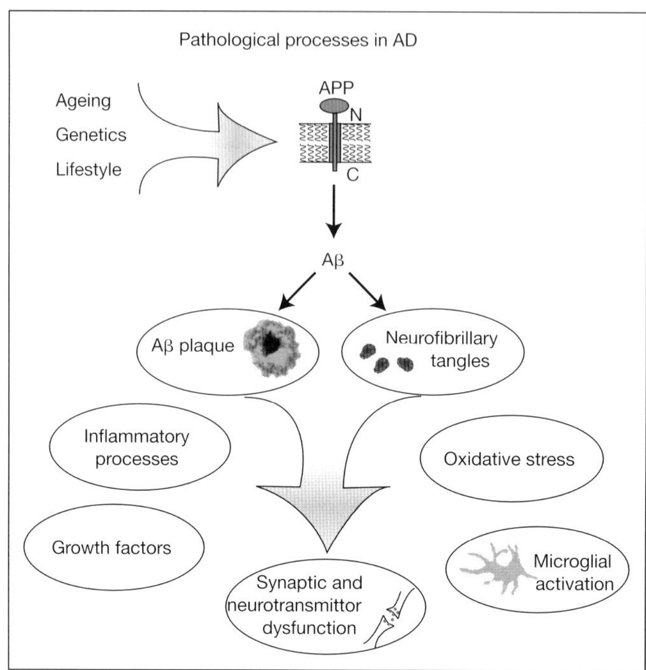


**Figure 10.1** Schematic picture of the suggested pathological processes in AD. Age, genetics and lifestyle are all important factors that might determine the risk of developing AD. The increased production of Aβ causes accumulation of Aβ into plaques and hyperphosphorylation of tau, which eventually leads to synaptic and neurotransmittor dysfunction as well as microglia activation, inflammatory processes, oxidative stress and disturbances in the release of growth factors.

composed of different α subunits or both α and β subunits; each combination appears to dictate particular pharmacological and physiological functions [9, 11].

The most abundant nAChR subtype is the α4-nAChR subtype, but also the α3- and α7-nAChRs subtypes are common in the human brain. The α4β2-nAChR binds nicotine with high affinity, while the α7-nAChR subtype binds α bungarotoxin [8]. The α4β2-nAChR channels recognize and bind agonists with high affinity and are not as rapidly desensitized as the α7-nAChRs, which have a high $Ca^{2+}$ permeability, short open time and recognize and bind with low affinity all nicotinic agonists [12]. It has been proposed that the influx of $Ca^{2+}$ regulated by nAChR activation may elicit a number of downstream intracellular events, including activation of protein kinases, initiation of immediate early genes and new protein synthesis, ultimately leading to changes in synaptic plasticity and neuronal remodelling. A single neurone often expresses several nAChR subtypes. Both the α4β2- and α7-nAChR subtypes are present in neurones of other systems including the glutamatergic, dopaminergic, serotonergic, noradrenergic and GABAergic neurotransmitter systems [13–17].

The nAChR subtypes studied in human post-mortem brain indicate a different regional distribution for the α4β2- and α7-nAChR subtypes. The α4- and α7-receptor subtypes, measured by [$^{3}$H]nicotine, [$^{3}$H]cytisine and [$^{3}$H]epibatidine binding in human post-mortem brain tissue, showed abundant binding in cortical regions with different laminar distributions [18], whereas the α7-receptor subtypes, measured by [$^{125}$I]α bungarotoxin binding, show high density in the hippocampus [19]. Recently, it has been shown that the α7-nAChRs are not only distributed on neuronal cells but also in glial cells, thus the nAChRs may have a different role in these type of tissues [20–22].

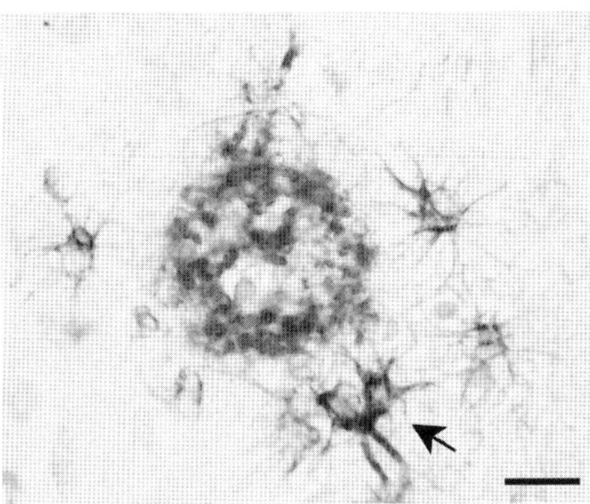

**Figure 10.2** α7-nAChRs are present on astrocytes, surrounding the plaques. Double immunolabelling for Aβ- and α7-nAChRs shows α7-nAChR positive astrocytes surrounding neuritic plaques. Scale bar = 20 μm. Reproduced with permission from [22].

There is a significant loss of nAChRs in the human brain during normal ageing. Receptor binding analysis in post-mortem brain tissue obtained from subjects with no neurological or psychiatric history have revealed an 80% reduction in nAChRs in the cortex between 56 and 85 years of age [19].

## NICOTINIC RECEPTOR CHANGES IN AD

There is a widespread reduction in the $\alpha_4$-nAChR subtype but also of the $\alpha_3$ in AD brains. Also the expression of the α7-nAChR is changed, but to a smaller extent, although an increase in mRNA encoding the α7-nAChR subtype was observed in hippocampus in post-mortem brain tissue from AD patients [23–25]. It has been unknown how these changes are associated with neurones and/or astrocytes. Ligand binding assays and Western blotting only provide information concerning the total binding capacity or total level of the protein, respectively, but give no information about the possible expression of the receptor proteins on astrocytes and neurones. When the presence of α7-nAChR was measured in neurones and astrocytes, respectively, a significant decrease was observed in the neurones while there was a significant increase in astrocytes [22]. The decrease in receptors on neurone may thus be levelled out by the increases in α7 on astrocytes of AD brain [22] (Figure 10.2), when receptors are quantified by binding studies in homogenates. The amyloid precursor protein (APP) 670/671 (Swedish) mutation (APPswe) [26], produces more $A\beta_{1-42}$ and subsequently larger plaques compared to sporadic AD [27, 28]. Although receptor analysis in post-mortem tissue from AD patients with the Swedish mutation (APPswe) showed similar reductions in nAChR binding sites as in sporadic AD [29], the loss in nAChRs was more pronounced in APP 670/671 brain due to the younger age-matched controls compared to sporadic AD. An elevated total number of astrocytes were observed in the hippocampus and temporal cortex of both APPswe and sporadic AD patients, while the increase in the level of expression of α7-nAChRs on astrocytes was more pronounced in the Swedish mutation than in the sporadic AD brain [22]. In addition, a reduction in nAChRs has also been found in non-neuronal peripheral cells, lymphocytes, from AD patients at both mRNA and binding site level [24, 30].

It has been possible to visualize the nAChRs by using $^{11}$C-nicotine and positron emission tomography (PET). A lower $^{11}$C-nicotine binding has been observed in cortical brain regions and hippocampus of AD patients compared to age-matched controls [31]. When a kinetic model is used for measuring the $^{11}$C-nicotine binding a positive correlation is observed between cognition (measured as Mini-mental State Examination [MMSE]) and $^{11}$C-nicotine binding in the temporal cortex [31]. Recently, a new amyloid PET ligand, the Pittsburgh Compound-B (PIB), has shown promising results in visualizing amyloid in AD patients [32, 33]. In cortical regions, such as the temporal–parietal association cortex, where there is a lower $^{11}$C-nicotine uptake and also lower cerebral glucose metabolism ($^{18}$F-FDG uptake) an increased retention is observed for $^{11}$C-PIB as a sign of high amyloid. PIB imaging will be a valuable tool for studies of anti-amyloid drug effects.

## APP/Aβ MECHANISMS IN AD

Aβ is produced via proteolytic processing of the APP. There are two variants of Aβ ($Aβ_{1-40}$ and $Aβ_{1-42}$). Ninety per cent of the Aβ produced is $Aβ_{1-40}$, but $Aβ_{1-42}$ is more prone to aggregate as fibrils [34]. $Aβ_{1-42}$ is the major Aβ species found in cerebral plaques [35]. Aβ has been identified in humans in a fibrilar form within the plaques [36], but also in a soluble form as stable dimers [37, 38]. It has been shown that soluble Aβ has a synaptotoxic effect at early age, prior to plaque formation, in the brain of different animal models of AD [4, 39, 40]. There is also evidence that soluble oligomers of Aβ, but not monomers or insoluble Aβ fibrils, may be responsible for synaptic dysfunction in AD patients [3, 41, 42].

One of the major targets in treatment strategies today is to lower the Aβ load in the AD brain [43] and by affecting the production, aggregation or clearance of Aβ, a modifying effect on disease progression is expected. One strategy for the development of anti-amyloid drugs is to block the production of Aβ. This effect might be obtained by inhibiting β- or γ-secretase activities, or by stimulating α-secretase activity [44, 45]. Blocking the aggregation of Aβ or enhancing the clearance of Aβ are other possible therapeutic strategies. Immune-based therapies directed against the Aβ peptide have been shown to ameliorate Aβ pathology and reverse cognitive behavioural deficits in transgenic mice models [46–50]. Based on the successful clearance of Aβ, an active immunization trial was performed in AD patients. However, the trial was terminated due to the development of meningoencephalitis in a subset of AD patients [51]. Brain autopsies of a few patients who died since receiving the vaccine showed lower-than-expected levels of plaques, while no reduction of Aβ in the vessels or tau pathology was found [52, 53]. Greater decrease in brain volume and greater ventricular enlargement, as well as a reduction of cerebrospinal fluid (CSF) tau, in the antibody responders compared to placebo patients have been reported, while the cognitive improvements were modest [54, 55]. As a result, passive immunization with anti-Aβ monoclonal antibodies has been suggested as a potentially safer alternative [56].

## NEUROPROTECTIVE MECHANISMS AND THE nAChRs

The protection of neurones and their synapses against damage and death with preservation of function in neurodegenerative diseases, such as AD, is of great therapeutic importance. Since nAChRs play a role in cognition and their expression is adversely affected by cholinergic degeneration, a link between nAChR expression/function and other pathological features of AD, such as Aβ deposition/toxicity, might be plausible. Experimental *in vitro* studies have shown neuroprotective effects *via* the nAChRs (Table 10.1). It has been demonstrated that oestrogen exerts neuroprotective properties via the α7-nAChRs and there is promotion of additional neuroprotection by cholinesterase inhibitors like tacrine and donepezil [57].

Nicotine has been shown to protect against cytotoxicity induced by excitotoxins and Aβ in both *in vitro* and *in vivo* systems [58]. Several studies suggest that both the α7- and the α4-nAChRs are involved in this neuroprotection. Selective nAChR agonists are candidates for symptomatic and neuroprotective AD therapy [7] and numerous investigations, both *in vivo* and *in vitro*, indicate that nicotine can enhance neurone survival in response to a range of neurotoxic insults. nAChR stimulation has been shown to increase neurotrophic factors in the

**Table 10.1** Neuroprotective effects via the nAChRs in cell lines

| *Model system* | *Drug* | *Toxic insult* | *Neuroprotective effect* | *Reference* |
|---|---|---|---|---|
| PC12 cells | Tacrine/ donepezil/ oestrogen | Aβ | ↓ cell death via nAChRs | [57, 83] |
| SH-SY5Y cells | Galantamine | Aβ or okadaic acid | ↓ Aβ or okadaic acid toxicity via α7-nAChR and PI3K-Akt pathway | [84] |
| SH-SY5Y cells | Donepezil | Aβ or okadaic acid | ↓ Aβ or okadaic acid toxicity via α7-nAChR and PI3K-Akt pathway | [84] |
| SH-SY5Y cells | Galantamine | Aβ or thapsigargin | Prevention of apoptotic cell death via α7-nAChRs | [85] |
| Primary rat cortical neurones | Galantamine | Aβ + glutamate | ↓ Aβ enhanced glutamate toxicity via α7-nAChR to PI3K cascade | [86] |
| Primary rat cortical culture | Donepezil | Glutamate | ↑ cell viability via both the α4- and α7-nAChRs | [87] |
| Human cortical neurones | Nicotine | Aβ + glutamate | ↓ Aβ enhanced glutamate toxicity via α7-nAChR to PI3K cascade | [88] |
| Primary rat cortical neurones | Nicotine | Glutamate | ↓ glutamate excitotoxicity via nAChRs | [89] |
| Primary rat cortical neurones | Nicotine | Aβ | ↓ of Aβ excitotoxicity via α7-nAChRs | [62] |
| Rat hippocampal culture | Nicotine | Aβ excitotoxicity | ↓ of Aβ via nAChRs | [90] |
| Differentiated PC12 cells | Nicotine | NGF and serum deprivation | ↑ cell viability via α7-nAChRs | [91] |

brain, increase the expression of nerve growth factor (NGF) receptors [6], and to protect neural cells against glutamate-induced toxicity [59]. nAChR stimulation also offers protection against trophic factor-deprivation-induced toxicity [60, 61] and Aβ-induced toxicity [62]. It has been suggested that stimulation of the α4β2-nAChRs and the α7-nAChRs may be responsible for neuroprotective effects against Aβ cytotoxicity [62, 63].

Due to these observations in experimental studies, it has been suggested that the α7-nAChRs might be a potential therapeutic target for treatment of neurodegenerative disorders. Epidemiological studies have indicated that tobacco smoking may be associated with a reduced risk of developing AD and a delayed onset of familial AD, although these findings are controversial (for review, see [64]). Post-mortem investigations have shown reduced levels of Aβ in smoking AD patients and controls [65–68]. Recent studies in the Tg2576 (APPswe) transgenic mice have revealed that both short- (10 days) and long-term treatment (5.5 months) with nicotine drastically reduce the levels of aggregated (guanidinium-soluble) $A\beta_{1-40}$ and $A\beta_{1-42}$ by 40–80% in the brain of these mice [66, 69, 70] (Figure 10.3). Treatment with nicotine for 10 days also resulted in less GFAP immunoreactive astrocytes around the plaques, increased levels of synaptophysin and increased number of

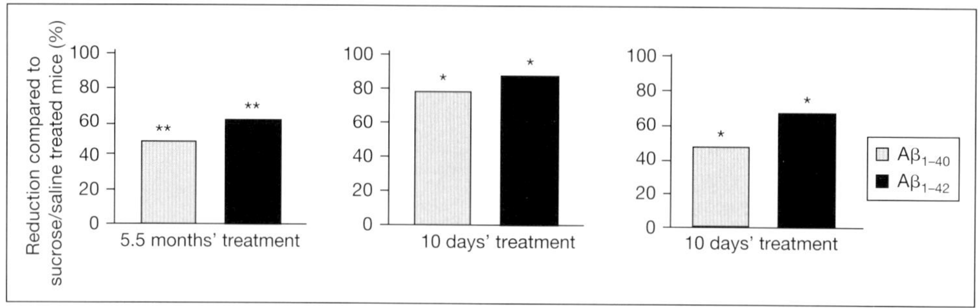


**Figure 10.3** The effect of nicotinic treatment on the Aβ levels in APPswe transgenic mice. (A) Reduction (%) in guanidinium soluble $A\beta_{1-40}$ and $A\beta_{1-42}$ levels following treatment with nicotine for 5.5 months (compared to sucrose treated animals) and 10 days (compared to saline treated animals) respectively. Reproduced with permission from reference [69]. $*P < 0.05$, $**P < 0.01$. Student t-test (from refs [69] and [75]). Non-parametric Kruskal-Wallis test followed by Mann-Whitney test (from ref [70]).

α7-nAChRs in the cortex of APPswe transgenic mice [70]. On the contrary, chronic nicotine treatment (5 months) in the triple transgenic mouse model, expressing $PS1_{M146V}$, APPswe and $tau_{P301L}$ (3×Tg-AD mice) resulted in an increase in hyperphosphorylation and aggregation of tau [71]. Nicotine has also been shown to increase tau in cell cultures [72]. Thus, the different effects observed on Aβ and tau following nicotine exposure call for further studies when considering nicotinic agonists as a possible therapy for AD.

It is important to determine whether the clearance of Aβ might be due to the β-sheet breaking activity of nicotine or whether nicotine can activate astrocytes, and thereby promote increased clearance of Aβ. It was recently demonstrated that L-(-)-nicotine not only inhibits the aggregation of $A\beta_{1-40}$ and $A\beta_{1-42}$, but can also disaggregate fibrils preformed from both of these peptides [73]. Furthermore, it has also been shown that both enantiomers of nicotine (D-(+)- and L-(-)-nicotine) can affect the early stages of Aβ aggregation, delaying oligomerization and fibril formation and thereby maintaining a population of less toxic Aβ species [74]. This suggests that this effect might not be due to a specific binding interaction between nicotine and Aβ, as previously thought, but could be due instead to a weaker, relatively non-specific binding or it could be due to the anti-oxidant or metal-chelating properties of nicotine. Since nicotine does not change the activities of cortical α-, β- or γ-secretase in APPswe transgenic mice or non-transgenic controls [75], and the levels of intracellular Aβ were not reduced [70], it is tempting to suggest that the action of nicotine (or one of its metabolites) might primarily be via degradation of insoluble Aβ deposits, rather than affecting the accumulation of the peptide. Further studies of the interaction of intracellular and extracellular Aβ at synapses as well as activation of α7-nAChRs in microglial cells may lead to a better understanding of the interactive effect of nicotine on AD pathology and may promote new therapeutic strategies for the disease.

## INTERACTION BETWEEN Aβ AND α7-nAChRs

Several experimental studies suggest that there is an interaction between Aβ and the α7-nAChRs in AD. A possible mechanism for how the α7-nAChRs can regulate the accumulation and formation of Aβ plaques in the brain and thereby play an important role in AD pathogenesis is as follows: $A\beta_{1-42}$ binds with high affinity to the α7-nAChRs and thereby a gradual intracellular accumulation of $A\beta_{1-42}$ by endocytosis occurs [76–79].

The binding of the $A\beta_{1-42}$ peptide to the receptor results in the formation of an $A\beta_{1-42}$/α7-nAChR complex, which might be an important step in the accumulation of $A\beta_{1-42}$ in the

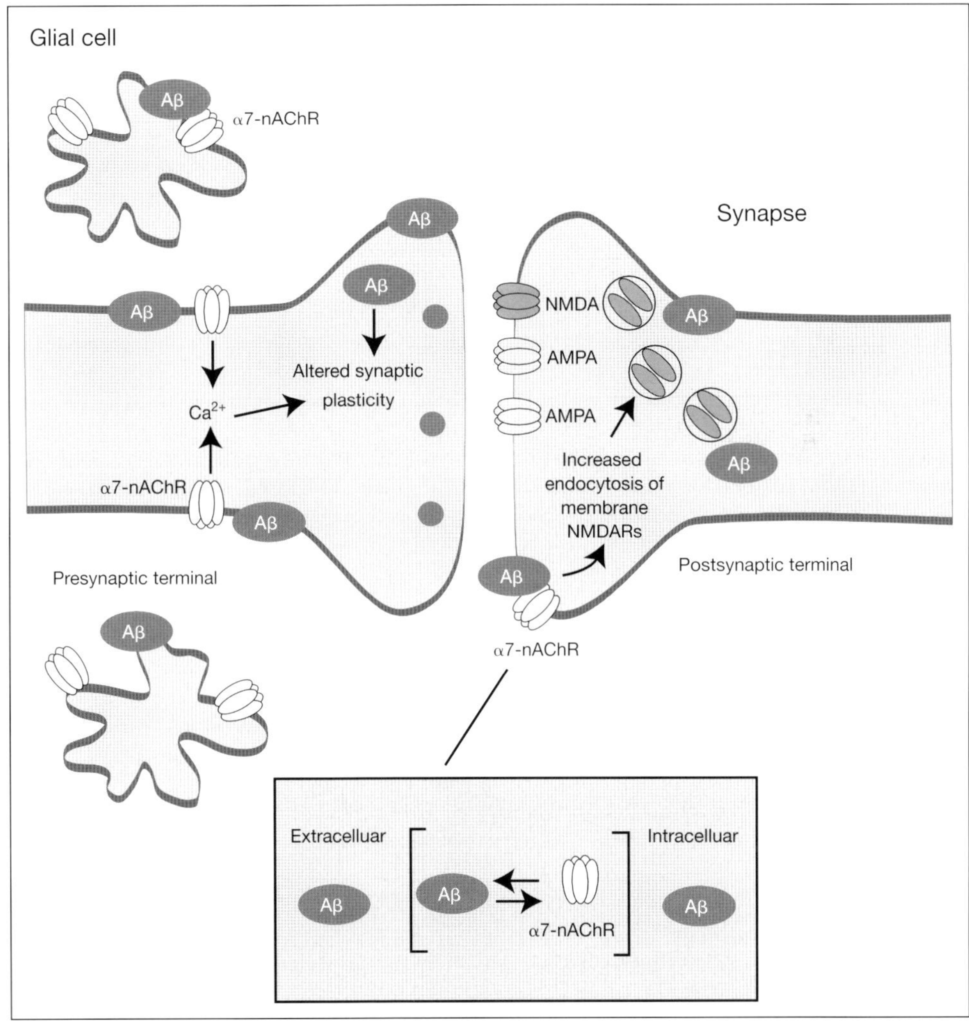


**Figure 10.4** Schematic picture of tentative interactions between Aβ- and α7-nAChRs. Several studies have shown a direct binding between Aβ and the α7-nAChR. The binding of Aβ peptide to the α7-nAChR results in the formation of an Aβ/α7 nAChR complex, which might be an important step in the accumulation of Aβ in the neurones [77]. It is also plausible that Aβ could activate intracellular signalling pathways, like the ERK2 MAPK cascade, which causes an influx of $Ca^{2+}$ into the cell leading to altered synaptic plasticity [76]. Furthermore, it has been proposed that Aβ might directly modulate the nAChRs by blocking the α7-nAChR-like currents in hippocampal interneurones [78]. Aβ may, by binding to α7-nAChRs, impair glutamatergic transmission, compromise synaptic function and reduce LTP and thereby promoting endocytosis of NMDA receptors [82]. The elevated expression of α7-nAChR on astrocytes might participate in Aβ cascade and formation of neuritic plaques [22].

neurones [77]. The consequence of accumulated $A\beta_{1-42}$ in the cell will eventually result in the cell undergoing lysis, following a selective loss of neurones and dispersal of their cytoplasmic contents, including the accumulated $A\beta_{1-42}$, into the surrounding extracellular space to form amyloidogenic plaques that disrupt neural and synaptic function in the brain (for review, see [80]). The $A\beta_{1-42}$/α7-nAChR complex is expected to be most abundant on neurones particularly those with a high α7-nAChR expression (e.g. cortical pyramidal cells).

It is also plausible that Aβ has a direct interaction with the nAChRs and that the $A\beta_{1-42}$ thereby could activate intracellular signalling pathways, like the ERK2 MAPK cascade, which causes an influx of $Ca^{2+}$ into the cell and leads to an increase in the α7-nAChRs in the hippocampus [76]. Furthermore, it has been proposed that $A\beta_{1-42}$ might directly modulate the nAChRs by blocking the α7-nAChR-like currents in hippocampal interneurones [78]. Figure 10.4 is a schematic picture of the possible interactions and consequences between Aβ and the α7-nAChRs.

A direct involvement of glial cells, notably astrocytes and microglia, has been apparent in plaque formation in AD brains. The α7-nAChRs are expressed on glial cells [20–22] and the elevated expression of α7-nAChR on astrocytes might participate in the Aβ cascade and the formation of neuritic plaques. Thus, the $A\beta_{1-42}$ peptide is abundant in astrocytic intracellular deposits and in amyloid plaques throughout AD brains. The detection of microglial cells, astrocyte processes and choline acetyltransferase- (ChAT-) positive fibres around β-amyloid plaques in transgenic APPswe mice suggest a close connection between cholinergic terminals and microglial cells [81].

Several lines of evidence suggest that the Aβ toxicity might be related to elevated levels of glutamate and/or over-activity of the NMDA receptors. The observation that Aβ reduces long-term potentiation (LTP) and facilitates long-term depression suggests a role for Aβ in regulating trafficking of glutamate receptors. A signalling pathway, where $A\beta_{1-42}$ may impair glutamatergic transmission, compromize synaptic function and reduce LTP by binding to α7-nAChRs thereby promoting endocytosis of NMDA receptors in cortical neurones, was recently reported [82]. Neuronal cell cultures from APPswe transgenic mice showed a reduction in surface-expressed NMDA receptors, while no change was observed in total receptor numbers [82].

The nAChRs (especially the α7 subtype) seem, according to the literature, to be of importance in neuroprotection. Whether the beneficial effects of nicotine in experimental studies reflect a possible pharmacological approach in the treatment of AD and the effect on cognition when Aβ is reduced, remains to be further studied. According to the hypothesis that Aβ binds to the α7-nAChR subtype, an α7 nicotinic antagonist might be of preference to reduce the Aβ levels in the AD brain. Furthermore, the observation that nicotine can dramatically decrease parenchymal Aβ and, in contrast to Aβ vaccination, is also able to reduce Aβ deposits associated with blood vessels, might be of importance for new therapeutic strategies. Increased understanding of the neuroprotective mechanisms and beneficial effects of nicotine, its interaction with Aβ (directly or *via* the nicotinic receptors) and the effect of Aβ on neurotransmission in the brain will eventually lead to a beneficial treatment of AD.

## ACKNOWLEDGEMENTS

Mrs. Marianne Grip is acknowledged for her professional help with the illustrations. Financial support was provided by the Swedish Research Council (project no. 05817).

## REFERENCES

1. Mattson MP. Pathways towards and away from Alzheimer's disease. *Nature* 2004; 430:631–639.
2. Davis JN 2nd, Chisholm JC. The 'amyloid cascade hypothesis' of AD: decoy or real McCoy? *Trends Neurosci* 1997; 20:558–559.
3. Hartley DM, Walsh DM, Ye CP *et al*. Protofibrillar intermediates of amyloid beta-protein induce acute electrophysiological changes and progressive neurotoxicity in cortical neurons. *J Neurosci* 1999; 19:8876–8884.
4. Hsia AY, Masliah E, McConlogue L *et al*. Plaque-independent disruption of neural circuits in Alzheimer's disease mouse models. *Proc Natl Acad Sci USA* 1999; 96:3228–3233.
5. Klein WL, Krafft GA, Finch CE. Targeting small Abeta oligomers: the solution to an Alzheimer's disease conundrum? *Trends Neurosci* 2001; 24:219–224.

6. Terry AV Jr, Clarke MS. Nicotine stimulation of nerve growth factor receptor expression. *Life Sci* 1994; 55:PL91–PL98.
7. Nordberg A. Toward an early diagnosis and treatment of Alzheimer's disease. *Int Psychogeriatr* 2003; 15:223–237.
8. Paterson D, Nordberg A. Neuronal nicotinic receptors in the human brain. *Prog Neurobiol* 2000; 61:75–111.
9. Pereira EF, Hilmas C, Santos MD *et al.* Unconventional ligands and modulators of nicotinic receptors. *J Neurobiol* 2002; 53:479–500.
10. Karlin A. Emerging structure of the nicotinic acetylcholine receptors. *Nat Rev Neurosci* 2002; 3:102–114.
11. Clementi F, Fornasari D, Gotti C. Neuronal nicotinic acetylcholine receptors: from structure to therapeutics. *Trends Pharmacol Sci* 2000; 21:35–37.
12. Albuquerque EX, Alkondon M, Pereira EF *et al.* Properties of neuronal nicotinic acetylcholine receptors: pharmacological characterization and modulation of synaptic function. *J Pharmacol Exp Ther* 1997; 280:1117–1136.
13. Cucchiaro G, Commons KG. Alpha 4 nicotinic acetylcholine receptor subunit links cholinergic to brainstem monoaminergic neurotransmission. *Synapse* 2003; 49:195–205.
14. Fabian-Fine R, Skehel P, Errington ML *et al.* Ultrastructural distribution of the alpha7 nicotinic acetylcholine receptor subunit in rat hippocampus. *J Neurosci* 2001; 21:7993–8003.
15. Hill JA Jr, Zoli M, Bourgeois JP *et al.* Immunocytochemical localization of a neuronal nicotinic receptor: the beta 2-subunit. *J Neurosci* 1993; 13:1551–1568.
16. Lambe EK, Picciotto MR, Aghajanian GK. Nicotine induces glutamate release from thalamocortical terminals in prefrontal cortex. *Neuropsychopharmacology* 2003; 28:216–225.
17. Wonnacott S. Presynaptic nicotinic ACh receptors. *Trends Neurosci* 1997; 20:92–98.
18. Sihver W, Gillberg PG, Nordberg A. Laminar distribution of nicotinic receptor subtypes in human cerebral cortex as determined by [3H](-)nicotine, [3H]cytisine and [3H]epibatidine in vitro autoradiography. *Neuroscience* 1998; 85:1121–1133.
19. Marutle A, Warpman U, Bogdanovic N *et al.* Regional distribution of subtypes of nicotinic receptors in human brain and effect of aging studied by (+/−)-[3H]epibatidine. *Brain Res* 1998; 801:143–149.
20. Graham AJ, Ray MA, Perry EK *et al.* Differential nicotinic acetylcholine receptor subunit expression in the human hippocampus. *J Chem Neuroanat* 2003; 25:97–113.
21. Teaktong T, Graham AJ, Johnson M *et al.* Selective changes in nicotinic acetylcholine receptor subtypes related to tobacco smoking: an immunohistochemical study. *Neuropathol Appl Neurobiol* 2004; 30:243–254.
22. Yu WF, Guan ZZ, Bogdanovic N *et al.* High selective expression of alpha7 nicotinic receptors on astrocytes in the brains of patients with sporadic Alzheimer's disease and patients carrying Swedish APP 670/671 mutation: a possible association with neuritic plaques. *Exp Neurol* 2005; 192:215–225.
23. Guan ZZ, Zhang X, Ravid R, Nordberg A. Decreased protein levels of nicotinic receptor subunits in the hippocampus and temporal cortex of patients with Alzheimer's disease. *J Neurochem* 2000; 74:237–243.
24. Hellström-Lindahl E, Mousavi M, Zhang X *et al.* Regional distribution of nicotinic receptor subunit mRNAs in human brain: comparison between Alzheimer and normal brain. *Brain Res Mol Brain Res* 1999; 66:94–103.
25. Nordberg A, Winblad B. Reduced number of [3H]nicotine and [3H]acetylcholine binding sites in the frontal cortex of Alzheimer brains. *Neurosci Lett* 1986; 72:115–119.
26. Mullan M, Crawford F, Axelman K *et al.* A pathogenic mutation for probable Alzheimer's disease in the APP gene at the N-terminus of beta-amyloid. *Nat Genet* 1992; 1:345–347.
27. Kalaria RN, Cohen DL, Greenberg BD *et al.* Abundance of the longer A beta 42 in neocortical and cerebrovascular amyloid beta deposits in Swedish familial Alzheimer's disease and Down's syndrome. *Neuroreport* 1996; 7:1377–1381.
28. Citron M, Oltersdorf T, Haass C *et al.* Mutation of the beta-amyloid precursor protein in familial Alzheimer's disease increases beta-protein production. *Nature* 1992; 360:672–674.
29. Marutle A, Warpman U, Bogdanovic N *et al.* Neuronal nicotinic receptor deficits in Alzheimer patients with the Swedish amyloid precursor protein 670/671 mutation. *J Neurochem* 1999; 72:1161–1169.
30. Adem A, Nordberg A, Bucht G *et al.* Extraneural cholinergic markers in Alzheimer's and Parkinson's disease. *Prog Neuropsychopharmacol Biol Psychiatry* 1986; 10:247–257.
31. Nordberg A, Lundqvist H, Hartvig P *et al.* Kinetic analysis of regional (S)(-)11C-nicotine binding in normal and Alzheimer brains – in vivo assessment using positron emission tomography. *Alzheimer Dis Assoc Disord* 1995; 9:21–27.
32. Klunk WE, Engler H, Nordberg A *et al.* Imaging brain amyloid in Alzheimer's disease with Pittsburgh Compound-B. *Ann Neurol* 2004; 55:306–319.

33. Nordberg A. Is amyloid plaque imaging the key to monitoring brain pathology of Alzheimer's disease in vivo? *Eur J Nucl Med Mol Imaging* 2004; 31:1540–1543.
34. Selkoe DJ. Alzheimer's disease: genes, proteins, and therapy. *Physiol Rev* 2001; 81:741–766.
35. Iwatsubo T, Odaka A, Suzuki N *et al.* Visualization of A beta 42(43) and A beta 40 in senile plaques with end-specific A beta monoclonals: evidence that an initially deposited species is A beta 42(43). *Neuron* 1994; 13:45–53.
36. Terry RD, Gonatas NK, Weiss M. The ultrastructure of the cerebral cortex in Alzheimer's disease. *Trans Am Neurol Assoc* 1964; 89:12.
37. Kuo YM, Emmerling MR, Vigo-Pelfrey C *et al.* Water-soluble Abeta (N-40, N-42) oligomers in normal and Alzheimer disease brains. *J Biol Chem* 1996; 271:4077–4081.
38. Roher AE, Chaney MO, Kuo YM *et al.* Morphology and toxicity of Abeta-(1–42) dimer derived from neuritic and vascular amyloid deposits of Alzheimer's disease. *J Biol Chem* 1996; 271:20631–20635.
39. Mucke L, Masliah E, Yu GQ *et al.* High-level neuronal expression of abeta 1–42 in wild-type human amyloid protein precursor transgenic mice: synaptotoxicity without plaque formation. *J Neurosci* 2000; 20:4050–4058.
40. Unger C, Hedberg MM, Mustafiz T *et al.* Early changes in Abeta levels in the brain of APPswe transgenic mice – implication on synaptic density, alpha7 neuronal nicotinic acetylcholine- and N-methyl-D-aspartate receptor levels. *Mol Cell Neurosci* 2005; 30:218–27.
41. Kayed R, Head E, Thompson JL *et al.* Common structure of soluble amyloid oligomers implies common mechanism of pathogenesis. *Science* 2003; 300:486–489.
42. Lambert MP, Barlow AK, Chromy BA *et al.* Diffusible, nonfibrillar ligands derived from Abeta1–42 are potent central nervous system neurotoxins. *Proc Natl Acad Sci USA* 1998; 95:6448–6453.
43. Cummings JL. Alzheimer's disease. *N Engl J Med* 2004; 351:56–67.
44. Citron M. Strategies for disease modification in Alzheimer's disease. *Nat Rev Neurosci* 2004; 5:677–685.
45. Wolfe MS. Therapeutic strategies for Alzheimer's disease. *Nat Rev Drug Discov* 2002; 1:859–866.
46. Bard F, Cannon C, Barbour R *et al.* Peripherally administered antibodies against amyloid beta-peptide enter the central nervous system and reduce pathology in a mouse model of Alzheimer disease. *Nat Med* 2000; 6:916–919.
47. DeMattos RB, Bales KR, Cummins DJ *et al.* Peripheral anti-A beta antibody alters CNS and plasma A beta clearance and decreases brain A beta burden in a mouse model of Alzheimer's disease. *Proc Natl Acad Sci USA* 2001; 98:8850–8855.
48. Janus C, Pearson J, McLaurin J *et al.* A beta peptide immunization reduces behavioural impairment and plaques in a model of Alzheimer's disease. *Nature* 2000; 408:979–982.
49. Morgan D, Diamond DM, Gottschall PE *et al.* A beta peptide vaccination prevents memory loss in an animal model of Alzheimer's disease. *Nature* 2000; 408:982–985.
50. Schenk D, Barbour R, Dunn W *et al.* Immunization with amyloid-beta attenuates Alzheimer-disease-like pathology in the PDAPP mouse. *Nature* 1999; 400:173–177.
51. Orgogozo JM, Gilman S, Dartigues JF *et al.* Subacute meningoencephalitis in a subset of patients with AD after Abeta42 immunization. *Neurology* 2003; 61:46–54.
52. Nicoll JA, Wilkinson D, Holmes C *et al.* Neuropathology of human Alzheimer disease after immunization with amyloid-beta peptide: a case report. *Nat Med* 2003; 9:448–452.
53. Ferrer I, Boada Rovira M *et al.* Neuropathology and pathogenesis of encephalitis following amyloid-beta immunization in Alzheimer's disease. *Brain Pathol* 2004; 14:11–20.
54. Fox NC, Black RS, Gilman S *et al.* Effects of Abeta immunization (AN1792) on MRI measures of cerebral volume in Alzheimer disease. *Neurology* 2005; 64:1563–1572.
55. Gilman S, Koller M, Black RS *et al.* Clinical effects of Abeta immunization (AN1792) in patients with AD in an interrupted trial. *Neurology* 2005; 64:1553–1562.
56. Schenk D. Amyloid-beta immunotherapy for Alzheimer's disease: the end of the beginning. *Nat Rev Neurosci* 2002; 3:824–828.
57. Svensson AL, Nordberg A. Beta-estradiol attenuate amyloid beta-peptide toxicity via nicotinic receptors. *Neuroreport* 1999; 10:3485–3489.
58. O'Neill MJ, Murray TK, Lakics V *et al.* The role of neuronal nicotinic acetylcholine receptors in acute and chronic neurodegeneration. *Curr Drug Targets CNS Neurol Disord* 2002; 1:399–411.
59. Akaike A, Tamura Y, Yokota T *et al.* Nicotine-induced protection of cultured cortical neurons against N-methyl-D-aspartate receptor-mediated glutamate cytotoxicity. *Brain Res* 1994; 644:181–187.
60. Marin P, Maus M, Desagher S *et al.* Nicotine protects cultured striatal neurones against N-methyl-D-aspartate receptor-mediated neurotoxicity. *Neuroreport* 1994; 5:1977–1980.

61. Yamashita H, Nakamura S. Nicotine rescues PC12 cells from death induced by nerve growth factor deprivation. *Neurosci Lett* 1996; 213:145–147.
62. Kihara T, Shimohama S, Sawada H *et al.* Nicotinic receptor stimulation protects neurons against beta-amyloid toxicity. *Ann Neurol* 1997; 42:159–163.
63. Kihara T, Shimohama S, Urushitani M *et al.* Stimulation of alpha4beta2 nicotinic acetylcholine receptors inhibits beta-amyloid toxicity. *Brain Res* 1998; 792:331–334.
64. Kukull WA. The association between smoking and Alzheimer's disease: effects of study design and bias. *Biol Psychiatry* 2001; 49:194–199.
65. Court JA, Johnson M, Religa D *et al.* Attenuation of Abeta deposition in the entorhinal cortex of normal elderly individuals associated with tobacco smoking. *Neuropathol Appl Neurobiol* 2005; 31:522–535.
66. HellströmLindahl E, Mousavi M, Ravid R, Nordberg A. Reduced levels of Abeta 40 and Abeta 42 in brains of smoking controls and Alzheimer's patients. *Neurobiol Dis* 2004; 15:351–360.
67. Perry E, Martin-Ruiz C, Lee M *et al.* Nicotinic receptor subtypes in human brain ageing, Alzheimer and Lewy body diseases. *Eur J Pharmacol* 2000; 393:215–222.
68. Ulrich J, Johannson-Locher G, Seiler WO *et al.* Does smoking protect from Alzheimer's disease? Alzheimer-type changes in 301 unselected brains from patients with known smoking history. *Acta Neuropathol (Berl)* 1997; 94:450–454.
69. Nordberg A, HellströmLindahl E, Lee M, *et al.* Chronic nicotine treatment reduces beta-amyloidosis in the brain of a mouse model of Alzheimer's disease (APPsw). *J Neurochem* 2002; 81:655–658.
70. Unger C, Svedberg MM, Yu WF *et al.* Effect of Subchronic treatment of memantine, galantamine and nicotine in the brain of APPswe transgenic mice. *J Pharmacol Exp Ther* 2006; 317:30–36.
71. Oddo S, Caccamo A, Green KN *et al.* Chronic nicotine administration exacerbates tau pathology in a transgenic model of Alzheimer's disease. *Proc Natl Acad Sci USA* 2005; 102:3046–3051.
72. Hellström-Lindahl E, Moore H *et al.* Increased levels of tau protein in SH-SY5Y cells after treatment with cholinesterase inhibitors and nicotinic agonists. *J Neurochem* 2000; 74:777–784.
73. Ono K, Hasegawa K, Yamada M *et al.* Nicotine breaks down preformed Alzheimer's beta-amyloid fibrils in vitro. *Biol Psychiatry* 2002; 52:880–886.
74. Moore SA, Huckerby TN, Gibson GL *et al.* Both the D-(+) and L-(−) enantiomers of nicotine inhibit Abeta aggregation and cytotoxicity. *Biochemistry* 2004; 43:819–826.
75. Hellström-Lindahl E, Court J, Keverne J *et al.* Nicotine reduces A beta in the brain and cerebral vessels of APPsw mice. *Eur J Neurosci* 2004; 19:2703–2710.
76. Dineley KT, Westerman M, Bui D *et al.* Beta-amyloid activates the mitogen-activated protein kinase cascade via hippocampal alpha7 nicotinic acetylcholine receptors: In vitro and in vivo mechanisms related to Alzheimer's disease. *J Neurosci* 2001; 21:4125–4133.
77. Nagele RG, D'Andrea MR, Anderson WJ *et al.* Intracellular accumulation of beta-amyloid(1–42) in neurons is facilitated by the alpha 7 nicotinic acetylcholine receptor in Alzheimer's disease. *Neuroscience* 2002; 110:199–211.
78. Pettit DL, Shao Z, Yakel JL. beta-Amyloid(1–42) peptide directly modulates nicotinic receptors in the rat hippocampal slice. *J Neurosci* 2001; 21:RC120.
79. Wang HY, Lee DH, D'Andrea MR, *et al.* beta-Amyloid(1–42) binds to alpha7 nicotinic acetylcholine receptor with high affinity. Implications for Alzheimer's disease pathology. *J Biol Chem* 2000; 275:5626–5632.
80. Cuello AC. Intracellular and extracellular Abeta, a tale of two neuropathologies. *Brain Pathol* 2005; 15:66–71.
81. Luth HJ, Apelt J, Ihunwo AO *et al.* Degeneration of beta-amyloid-associated cholinergic structures in transgenic APP SW mice. *Brain Res* 2003; 977:16–22.
82. Snyder EM, Nong Y, Almeida CG *et al.* Regulation of NMDA receptor trafficking by amyloid-beta. *Nat Neurosci* 2005; 8:1051–1058.
83. Svensson AL, Nordberg A. Tacrine and donepezil attenuate the neurotoxic effect of A beta(25–35) in rat PC12 cells. *Neuroreport* 1998; 9:1519–1522.
84. Arias E, Gallego-Sandin S, Villarroya M *et al.* Unequal neuroprotection afforded by the acetylcholinesterase inhibitors galantamine, donepezil, and rivastigmine in SH-SY5Y neuroblastoma cells: role of nicotinic receptors. *J Pharmacol Exp Ther* 2005; 315:1346–1353.
85. Arias E, Ales E, Gabilan NH *et al.* Galantamine prevents apoptosis induced by beta-amyloid and thapsigargin: involvement of nicotinic acetylcholine receptors. *Neuropharmacology* 2004; 46:103–114.
86. Kihara T, Sawada H, Nakamizo T *et al.* Galantamine modulates nicotinic receptor and blocks Abeta-enhanced glutamate toxicity. *Biochem Biophys Res Commun* 2004; 325:976–982.

87. Takada Y, Yonezawa A, Kume T *et al*. Nicotinic acetylcholine receptor-mediated neuroprotection by donepezil against glutamate neurotoxicity in rat cortical neurons. *J Pharmacol Exp Ther* 2003; 306:772–777.
88. Kihara T, Shimohama S, Sawada H *et al*. alpha 7 nicotinic receptor transduces signals to phosphatidylinositol 3-kinase to block A beta-amyloid-induced neurotoxicity. *J Biol Chem* 2001; 276:13541–13546.
89. Shimohama S, Akaike A, Kimura J. Nicotine-induced protection against glutamate cytotoxicity. Nicotinic cholinergic receptor-mediated inhibition of nitric oxide formation. *Ann N Y Acad Sci* 1996; 777:356–361.
90. Zamani MR, Allen YS, Owen GP *et al*. Nicotine modulates the neurotoxic effect of beta-amyloid protein(25–35) in hippocampal cultures. *Neuroreport* 1997; 8:513–517.
91. Jonnala RR, Buccafusco JJ. Relationship between the increased cell surface alpha7 nicotinic receptor expression and neuroprotection induced by several nicotinic receptor agonists. *J Neurosci Res* 2001; 66:565–572.

# 11

# Butyrylcholinesterase

*M. R. Farlow*

## INTRODUCTION

Acetylcholine is a neurotransmitter with major roles in learning and memory in both mice and men. Deficits in cognitive functioning are a major feature in Alzheimer's disease (AD). Up to 90% of cholinergic neurones may be lost as the illness progresses [1]. The most successful symptomatic approach to treating cognitive symptoms in AD is focused on raising levels of acetylcholine, primarily by blocking the enzymes (cholinesterases) that metabolize this neurotransmitter.

Two major forms of cholinesterase are found in the brain and spinal cord. The most common form, acetylcholinesterase (AChE), is responsible for 90–95% of activity in the central nervous system in normal individuals, while butyrylcholinesterase (BuChE) is responsible for almost all of the remainder [2]. Butylcholine is not a substrate normally present in mammalian brain, but rather a synthetic chemical that allows initial differentiation of BuChE. AChE and BuChE share 65% sequence homology, but the encoding genes are at entirely different sites on chromosomes 7 (7q22) and 3 (3q26), respectively [3]. Both AChE and BuChE are very efficient at hydrolysing acetylcholine and are both thought to have parallel functions in hydrolysing this neurotransmitter at the synapse [4]. It has been suggested that the primary physiological role of BuChE is to hydrolyse excess acetylcholine [5]. Support for this hypothesis comes from experiments demonstrating that BuChE in brain clearly hydrolyses acetylthiocholine (a surrogate for acetylcholine that can be easily measured) in the presence of an acetycholine-specific inhibitor [4]. AChE has greater catalytic activity at low concentrations of acetylcholine and the activity of BuChE is greater at much higher concentrations of this neurotransmitter [3, 6]. Both of these enzymes have a deep hydrophobic gorge where acetycholine is thought to enter by diffusion and to be cleaved. Differences in several amino acids in this gorge are thought to underlie the ability of BuChE to hydrolyse several different molecules beyond acetylcholine [7]. A peripheral anionic site also exists for both enzymes and weaker affinity of this site for many ligands may contribute to the greater diversity of molecules that are hydrolysed by BuChE. AChE is also more specific for acetylcholine than BuChE, but BuChE also metabolizes a number of other neuroactive peptides [7]. Classically AChE is thought to be produced primarily by neurones and to be active chiefly at the synapse, playing a major role in regulating neurotransmission.

BuChE is synthesized in many tissues including heart, lungs, liver and brain. In the brain it is predominantly produced by glial cells and it has been demonstrated to have other less well-known actions including roles in modulating lipid metabolism, myelin maintenance, inflammation, and in regulation of amyloid precursor protein (APP) processing [8–12]. It has become clear from recent neuropathological studies that substantial amounts of BuChE activity

**Martin R. Farlow**, MD, Professor and Vice Chairman for Research, Department of Neurology, Indiana University School of Medicine, Indianapolis, Indiana, USA

are present in the hippocampus, amygdala and other neocortical areas which are known to receive cholinergic input. Much of the enzyme is located in glia, but it diffuses to the synapse where it appears to be enzymatically active and capable of hydrolysing acetylcholine.

## CHANGES IN BuChE WITH AGEING AND DEMENTIA

BuChE activity in the brain progressively increases past the age of 60 years in an age-dependent manner [5].

Alternative splicing for both AChE and BuChE, each of which is encoded by a different single gene, gives multiple forms including; an asymmetric form of AChE with tail that anchors to cell membranes and globular forms G1, G2, and G4 with one, two, and four active catalytic sites, respectively [13]. In an analogous manner, BuChE is also found in G1, G2 and G4 forms [2]. The G4 form of AChE which is predominantly at the synapse in the normal brain may be reduced in AD by as much as 90% in some areas of the brain. This reduction is primarily due to loss of the G4 form at presynaptic sites of cholinergic synapses in the brain [14]. Overall AChE levels in AD progressively decline with worsening disease stage by 50–67% in different regions of the brain (Figure 11.1) [2, 15]. The G4 form of BuChE which is of glial origin, maintains stable levels or is mildly reduced, while the G1 form increases by as much as 30–60% with the percentages going up with worsening disease stage [2, 14]. In areas of the cortex affected by AD, the ratio of BuChE to AChE has been shown to increase from 0.5 to as much as 11 [16]. This increase may relate to proliferation of glial cells. These changes suggest BuChE may become a more significant target for drug therapy as the illness worsens, particularly in older patients and in those entering the moderate to severe stages of AD.

In both normal and AD brains, AChE-positive glia are found widely throughout the cortex and white matter, while BuChE is localized to capillary endothelial cells and glia. These glia are found predominantly in the deep cortical layers and in the subcortical white matter [4, 17]. In normal brains the ratio of BuChE-positive glia to AChE-positive glia are highest in the entorhinal and in frontotemporal cortices (two areas very susceptible to AD) [18]. In AD brain, glial BuChE/AChE ratios are increased in these areas, but this increase does not occur in other areas of the brain. Most investigators believe reactive gliosis occurs around plaques, but it is also possible that glia in AD exacerbate amyloid β (Aβ) deposition by their secretion of cytokines [18, 19]. Certainly, increased secretion of BuChE from glia may worsen cholinergic transmission by further driving down levels of acetylcholine.

Although AChE-positive neurones are predominant, BuChE-positive neurones are located in all brain regions that receive cholinergic innervation with particularly large numbers of these neurones being located in amygdala, hippocampus, and thalamus [6, 20–22].

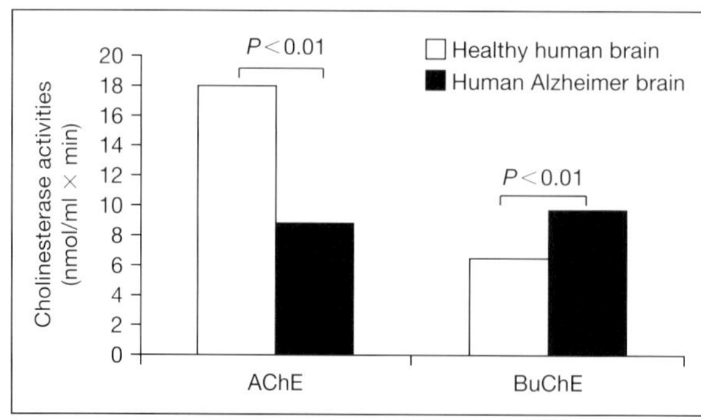


**Figure 11.1** AChE activity decreases, and relative BuChE activity increases in the AD brain. With permission from [2].

## ANATOMICAL–BEHAVIOURAL CORRELATIONS

Neuronal losses in the specific distributions of BuChE-staining neurones, particularly in subcortical nuclei and the regions they project, to have previously been associated with specific cognitive and or behavioural deficits. The variable presence of BuChE at high levels in greater numbers of neurones in specific areas of the brain and its greater activity in the presence of high concentrations of acetylcholine as compared to AChE, also suggests that it may have dampening or modulating effects on specific cognitive or behavioural modalities. For example, BuChE-staining neurones are found in particularly high numbers in thalamic nuclei that project to the prefrontal cortex [22]. These nuclei include the medial dorsal nucleus which projects to both prefrontal and cingulate cortices and is involved in working memory and planning, and the pulvinar nucleus which is involved in visual attention. These deficits are central to the AD process.

Though hypothetical, the specific geographical distribution where BuChE-staining in the brain neurones are located suggests specific aspects of cognitive and behavioural functioning in AD may be more benefited by BuChE inhibition than others, a concept supported by preliminary data in following sections.

## BuChE AND PLAQUE FORMATION

In the brains of patients with AD, there is evidence that BuChE decorates the cortical and subcortical plaques, which are composed predominantly of Aβ protein, a hallmark feature of the illness. BuChE is also found in close association with neurofibrillary tangles, the other major neuropathological feature which defines AD (Figure 11.2) [23]. The presence of BuChE, as detected by immunostaining, increases both with the numbers of plaques and

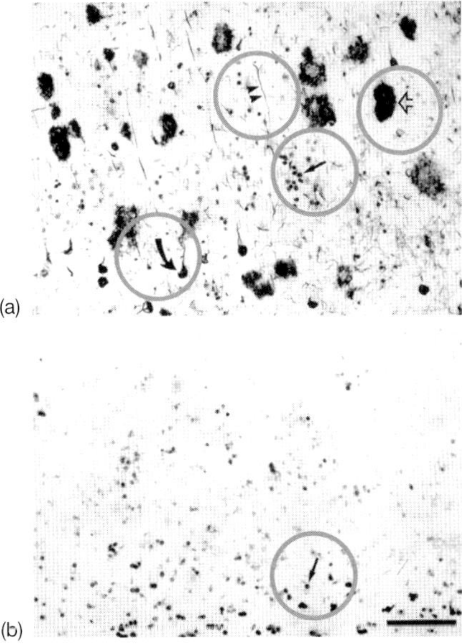


**Figure 11.2** BuChE activity increases in the AD brain, compared with healthy controls. (a) BuChE staining in the temporal cortex of a 71-year-old patient with AD. BuChE is found in plaques (⇦), tangles (⇦), dystrophic neuritis (△△), and glia (→) (b) BuChE staining in an 89-year-old non-demented individual. BuChE staining is limited to the glia (→). With permission from [23].

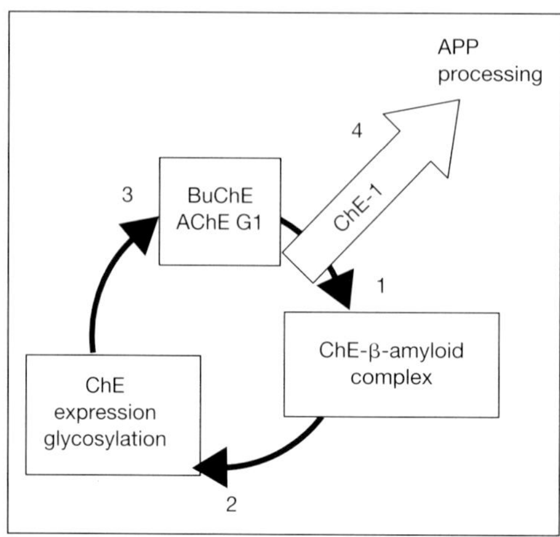


**Figure 11.3** BuChE/AChE in the life cycle of the amyloid plaques. 1. BuChE/AChE co-localise with Aβ and may accelerate β-amyloid formation and deposition in AD brain; 2. In turn, β-amyloid protein regulates ChE expression, assembly and glycosylation; 3. Increased levels of BuChE as disease progresses, augmenting the cycle; 4. Inhibition by ChE-Is may influence β-amyloid deposition and may influence APP processing. Adapted with permission from [25].

with the clinical disease stage [23]. Studies investigating plaque maturation suggest little BuChE is present initially associated with diffuse deposits of Aβ (early stage plaques), but BuChE staining becomes more prominent as the plaques become more mature exhibiting a compact amyloid core [24].

Histochemistry comparing adjacent brain tissue sections, looking at both BuChE and the Aβ protein, has suggested that in diffuse or primitive plaques, most of the BuChE is located over plasma membranes of healthy-appearing cellular processes. In more extensive plaques, BuChE begins to decorate amyloid filaments [23]. BuChE-containing plaques almost all bind thioflavin and 93% of all thioflavin-staining plaques were found to contain BuChE. In classic neuronal plaques, BuChE is found colocalized with the amyloid filaments as well as the plaque core suggesting that BuChE may play a role in plaque maturation (Figure 11.3) [2, 25].

The predominant structural form of cholinesterase for both AChE and BuChE that aggregates with Aβ plaques is the G1 form [2, 23]. The level of G1 BuChE increases in a manner that correlates directly with the deposition of amyloid deposition in neocortical plaques (Figure 11.4) [2, 23].

In tissue culture studies, where Aβ protein is in the medium when BuChE is added, the neurotoxic effects of the Aβ protein are amplified. This provides further evidence suggesting that BuChE plays a role in the toxic cascade of events that underlies the neuropathological features of AD and the potential for a BuChE inhibitor to have therapeutically useful effects in reducing neurodegeneration [26].

## ANIMAL STUDIES AND BuChE INHIBITION

Supporting evidence that strongly suggests BuChE plays a significant role in cholinergic neurotransmission comes from studies in mice where AChE has been selectively knocked out. These mice have functional cholinergic systems with BuChE substituting for the actions of AChE [27–29].

In these knockout mice, staining for the enzyme, choline acetyltransferase (ChAT), was present in the same distributions as in normal mice, suggesting that AChE is not necessary

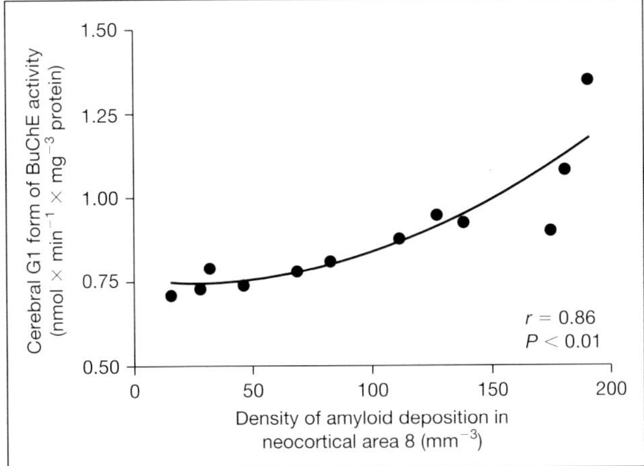


**Figure 11.4** Correlation between G1 BuChE activity and neocortical amyloid deposition. Adapted with permission from [2].

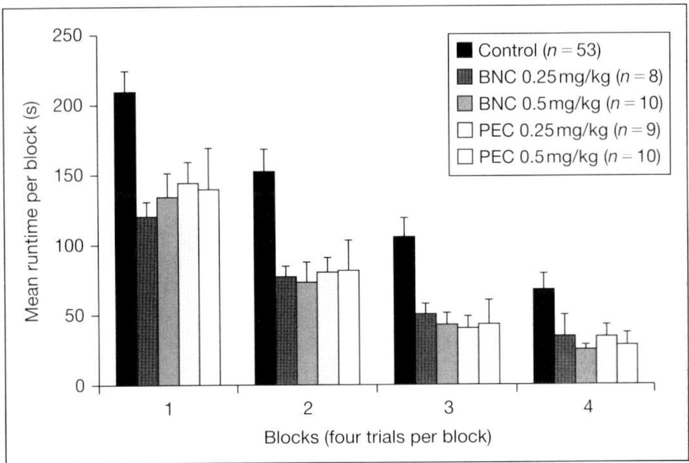


**Figure 11.5** Mean (± SEM) number of errors made ($P < 0.05$ for PEC 0.5, BNC 0.25, 0.5 mg/kg vs. control) in BNC- and PEC-treated groups of aged rats relative to controls, during acquisition training in the 14-unit T-maze. With permission from [30].

for the maintenance of the cholinergic system and that BuChE can substitute for its functions at the synapse throughout the brain allowing relatively normal functioning.

Despite low levels of BuChE in the rat brain, cortical perfusion with a selective inhibitor for BuChE has led to a 15-fold increase in acetylcholine, further suggesting this enzyme may have greater influence on cortical neurotransmission than generally recognized [17].

BuChE-specific inhibitors in mouse studies have been demonstrated to improve cognitive functioning of the animals in several specific tasks or learning paradigms [30].

It is of interest that treatment with the BuChE inhibitor, bisnorcymserine, resulted in fewer errors in aged rats running a 14-unit maze. These animals had increased levels of acetylcholine despite the fact that far fewer neurones in rat brain are positive for BuChE [30] (Figure 11.5). In brain slices from rats, treatment with a BuChE inhibitor improves long-term potentiation. In summary, mouse and rat studies strongly support that BuChE may play a larger role than previously thought in cholinergic functioning and that BuChE inhibitors may have a greater ability to increase levels of acetylcholine than would be predicted from the low levels of BuChE present in these animals.

## NON-SYNAPTIC ACTIONS OF BuChE

Both AChE and BuChE appear to have a number of non-synaptic mechanisms of action including: effects on Aβ processing, inflammation, lipid metabolism, as well as tau phosphorylation and even regional cerebral blood flow [5, 12, 31, 32].

Cerebral vasculature has extensive cholinergic innervation that plays a role in regulating cerebral blood flow [33]. Both inhibition of AChE and BuChE have been demonstrated to increase blood flow in the cortex and there is also evidence that metabolism of glucose is increased by cholinesterase inhibitors [34–38]. These improvements in blood flow and potentially even metabolism are another method by which these drugs may improve cognitive symptoms in AD [30, 39].

BuChE may play a role in neurofibrillary tangle formation. In the temporal cortex obtained after death from 30 prospectively studied patients with either AD or diffuse Lewy body dementia and genotyped for the K variant of BuChE, individuals with one or more K alleles (associated with 30% less BuChE activity) had 42% less phosphorylated tau in the temporal cortex [40]. These data suggest a relationship between BuChE activity and tau phosphorylation, and further that the reduced levels of activity found in patients with the K-variant polymorphism, or inhibition of BuChE by targeted drugs may slow or reduce rates of disease progression.

Finally, in transgenic mice (Swedish + Presenilin 1), treatment with the BuChE inhibitor, phenylethylcymserine, significantly decreased both $A\beta_{1-40}$ and $A\beta_{1-42}$

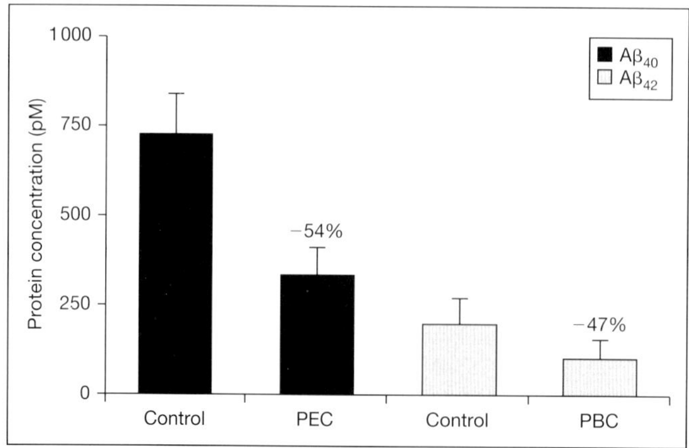


**Figure 11.6** Reductions in brain levels of $A\beta_{40}$ and $A\beta_{42}$ in Tg mice overexpressing human Aβ, after daily treatment with PEC or vehicle control ($P < 0.05$ PEC vs. control, Student's *t* test). With permission from [30].

levels, actions that theoretically could reduce long-term rates of Aβ deposition and AD (Figure 11.6) [30].

## BuChE AND THE CHOLINESTERASE INHIBITORS

Available cholinesterase inhibitors that are currently in clinical use, or that have been tested in humans, are listed in Table 11.1 [41, 47]. Rivastigmine has the most inhibitory activity for BuChE of the drugs currently used in clinical practice, though tacrine (a drug no longer much used because of short half-life and hepatotoxicity) had approximately equivalent levels of inhibition for BuChE. Several new selective drugs for BuChE inhibition have been developed (e.g. cymserine and phenylethylcymserine) but whether they have clinical efficacy in AD when given as monotherapy and/or whether their use in combination with AChE inhibitors provides any additional benefits is unknown [30].

The characteristics of cholinesterase inhibitors available and currently used in clinical practice differ markedly in their selectivity, or lack thereof, for AChE and BuChE as well as the different forms of these enzymes (*Table 11.2*) [48]. Because of differences in metabolism, central nervous system (CNS) penetration, plasma binding etc., *in vitro* studies of selectivity may not give an accurate representation of these drugs' *in vivo* selectivity and potency in the human brain.

Two potential methods to overcome these obstacles are to obtain cerebrospinal fluid (CSF) before and after dosing and/or performing brain neuroimaging using positron emission tomography (PET) ligands for AChE or BuChE as will be further detailed in the next two sections.

## CHOLINESTERASE AND CSF STUDIES

It has been reported that CSF AChE activity increases with age in normal subjects, while it remains stable in AD patients not taking cholinesterase inhibitors over 12 months [49]. Other investigators have suggested that AChE activity declines while that of BuChE increases in patients with AD [2].

In general, CSF measurements of BuChE and AChE activities and their inhibition have certainly demonstrated that activities of these enzymes are being affected by different cholinesterase inhibitors, but with wide variability in the methodologies employed, including sampling times after dose, measurement of levels of enzyme vs. functional activity, and finally differences in the mechanisms of action of these drugs (i.e. donepezil and galantamine ionically bind to cholinesterases while rivastigmine binds covalently), as well as factors such as diurnal effects, all are confounds that have made it difficult to interpret CSF BuChE- and AChE-inhibition data with confidence.

## BRAIN CHOLINESTERASE AND NEUROIMAGING STUDIES

The effects of cholinesterase inhibition can be measured in the living human brain using PET/MRI by measuring the uptake of a radiolabelled BuChE substrate analogue, *N*-[$^{11}$C]methyl-piperidyl-n-butyrate [50]. In normal individuals studies with this compound have recently demonstrated that most BuChE activity is in cerebellum, striatum, thalamus and hippocampus. When rivastigmine is administered in patients with AD, this ligand showed a marked decrease in BuChE activity consistent with inhibition not only in the hippocampus but also temporal, frontal and parietal regions [50].

A BuChE PET ligand study in subjects with AD treated with rivastigmine, which inhibits both cholinesterases, showed 50% inhibition of BuChE in both the hippocampus and cortex, while inhibition of binding by donepezil as expected was negligible [50]. Further studies with such ligands may help to clarify the longer term implications of BuChE as well as the consequences of long-term inhibition of this enzyme in disease progression.

**Table 11.1** Overview of pharmacological characteristics of cholinesterase (ChE) inhibitors (adapted with permission from [41, 48])

| | *Donepezil* | *Rivastigmine* | *Galantamine* |
|---|---|---|---|
| Chemical class | Piperidine | Carbamate | Tertiary alkaloid |
| Inhibition of ChE enzymes | Non-competitive, rapidly reversible (<1 ms) of AChE | Non-competitive, very slowly reversible (~6–8 h) of both BuChE and AChE | Competitive, rapidly reversible (<1 ms) of AChE |
| Site of inhibition of enzyme | Covers catalytic gorge and peripheral anionic site, binding to choline anionic site | Catalytic binding site | Choline anionic site and target catabolic binding site |
| Increased activity/levels of target enzymes during long-term treatment[1,2] | 5–10 mg/day: ~3-fold increase in AChE levels over 6–12 months[1] | 3–12 mg/day – sustained decrease in AChE and BuChE activity over 12 months[2] | 24–32 mg/day: ~2-fold increase in AChE levels over 6 months[1] |
| Brain vs. peripheral selectivity | Uncertain | Yes | None |
| Preferential isoform selectivity[3,4,5] | None in most studies[3,4], G1 in one[5] | G1 (or AChE-R)[3,4] | None[4] |
| Allosteric modulation of nicotinic receptor[6] | No | No | Particular subtypes (e.g. $\alpha_4/\beta_2$) *in vitro* |
| Metabolism | CYP2D6 and 3A4 | AChE and BuChE | CYP2D6 and 3A4 |
| Plasma protein binding | ~96% | ~40% | ~20% |

AChE = acetylcholinesterase; BuChE = butyrylcholinesterase; CYP450 = cytochrome P450; nAChR = nicotinic Ach receptor.
[1][42], [2][43], [3][44], [4][45], [5][46], [6][47].

**Table 11.2** *In vitro* selectivity ($IC_{50}$; nmol/l) cholinesterase inhibitors in humans (adapted with permission from [16])

| *Compound ($IC_{50}$)* | *AChE*[1] | *BuChE*[2] | *BuChE/AChE*[3] | *Clinical dose (mg/day)* |
|---|---|---|---|---|
| BW 284 C51 | 18.8 | 48 000 | 2553 | |
| Huperzine A | 47 | 30 000 | 638 | 0.15–0.8 |
| Donepezil | 22 | 4150 | 189 | 5–10 |
| Phenserine | 22 | 1560 | 71 | |
| Metrifonate | 800 | 18 000 | 22.5 | 25–80 |
| Galantamine | 800 | 7300 | 9 | 30 |
| Rivastigmine | 48 000 | 54 000 | 1.1 | 6–12 |
| Physostigmine | 28 | 16 | 0.6 | 36 |
| Tacrine | 190 | 47 | 0.25 | 80–160 |
| Eptastigmine | 20 | 5 | 0.25 | 45–60 |
| Cymserine | 758 | 50 | 0.07 | |
| Iso-ompa | 34 000 | 980 | 0.03 | |
| Hetopropazine | 260 000 | 300 | 0.001 | |
| Phenylethylcymserine | 30 000 | 6 | 0.0002 | |
| Bambuterol | 30 000 | 3 | 0.0001 | |
| MF-8622 | 100 000 | 9 | 0.00009 | |

AChE = acetylcholinesterase; BuChE = butyrylcholinesterase; $IC_{50}$ = concentration of drug required to inhibit enzyme activity by 50%

[1]In human erythrocytes.

[2]In human plasma.

[3]The higher the ratio the higher the selectivity of the drug for AChE.

## GENETICS OF BuChE

The gene for BuChE is located on chromosome 3 at q26.1–q26.2 and has several polymorphisms that include silent alleles, atypical (dibacaine-resistant, fluoride-1 and -2(fluoride-resistant) and the K, J and H variants. The last three variants reduce activity of the encoded-for enzyme. The atypical allele is found in approximately 4% of Caucasians and is associated with hypersensitivity to succinylcholine [51].

The BuChE-K polymorphism is a single point mutation with substitution of the amino acid alanine with threonine at position 539 of this 574 amino acid protein that acts genetically as a recessive gene. Approximately one-third of the Caucasian population carries this polymorphism and when an individual is homozygous, there is 30% reduction in BuChE activity [49, 51]. The BuChE-A polymorphism occurs in approximately 6% of the population and consists of a single point modification with substitution of asparagine for glycine at position 70 and as this polymorphism is determinant, individuals inheriting either one or two copies have a 30–40% reduction in enzymic activity [49].

The possible role of the BuChE variants in AD, such as protecting function in particular clinical domains, delaying disease progression and or differentially predicting response to cholinesterase inhibition therapy, are still being determined. Data from available studies are discussed in the next section.

## CLINICAL ASSOCIATIONS OF BuChE-K AND -A

Several recent studies have suggested that BuChE-K and -A may be associated with different patterns of cognitive deterioration, greater risk for disease and or lesser rates of disease progression.

A small study in subjects with AD tested by computerized battery suggested that individuals with BuChE-A or -K have better reaction time and or attention than those who inherit normal or wild-type BuChE (Figure 11.7) [49].

Limited evidence supports a link between the K-variant and the diagnosis of AD. Of 21 case-controlled studies reported to date, eight have demonstrated significant positive associations, though a meta-analysis of all three studies gave an odds ratio of approximately 1, suggesting that there is no increased risk of developing AD associated with this particular polymorphism [51]. However, stratified sub-meta-analyses suggested that there is an association between the BuChE-K variant and AD in males 75 years or older who also carry the ApoE-ε4 polymorphism. This subgroup represents approximately 9% of the elderly male population [51].

Cognitive decline has been investigated over 2–3 years in patients who have dementia with Lewy bodies and moderate to severe stage AD using the Cambridge Cognitive Examination (CAMCOG). Wild-type patients deteriorated significantly more rapidly than patients carrying either one or two K alleles ($P = 0.04$) (Figure 11.8) [49, 52].

Two recent clinical trials have suggested that patients with dementia and the K variant or the atypical variant of BuChE (both with lower levels of BuChE) had slower rates of disease progression as measured by lesser rates of decline in cognitive functioning, with the effect being significant and of greatest magnitude in those with the most severe disease [49, 53]. These trial results would be consistent with the increase in brain BuChE levels and activity that occur during the moderate to severe stages of AD associated with increased numbers of BuChE-positive plaques. Increased levels of the enzyme would naturally magnify functional differences associated with these polymorphisms.

In summary, evidence to date does suggest greater attention and faster reaction time in BuChE-A and -K subjects and lesser rates of disease progression, but is inconclusive regarding initial risk for developing AD.

## BuChE INHIBITION AND COGNITION

Data from the BuChE-K studies that suggest patients with this allelic variant with AD may deteriorate more slowly and mouse and rat studies treated with BuChE inhibitors that show

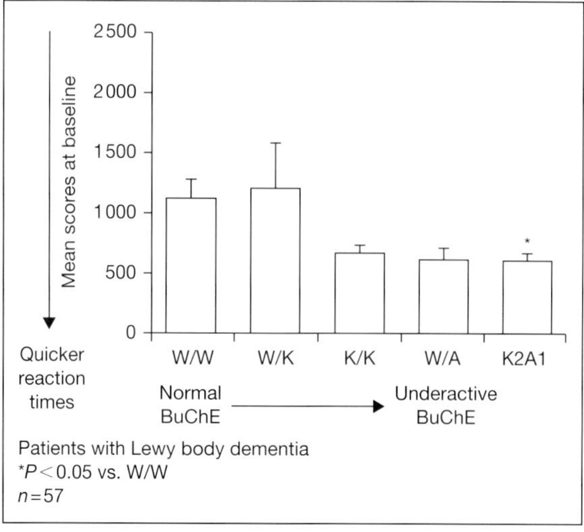


**Figure 11.7** Greater attentional performance (choice reaction time) with decreased BuChE activity. Adapted with permission from [49].

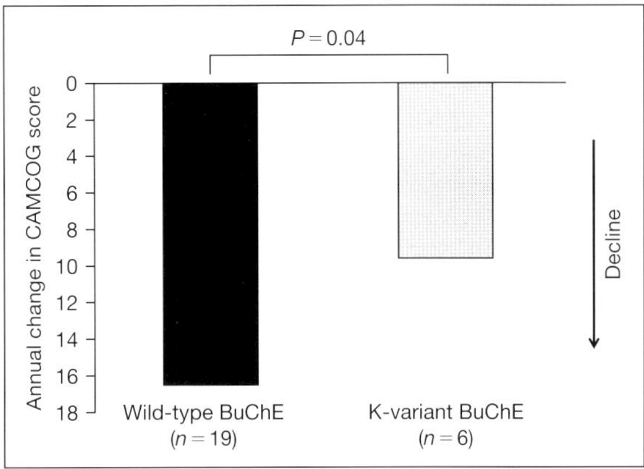


**Figure 11.8** Carriers of 'less active' BuChE have slower disease progression. CAMCOG = Cambridge Cognitive Examination. With permission from [52].

improvement in mouse task-performing abilities after treatment, both suggest lowered levels of BuChE activity might be therapeutically beneficial to the AD patient.

Indeed, improvement in cognitive functioning after treatment with a cholinesterase inhibitor may correlate best with inhibition of BuChE activity in the central nervous system [54]. Eighteen patients with mild to moderate stage AD were titrated up to steady-state doses of 1, 2, 3, 4, 5 or 6 mg BID of rivastigmine. Cognition was measured using a Computerized Neuropsychological Test Battery (CNTB) before and after dosing. Levels of inhibition of AChE but not BuChE were inhibited in a dose-dependent manner. However, improvement in the CNTB Summary Score correlated with both inhibition of AChE activity ($r = -0.56$) and BuChE activity ($r = -0.63$) (Figure 11.9), but individual subjects that showed improvement in speed, attention and the memory-related testing, all significantly correlated with inhibition of BuChE, but not AChE [54]. No correlations between these cognitive tests were seen for levels of inhibition of either of these forms of cholinesterase in plasma. This evidence further suggests that inhibition of BuChE in the central nervous system (as by rivastigmine in this study) may be a therapeutically beneficial mechanism that is clinically useful in treating AD.

As detailed above, both basic and clinical lines of evidence suggest that inhibition of BuChE may improve symptoms and or delay progression in AD. Optimal therapy may require inhibition of both AChE and BuChE to better improve cholinergic deficits.

## SUMMARY

BuChE in the brains of patients with AD is a potential target for therapy. Neuroanatomical studies suggest this enzyme is present in significant levels in areas of the brain known to deteriorate with this illness. BuChE is present and functions to hydrolyse AChE at the synapse for many subcortical nuclei and is present in NFT and also found in increasing concentrations in β-amyloid plaques as they mature. Genetic studies suggest that the BuChE-K variant is associated in patients affected by AD with greater attention and motor speed as well as slower rate of disease progression. Knockout animals for AChE enzyme still survive quite well, suggesting BuChE can largely compensate for its absence at the synapse in these animals. Further studies with BuChE inhibitors in aged rats and transgenic AD mice suggest these drugs improve task performance in various different testing paradigms.

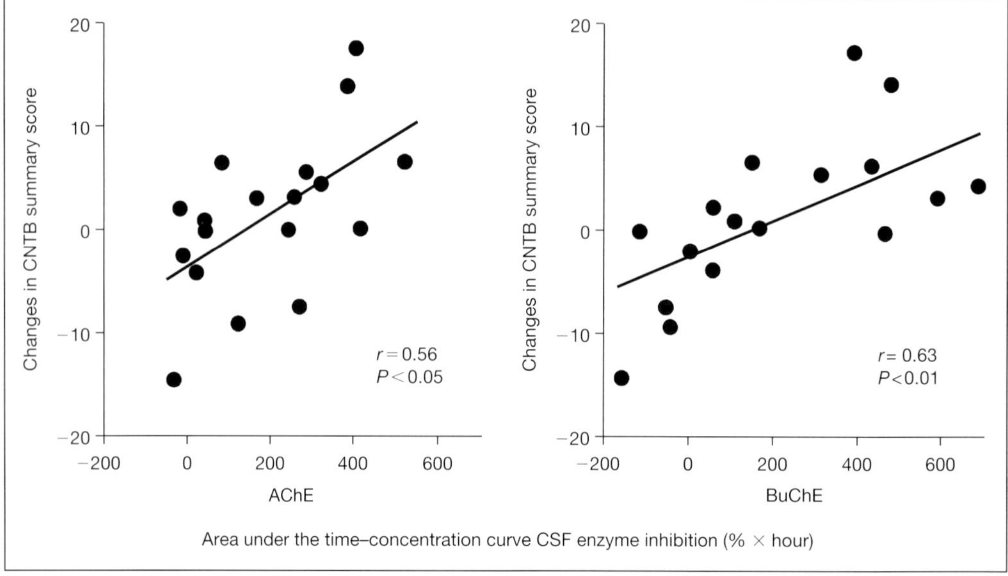


**Figure 11.9** Dual inhibition of AChE and BuChE with rivastigmine was significantly correlated with cognitive improvements. CNTB = Computerised Neuropsychological Test Battery. With permission from [16, 54].

Preliminary data suggest but do not prove that BuChE inhibition by rivastigmine (a drug which inhibits both AChE and BuChE), in patients with mild to moderate stage AD, potentially confers benefits in domains such as attention and behavioural abnormalities. It remains difficult to establish that the preclinical data, where multiple convergent lines of evidence suggest BuChE may play a significant role in the disease process for AD, to establish whether available drugs such as rivastigmine, that inhibit both AChE and BuChE are capable of providing additional beneficial actions through inhibition of BuChE, or whether this effect is incidental and not clinically significant. Future studies of a pure BuChE inhibitor in patients with AD would be the most effective and convincing approach to clarify this issue.

## REFERENCES

1. Davies KL, Maloney AJ. Selective loss of central cholinergic neurons in Alzheimer's disease. *Lancet* 1976; 2:1403.
2. Arendt T, Bruckner MK, Lange M *et al.* Changes in acetylcholinesterase and butyrylcholinesterase in Alzheimer's disease resemble embryonic development – a study of molecular forms. *Neurochem Int* 1992; 21:381–396.
3. Soreq H, Zakut H. *Human Cholinesterases and Anticholinesterases*. Academic Press, New York, 1993.
4. Mesulam M-M, Guillozet A, Shaw P *et al.* Widely spread butyrylcholinesterase can hydrolyze acetylcholine in the normal and Alzheimer brain. *Neurobiol Dis* 2002; 9:88–93.
5. Grieg NH, Sambamburti K, Yu Q *et al.* Butyrylcholinesterase: its selective inhibition and relevance to Alzheimer disease therapy. In: Giacobini E (ed). *Butyrylcholinesterase: Its Function and Inhibitors*. Martin Dunitz, London, 2003, pp 69–90.
6. Mesulam M-M. Neuroanatomy of cholinesterases in the normal human brain and in Alzheimer's disease. In: Giacobini E (ed). *Cholinesterases and Cholinesterase Inhibitors*. Martin Dunitz, London, 2000, pp 121–138.
7. Taylor P, Radic Z. The cholinesterases: from genes to proteins. *Annu Rev Pharmacol Toxicol* 1994; 34:281–320.

8. Robitzki A, Doll F, Riechter-Landeberg C *et al.* Regulation of the rat oligo-dendroglia cell line OLN-93 by antisense transfection of butyrylcholinesterase. *Glia* 2000; 31:195–205.
9. von Bernhardi R, Ramirz G, De Ferrari GV *et al.* Acetylcholinesterase induces the expression of the beta-amyloid precursor protein in glia and activates glial cells in culture. *Neurobiol Dis* 2003; 14:447–457.
10. Small DH, Michaulson S, Sberna G. Non-classical actions of cholinesterase: role in cellular differentiation, tumourigenesis and Alzheimer's disease. *Neurochem Int* 1996; 28:453–483.
11. Reale M, Iarlori C, Gambi F *et al.* Treatment with an acetylcholinesterase inhibition in Alzheimer patients modulates the expression and production of the pro-inflammatory and anti-inflammatory cytokines. *J Neuroimmunol* 2004; 148:162–171.
12. Abbott CA, Mackness MI, Kumar S *et al.* Relationship between serum butyrylcholinesterase activity, hypertriglyceridemia and insulin sensitivity in diabetes mellitus. *Clin Sci* 1993; 85:77–81.
13. Mussoulic J, Auselmot A, Bon S *et al.* The polymorphism of acetylcholinesterase: post-translational processing, quaternary associations and localization. *Chem Biol Interact* 1999; 119–120:29–42.
14. Siek GC, Katz LS, Fishman EB *et al.* Molecular forms of acetylcholinesterase in subcortical areas of normal and Alzheimer disease brain. *Biol Psychiatry* 1990; 27:573–580.
15. Perry EK, Tomlinson BE, Blessed G *et al.* Correlation of cholinergic abnormalities with senile plaques and mental scores in senile dementia. *Br Med J* 1978; 2:1457–1459.
16. Giacobini E. Selective inhibitors of butyrylcholinesterase: a valid alternative for therapy of Alzheimer's disease? *Drugs Aging* 2001; 18:891–898.
17. Giacobini E, Holmstedt B. Cholinesterase: new roles in brain function and in Alzheimer's disease. *Neurochem Res* 2003; 28:515–522.
18. Meda L, Baron P, Scarlato G. Glial activation in Alzheimer's disease: the role of A-beta and its associated proteins. *Neurobiol Aging* 2001; 22:885–893.
19. Wright CI, Geula C, Mesulam MM. Neurological cholinesterases in the normal brain and in Alzheimer's disease: relationship to plaques, and patients on selective vulnerability. *Ann Neurol* 1993; 34:373–384.
20. Darvesh S, Walsh R, Kumar R *et al.* Inhibition of human cholinesterases by drugs used to treat Alzheimer's disease. *Alzheimers Dis Assoc Disord* 2003; 17:111–126.
21. Darvesh S, Grantham DL, Hopkins DA. Distribution of butyrylcholinesterase in the human amygdala and hippocampal formation. *J Comp Neurol* 1998; 393:374–390.
22. Darvesh S, Hopkins DA. Differential distribution of butyrylcholinesterase and acetylcholinesterase in the human thalamus. *J Comp Neurol* 2003; 463:25–43.
23. Guillozet A, Smiley JF, Mash DC *et al.* Butyrylcholinesterase in the life cycle of amyloid plaques. *Ann Neurol* 1997; 42:909–918.
24. Mesulam M, Geula C. Butyrylcholinesterase reactivity differentiates the amyloid plaques of aging from those of dementia. *Ann Neurol* 1994; 36:722–727.
25. Giacobini E. Cholinesterase inhibitors: from the Calabar bean to Alzheimer therapy. In: Giacobini E (ed). *Cholinesterases and Cholinesterase Inhibitors.* Martin Dunitz, London, 2000, pp 181–226.
26. Barber KL, Mesular MM, Kraft GA, Klein WL. Butyrylcholinesterase alters the aggregate of β-amyloid. *Proc Soc Neurosci* 1996; 72:1172.
27. Duysen EG, Stribley JA, Fry DL *et al.* Rescue of the acetyl cholinesterase knockout mouse by feeding a liquid diet; phenotype of the adult acetylcholinesterase deficient mouse. *Brain Res Dev Brain Res* 2002; 137:43–54.
28. Xie W, Stribley JA, Chatonnet A *et al.* Postnatal development delay and super sensitivity to organophosphate in gene-targeted mice lacking acetylcholinesterase. *J Pharmacol Exp Ther* 2000; 293:896–902.
29. Mesulam M-M, Guillozet A, Shaw P *et al.* Acetylcholinesterase knockouts establish central pathways and can use butyrylcholinesterase to hydrolyze acetylcholine. *Neuroscience* 2002; 9:627–639.
30. Greig N, Utsuki T, Ingram D *et al.* Selective butyrylcholinesterase inhibition elevates brain acetylcholine, augments leucine and lowers Alzheimer β-amyloid peptide in rodent. *Proc Natl Acad Sci VSA* 2005; 102–147:17213–17218.
31. Rustemeijer C, Schouten JA, Voerman HJ *et al.* Is pseudo cholinesterase activity related to markers of triacyl glycerol synthesis in Type II diabetes mellitus? *Clin Sci* 2001; 101:29–35.
32. Ballard CG, Perry EK. The role of butyrylcholinesterase in Alzheimer's disease. In: Giacobini E (ed). *Butyrylcholinesterase: its functions and inhibitors.* Martin Dunitz, London, 2003, pp 123–311.
33. Toda N, Okamura T. The pharmacology of nitric oxide in the peripheral nervous system of blood vessels. *Pharmacol Rev* 2003; 55:271–324.

34. Kasa P, Papp H, Kasa P Jr *et al.* Donepezil dose-dependently inhibits acetylcholinesterase activity in various areas and in the presynaptic cholinergic and the post synaptic cholinceptive enzyme-positive structures in the human and rat brain. *Neuroscience* 2000; 101:89–100.
35. Lojkowska W, Ryglewicz D, Jedizejczak T *et al.* The effect of cholinesterase inhibitors on the regional blood flow in patients with Alzheimer's disease and vascular dementia. *J Neurobiol Sci* 2003; 24:119–126.
36. Vemncri A, Shanks MF, Staff RT *et al.* Cholinesterase inhibition increases regional blood flow and restores function in Alzheimer's disease. *Neuro Rep* 2002; 13:83–87.
37. Potkin SG, Anand P, Fleming K *et al.* Brain metabolic and clinical effects of rivastigmine in Alzheimer's disease. *Int J Neuropsychopharmacol* 2001; 4:223–230.
38. Stefanova E, Blennow K, Almkuist O *et al.* Cerebral glucose metabolism, cerebrospinal fluid-B-amyloid 1–42 (CSF AB42), tau and apolipoprotein E genotype in long-term rivastigmine and tacrine-treated Alzheimer's disease in patients. *Neurosci Lett* 2003; 338:159–163.
39. Tsukuda H, Kakiuchi T, Ando I *et al.* Functional activation of cerebral blood flow abolished by scopolamine is reversed by cognitive enhancers associated with cholinesterase inhibition: a positron emission tomography study in unanesthetized monkeys. *J Pharmacol Exp Ther* 1997; 281:1408–1414.
40. Ballard C, Morris C, Kalavia R *et al.* The K-variant of the butyrylcholinesterase gene is associated with reduced phosphorylation of Tau in dementia patients. *Dement Geriatr Cogn Disord* 2005; 19:357–360.
41. Poirier J. Evidence that the clinical effects of cholinesterase inhibitors are related to potency and targeting of action. *Int J Clin Pract* 2002; (suppl 127):6–19.
42. Davidsson P, Blennow K, Andreasen N *et al.* Differential increase in cerebrospinal fluid-acetylcholinesterase after treatment with different AChE inhibitors. *Neurol Sci* 2002; 23(suppl 2): S95–S96.
43. Darren-Shori T, Alkvist O, Guan ZZ *et al.* Sustained cholinesterase inhibition in Alzheimer's disease patients receiving rivastigmine for 12 months. *Neurology* 2002; 29:563–572.
44. Enz A, Amstutz R, Boddeke H *et al.* Brain selective inhibition of acetylcholinesterase: a novel approach to therapy for Alzheimer's disease. *Prog Brain Res* 1991; 98:431–438.
45. Rakonczay Z. Potencies and selectivities of inhibitors of acetylcholinesterase and its molecular forms in normal and Alzheimer's disease brain. *Acta Biol Hung* 2003; 54:183–189.
46. Zhao Q, Tang XC. Effects of huperzine A on acetylcholinesterase isoforms in vitro: comparison with tacrine, donepezil, rivastigmine and physostigmine. *Eur J Pharmacol* 2002; 455:101–107.
47. Samochocki M, Zerlin M, Jostock R *et al.* Galantamine is an allosterically potentiating ligand of the human $\alpha 4/\beta 2$ nAChR. *Acta Neurol Scand* 2000; (suppl 176):68–73.
48. Lane RM, Potkin SG, Enz A. Targeting acetylcholinesterase and butyrylcholinesterase in dementia. *Int J Neuropsychopharmacol* 2005; 9:1–25.
49. O'Brien KK, Saxby BK, Ballard CG *et al.* Regulation of attention and response to therapy in dementia by butyrylcholinesterase. *Pharmacogenetics* 2003; 13:231–239.
50. Rinne U. Effects of rivastigmine and donepezil on brain butyrylcholinesterase activity in patients with Alzheimer's disease. *Neurobiol Aging* 2004; 25(suppl 1):1–32.
51. Lehmann, D. The genetics of butyrylcholinesterase and Alzheimer's disease. *Alzheimer Insights Online* 2002; 7:1–8.
52. Ballard CG, McKeith IG, O'Brien KK *et al.* Regulation and attention and rate of progression of cognitive deficits by butyrylcholinesterase in DLB and moderate/severe Alzheimer's disease. *Neurology* 2002; 58(suppl 3):A42.
53. Holmes C, Ballard C, Lehmann D. Rate of progression of cognitive decline in Alzheimer's disease: effect of butyrylcholinesterase K gene variation. *J Neurol Neurosurg Psychiatry* 2005; 76:640–643.
54. Giacobini E, Spiegel R, Veroff AE *et al.* Inhibition of acetyl- and butyryl-cholinesterases in the cerebrospinal fluid of patients with Alzheimers disease by rivastigmine: correlation with cognitive benefits. *J Neural Transm* 2002; 109:1053–1065.

# 12

# Sex hormones in the treatment of Alzheimer's disease

*D. Ames, K. Draper*

## INTRODUCTION

It has been proposed that the sex hormones oestrogen and testosterone both may have effects on cognitive function, including the possible prevention or amelioration of the symptoms of Alzheimer's disease (AD) [1, 2]. In addition, it has been suggested [3] that oestrogen may moderate symptoms of aggression exhibited by men and women affected by dementia. Finally, recent research has raised the possibility that gonadatropins may accelerate the process of cellular death in AD [4], and that for this reason gonadatropin antagonists may be putative disease-modifying agents in AD. This chapter will address the possible roles of sex hormones in the prevention and treatment of AD.

## HORMONE REPLACEMENT THERAPY WITH OESTROGEN AND THE PREVENTION OF ALZHEIMER'S DISEASE – THE EPIDEMIOLOGICAL EVIDENCE

Oestrogen promotes the sprouting of neurones, enhances cholinergic activity, increases neuronal plasticity in rats, reduces oxidative stress, contributes to the regulation of apolipoprotein E expression and decreases β amyloid levels in human plasma [1]. Therefore it is sensible to examine whether there is epidemiological evidence to suggest that women taking hormone replacement therapy (HRT), which includes oestrogen after the menopause show evidence of any protective effect on cognitive capacity.

Twelve case–control and four cohort studies which address this issue are available [5–20]. None has found an increased risk of AD to be associated with the use of oestrogen, and four of the case–control and three of the cohort studies found an association between oestrogen use and diminished risk of AD. Systematic reviews of the topic indicate a possible reduction in risk of AD of the order of 10–60% among those taking post-menopausal oestrogen replacement [1, 21, 22]. However, selection bias and confounding factors may account for some or all of this apparent but modest reduction in risk for AD among those taking oestrogen. Oestrogen use is more common among educated women of high social class who tend to score better on cognitive tests than do uneducated women of low social class. Women with cognitive impairment may be less able correctly to recall past oestrogen use than cognitively intact subjects, and women with risk factors for the development of dementia such as diabetes, hypertension

**David Ames**, BA, MD, FRCPsych, FRANZCP, Professor of Psychiatry of Old Age, University of Melbourne Academic Unit for Psychiatry of Old Age, St George's Hospital, Kew, Victoria, Australia

**Kristy Draper**, BA (Hons), Research Assistant, Academic Unit for Psychiatry of Old Age, Department of Psychiatry, The University of Melbourne, Melbourne, Australia

and a history of previous strokes are less likely to receive an HRT prescription from their doctor than healthier individuals who do not manifest these risk factors.

Although epidemiological studies point to a possible weak protective effect against AD conveyed by the use of exogenous oestrogen after the menopause, the only way to tell if this is really the case would be to conduct an adequately powered prospective randomized placebo-controlled trial of the use of post-menopausal oestrogen in a large cohort of healthy women and to observe the rate at which participants in the two arms develop dementia in general and AD in particular.

## PREVENTION OF ALZHEIMER'S DISEASE WITH HRT – PROSPECTIVE TRIALS

In the Women's Health Initiative Memory study (WHIMS) randomized controlled trial, 2229 women were treated with either placebo or conjugated equine oestrogen plus methoxyprogesterone acetate (HRT) for a mean period of 4 years. Twice as many women in the treatment as in the placebo arm (40 vs. 21; hazard ratio (HR) 2.0; 95% confidence interval [CI] 1.2–3.5) developed dementia. Exactly half the dementias in the treatment group and 11 of those in the placebo group (57%) were thought to be due to AD [23]. Another arm of the study randomized women either to oestrogen alone or placebo and followed them for 5 years [24]. Of 1464 randomized to oestrogen treatment 28 developed dementia compared to 19/1483 on placebo, a result which could have been consistent with no increased risk in the treatment group (HR 1.5; 95% CI 0.8–2.7), but nevertheless showed the same direction of trend as was seen in the HRT arm. When the development of mild cognitive impairment (MCI) [25] was considered together with the incidence of dementia over 5 years the result almost achieved significance with a hazard ratio of 1.4 (95% CI 1.0–1.9), and significance was achieved in relation to the risk of developing dementia when women on either HRT or oestrogen alone were compared with those on placebo (HR 1.8; 95% CI 1.2–2.6) [24]. These results may have been accounted for by the larger number of women in the treatment group (146/2229) vs. the placebo group (119/2303) who had low cognitive scores on the Modified Mini-mental State Examination at baseline, but the fact that women on any type of hormonal therapy in the WHIMS study were more likely to experience a stroke than those on placebo is likely to put paid to future studies of this type. Put simply, the established risk of adverse health consequences from taking post-menopausal oestrogen [26, 27] is too great to justify putting the health of a substantial number of older women at risk in order to get better data on the (at best) weak potential of oestrogen to protect against the development of AD [1].

There may, however, be room for a slight degree of optimism in relation to raloxifene, a selective oestrogen receptor modulator, used to prevent and treat osteoporosis. In a three-year study of 5386 osteoporotic women (mean age 66 years) treated for the prevention of vertebral fractures with raloxifene 120 mg or 60 mg per day or placebo, the risk of developing MCI (181 cases; relative risk [RR] 0.67; 95% CI 0.46–0.98), AD (36 cases; RR 0.52; 95% CI 0.22–1.21) or any cognitive impairment (233 cases including 16 with non-AD dementia; RR 0.73; 95% CI 0.53–1.01) was lower for those taking 120 mg per day of raloxifene than for women on placebo, though no significant difference in risk was seen for those taking only 60 mg raloxifene daily compared to women prescribed placebo [28]. Although the results show only a possible weak protective effect and could have arisen by chance, there may be grounds for larger, longer studies in groups of women at higher risk for the development of AD than this cohort, who were at very low risk for cognitive decline. The paper reporting these findings gives no data on any adverse events occurring in the cohort [28].

## TREATMENT OF ESTABLISHED AD WITH OESTROGEN

Three randomized trials treating respectively 40 [29], 50 [30] and 120 [31] women affected by AD with either oestrogen or placebo for between 12 weeks and 1 year all report negative outcomes. Another study reported equivalent outcomes for 26 women treated with tacrine for 6 months as opposed to 29 given HRT, but as there was no placebo arm it is impossible to know whether either group derived appreciable benefit from medication [32]. Commentaries seeking to explain away these negative findings reek of special pleading [33]. The clear conclusion to be drawn from this limited literature is that there is no evidence that oestrogen is useful in treating established AD.

## OESTROGEN AS THERAPY FOR AGGRESSION IN PATIENTS WITH DEMENTIA

Men with or without dementia tend to be more aggressive than women, and reducing serum testosterone levels may reduce the expression of aggressive behaviours. Doing this by the administration of oestrogen prevents oestrogen depletion within the brain (testosterone is aromatized to oestrogen in the brain) and may prevent any negative consequences of oestrogen depletion upon cognitive function [3].

Trials of oestrogen therapy for aggression among people with dementia report varying findings. Among 13 women and 2 men treated for 4 weeks with increasing doses of conjugated equine oestrogen, total aggression and physical aggression scores fell significantly [34], and in a prospective study of 18 women, those who had never received postmenopausal oestrogen scored higher on an aggression rating scale than subjects who had received oestrogen after the menopause [35]. However, the longest study of this type, which randomized 27 aggressive men who had dementia to treatment with transdermal oestrogen patches or placebo, found no significant difference between the two treatment groups in the expression of aggressive behaviour over 8 weeks, though there was significant aggressive 'rebound' and an increase in benzodiazepine administration for individuals who had received active therapy in the 2 weeks after oestrogen treatment was ceased [3]. No significant adverse events such as gynaecosmastia, oedema, thrombophlebitis, rise in blood pressure or weight gain were seen during this short study, but the potential of oestrogen to produce unwanted feminization in males over a longer term of administration argues in favour of any future studies of this type being confined to women alone. At present the available trial results are too sparse to allow any definite conclusions about the possible utility of this novel approach to treating aggression in those with dementia to be drawn.

## THE EFFECTS OF TESTOSTERONE ON MALE PATIENTS WITH AD

Male ageing is associated with a steady decline in testosterone levels [2]. Testosterone reduces formation of β amyloid from amyloid precursor protein and decreases the phosphorylation of tau protein in experimental models [2]. Middle-aged men who later develop AD have been reported to have lower levels of testosterone than those who did not develop the illness [2]. A number of studies have reported an association between levels of testosterone and spatial function, verbal and visual memory in old men [2]. Small, placebo-controlled trials of testosterone supplementation appeared to improve spatial cognition and working memory [36]. However, a 6 month double-blind placebo-controlled trial of testosterone replacement in 16 AD subjects and 22 healthy elderly male controls failed to show significant benefits to cognition for the treated group, though caregiver reports on quality of life suggested some modest benefits were achieved by testosterone administration [2]. Testosterone was well-tolerated in the latter study, though it has the potential to produce adverse effects. On the basis of this small evidence base, it would be inappropriate to prescribe testosterone supplementation for men with AD.

## GONADOTROPINS AND AD

The hypothalamic–pituitary–gonadal (HPG) axis controls the production and release of oestrogen and testosterone with the hypothalamus increasing the secretion of gonadotrophin-releasing hormone (GnRH), which stimulates the anterior pituitary to release the gonadotropins, luteinizing hormone (LH) and follicle stimulating hormone (FSH). A negative feedback mechanism controls gonadal hormone production by inhibiting the hypothalamic secretion of GnRH, which modulates the levels of the circulating hormones. Following menopause loss of the negative feedback provided by oestrogen on gonadotropin production results in an increase in the serum concentrations of LH and FSH respectively [37, 38]. Likewise, during andropause, men experience increases in LH and FSH [39]. The possibility that increased gonadotropin levels rather than hormone levels may explain the neurobiological and biochemical changes associated with AD requires further investigation.

Evidence for the possible role of gonadotropins in AD comes from two studies in which AD patients had twice the concentration of circulating gonadotropins above that of the already elevated concentrations found in age-matched controls [4, 40]. Furthermore, other studies have shown that the highest density of LH receptors in the brain is within the hippocampus [41–43] and that LH accumulates intracellularly within the pyramidal neurones of AD brains compared to age-matched control brains [44]. If elevated gonadotropin levels do underlie the neurobiological and chemical changes associated with AD then drugs that inhibit their synthesis and secretion should have an effect on the progression of AD. Leuprolide acetate is a currently marketed GnRH analogue used for treatment of advanced prostate cancer that causes an initial increase in serum gonadotropin levels followed by a precipitous decline. This decline occurs as a result of the downregulation and desensitization of the pituitary GnRH receptors.

Anecdotal reports of slowed progression of AD in individuals treated for prostate cancer with leuprolide provided some impetus for an unpublished phase II study in which 100 men and 100 women with AD were treated with leuprolide or placebo for 12 months. As those who received active treatment tolerated it well and declined more slowly than those on placebo, a large international multicentre study funded by the US based Voyager company is now underway to test the hypothesis that individuals treated with leuprolide implants and concomitant cholinesterase therapy will show a significant amelioration of their cognitive decline compared to AD patients treated with cholinesterase inhibitors alone. Results should be available by 2008.

## SUMMARY

As has happened before in the history of research on AD, encouraging epidemiological findings have not yet been translated into effective therapy to prevent AD or ameliorate the course of established disease. Raloxifene and leuprolide show some promise, but at present any woman considering the consumption of post-menopausal oestrogen with its attendant risks should weigh up the potential benefits upon her bones and gynaecological apparatus well ahead of any putative and unproven benefits on cognition. The possibility that oestrogen taken after the menopause may raise the risk of contracting dementia cannot be excluded. Testosterone should only be prescribed for the treatment of AD as part of evaluative ethics committee approved trials.

## REFERENCES

1. Almeida OP, Flicker L. Association between hormone replacement therapy and dementia. Is it time to forget? *Int Psychogeriatr* 2005; 17:155–164.
2. Lu PH, Masterman DA, Mulnard R *et al.* Effects of testosterone on cognition and mood in male patients with mild Alzheimer disease and healthy elderly men. *Arch Neurol* 2006; 63:1–9.
3. Hall KA, Keks NA, O'Connor DW. Transdermal estrogen patches for aggressive behavior in male patients with dementia: a randomized, controlled trial. *Int Psychogeriatr* 2005; 17:165–178.
4. Bowen RL, Isley JP, Atkinson RL. An association of elevated serum gonadotropin concentrations and Alzheimer disease? *J Neuroendocrinol* 2000; 12:351–354.

5. Heyman A, Wilkinson WE, Stafford JA, Helsm MJ, Sgmon AH, Weinburg T. Alzheimer's disease: a study of epidemiological aspects. *Ann Neurol* 1984; 15:335–341.
6. Amaducci LA, Fratiglioni L, Rocca WA *et al.* Risk factors for clinically diagnosed Alzheimer's disease: a case-control study of an Italian population. *Neurology* 1986; 36:922–931.
7. Broe GA, Henderson AS, Creasey H *et al.* A case-control study of Alzheimer's disease in Australia. *Neurology* 1990; 40:262–267.
8. Graves AB, White E, Koepsell TD *et al.* A case-control study of Alzheimer's disease. *Ann Neurol* 1990; 28:766–774.
9. Brenner DE, Kukull WA, Stergachis A *et al.* Postmenopausal estrogen replacement therapy and the risk of Alzheimer's disease: a population-based case-control study. *Am J Epidemiol* 1994; 140:262–267.
10. Henderson VW, Paganini-Hill A, Emanuel CK, Dunn ME, Buckwalter JG. Estrogen replacement therapy in older women. Comparisons between Alzheimer's disease cases and nondemented control subjects. *Arch Neurol* 1994; 51:896–900.
11. Mortel KF, Meyer JS. Lack of postmenopausal estrogen replacement therapy and the risk of dementia. *J Neuropsychiatry Clin Neurosci* 1995; 7:334–337.
12. Paganini-Hill A, Henderson VW. Estrogen replacement therapy and risk of Alzheimer's disease. *Arch Intern Med* 1996; 156:2213–2227.
13. Harwood DG, Barker WW, Loewenstein *et al.* A cross-ethnic analysis of risk factors for AD in white Hispanics and white non-Hispanics. *Neurology* 1999; 52:551–556.
14. Waring SC, Rocca WA, Petersen RC, O'Brien PC, Tangalos EG, Kokmen E. Postmenopausal estrogen replacement therapy and risk of AD: a population-based study. *Neurology* 1999; 52:965–970.
15. Slooter AJ, Bronzova J, Witteman JC, Van Broeckhoven C, Hofman A, van Duijn CM. Oestrogen use and early onset Alzheimer's disease: a population-based study. *J Neurol Neurosurg Psychiatry* 1999; 67:779–781.
16. Seshadri S, Zornberg GL, Derby LE, Myers MW, Jick H, Drachman DA. Postmenopausal estrogen replacement therapy and the risk of Alzheimer's disease. *Arch Neurol* 2001; 58:435–440.
17. Tang MX, Jacobs D, Stern Y *et al.* Effect of oestrogen during menopause on risk and age at onset of Alzheimer's disease. *Lancet* 1996; 348:429–432.
18. Kawas C, Resnick S, Morrison A *et al.* A prospective study of estrogen replacement therapy and the risk of developing Alzheimer's disease: the Baltimore Longitudinal study of ageing. *Neurology* 1997; 48:1517–1521.
19. Zandi PP, Carlson MC, Plassman BL *et al.* Hormone replacement therapy and incidence of Alzheimer disease in older women: the Cache County study. *JAMA* 2002; 288:2123–2129.
20. Lindsay J, Laurin D, Verreault D *et al.* Risk factors for Alzheimer's disease: a prospective analysis from the Canadian study of health and aging. *Am J Epidemiol* 2002; 156:445–453.
21. LeBlanc ES, Janowsky J, Chan BKS, Nelson HD. Hormone replacement therapy and cognition: systematic review and meta-analysis. *JAMA* 2001; 285:1489–1499.
22. Yaffe K, Sawaya G, Lieberburg I, Grady D. Estrogen therapy in postmenopausal women. Effects on cognitive function and dementia. *JAMA* 1998; 279:688–695.
23. Shumaker SA, Legault C, Rapp SR *et al.* Estrogen plus progestin and the incidence of dementia and mild cognitive impairment in postmenopausal women: Women's Health Initiative Memory Study. *JAMA* 2003; 291:2947–2958.
24. Shumaker SA, Legault C, Kuller L *et al.* Conjugated equine estrogen and incidence of probable dementia and mild cognitive impairment in postmenopausal women: Women's Health Initiative Memory Study. *JAMA* 2004; 291:2947–2958.
25. Petersen RC, Doody R, Kurz A *et al.* Current concepts in mild cognitive impairment. *Arch Neurol* 2001; 58:1985–1992.
26. Writing Group for the Women's Health Initiative Investigators. Risks and benefits of estrogen plus progestin in healthy postmenopausal women: principal results from the Women's Health Initiative randomised controlled trial. *JAMA* 2002; 288:321–333.
27. Women's Health Initiative Steering Committee. Effects of conjugated equine estrogen in postmenopausal women with hysterectomy: the Women's health initiative randomised controlled trial. *JAMA* 2004; 291:1701–1712.
28. Yaffe K, Krueger K, Cummings SR *et al.* Effect of raloxifene on prevention of dementia and cognitive impairment in older women: the multiple outcomes of raloxifene evaluation (MORE) randomized trial. *Am J Psychiatry* 2005; 162:683–690.
29. Henderson VW, Paganini-Hill A, Miller BL *et al.* Estrogen for Alzheimer's disease in women: randomized, double-blind placebo-controlled trial. *Neurology* 2000; 54:295–301.

30. Wang PN, Liao SQ, Liu RS *et al.* Effects of estrogen on cognition, mood, and cerebral blood flow in AD. *Neurology* 2000; 54:2061–2066.
31. Mulnard RA, Cotman CW, Kawas C *et al.* Estrogen therapy for treatment of mild to moderate Alzheimer disease: a randomized controlled trial. *JAMA* 2000; 283:1007–1015.
32. Yoon B-K, Kim DK, Kang Y, Kim J-W, Shin M-H, Na DL. Hormone replacement therapy in postmenopausal women with Alzheimer's disease: a randomized, prospective study. *Fertil Steril* 2003; 79:274–280.
33. Marder K, Sano M. Estrogen to treat Alzheimer's disease: too little, too late? So what's a woman to do? *Neurology* 2000; 54:2035–2037.
34. Kyomen HH, Satlin A, Hennen J, Wei JY. Estrogen therapy and aggressive behavior in elderly patients with moderate-to-severe dementia. *Am J Geriatr Psychiatry* 1999; 7:339–348.
35. Wiseman EJ, Souder E, Liem PH. Estrogen use and psychiatric symptoms in women with dementia. *Clin Gerontol* 1997; 18:81–82.
36. Cherrier MM, Matsumoto AM, Amory JK *et al.* Testosterone improves spatial memory in men with Alzheimer disease and mild cognitive impairment. *Neurology* 2005; 64:2063–2068.
37. Couzinet B, Schaison G. The control of gonadotrophin secretion by ovarian steroids. *Human Reprod* 1993; 2(suppl):97–101.
38. Chakravarti S, Collins WP, Forecast JD, Newton JR, Oram DH, Studd JW. Hormonal profiles after the menopause. *Br Med J* 1976; ii:784–787.
39. Neaves WB, Johnson L, Porter JC, Parker CR Jr, Petty CS. Leydif cell numbers, daily sperm production and serum gonadotrophin levels in ageing men. *J Clin Endocrinol Metab* 1984; 59:756–763.
40. Short RA, Bowen RL, O'Brien PC, Graff-Radford NR. Elevated gonadotrophin levels in patients with Alzheimer's disease. *Mayo Clin Proc* 2001; 76:906–909.
41. Lei ZM, Rao CV, Kornyei JL, Licht P, Hiatt ES. Novel expression of human chorionic gonadotrophin/luteinizing hormone receptor gene in brain. *Endocrinology* 1993; 132:2262–2270.
42. Al-Hader AA, Lei ZM, Rao CN. Novel expression of functional luteinizing hormone/chorionic gonadotrophin receptors in cultural glial cells from neonatal rat brains. *Biol Reprod* 1997; 56:501–507.
43. Al-Hader AA, Lei ZM, Rap CV. Neurons from foetal rat brains contain functional luteinizing hormone/chorionic gonadotrophin receptors. *Biol Reprod* 1997; 56:1071–1076.
44. Bowen RL, Smith MA, Harris PLR *et al.* Elevated luteinizing hormone expression co-localises with neurons vulnerable to Alzheimer's disease pathology. *J Neurosci Res* 2002; 70:514–518.

# 13

# Allosteric sensitization of brain nACh receptors as a treatment strategy in Alzheimer's dementia

*A. Maelicke*

## INTRODUCTION

The classical 'cholinergic hypothesis' of Alzheimer's disease (AD) suggests a neurodegenerative loss of cholinergic neurotransmission that is caused by insufficient synthesis of acetylcholine (ACh) and a concomitant deficit in this neurotransmitter [1, 2]. The ACh deficit then is supposed to induce an impairment of mainly muscarinic cholinergic neurotransmission [3]. More recent studies have demonstrated, however, that the deficit in ACh content of the brain is much less significant than originally assumed, at least in the early and moderate stages of AD [4], and that instead the neurodegenerative process is accompanied by a severe and selective loss of nicotinic ACh receptors (nAChR) (reviewed in [5–7]). As a consequence of these findings, the focus of cholinergic therapies in AD has moved from simple attempts to increase ACh levels in the brain [8–10] to a selective enhancement of impaired nicotinic cholinergic neurotransmission [11, 12]. A recent approach in this area is the application of allosteric potentiating ligands (APL) of nAChR [13, 14], such as the plant alkaloid galantamine and related compounds [15]. Here, we discuss the history and basis of this therapeutic approach, compare it to other cholinergic treatments, and report on recent developments in this area.

## NICOTINIC ACETYLCHOLINE RECEPTORS; DISTRIBUTION, FUNCTION, PATHOLOGY AND INVOLVEMENT IN CELL SURVIVAL AND CELL DEATH

### *DISTRIBUTION AND FUNCTION OF HUMAN BRAIN NICOTINIC ACETYLCHOLINE RECEPTORS*

Nicotinic ACh receptors (nAChR) are widely distributed on neurones and glial cells throughout the central nervous system [5–7, 16, 17]. Neuronal nAChRs are located not only at postsynaptic locations to cholinergic nerve endings but also at pre-synaptic and peri-synaptic locations of neurones that belong to synapses controlled by other neurotransmitters, e.g. glutamate, γ-aminobutyrinic acid (GABA), dopamine, noradrenaline and serotonin [16]. While all nicotinic receptors are ACh-gated cation channels, the various subtypes differ in their ligand binding affinities, and in their cation selectivities, permeabilities and channel kinetics [18]. Thus, the homopentameric α7-nAChR has a relatively low affinity for agonists such as nicotine, cytosine and epibatidine, and has high $Ca^{2+}$ permeability, and rapid channel desensitization. Receptors containing α4 and β2 subunits have relatively high affinity for the above-mentioned agonists, preferentially permeate $Na^+$ and $K^+$, and desensitize more

**Alfred Maelicke**, PhD, Professor and CEO, Galantos Pharma GmbH, Mainz, Germany

slowly [19]. Other less prominent nAChR subunits found in the human brain are α3, α5, α6 and β4 may form functional receptor channels on their own or in combination with α4 and/or β2 subunits [20]. The functional significance of the various subtypes and their differential distribution in the brain are not yet fully understood. However, some subtypes seem to be selectively associated with particular neurotransmitter systems, e.g. the α6 subunits with the catecholaminergic system. The $Ca^{2+}$ permeating α7-nAChR channels seem to be located more prominently in pre-synaptic and peri-synaptic locations where they are involved in modulating transmitter release and action potentials (reviewed in [18, 21]). Moreover, α7-nAChRs seem to play an important role in development and plasticity of the central nervous system [22–24], intracellular regulation of a variety of processes, including glucose uptake, energy metabolism and apoptosis [25–27]. The link between nicotinic receptors on the one hand, and reduced glucose uptake and energy metabolism on the other hand, has led to the suggestion that AD may be a neuro-endocrine disorder, resembling a unique form of diabetes mellitus and progressing with accompanied neuro-degeneration [26]. Recently, the expression of several nAChR subunits, including the α7 subunit, has also been observed on brain astrocytes, and there is strong indication of an involvement of these receptors in the regulation of cell survival and programmed cell death [28].

## NICOTINIC ACETYLCHOLINE RECEPTORS IN COGNITION: LOSS OF nAChRs IN AGEING AND DISEASE

It has long been recognized that not only muscarinic antagonists such as scopolamine but also nicotinic antagonists can induce cognitive impairment in humans [29]. Moreover, nicotine and other nicotinic agonists have been shown to improve cognition both in healthy volunteers and in Alzheimer patients [30]. More recently, it has been demonstrated that nicotinic agonists facilitate induction of long-term potentiation (LTP), a cellular mechanism believed to underlie learning and memory [31], and that the effect can be blocked by various nicotinic antagonists [32, 33]. Presently, intensive research focuses on the questions of whether agonist-induced activation of α7-nAChR may account for the memory-enhancing properties of nicotine and other nicotinic agonists ([34] and references therein). These findings support the notion that in AD a loss of nicotinic receptors may underlie the cognitive impairment that is the established lead clinical symptom of the disease.

During the past two decades, extensive neuro-anatomical studies have established [5, 7, 17, 35–37] that AD is associated with a dramatic loss of nicotinic receptors, i.e. (i) related to the severity of the disease at the time this loss can be measured, i.e. in autopsied brain tissue after death of the patient, and (ii) significantly larger than the loss of nicotinic receptors associated with normal ageing. From these data, ageing and AD appear to represent a continuum in the sense that Alzheimer's may be considered an accelerated ageing process [38]. A similar view of the aetiology of AD has been proposed on the basis of the enhanced amyloid load and early onset of senile dementia that is observed in patients with Down's syndrome.

## RELATIONSHIP OF NICOTINIC RECEPTOR EXPRESSION TO OTHER PATHOLOGIES AND MARKERS OF AD

Independently of the nAChR deficit in AD described above, the most prominent markers of the disease remain amyloid plaques, neurofibrillary tangles and inflammatory events, and the main approaches to causal AD therapy continue to focus on lowering the β-amyloid (Aβ) load in the brain. Interestingly in this regard, an increasing body of recent reports suggests links between nicotinic receptor loss, Aβ load, inflammatory responses, and growth factor deficits.

In 1994, it was reported that amyloid peptides can inhibit nicotine-induced $Ca^{2+}$ currents into cells that express nicotinic receptor channels [39]. In particular, the $A\beta_{1-42}$ peptide, the most prominent component of amyloid plaques, tightly binds to α7 nicotinic receptors thereby activating them at low concentrations, and inactivating them (probably by desensitization) at high concentrations, just as classical low molecular weight agonists such as nicotine, do. A certain level of α7-nAChR activity may foster cell survival whereas inactivation of nAChRs, e.g. by desensitization, may induce apoptotic death of cells expressing these receptors, possibly by disturbing intracellular $Ca^{2+}$ homoeostasis or other second messenger mechanisms [40, 41]. Nicotine is able to compete with Aβ in binding to nicotinic receptors, and in this way the drug appears to protect against Aβ-induced neurotoxicity [39, 40].

In view of the above findings, it appears noteworthy that co-localization of amyloid plaques and nicotinic receptors has been observed in Alzheimer brain neurones and in SK-N-MC cells transfected with α7-nAChR [42, 43], and enhanced α7-nAChR expression has been observed in amyloid precursor protein (APP) transgenic mice [44]. Furthermore, elevated brain α7-nAChR may couple the Aβ pathway to mitogen-activated protein kinase [44] and to Aβ internalization [45].

In addition to an elevated amyloid load, inflammatory events are believed to play a major role in neuro-degeneration and also in normal ageing [46–49]. Cytokine activation of astrocytes may lead to enhanced Aβ production and plaque formation [50, 51]. Nicotinic receptors have been shown to be expressed on astrocytes from rat brain and human brain [52, 53]. Because in the peripheral nervous system nicotinic receptors are involved in the regulation of tumour necrosis factor release, enhanced expression of α7-nAChR on astrocytes in AD patients may be a protective measure, as it could inhibit release of inflammatory mediators into the cerebrospinal fluid space. Consistent with this idea, enhanced astroglial expression of α7-nAChRs in the hippocampus has recently been observed [54].

Nicotinic receptor activation by agonist can modulate the expression of growth factors *in vivo*, such as basic fibroblast growth factor-2, brain-derived neurotrophic factor and nerve growth factor (NGF), the latter two factors of which have been reported to modulate APP expression and Aβ production [55–58]. Furthermore, nicotine-induced activation of the α7-nAChR has been shown to increase the expression of the high affinity receptor for NGF, TrkA [59], a loss of which is believed to be one of the earliest markers of neuronal dysfunction. In an animal model of NGF deprivation, nicotinic enhancement is able to reduce degeneration and cell death of neurones, formation of plaques and cognitive impairment [60].

Even though a considerable body of data strongly suggests that nicotinic receptors may represent essential elements of brain plasticity and cell survival, their exact involvement in AD pathology and neuro-protective mechanisms remains to be fully elucidated. Moreover, it seems possible that neuro-toxic and neuro-protective effects may be mediated by the same subtype(s) of nAChR depending on the dose of agonist applied and the time of exposure to the particular agonist [61], just as has been shown for the differential control of synaptic function by nicotinic receptors [62].

In summary, nAChRs are widely distributed in the human brain. In addition to their classical location in post-synaptic areas to cholinergic neurones, they are also expressed in pre-synaptic and peri-synaptic locations of many non-cholinergic neurones where they are involved in the regulation of neurotransmitter release, synaptic strength and action potential propagation. Nicotinic receptors are also expressed on glial cells. In addition to acting as excitatory cation channels, they are often coupled to various second messenger systems and intracellular signalling cascades, making them versatile control elements of synaptic and cellular plasticity. The $Ca^{2+}$ permeating α7 subtype of nAChR seems to be the most important one for the regulation of plasticity, as it has low affinity for the natural transmitters ACh and choline, and therefore is particularly capable of responding to longer lasting tonic changes in neurotransmitter.

There is a consistent and severe loss of nAChR in AD and other neurological and psychiatric diseases. No such deficits have been observed for muscarinic ACh receptors or any

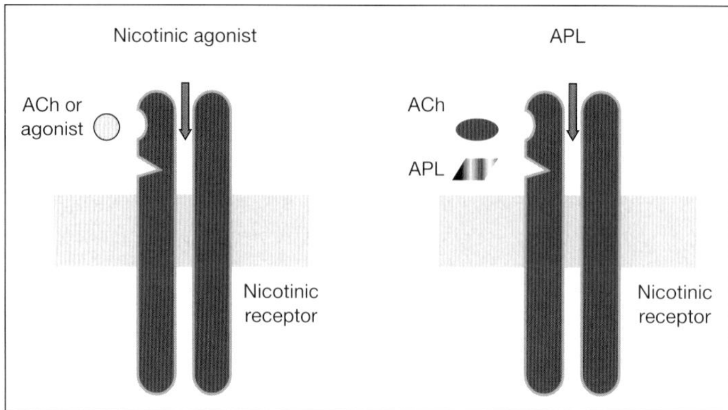


**Figure 13.1** Differences between a nicotinic agonist and an allosteric modulator of nicotinic receptors. Classical nicotinic agonists bind to the same site on the receptor as ACh does. In this way they mimic the functional activities of ACh, in the sense that they can also induce openings of the receptor channel and, at elevated concentrations, induce inactivation by desensitization of the receptor. In *allosteric modulation*, the modulator binds to a different binding site to the one used by the natural agonist. The allosteric modulator has little, if any, effect on channel activity when bound in the absence of ACh or agonist. However, when the modulator and agonist bind simultaneously to their respective binding sites on the receptor, there is a large amplification in the agonist's ability to increase ionic conductance. The result is a *potentiation* of the receptor's response to agonist. ACh = acetylcholrine, APL = allosteric potentiating ligands.

other neurotransmitter receptor system in the human brain. The loss of nicotinic receptors is particularly evident near plaques and tangles which are the classical neuro-anatomical markers of AD. There is mounting evidence of a correlation between the various markers of the disease, including a direct and antagonistic interaction of Aβ peptides with at least the α7 nicotinic receptor. These findings argue for a selectively nicotinic drug therapy for senile dementia, as has been proposed recently [12, 14] and will be discussed in the following subchapter.

## ALLOSTERIC SENSITIZATION OF NICOTINIC ACETYLCHOLINE RECEPTORS

### *MECHANISM OF ALLOSTERIC SENSITIZATION*

APL are a distinct class of nicotinic receptor ligands that are defined by their action as follows: They 'significantly increase the frequency of opening of nicotinic receptor channels and potentiate agonist-activated currents' [13]. APLs are in several respects different from classical agonists: Firstly, they bind to an allosteric binding site, i.e. a site on the nAChR that is separate from the classical binding sites for ACh and its agonists and antagonists (Figure 13.1). Separate locations of the ACh and APL sites have been proven by photoaffinity labelling [63], the existence of site-selective monoclonal antibodies [64] and site-directed mutagenesis of nAChR, in combination with channel activity measurements [65]. Secondly, while APLs have little, if any, agonistic activity on their own [66, 67], they are capable of enhancing (potentiating) the channel activity induced by ACh and other nicotinic agonists [13, 68, 69] (Figure 13.2). In whole-cell current electrophysiological studies, the APL action produces a shift to the left and an increase in the slope of the agonist dose–response curve [69]. The APL effect neither is additive nor competitive to nicotinic agonist binding and response, and it is completely lost when the APL site is blocked by a site-specific antibody [64, 69], or is mutated away [65].

The action of APL may be described as (i) allosteric enhancement of the binding affinity of agonist to nicotinic receptors, and (ii) increase in the probability of agonist-induced channel

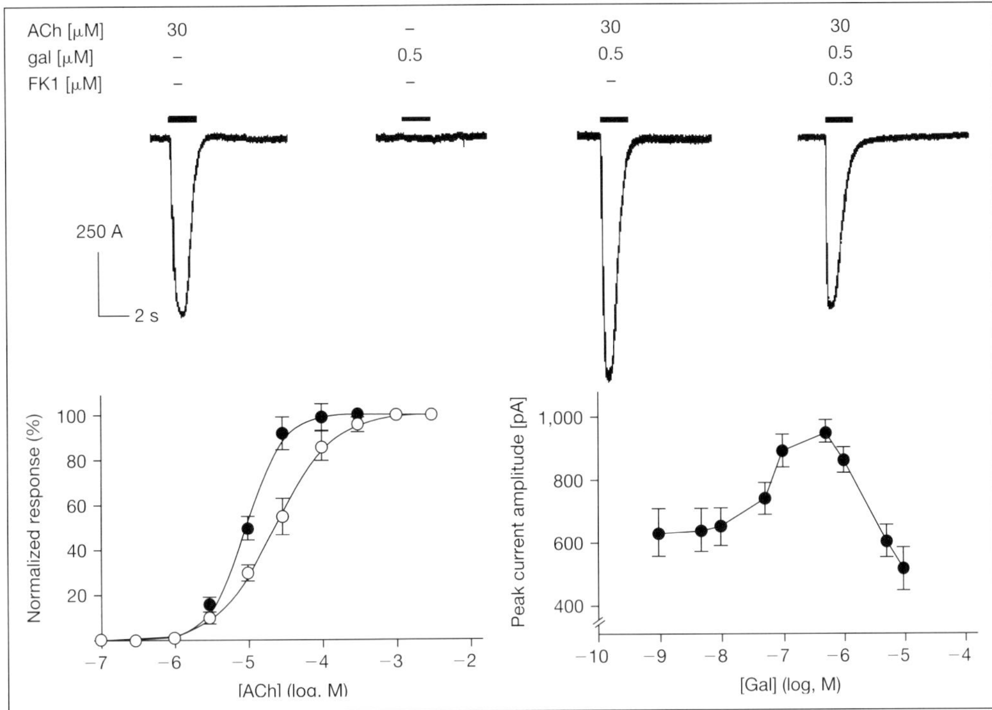


**Figure 13.2** Nicotinic enhancement by APL; facilitated activation of nicotinic receptors. Upper, first trace: In HEK-293 cells that ectopically express the human $\alpha4\beta2$-nAChR, (30 μM) ACh induces whole-cell inward currents of distinct amplitude. Second trace: 0.5 μM of the APL galantamine do not produce any significant whole-cell current. Third trace: When applied together, ACh and APL produce a current of larger amplitude than in the absence of APL. Fourth trace: When the APL site is selectively blocked by the monoclonal antibody FK1, the APL cannot act potentiating, and the amplitude of ACh-induced inward current is the same as in the absence of APL. Lower left: In the presence of APL, the dose–response curve for ACh is shifted to the left, and the slope of the sigmoid curve is increased. Right: The curve displays the inward currents induced by 30 μM ACh in the presence of different concentrations of APL. There is an intermediate concentration range in which the APL produces potentiation followed, at higher concentrations, by a range in which the APL effect decreases and eventually disappears completely. Gal = galantamine.

opening, or both. The first effect is demonstrated by the left shift, in the presence of APL, of the agonist dose–response curves (Figure 13.2), the second one by the enhanced single-channel activity produced by a given concentration of the agonist in the presence of APL [66]. A third effect is the increase in slope of the dose–response curve for agonist (Figure 13.2), which may be seen as an APL-induced increase in the cooperativity of agonist sites, or subunits, or both of the nAChR. Taken together, nicotinic APLs enhance the sensitivity to agonist of the nAChR, and thereby enhance the probability of agonist-induced channel opening. The APL action may be envisaged as a conformational shift of the receptor *in the direction of* the open channel conformation, albeit with a rather low probability of reaching that conformation in the absence of agonist. However, the APL-induced conformational shift may *prepare the channel for opening events*, in the sense that it facilitates full channel opening by agonist. Such allosterically sensitizing agents have been described previously for other neurotransmitter systems; e.g. the benzodiazepines may be regarded as APLs of $GABA_A$ receptor channels [70].

On the basis of amino acid sequence comparisons, it is likely that all nicotinic receptor α-subunits express APL binding sites, as the sequence of regions participating in the formation

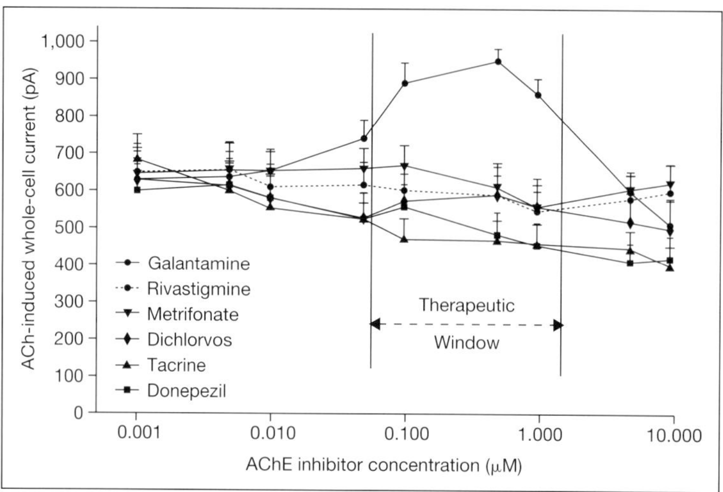


**Figure 13.3** Galantamine but not rivastigmine, metrifonate, tacrine and donepezil acts as a nicotinic APL. The effects of various doses of the AChE inhibitors galantamine, rivastigmine, metrifonate, tacrine and donepezil on ACh (100 μM)-induced whole-cell responses recorded from HEK-293 cells expressing the human α4β2-nAChR were determined. In the concentration range tested, none of the AChE inhibitors, with the exception of galantamine, significantly affects ACh-induced currents. In dramatic contrast, galantamine enhances the ACh-induced response in a window of concentrations [110].

of the APL site are highly conserved [63, 64]. Pathogenic mutations in the APL site may produce clinical symptoms of disease, and/or accelerate the appearance of clinical symptoms, as has been shown for a muscle disease in which nAChR is involved, but so far not yet for AD.

The ability of nicotinic APL to facilitate agonist-induced receptor channel opening also applies to desensitized receptor channels. Thus, under conditions of chronic desensitization in the presence of agonist, application of an appropriate concentration of APL may induce spontaneous channel openings, as can be demonstrated in single-channel recordings and, to a lesser extent, also in ion flux measurements and whole cell recordings [71]. These findings have led us to suggest that desensitization can be regarded as an incapability of the ACh/agonist site to open the channel gate(s), rather than a receptor channel conformation in which the channel is collapsed or otherwise incapable of ion permeation [71]. It has not escaped our attention that the ability to re-activate desensitized nAChR may have useful applications for nicotinic APL in the treatment of human intoxication by overdoses of AChE inhibitors and nicotinic agonists. Such applications are in progress.

During the past several years, a considerable number of compounds with APL activity have been identified. They include acetylcholinesterase inhibitors, such as physostigmine and galantamine [66], but also compounds without such inhibitory activity, such as codeine [15, 66]. Most AChE inhibitors presently employed in the treatment of AD do not act as nicotinic APL (Figure 13.3, [15, 66]). Endogenous compounds displaying nicotinic APL activity are the neurotransmitter serotonin [13] and the GPI-anchored peptide hNARS (human nAChR sensitizer), which originally was cloned and sequenced in our laboratories and is a sequence-identical analogue to the murine Lynx 1 protein [72, 73]. HNARS/lynx 1 is structurally related to large snake venom neurotoxins, such as α-cobratoxin [74], it is expressed by large projection neurones in the hippocampus, cerebral cortex and cerebellum, and it potentiates agonist-induced activation of α4β2-nAChR [73] and other receptor subtypes (unpublished results from our laboratory). There is indication for serotonin and hNARS that, depending on their local concentrations and other conditions, they can act potentiating and inhibitory [75]. The existence of endogenous APL suggests that modulatory mechanisms of this kind are of importance for brain physiology, e.g. expression of plasticity and chemical network interactions [76]. On a different level, the existence of hNARS may have solved the question of how snake toxins have developed during evolution: apparently, nature has tailored these toxins to the endogenous peptide ligand(s), such as hNARS, and has modified them to become high-affinity antagonists instead of remaining modulatory ligands. This may have been an easy task for evolution because the APL site and the ACh site are neighbouring and partially overlapping regions on nicotinic receptors [64, 65], and few amino acid exchanges are required to shift the site specificity of the peptide. This aspect is noteworthy also in the context of α7-nAChR antagonism of Aβ peptides, and the involvement of some AChE endogenous sequences in amyloid plaque formation. They all indicate the existence of peptide sequence motifs that may be expressed in a variety of proteins that are involved in the modulatory control of nicotinic function.

## *HISTORY OF THE DISCOVERY OF THE MECHANISM OF ALLOSTERIC SENSITIZATION OF nAChR, AND OF GALANTAMINE AS A PROTOTYPIC APL*

Almost 30 years ago, in 1977, Katz and Miledi [77] observed that the classical cholinesterase inhibitor physostigmine had an additional mode of action, namely weak agonistic activity on nicotinic receptors from frog muscle. These findings were confirmed 2 years later by Bloch and Stallcup for mammalian muscle. Expanding on these initial observations, Edson Albuquerque and colleagues then showed in the 80s that several more carbamate type cholinesterase inhibitors were capable of inducing single-channel currents typical for agonist-induced nAChR channel activity at endplates, at concentrations as low as 0.1 μM [78]. Again a few years later, we repeated these studies using *Torpedo* electric fish nAChR-rich membranes and a biochemical ion flux approach. After confirming the data obtained by the Albuquerque laboratory, we proceeded to discover that physostigmine actually did not act as a classical competitive agonist of ACh but rather as a non-competitive agonist [71, 79]. Thus, the carbamate was capable of activating, albeit at rather low efficacy, the nAChR channel, even when the ACh binding sites were blocked by α-neurotoxin or tubocurarine, or when the nAChR was desensitized by pre-incubation with high concentrations of ACh. In further studies, both ion flux and electrophysiological studies, and using various animal species and preparations, we then discovered that the studied carbamate anti-cholinesterases were non-competitive agonists of only very low channel activating efficacy [80] and that their main action was an allosteric potentiating (APL) effect on nicotinic receptor activation by agonist [13, 15, 18, 67, 69]. In addition to their APL activity, the carbamates all acted at higher concentrations as direct channel blockers, suggesting the presence of yet another allosteric site on the receptor, probably being located within the channel moiety [80]. The distinct location of the APL site was elucidated by biochemical, immunological and molecular genetic approaches [63–65]. Together with the Albuquerque laboratory we then proceeded to analyse its physiological and patho-physiological significance [12, 62, 67, 69].

After a seminar delivered in 1993 to members of the CNS department of Boehringer-Ingelheim, a German pharmaceutical company, one of their research scientists, Karl-Heinz Weber, drew my attention to a cholinesterase inhibitor that was at that time in development as a drug candidate for AD. In his hands, this compound had only rather weak anti-cholinesterase activity, but nevertheless appeared to have similar therapeutic efficacy as much stronger anti-cholinesterases under development elsewhere. He suggested that we should test this weak cholinesterase blocker, galantamine, in our system and, sure enough, we discovered within a very short time that galantamine was much more powerful as a nicotinic APL than as an esterase inhibitor [13, 15]. Following these developments, we then focused our studies on the pharmacology of this APL that is available from various plants as well as synthetically, and which meanwhile has been approved in many countries as a drug treatment for Alzheimer's dementia.

Galantamine has come to the attention of modern medicine as the main component of an extract from the bulbs of snowdrops (*Galanthus nivalis*) that is used in the Caucasian alps and in Bulgaria as a 'remedy against old age'. An extract from a similar plant was already described by the Greek poet Homer in his epic *The Odyssey*. Therein it was used by Odysseus as an antidote to intoxication by an anti-cholinergic agent thought to have been used by Circe to induce amnesia in his crew members. It is believed that Homer's 'Moly' or μωλυ and *Galanthus nivalis* are the same plant [81], or are from the same family of plants. The cognition enhancing effect of galantamine, the main alkaloid from *Galanthus nivalis*, has been described as early as 1977 [82]. Notwithstanding this fact and the widespread common knowledge on the properties of galantamine in Europe and Asia, a US patent has been granted in 1987 for the use of the compound as an anti-dementia drug [83]. The real breakthrough for galantamine as a drug, however, is attributed to the total chemical synthesis by Ulrich Jordis and colleagues from Vienna Technical University, and their 1994 patent (reviewed in [84]). After the chemical synthesis procedure of galantamine had made feasible the production of ton-amounts of the compound, it became one of the three leading drugs in the treatment of AD [85].

## ADVANTAGEOUS PROPERTIES OF APLS, AS COMPARED TO OTHER CHOLINERGIC THERAPIES

The classical approach to cholinergic therapy of senile dementia is inhibition of AChE [1, 2, 8–10], the enzyme that inactivates ACh by hydrolysis to choline and acetate. There are at least two drawbacks associated with this therapeutic approach: (i) nAChR desensitization, if AChE inhibition is too strong and/or too long-lasting, and (ii) upregulation of AChE expression, if inhibition is too long-lasting, as is the case in continuous treatment of dementia by AChE inhibitors.

Under physiological conditions, binding of ACh to nAChR induces channel opening events, and the enzyme AChE terminates these events by hydrolytically liberating the synaptic cleft from the enhanced levels of ACh required for nAChR activation. These cycles of pre-synaptic ACh release, activation of nAChRs, and rapid removal of ACh allow for chemo-electric excitation of the post-synaptic cell, and at the same time, avoid excessive (excitotoxic) cation fluxes into the receiving cell. As a further means of protecting the receiving cell from cytotoxic cation influx due to excessive nAChR activation, the receptor channel closes spontaneously if synaptic ACh levels remain high for too long periods of time (50 ms or more), as is the case under conditions of too strong and/or long-lasting inhibition of AChE. This mechanism of spontaneous inactivation of nAChR under conditions of long-lasting high ACh levels is called desensitization. In cholinergic therapy of AD, nAChR desensitization must be avoided, as it is detrimental to the intended cholinergic enhancement. Consequently, the potency of AChE inhibitors to be used in therapy is limited to levels that are capable of producing sufficient cholinergic enhancement, but, at the same time, do not induce significant levels of desensitization of nAChR. Such conditions are difficult to adjust by drugs that act as so-called 'covalent AChE inhibitors', as are carbamates and organophosphates, such as rivastigmine and metrifonate. In these cases, the esters formed between the acids of the inhibitors and the active serine residue in the active site of the enzyme dissociate only rather slowly, thereby delaying liberation of the enzyme. Thus, reversible rather than covalent AChE inhibitors are recommended as drugs for AD treatment. Of these, the drug donepezil [86, 87] has significantly higher potency as AChE inhibitor than galantamine, and also produces longer-lasting inhibition.

To maintain the physiologically required balance between transiently elevated ACh levels for nAChR activation and rapid inactivation of ACh after each excitatory event, the local expression levels of nAChR and AChE are tightly controlled by a feedback mechanism. Thus, if between excitatory events the ACh levels do not rapidly drop to basal levels, AChE expression is upregulated [88]. AChE inhibitors, when applied chronically, are therefore very likely to induce some upregulation of AChE expression. Because inhibitory potency and ability of an esterase inhibitor to enhance enzyme expression parallel each other, this effect further limits the usefulness of more potent AChE inhibitors in the treatment of senile dementias.

For the above reasons, donepezil probably is an optimally balanced AChE inhibitor for the treatment of AD [89], as its inhibitory potency is high enough to produce the wanted cholinergic enhancement, but it is not so high that it produces significant nAChR desensitization and/or AChE upregulation at the present dosing regimen. As shown in Figure 13.3 and repeatedly reported in the literature, donepezil does not act as nicotinic APL [14, 15, 69]. The therapeutic potency of this drug therefore appears to originate solely and specifically from AChE inhibition.

The assessment of AChE inhibition in drug treatment of AD should not be closed without alluding to the fact that not only ACh but also choline is a natural neurotransmitter, meaning that the levels of choline in the human brain, and their modulation, may be of more physiological significance than is so far generally assumed.

About 25 years ago, choline was reported to stimulate catecholamine secretion by interacting with nAChRs on adrenal medullary chromaffin cells [90]. However, it took a further 15 years until choline was recognized as a full agonist of the $\alpha$7-nAChR of hippocampal neurones [91] and various ectopically expressed nAChR subtypes [92, 93]. Choline is roughly one order of magnitude less potent as agonist than is ACh [91]. As a consequence, $\alpha$7-nAChRs recover much faster from desensitization by choline than by ACh [94], making choline a protective agent against excessive desensitization induced by high affinity agonists, such as ACh. Based on these and other data it has been speculated that early in evolution choline rather than ACh was the natural neurotransmitter [95]. As most $\alpha$7-nAChRs are located a considerable distance from ACh release sites, and given the ubiquitous distribution of cholinesterases in the brain, it is probable that choline still serves as the primary endogenous agonist for activation of extra-synaptic $\alpha$7-nAChR.

Earlier in this chapter, we mentioned evidence suggesting that nicotinic receptor activation is capable of inducing LTP [31–33]. It is noteworthy in this regard that choline has many features attributed to a 'retrograde messenger'. Because synaptic choline levels build up proportionally to the frequency of ACh release events, a correlation is produced between synaptic use and enhanced choline levels. Enhanced choline levels can increase the activation of pre-synaptic nAChRs and thereby can enhance pre-synaptic transmitter release. Such a feedback loop can produce enhanced synaptic activity under conditions of enhanced usage of the particular synapse, just as has been proposed as a pre-synaptic mechanism of LTP induction. Fluctuating choline levels in the brain may therefore be an essential element of brain plasticity in general, and learning and memory acquizition in particular.

Because tonic levels of choline may therefore be an essential modulatory element of synaptic and extra-synaptic nicotinic transmission [72], this is a strong general argument against using AChE inhibitors in the treatment of cognitive impairment in humans.

Potent nicotinic agonists such as nicotine and epibatidine, and low affinity agonists such as ABT-418, have so far not proven to be successful treatments for AD, as they all have the disadvantage of not being inactivated fast enough, e.g. by enzymatic attack, as ACh is. Consequently, they are all likely to produce some level of nAChR desensitization when applied chronically and at levels that suffice to produce significant initial activation of nAChR [12, 14, 96].

In contrast to compounds that act on the ACh sites on nicotinic receptors, allosterically acting ligands do not directly interfere with the physiological activation/inactivation cycles of nicotinic receptors. Allosterically acting compounds therefore are less prone to producing disturbances in physiological mechanisms but rather are capable of modulating these in a non-pathological fashion. Compounds that act in this fashion are endogenous and exogenous APLs: $Ca^{2+}$, steroids, ATP, arachidonic acid, kynurenic acid and others [95]. While these other nAChR ligands are also of considerable pharmacological interest, we shall focus in this review exclusively on nicotinic APL.

Nicotinic APLs, in contrast to nicotinic agonists and to anti-cholinesterase-induced artificially enhanced levels of ACh, do not interfere with or pathologically modify the physiological events of nAChR activation and inactivation; rather they modulate these [12, 96]. Moreover, APLs do not enhance but rather reduce desensitization by agonist or excessive ACh [71].

Summarizing this subchapter, selective nicotinic cholinergic therapy by means of treatment with APL appears to have several advantages over classical cholinergic enhancement therapy using AChE inhibitors or nicotinic agonists. APL treatment is not accompanied by significant risks of (i) nAChR desensitization due to chronically elevated levels of ACh resulting from too strong AChE inhibition, (ii) nAChR desensitization due to chronically elevated doses of exogenous nicotinic agonists, (iii) upregulation of AChE expression resulting from chronic inhibition of AChE. Optimal therapeutic benefit should be achieved in particular by nicotinic APLs that do not act at all as cholinesterase inhibitors, as they would act selectively nicotinic and hence would not cause any muscarinic ('anti-cholinergic') side-effects due to enhanced stimulation, by elevated ACh levels, of muscarinic receptors [97]. As there also exists endogenous nicotinic APL, a treatment with exogenous APL probably is mimicking natural modulation by nicotinic receptors of synaptic activity in the human brain.

## *THERAPEUTIC EFFECTS TO BE EXPECTED FROM APL TREATMENT; PRE-CLINICAL AND CLINICAL DATA ON GALANTAMINE*

Nicotinic APLs selectively enhance nicotinic cholinergic neurotransmission which is severely impaired in AD. In addition, by sensitization of pre-synaptic nicotinic receptors, nicotinic APL may positively modulate other (non-cholinergic) neurotransmitter systems, such as those for glutamate, GABA, noradrenaline, serotonin and dopamine (Figures 13.4, 13.5) [98–100]. Cholinergic, glutamatergic and GABAergic dysfunctions have been shown to be associated with cognitive decline and behavioural changes in AD patients [101, 102]. As one possible scenario in AD, reduced expression of pre-synaptic nAChRs could limit or even abolish the modulatory control of glutamate release which is a prerequisite for the learning paradigm LTP [12, 72, 96]. In addition, because $\alpha$7-nAChR can be activated by choline [91, 103], choline may act as a retrograde messenger in LTP [76]. In a similar fashion, an AD-associated loss of pre-synaptic nAChR (Figure 13.6) could also impair nicotinic modulatory control of the GABAergic and serotonergic systems, thereby leading to non-cognitive (behavioural) symptoms, as observed in AD patients. Nicotinic APLs, by sensitizing the remaining nicotinic receptors, should therefore also produce symptomatic benefits in behaviour.

Further benefits due to APL-enhanced nicotinic neurotransmission may be an increase in the number of expressed nicotinic receptors [104], and a slowing-down of neuro-degeneration, as could be due, among other effects, to protection by enhanced nAChR activation against $\beta$-amyloid induced neuronal death [105].

Galantamine is the only nicotinic APL that is approved by the health authorities of various countries for treatment of AD. The $EC_{50}$ for the action of galantamine on human brain nAChR is approximately 0.1 $\mu$g/ml [69]. In addition to being an APL, galantamine is also a moderate inhibitor of AChE, with an $IC_{50}$ of approximately 1 $\mu$g/ml. Depending on the system studied, galantamine inhibits the esterase 4–50 times less potently than donepezil [87, 106, 107], clearly suggesting that the therapeutic effects of galantamine in AD are not only mediated by AChE inhibitory activity but are rather due to the action as APL, i.e. allosteric sensitization of nicotinic receptors [12, 96]. In fact, the therapeutic effects of galantamine on cognitive function are rather similar, if not better, than those reported for

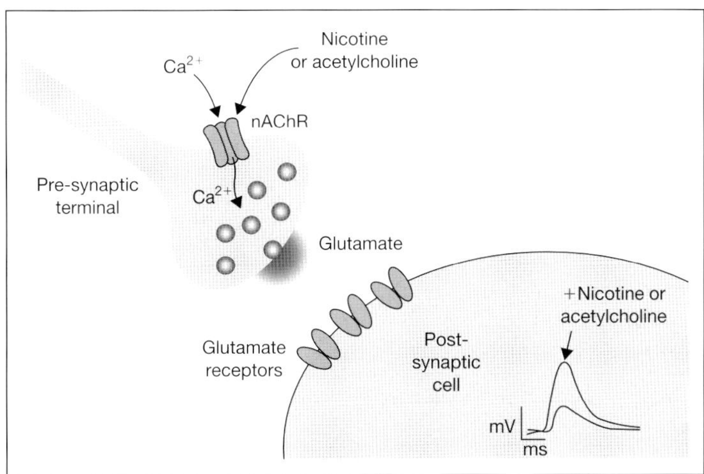


**Figure 13.4** Pre-synaptic nicotinic acetylcholine receptors are capable of modulating transmitter release; a schematic representation. The synapse shown is supposed to be glutamatergic, in that glutamate is stored in the pre-synaptic vesicles and is released following an action potential-induced activation of voltage-gated $Ca^{2+}$ channels, enhanced influx of $Ca^{2+}$ into the pre-terminal and thereby induced glutamate release into the synaptic cleft. Following diffusion through the cleft, glutamate binds to the post-synaptic glutamate receptors which results in an excitatory post-synaptic potential (EPSP). If pre-synaptic nAChRs are activated at the same time as when the action potential arrives at the terminal, there is an enhanced influx of $Ca^{2+}$ into the pre-terminal. Accordingly, more vesicles will fuse with the plasma membrane and more glutamate will be released. This will in turn produce a larger post-synaptic EPSP, i.e. an enhanced synaptic activity. In this way, pre-synaptic nAChR can provide 'plasticity' to otherwise rather stereotypic synaptic responses. Enhanced plasticity of glutamatergic, cholinergic and dopaminergic synapses may have a beneficial effect on learning and memory acquisition, whereas enhanced plasticity of GABA ($\gamma$-aminobutyric acid)-ergic and serotonergic synapses may positively affect anxiety and other behavioural symptoms [98, 115].

donepezil and other more potent esterase inhibitors [85, 108]. Pre-clinical studies on memory acquizition have provided direct evidence in favour of a positive correlation between nicotinic enhancement and cognitive function [109]. The other presently approved cholinesterase inhibitors do not act as nicotinic APLs (Figure 13.3, [110]).

When comparing the mechanisms of action and the therapeutic benefits of AChE inhibitors and APL, it should not be overlooked that AChE inhibitors produce both muscarinic and nicotinic enhancement, as the elevated levels of ACh work on both types of ACh receptors. It is therefore not surprising that some of the therapeutic effects observed with APLs have also been described for AChE inhibitors. However, there exist very significant differences between the two types of AD therapy in that, in principle, APLs act selectively nicotinic, whereas AChE inhibitors act both, nicotinic and muscarinic. Consequently, nicotinic APLs should display only nicotinic benefits and adverse side-effects, whereas AChE inhibitors should additionally display muscarinic side-effects (and, if they existed, muscarinic benefits). As it is assumed that most 'anti-cholinergic' side-effects produced in the brain are of muscarinic nature [97], APL therapy should therefore be associated, in principle, with a more benign side-effect profile. In the case of the APL galantamine, this picture is obscured though by the facts that galantamine (i) exhibits additional modest AChE inhibitory activity, and (ii) does not penetrate well into the brain, resulting in excessive peripheral side-effects (see discussion in section: What can be improved?). This situation may well have hampered full recognition of the advantages of AD therapy using nicotinic APL.

During the past several years, much attention has been focused on possible 'neuroprotective' effects of presently available anti-dementia drugs. Neuro-protection includes a

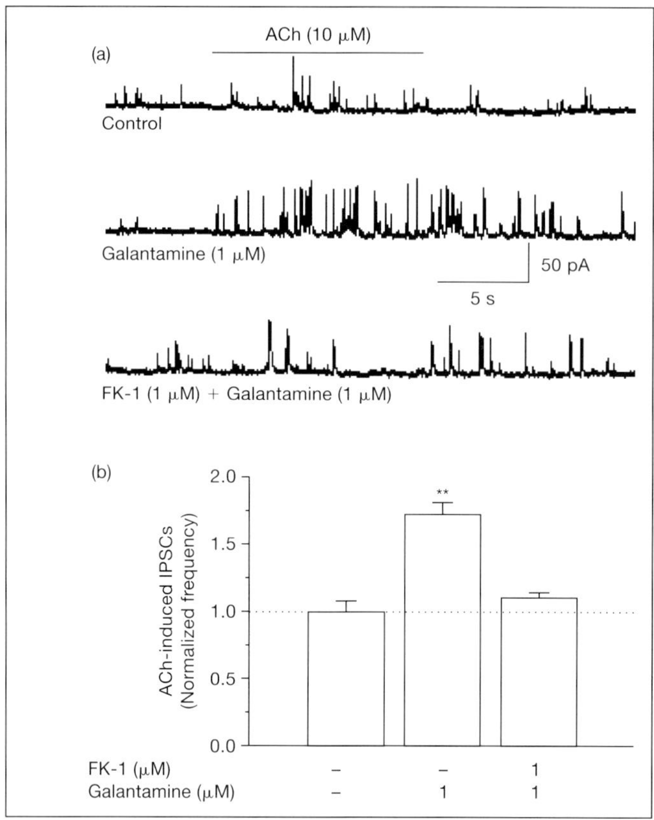


**Figure 13.5** Galantamine enhances acetylcholine-triggered release of GABA from human cortical slices. Samples of electrical traces produced by ACh-induced GABA release in fresh human cortical slices are shown. The upper trace is a typical example of a release pattern produced after application of 10 μM ACh onto the slices. The second trace exemplifies patterns observed in the presence of 1 μM galantamine. Typically, more frequent and larger release events are seen. When the monoclonal antibody FK-1 is applied prior to the application of galantamine (third trace), the release pattern resembles the one of the control experiment (upper trace). Because FK-1 selectively blocks the binding site for galantamine, without any effect on the ACh binding site on nicotinic receptors, this finding demonstrated that the enhanced release of GABA in the presence of galantamine results from the action of the drug on pre-synaptic nAChRs. The effect disappears when the binding site for galantamine is blocked, as in this case by the site-specific antibody FK-1 [98].

wide range of aspects, from protection against the action of neurotoxins through inhibition of apoptosis and recovery of a normal metabolic state of cells to synaptic and neuronal sprouting, formation, removal and stabilization of synaptic contacts and genesis of neurones. Galantamine has been shown *in vitro* and in animal models to be capable of inducing some such neuro-protective effects [40, 41, 43, 60, 105, 111]. Based on these data, a pathology cascade can be envisaged (Figure 13.7), with galantamine-induced sensitization of nAChR beneficially interfering at the levels of nAChR inhibition by Aβ, nAChR-induced loss of function in other transmitter systems, nAChR loss, and apoptosis.

Most of the studied neuro-protective effects of galantamine seem to be mediated by α7-nAChR, the subtype that has the highest $Ca^{2+}$ permeability of all nicotinic receptors and seems to be associated with many modulatory activities in the CNS (Figure 13.4). Interestingly, activation of this receptor may also affect neurogenic vasodilation, with

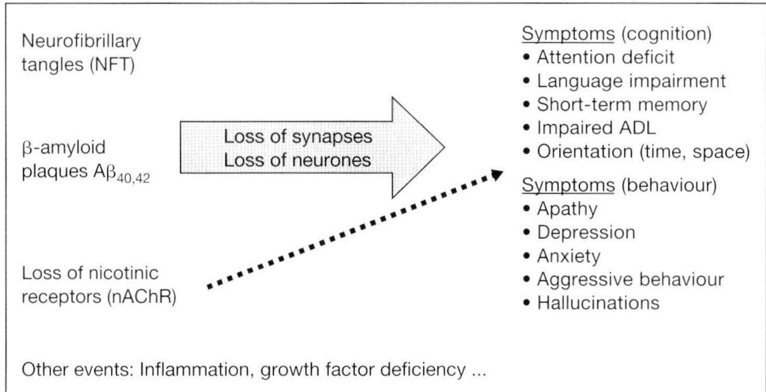


**Figure 13.6** Schematic representation of major pathologies in AD and their possible relationship to clinical symptoms of the disease. Because amyloid plaques and neurofibrillary tangles do not by themselves produce changes in cognition and behaviour, there must exist pathology pathways from these putative causes to the clinical symptoms observed. A general assumption is that that plaques and tangles, in some way or other, are neurotoxic, in the sense that synapses and even whole neurones become lost during the progression of AD, with the concomitant induction of functional deficits in the respective neurotransmitter systems. In contrast to plaques and tangles, a deficit in nicotinic receptors can directly affect cognition and behaviour, as nicotinic receptors are also important elements of modulation of non-cholinergic neurotransmission (see Figure 13.5).

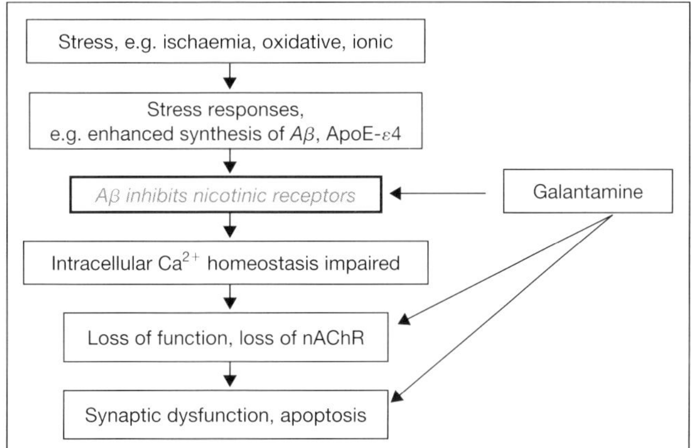


**Figure 13.7** A putative pathology cascade of AD, and how it may be affected by the APL galantamine. Enhanced synthesis of Aß peptides has been identified as a major cellular response to various types of stress. As one activity of Aß recently identified, it is capable of inhibiting α7-nAChR, by competing with ACh in binding and activation of the receptor. In this way, intracellular $Ca^{2+}$ currents may be perturbed, and this may induce synaptic dysfunction and eventually apoptosis of nAChR-expresing cells. Galantamine can interfere with this pathology cascade at various levels, by reducing inactivation of nAChR by Aß, and in this way also reducing the secondary effects of Aβ-induced toxicity, and by reducing or halting apoptosis. These data suggest neuro-protective properties of galantamine. For further details, see text.

perivascular sympathetic nerve $Ca^{2+}$-influx leading to noradrenaline release, subsequent β-adrenoreceptor activation and NO release [112]. These findings suggest a link between the nAChR deficit in AD and cerebrovascular risk factors of AD.

The safety and efficacy of galantamine for treatment of mild to moderate AD has been demonstrated in several randomized, double-blind, placebo-controlled studies, and in extended open-label studies. In systematic reviews by the Cochrane library on clinical effectiveness of donepezil, rivastigmine and galantamine, the latter drug demonstrated superior, or at least similar, efficacy vs. donepezil and superior efficacy vs. rivastigmine [85]. Interestingly, there were no significant differences in results between the galantamine doses of 16 and 24 mg/day. In a head-to-head study of galantamine vs. donepezil [112], galantamine performed better in several primary and secondary outcome measures, suggesting that the drug is presently the best available cholinergic treatment for AD. Furthermore, long-term open-label studies [113] and a recent study on the delay of institutionalization of AD patients as a function of time of treatment with galantamine, showed encouraging results in that they both suggested delays by at least 1 year in disease progression. This may look like a rather small improvement but must be seen in the context of the fact that clinical symptoms of AD begin to occur only after all markers of AD are well developed, meaning that the pathology of the underlying neuro-degeneration has already progressed for many years and has entered a terminal stage. It has been suggested that at the time when treatment is usually initiated, the concentration of nAChR in the brain has already dropped to less than one-third of what it was at middle age.

Taken together, the available clinical data clearly show that the presently approved cholinergic drugs are efficacious and safe. However, they are far from being a fully satisfactory treatment for AD, as only a fraction of patients responds at all, and galantamine and related drugs do not halt or reverse the progression of neuro-degeneration to any significant extent. This may also be the reason why less than 20% of all patients diagnosed with AD are presently treated with the approved drugs [85]. As a consequence of the limited performance of cholinergic therapies, a considerable number of other treatment strategies are under development and have progressed quite well (see other chapters in this volume). The question therefore arises whether cholinergic enhancement therapies and, in particular, selective nicotinic enhancement by APL, will have a place in future drug treatment of senile dementia.

## TOWARDS IMPROVED GALANTAMINE DERIVATIVES AND ANALOGUES FOR THE TREATMENT OF AD

### *WHAT CAN BE IMPROVED?*

We have already alluded to the different cholinergic therapy approaches available, and to their advantages and limits. Assuming that the key purpose of cholinergic therapies should be a reduction of the nicotinic cholinergic deficit in AD [12], the properties of available drug classes can be summarized as follows:

*Nicotinic agonists*: Because they usually are not substrates of AChE and hence their levels in the brain do not rapidly return to basal levels, they carry a high risk of nAChR desensitization and hence will probably remain unsuited for AD treatment. It should be remembered in this context that nicotine has long been recognized as highly toxic to human beings and that its common use as an insecticide in poultry farms was discontinued decades ago.

*AChE inhibitors*: For these an optimal balance between therapeutic efficacy on the one hand and risks of receptor desensitization and AChE upregulation on the other hand, has already been found. Significantly more potent AChE inhibitors than presently approved for AD treatment are likely to produce unfavourable side-effect profiles and human toxicity, which is why most recent clinical developments of stronger AChE inhibitors have been discontinued.

*Nicotinic APLs*: These novel ligands were discovered by serendipity [79], and their potential as drugs continues to be unveiled [12–15, 18, 40–44, 60–62, 69, 90, 91, 95, 96, 98–100, 103–105, 109]. They do not carry a similar risk of receptor desensitization at elevated concentration levels or higher potency, to nicotinic agonists and potent AChE inhibitors, and they also do not carry a risk of inducing AChE upregulation when chronically applied, as the more potent AChE inhibitors do. The identification and development of nicotinic APLs with higher efficacy and improved AE profile when compared with the presently available galantamine.

## TOWARDS NOVEL NICOTINIC APLs AS DRUG TREATMENT IN AD

Development of nicotinic APL can take several directions. Setting out from galantamine as a suitable lead structure, three properties may be improved: (i) the activity as AChE inhibitor can be removed, reduced or enhanced; (ii) nAChR binding and sensitization can be made receptor subtype-specific and/or increased in efficacy; and (iii) pharmacokinetic properties can be improved. We have set out to develop four types of improved APL: (a) APL without any AChE inhibitory activity; (b) APL with higher potency in sensitizing nAChR; (c) APLs that act selectively on distinct subtypes of nAChRs; and (d) galantamine derivatives with improved blood–brain barrier permeability. Here we shall focus on the latter approach, as it permits an unusually fast time-to-market of improved galantamines.

Quite unusual for a drug that is of natural origin, galantamine has been brought to market without any chemical modification. This is more surprising, as there is ample opportunity for improvement, in particular in regard to blood–brain barrier penetration and to tissue distribution. The only improvement achieved so far in the area of pharmacokinetic properties since market introduction is the development of a once-a-day formulation using a prolonged-release micropore pellet [114] that produces slower and more even decay kinetics of galantamine's serum levels. In comparison to donepezil, the market leader in the class of esterase inhibitors, galantamine is considerably less hydrophobic and permeates the blood–brain barrier considerably less efficiently, with the result that only a small fraction of the drug reaches the target sites within the brain and produces there the wanted therapeutic benefit. A further disadvantage is the relatively short serum half-life of galantamine which, at least in part, is due to a quite large first-pass effect. Even though galantamine is routinely higher dosed than donepezil (16–24 mg/day in comparison to 5–10 mg/day), increased dosing is not sufficient to correct for the much less favourable brain-to-plasma ratio of the plant alkaloid. To deal with these limitations we have developed galantamine derivatives (international patents pending) that permeate much more efficiently through the blood–brain barrier and consequently should produce a more favourable brain-to-plasma ratio than is reported for the parent compound.

Some of our galantamine derivatives are designed as 'pro-drugs' in the sense that after having reached the brain, they are converted back to galantamine and act as such. Such compounds can be brought to market much faster than usual 'new chemical entities', as the acting molecule in the brain (galantamine) has been extensively tested and is approved by the health authorities for use in AD. By employing modifications that are known to be accepted by the human body without additional side-effects, or having 'Trojan horse' quality, this approach should allow a 'second generation galantamine' to reach market within 3–5 years. Such second generation galantamines should have a better efficacy-to-dose ratio than the original drug and hence should allow a significantly lower dosing regimen. Lower dosing should have at least two significant advantages: the drug should display much less adverse side-effects and, accordingly, the usual uptitration, over a period of 1–2 months, of the daily dose should become obsolete. These advantages of the novel drug candidates may finally unveil in full the advantages of APL as a treatment strategy for AD and may produce a breakthrough for this therapeutic approach.

In addition to pro-drugs of galantamine, we are developing new and more efficacious APLs of which only a few are derivatives of galantamine. We have developed pharmacophores for the interaction of drug candidates with nicotinic receptors and cholinesterases, and we select drug candidates on the basis of additional tests *in vitro* and in animal models. A particularly interesting aspect for candidate selection is the ability to act neuro-protectively. Drugs with neuro-protective properties may be able to slow down, halt or even reverse the course of AD, and hence could well compete with other therapeutic approaches that are aimed at alleviating the cause(s) or the risk factors of this devastating disease of old age.

## SUMMARY

There exists a strong scientific basis for the notion that nAChRs are essential elements of plasticity in cognition and behaviour, and also in the pathology of Alzheimer's dementia. The most recent approach to cholinergic therapy in AD is the application of nicotinic APLs, of which the plant alkaloid galantamine is a prototype. Some of the limiting properties of this drug can be easily alleviated by chemical modification, with the result that novel APLs with various optimized properties have already progressed well in development. Some of them should be more efficacious and selective than galantamine, others should have more pronounced neuro-protective properties. Based on these developments, cholinergic therapy may well continue to remain a cornerstone in AD therapy, even after completely different therapeutic approaches, as discussed in other chapters of this volume, have reached the patient. An important consideration in this regard is the property of cholinergic therapies to act directly on the immediate causes of clinical symptoms which are a request of impaired neurotransmission. Because other key events in AD pathology, e.g. amyloid plaque formation, neurofibrillary tangle formation and inflammatory events, are clinically non-symptomatic, there will remain a need for symptomatic therapy, even after the causes and risk factors of AD have been fully elucidated and can be treated or prevented. Symptomatic therapy using nicotinic APLs is able to rapidly reduce or alleviate many clinical symptoms of AD, particularly if APLs of higher efficacy and better blood–brain barrier penetration become available.

## REFERENCES

1. Bartus RT, Dean RL, Beer B, Lippa AS. The cholinergic hypothesis of geriatric memory dysfunction. *Science* 1982; 217:408–417.
2. Gallagher M, Colombo PJ. Ageing: the cholinergic hypothesis and cognitive decline. *Curr Opin Neurobiol* 1995; 6:161–168.
3. McKinney M, Coyle M. The potential for muscarinic receptor subtype-specific pharmacotherapy for Alzheimer's disease. *Mayo Clin Proc* 1991; 42:1225–1237.
4. Davis KL, Yamamura HL. Cholinergic underactivity in human memory disorders. *Life Sci* 1988; 23:1729–1734.
5. Nordberg A. Neuroreceptor changes in Alzheimer's disease. *Cerebrovasc Brain Metab Rev* 1992; 4:303–328.
6. Perry EK, Court JA, Piggott MA, Perry RH. Cholinergic components of dementia and aging. In: Huppert FA, Brayne C, O'Connor DW (eds). *Dementia and Normal Aging*. Cambridge University Press, 1994, pp 437–469.
7. Perry E, Martin-Ruiz C, Lee M *et al*. Nicotinic receptor subtypes in human brain ageing, Alzheimer's and Lewy body diseases. *Eur J Pharmacol* 2000; 393:215–222.
8. Davis KL, Mohs RC. Enhancement of memory by physostigmine. *N Engl J Med* 1979; 301:946–956.
9. Thal J, Fuld PA. Memory enhancement with oral physostigmine in Alzheimer's disease. *N Engl J Med* 1983; 308:708–718.
10. Becker E, Giacobini E. Mechanism of cholinesterase inhibition in senile dementia of the Alzheimer type. *Drug Dev Res* 1988; 12:163–195.
11. Arneric SP, Sullivan JP, Williams M. Neuronal nicotinic receptors; novel targets for central nervous system therapeutics. In: Bloom FE, Kupfer DJ (eds). *Psychopharmacology: The Fourth Generation of Progress*. Raven Press, New York, 1995, pp 95–110.

12. Maelicke A, Albuquerque EX. New approach to drug therapy in Alzheimer's dementia. *Drug Discov Today* 1996; 1:53–59.
13. Schrattenholz A, Pereira EFR, Methfessel C *et al.* Agonist responses of neuronal nicotinic acetylcholine receptors are potentiated by a novel class of allosterically acting ligands. *Mol Pharmacol* 1996; 49:1–6.
14. Maelicke A. Allosteric modulation of nicotinic receptors as a treatment strategy for Alzheimer's disease. *Dement Geriatr Cogn Disord* 2000; 11:11–18.
15. Maelicke A., Samochocki M, Jostock R *et al.* Allosteric sensitization of nicotinic receptors by galantamine, a new treatment strategy for Alzheimer's disease. *Biol Psychiatry* 2001; 49:279–288.
16. Paterson D, Nordberg A. Neuronal nicotinic receptors in the human brain. *Prog Neurobiol* 2000; 61:75–111.
17. Court J, Martin-Ruiz C, Piggott M *et al.* Nicotinic receptor abnormalities in Alzheimer's disease. *Biol Psychiatry* 2001; 49:175–184.
18. Albuquerque EX, Alkondon M, Pereira EF *et al.* Properties of neuronal nicotinic acetylcholine receptors; pharmacological characterization and modulation of synaptic function. *J Pharmacol Exp Ther* 1997; 280:1117–1136.
19. Alkondon M, Pereira EFR, Albuquerque EX. Alpha-bungarotoxin- and metyllycaconitine-sensitive nicotinic receptors mediate fast synaptic transmission in interneurons of hippocampal slices. *Brain Res* 1998; 810:257–263.
20. Lindstrom J. Neuronal nicotinic acetylcholine receptors. *Ion Channels* 1996; 4:377–450.
21. Lena C, Changeux JP. Allosteric nicotinic recptors, human pathologies. *J Physiol (Paris)* 1998; 92:63–74.
22. Dani JA. Overview of nicotinic receptors and their roles in the central nervous system. *Biol Psychiatry* 2001; 49:166–174.
23. McGehee DS. Nicotinic recptors and hippocampal synaptic plasticity…it's all in the timing. *Trends Neurosci* 2002; 25:171–172.
24. Shoop R, Chang K. Ellisman M, Berg D. Synaptically driven calcium transients via nicotinic receptors on synaptic spines. *J Neurosci* 2001; 21:771–781.
25. Duelli R, Staudt R, Grunwald F, Kuschinsky W. Increase of glucose transporter densities (GluT1 and GluT3) during chronic administration of nicotine in rat brain. *Brain Res* 1998; 782:36–42.
26. Rivera EJ, Goldin A, Fulmer N, Tavares R, Wands JR, de la Monte SM. Insulin and insulin-like growth factor expression and function deteriorate with progression of Alzheimer's disease: link to brain reductions in acetylcholine. *J Alzheimers Dis* 2005; 8:247–268.
27. Orr-Urtreger A, Broide RS, Kasten MR *et al.* Mice homozygous for the L250T mutation in the α7 nicotinic acetylcholine receptor show increased neuronal apoptosis and die within 1 day of birth. *J Neurochem* 2000; 74:2154–2166.
28. Sharma G, Vijayaraghavan S. Nicotinic cholinergic signalling in hippocampal astrocytes involves calcium-induced calcium release from intracellular stores. *Proc Natl Acad Sci USA* 2001; 98:4148–4153.
29. Newhouse PA, Potter A, Corwin J, Lenox R. Age-related effects of the nicotinic antagonist medamylamine on cognition and behaviour. *Neuropsychopharmacology* 1994; 10:93–107.
30. Newhouse PA, Potter A, Levin ED. Nicotinic system involvement in Alzheimer's and Parkinson's diseases. Implications for therapeutics. *Drugs Aging* 1997; 11:206–228.
31. Matsuyama S, Matsumoto A. Epibatidine induces long-term potentiation (LTP) via activation of α4β2 nicotinic acetylcholine receptors (nAChRs) in vivo in the intact mouse dendate gyrus; both α7 and α4β2 nAChRs are essential to nicotinic LTP. *J Pharmacol Sci* 2003; 93:180–187.
32. Ji D, Lape R, Dani JA. Timing and location of nicotinic activity enhances or depresses hippocampal synaptic plasticity. *Neuron* 2001; 31:131–141.
33. Mann EO, Greenfield SA. Novel modulatory mechanisms revealed by the sustained application of nicotine in the guinea pig hippocampus in vitro. *J Physiol* 2003; 551:539–550.
34. Levin ED. Nicotinic receptor subtypes and cognitive function. *J Neurobiol* 2002; 53:633–640.
35. Schroeder H, Giacobini E, Struble RG *et al.* Cellular distribution and expression of cortical acetylcholine receptors in aging and Alzheimer's disease. In: Growdon JH, Corkin S, Ritter-Walker E, Wurtman RJ (eds). *Aging and Alzheimer's Disease*. Ann NY Acad Sci, 1991, vol 640, pp 189–199.
36. Banerjee C, Nyengaard JR, Wevers A *et al.* Cellular expression of a7 nicotinic acetylcholine receptor protein in the temporal cortex in Alzheimer's and Parkinson's disease – a stereological approach. *Neurobiol Dis* 2000; 7:666–672.
37. Hellstrom-Lindahl E, Mousavi M, Zhang X *et al.* Regional distribution of nicotinic receptor subunit mRNA in human brain: Comparison between Alzheimer and normal brain. *Brain Res Mol Brain Res* 1999; 66:94–103.

38. Maelicke A. Biochemical aspects of the ageing brain. In: *Neuroworlds.* Fedrowitz J, Matejowski D, Kaiser G (eds). Campus Press, Frankfurt-New York, 1994, vol 3, pp 246–253.
39. Takenouchi T, Munekata E. Inhibitory effects of β-amyloid peptides on nicotine-induced Ca2+ influx in PC12h cells in culture. *Neurosci Lett* 1994; 173:147–150.
40. Kihara T, Shimohama S, Sawada H *et al.* α7 nicotinic receptor transduces signals to phosphatidylinositol 3-kinase to block a β-amyloid-induced neurotoxicity. *J Biol Chem* 2001; 276:13541–13546.
41. Arias E, Ales E, Gabilan NH *et al.* Galantamine prevents apoptosis induced by β-amyloid and thapsigargin. *Neuropharmacology* 2004; 46:103–114.
42. Wevers A, Monteggia L, Nowacki S *et al.* Expression of nicotinic acetylcholine receptor subunits in the cerebral cortex of Alzheimer's disease: histotopographical correlation with amyloid plaques and hyperphsophorylated tau protein. *Eur J Neurosci* 1999; 11:2551–2565.
43. Nagele RG, D'Andrea MR, Anderson WJ, Wang HY. Intracellular accumulation of beta-amyloid (1–42) in neurons is facilitated by the alpha 7 nicotinic acetylcholine receptor in Alzheimer's disease. *Neuroscience* 2002; 110:199–211.
44. Dineley KT, Xia X, Bui D *et al.* Accelerated plaque accumulation, associative learning deficits, and up-regulation of alpha 7 nicotinic receptor protein in transgenic mice co-expressing mutant human presenilin 1 and amyloid precursor proteins. *J Biol Chem* 2002; 277:22768–22780.
45. Shie FS, Le Boeuf RC, Jin LW. Early intraneuronal A beta deposition in the hippocampus of APP transgenic mice. *Neuroreprot* 2003; 14:123–129.
46. Butterfield DA, Griffin S, Munch G, Pasinetti GM. Amyloid beta-peptide and amyloid pathology are central to the oxidative stress and inflammatory cascades under which Alzheimer's disease brain exists. *J Alzheimers Dis* 2002; 4:193–201.
47. Weiner HL, Selkoe DJ. Inflammation and therapeutic vaccination in CNS diseases. *Nature* 2002; 420:879–884.
48. Grimble RF. Inflammatory response in the elderly. *Curr Opin Clin Nutr Metab Care* 2003; 6:21–29.
49. Chung HY, Kim HJ, Kim KW *et al.* Molecular inflammation hypothesis of aging based on the anti-aging mechanism of calorie restriction. *Microsc Res Tech* 2002; 59:264–272.
50. Potter H, Wefes IM, Nilsson LM. The inflammation-induced pathological chaperones ACT and apo-E are necessary catalysts of Alzheimer amyloid formation. *Neurobiol Aging* 2001; 22:923–930.
51. Schubert P, Ogata T, Marchini C, Ferroni S. Glia-related pathomechanisms in Alzheimer's disease: a therapeutic target? *Mech Ageing Dev* 2001; 123:47–57.
52. Hösli L, Hösli E, Maelicke A, Schroeder H. Peptidergic and cholinergic receptors on cultured astrocytes of different brain regions of the rat CNS. *Prog Brain Res* 1992; 94:317–329.
53. Graham A, Court JA, Martin-Ruiz CM *et al.* Immunohistochemical localization of nicotinic acetylcholine receptor subunits in human cerebellum. *Neuroscience* 2002; 113:493–507.
54. Teaktong T, Graham A, Court J *et al.* Alzheimer's disease is associated with a selective increase in alpha7 nicotinic acetylcholine receptor immunoreactivity in astrocytes. *Glia* 2003, 41:207–211.
55. Belluardo N, Blum M, Mudo G *et al.* Acute intermittent nicotine treatment produces regional increases of basic fibroblast growth factor messenger RNA and protein in the tel- and diencephalon of the rat. *Neuroscience* 1998; 83:723–740.
56. Maggio R, Riva M, Vaglini F *et al.* Nicotine prevents experimental parkinsonism in rodents and induces striatal increase of neurotrophic factors. *J Neurochem* 1998; 71:2439–2446.
57. Parain K, Murer MG, Yan Q *et al.* Reduced expression of brain-derived neurotrophic factor protein in Parkinson's disease substantia nigra. *Neuroreport* 1999; 10:557–561.
58. Ge YW, Lahiri DK. Regulation of promoter activity of the APP gene by cytokines and growth factors: implications in Alzheimer's disease. *Ann NY Acad Sci* 2002; 973:463–467.
59. Jonnala RR, Buccafusco JJ. Relationship between the increased cell surface alpha7 nicotinic receptor expression and neuroprotection induced by several nicotinic receptor agonists. *J Neurosci Res* 2001; 66:565–572.
60. Capsoni S, Ugolini G, Comparini A *et al.* Alzheimer-like neurodegeneration in aged antinerve growth factor transgenic mice. *Proc Natl Acad Sci USA* 2000; 97:6826–6831.
61. Liu Q, Kawai H, Berg DK. Beta-Amyloid peptide blocks the response of alpha 7-containing nicotinic receptors on hippocampal neurons. *Proc Natl Acad Sci USA* 2001; 98:4734–4739.
62. Alkondon M, Albuquerque EX. Nicotinic acetylcholine receptors α7 and α4β2 subtypes differentially control GABAergic input to CA1 neurons in rat hippocampus. *J Neurophysiol* 2001; 86:3043–3055.

63. Schrattenholz A, Godovac-Zimmermann J, Schaefer H *et al.* Photoaffinity labelling of Torpedo acetylcholine receptor by physostigmine. *Eur J Biochem* 1993; 216:671–677.
64. Schroeder B, Reinhardt-Maelicke S, Schrattenholz A *et al.* Monoclonal antibodies FK1 and WF6 define two neighboring ligand binding sites on Torpedo acetylcholine receptor α-peptide. *J Biol Chem* 1994; 269:10407–10416.
65. Ludwig J, Höffle A, Samochocki M *et al.* Localization by site-directed mutagenesis of the APL binding site on α7 nicotinic acetylcholine receptor extracellular domain. 2006; in preparation.
66. Storch A, Schrattenholz A, Cooper JC *et al.* Physostigmine, galantamine and codeine act as noncompetitive nicotinic agonists on clonal rat pherchromocytoma cells. *Eur J Pharmacol* 1995; 290:207–219.
67. Pereira EF, Reinhardt-Maelicke S, Schrattenholz A *et al.* Identification and functional characterization of a new agonist site on nicotinic acetylcholine receptors of cultured hippocampal neurons. *J Pharmacol Exp Ther* 1993; 265:1474–1491.
68. Albuquerque EX, Alkondon M, Pereira EF *et al.* Properties of neuronal nicotinic acetylcholine receptors: Pharmacological characterization and modulation of synaptic function. *J Pharmacol Exp Ther* 1997; 280:1117–1136.
69. Samochocki M, Hoeffle A, Fehrenbacher A *et al.* Galantamine is an allosterically potentiating ligand of neuronal nicotinic but not of muscarinic acetylcholine receptor. *J Pharmacol Exp Ther* 2003; 305:1024–1036.
70. McDonald RL, Twyman RE. Kinetic properties and regulation of GABA receptor channels. *Ion Channels* 1992; 3:315–343.
71. Kuhlmann J, Okonjo KO, Maelicke A. Desensitization is a property of the cholinergic binding region of the nicotinic acetylcholine receptor, not of the receptor-integral ion channel. *FEBS Lett* 1991; 279:216–218.
72. Miwa JM, Ibanez-Tallon I, Crabtree GW *et al.* Lynx 1, an endogenous toxin-like modulator of nicotinic acetylcholine receptors in the mammalian CNS. *Neuron* 1999; 23:105–114.
73. Ibanez-Tallon I, Miwa JM, Wang HL *et al.* Novel modulation of neuronal nicotinic acetylcholine receptors by association with the endogenous prototoxin lynx 1. *Neuron* 2002; 33:893–903.
74. Betzel C, Lange G, Pal GP *et al.* The refined crystal structure of a-cobratoxin from Naja naja siamensis at 2.4 A resolution. *J Biol Chem* 1991; 266:21530–21536.
75. Garcia-Colunga J, Miledi R. Blockade of mouse muscle nicotinic receptors by serotonergic compounds. *Exp Physiol* 1999; 84:847–864.
76. Maelicke A, Schrattenholz A, Schröder H. Modulatory control by noncompetitive agonists of nicotinic cholinergic neurotransmission in the central nervous system. *Semin Neurosci* 1995; 7:103–114.
77. Katz B, Miledi R. A re-examination of curare action at the motor endplate. *Proc R Soc Lond* 977; 196:59–72.
78. Shaw KP, Aracava Y, Akaike A *et al.* The reversible cholinesterase inhibitor physostigmine has channel-blocking and agonist effects on acetylcholine receptor ion channel complex. *Mol Pharmacol* 1985; 28:527–538.
79. Okonjo KO, Kuhlmann J, Maelicke A. A second pathway of activation of the nicotinic recptor ion channel. *Eur J Biochem* 1991; 200:671–677.
80. Maelicke A, Coban T, Schrattenholz A *et al.* Physostigmine and neuromuscular transmission. *Ann NY Acad Sci* 1993; 681:140–154.
81. Plaitakis A, Duvoisin RC. Homer's moly identified as *Galanthus nivalis L.*: Physiologic antidote to Stramonium poisoning. *Clin Neuropharmacol* 1983; 6:1–5.
82. Baraka A, Harik S. Reversal of central anticholinergic syndrome by galantamine. *JAMA* 1977; 238:2293–2294.
83. Davis B. Method of treating Alzheimer's disease. US patent 1987; US 4663318 A.
84. Marco-Contelles J, do Carmo Carreiras M, Rodriguez C *et al.* Synthesis and pharmacology of galantamine. *Chem Rev* 2006; 106:116–133.
85. Olin J, Schneider L. Galantamine for Alzheimer's disease (Cochrane Review). *Cochrane Lib* 2004; 2:35–51.
86. Rogers SL, Cooper NM, Sukovaty R *et al.* Pharmacokinetic and pharmacodynamic profile of donepezil HCl following multiple oral doses. *Br J Clin Phamacol* 1998; 46:7–12.
87. Geerts H, Guillaumat PO, Grantham C *et al.* Brain levels and acetylcholinesterase inhibition with galantamine and donepezil in rats, mice, and rabbits. *Brain Res* 2005; 1033:186–193.
88. Davidsson P, Blennow K, Andreasen N *et al.* Differential increase in cerebrospinal fluid-acetycholinesterase after treatment with acetylcholinesterase inhibitors in patients with Alzheimer's disease. *Neurosci Lett* 2001; 300:157–160.

89. Dooley M, Lamb HM. Donepezil; a review of its use in Alzheimer's disease. *Drugs Aging* 2000; 16:199–226.
90. Holz RW, Senter RA. Choline stimulates nicotinic receptors on adrenal medullary chromaffin cells to induce catecholamine secretion. *Science* 1981; 214:466–468.
91. Alkondon M, Pereira EFR, Cortes WS *et al.* Choline is a selective agonist of α7 nicotinic acetylcholine receptors in rat brain neurons. *Eur J Neurosci* 1997; 9:2734–2742.
92. Mandelzys A, De Koninck P, Cooper E. Agonist and toxin sensitivities of ACh-evoked currents on neurons expressing multiple nicotinic ACh receptor subunits. *J Neurophysiol* 1995; 74:1212–1221.
93. Sgard F, Charpantier E, Bertrand S *et al.* A novel human nicotinic receptors subunit, alpha 10, that confers functionality to the alpha 9 subunit. *Mol Pharmacol* 2002; 61:150–159.
94. Mike A, Castro NG, Albuquerque EX. Choline and acetylcholine have similar kinetic properties of activation and desensitization of the α7 nicotinic receptors in rat hippocampal neurons. *Brain Res* 2000; 882:155–168.
95. Pereira EFR, Hilmas C, Santos MD *et al.* Unconventional ligands and modulators of nicotinic receptors. *J Neurobiol* 2002; 53:479–500.
96. Maelicke A, Albuquerque EX. Allosteric modulation of nicotinic acetylcholine receptors as a treatment strategy for Alzheimer's disease. *Eur J Pharmacol* 2000; 393:165–170.
97. Mintzer J, Burns A. Anticholinergic side-effects of drugs in elderly people. *J Roy Soc Med* 2000; 93:457–462.
98. Santos MD, Alkondon M, Pereira EFR *et al.* The nicotinic allosteric ligand galantamine facilitates synaptic transmission in the mammalian central nervous system. *Mol Pharmacol* 2002; 61:1222–1234.
99. Alkondon M, Braga MF, Pereira EF *et al.* Alpha 7 nicotinic acetylcholinereceptors and modulation of GABAergic synaptic transmission in the hippocampus. *Eur J Pharamacol* 2000; 393:59–62.
100. Zhang L, Zhou FM, Dani JA. Cholinergic drugs for Alzheimer's disease enhance in vitro dopamine release. *Mol Pharmacol* 2004; 66:538–544.
101. Francis PT. Glutamatergic systems in Alzheimer's disease. *Int J Geriatr Psychiatry* 2003; 18:15–21.
102. Rissman RA, Mishizen-Eberz AL, Carter TL *et al.* Biochemical analysis of $GABA_A$ receptors subunits 1,5,12 in the hippocampus of patients with Alzheimer's disease neuropathology. *Neuroscience* 2003; 120:695–704.
103. Alkondon M, Pereira EFR, Eisenberg HM, Albuquerque EX. Choline and selective antagonists identify two subtypes of nicotinic acetylcholine receptors that modulate GABA release from CA1 interneurons in rat hippocampal slices. *J Neurosci* 1999; 19:2693–2705.
104. Perry DC, Davilla-Garcia MI, Stockmeier CA, Kellar KJ. Increased nicotinic receptors in brains from smokers: membrane binding and autoradiographic studies. *J Pharmacol Exp Ther* 1999; 289:1545–1552.
105. Kihara T, Shimohama S, Sawada H *et al.* Nicotinic receptor stimulation protects neurons against β-amyloid toxicity. *Ann Neurol* 1997; 42:159–163.
106. Thomsen T, Kaden B, Fischer JP *et al.* Inhibition of acetylcholine esterase activity in human brain tisue and erythrocytes by galantamine, physostigmine and tacrine. *Eur J Clin Biochem* 1991; 29:487–492.
107. Nordberg A, Svensson A. Cholinesterase inhibitors in the treatment of Alzheimer's disease: a comparison of tolerability and pharmacology. *Drug Saf* 1998; 19:465–480.
108. Doody RS. Current treatment for Alzheimer's disease: cholinesterase inhibitors. *J Clin Psychiatry* 2003; 64:11–17.
109. Woodruff-Pak DS, Vogel RW, Wenk GL. Galantamine; effect on nicotinic receptor binding, acetylcholine esterase inhibition and learning. *Proc Natl Acad Sci USA* 2001; 98:2089–2094.
110. Samochocki M, Zerlin M, Jostock R *et al.* Galantamine is an allosterically potentiating ligand of human α4β2 nAChR. *Acta Neurol Scand* 2000; 176:68–73.
111. Shaw S, Bencherif M, Marrero MB. Janus kinase 2, an early target of a7 nicotinic acetylcholine receptor in acute and chronic neurodegeneration. *Curr Drug Target CNS Neurol Disord* 2002; 1:399–411.
112. Li Y, Meyer EM, Walker DW *et al.* Alpha 7 nicotinic receptor activation inhibits ethanol-induced mitochondrial dysfunction, cytochrome c release and neurotoxicity in primary rat hippocampal neuronal cultures. *J Neurochem* 2002; 81:853–858.
113. Wilcock G, Howe I, Coles H *et al.* A long-term comparison of galantamine and donepezil in the treatment of Alzheimer's disease. *Drugs Aging* 2003; 20:777–89.
114. Brodaty H, Corey-Bloom J, Potocnik FC *et al.* Galantamine prolonged-release formulation in the treatment of mild to moderate Alzheimer's disease. *Geriatr Cogn Disord* 2005; 20:120–132..

# 14

# The utility of biomarkers in the diagnosis and monitoring of Alzheimer's disease

*C. W. Ritchie*

## INTRODUCTION

Alzheimer's disease (AD) is a disease defined by pathology but diagnosed by symptoms. These symptoms include cognitive, behavioural, functional and neuropsychiatric symptoms that are not absolutely correlated with the extent or distribution of the underlying pathology. It is sufficient for symptomatic treatments to have their efficacy and effectiveness measured solely by changes in these symptoms. Traditionally this has focused almost exclusively on cognition because of the assumption that the other symptoms are a consequence of this primary problem. There are limitations to a symptomatic approach to drug treatment and the current symptomatic treatments are of modest though important efficacy [1]. Current drug development programs are broken into two groups: those that are of predominantly better symptomatic treatments and those that are of potentially (Alzheimer's) disease-modifying treatments (ADMTs). The former could sensibly be classed as second generation symptomatic treatments and will rely predominantly on improving neurotransmission through direct interaction with neurotransmitters and receptors. These drugs will have a very important role in future management as it is likely that they will be used in combination with ADMTs.

ADMTs will primarily have an effect on the underlying pathology. This may mean that they have little measurable symptomatic effect early in treatment; their benefit will be in minimizing or preventing the inevitable decline associated with the progression of pathology and deteriorating clinical state.

No drug currently licensed is disease-modifying. Several targets are being pursued currently: secretase inhibitors (both γ and β), amyloid β (Aβ) aggregation inhibitors, monoclonal antibodies and tau phosphorylation inhibitors to name but a few (these and other targets are described in detail in chapter 8). The similarity between all of these targets is that if a drug does 'work', it will cause measurable change to either the phosphorylation of tau or the aggregation of Aβ. As a result, ADMTs can have their *in vivo* mechanism tested by measuring the drug's effect on biomarkers measurable downstream from principle AD pathology.

'Biomarkers' are biological markers of a disease. Concurrent to the development of ADMTs has been a parallel enquiry into the nature and behaviour of biomarkers in AD.

Biomarker research is firstly describing the natural history of biomarker change as disease advances to assess whether these tests are valid and follow an accepted scientific

**Craig W. Ritchie**, MB ChB, MRCPsych, MSc, Director of Clinical Trials, Metabolic and Clinical Trials Unit, Department of Mental Health Sciences, Royal Free and University College Medical School, London, UK

rationale. If they do, and they change with progression in AD, then this understanding of normal biomarker change can be used to measure a drug's effect on pathology *in vivo*, by describing the putative parameters of the placebo curve. Secondly these same biomarkers could be useful in earlier, potentially pre-clinical diagnosis of disease, potentially allowing ADMTs to be used at, what is presumed to be, the time when they will be of greatest clinical benefit.

This chapter will document the evidence to date with regard to biomarkers as diagnostic aids and secondly as potential markers of a drug's efficacy.

## BIOCHEMICAL AND GENETIC BIOMARKERS

The utility of a new test is measured against a gold standard test. In the case of AD, the 'gold standard' is only available post-mortem. Therefore to test any biomarker as a diagnostic test, the gold standard has to be the best available clinical research diagnosis: criteria for these exist (e.g. NINCDS-ADRDA [2]).

### *GENETIC RISK FACTORS AS DIAGNOSTIC TESTS*

Risk factor genes are examples of diagnostic biomarkers. The most investigated of these is apolipoprotein E (ApoE) on chromosome 19 [3], whereby presence of the $\varepsilon_4$ allele increases the risk of developing AD [4] though the predictive values of this test are such that it is of limited clinical utility [5]. Other putative risk factor genes which have been investigated are polymorphisms of the low-density lipoprotein receptor gene [6] and the $\alpha_2$-macroglobulin gene [7] both on chromosome 12 though with conflicting evidence of association with AD.

As an individual's genetic status is fixed, these tests have no utility to test the efficacy of an ADMT, though their gene product, e.g. ApoE, could be measured. They are of greater use in clinical trials as a pharmacogenetic test to determine if a drug's effect is influenced by an individual's ApoE status. This has been shown to be the case with early data from studies in AD of the peroxisome proliferator-activated receptor-$\gamma$ agonist rosiglitazone. This drug only showed efficacy in patients who did not carry the $\varepsilon_4$ allele [8].

### *BIOCHEMICAL BIOMARKERS AS DIAGNOSTIC TESTS*

There needs to be a clear understanding in any work investigating AD diagnostic markers of the relationship between pathological changes and alterations in biomarkers and clinical symptoms. In the case of ApoE, this biomarker has been present lifelong, but does not usually have its effect for over 60 years. An ideal biomarker would be abnormal or become abnormal only in the period immediately preceding the earliest clinical symptoms so that interventions can be used rationally and parsimoniously.

Non-genetic biomarker tests can be subdivided into biochemical biomarkers and radiological biomarkers (Figure 14.1).

Biomarkers can be measured in one of two body fluids; plasma and cerebrospinal fluid (CSF). It is intuitive that CSF markers will bear a closer relationship with what is going on intracerebrally than plasma markers, though taking samples of plasma is invariably more acceptable to the patient than a lumbar puncture (LP). If the benefits of CSF sampling in terms of diagnosis and monitoring disease progression are such, then it should become commonplace for LPs to be performed in clinical practice [9].

### *BIOCHEMICAL DIAGNOSTIC BIOMARKERS IN CSF*

#### *Tau and phosphorylated-tau*

The most investigated biomarker in CSF is the protein tau and phosphorylated tau (p-tau). The abnormal phosphorylation of the cytoskeletal protein tau is one of the characteristic

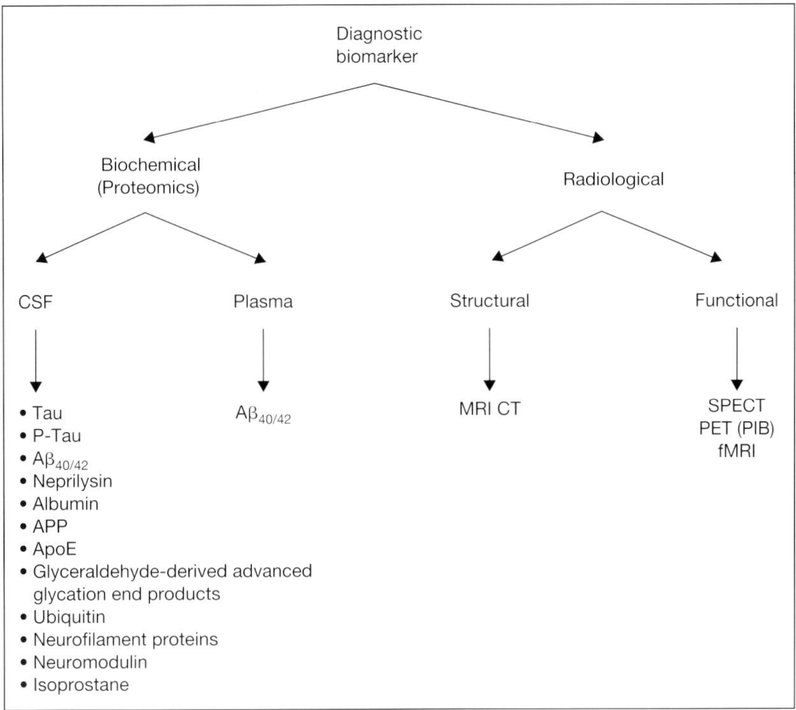


**Figure 14.1** Non-genetic diagnostic biomarkers.

pathological lesions in AD [10]. Axonal degeneration liberates tau and p-tau (as a marker of the abnormal phosphorylation of this protein in AD) into the extracellular space and hence into the CSF. From this, it could be predicted that people with AD would have higher levels of these markers than normal controls. This has been demonstrated with both total tau (t-tau) [11] and p-tau [12] with potentially greater specificity for AD with p-tau [13]. An elevation of p-tau has also been observed in more impaired mild cognitive impairment (MCI) patients whilst normal in less severe MCI cases [14]. The gathering and consensual evidence which shows that CSF markers can differentiate early and incipient AD from normal ageing, depression, alcohol dementia and Parkinson's disease, has led to a belief that CSF t-tau and p-tau should be used in the diagnosis of AD [15] especially with a view to the earliest possible treatment.

### *Amyloid beta (Aβ)*

The amyloid plaque in AD is formed from the aggregation of Aβ that is either 40 or 42 amino acids long. These proteins are derived from their parent amyloid precursor protein (APP) through the enzymic activity of the secretases β and γ. It is now considered that this aggregation represents a physiological reaction to increase in the levels of metal ions trafficked by $A\beta_{40}$ and $A\beta_{42}$ into plaque [16]. It is also considered that the initial elevated production of Aβ may be triggered by oxidative stress from mitochondrial sources [17] as Aβ has potent anti-oxidant properties [18]. It has consistently been shown that levels of Aβ in CSF are lower in patients with AD than in normal controls and this may also be associated with an increased mortality from the disease [19]. Low levels of CSF Aβ are consistent with the hypothesis that in AD a mechanism exists for sequestering Aβ into plaque. Higher levels in healthy individuals may reflect a normal, physiological increase in this anti-oxidant protein in response to increasing oxidative stresses derived from mitochondrial decay associated with normal ageing [20]. Cognitively normal older people who carry the ApoE-ε4 allele have been shown to have a lower level of CSF Aβ similar to levels seen in AD. In this sense, CSF Aβ may be a good biomarker for incipient disease [21].

#### *Other potential CSF biochemical biomarkers*

Numerous other biomarkers have been looked at in CSF. As work with these biomarkers is not as extensive or conclusive as it is with tau, p-tau and Aβ, conclusions about their utility as diagnostic markers is not yet available. These novel markers include the following:

CSF/serum albumin ratio, as a marker for blood–brain barrier damage, is used to exclude patients with concomitant cerebrovascular pathology and differentiate AD from vascular dementia [22].

Neprilysin is a metalloprotein involved in the normal metabolism of $A\beta_{40}$ and $A\beta_{42}$ whose activity decreases in AD and with normal ageing [23]. This enzyme has been shown to be lower in the CSF of patients with AD [24]. This enzyme is activated by zinc, though activity diminishes precipitously if zinc levels become too high. High cerebral zinc levels are associated with AD [25], which may mediate the decline in neprilysin activity in AD and hence levels of this enzyme in the CSF of patients with AD.

Other investigated biomarkers are the soluble fragment of APP found to be normal in some studies [26] but elevated [27] in others. ApoE, which may be reduced in the CSF of patients with AD and which perhaps reflects increased utilization in a neurodegenerative environment or sequestration into plaque [28]. Glyceraldehyde-derived advanced glycation end products may also be a promizing biomarker, though have not yet been fully characterized in AD [29]. Ubiquitin levels are increased in AD which hypothetically could lead to elevations in CSF [30], though there is little recent evidence to support this. There is also work that demonstrates increased levels of various neurofilament proteins [31], normality of neuromodulin or growth-associated protein GAP-43, as a marker for synaptic degeneration [32] though elevation of this marker in reaction to clioquinol [33] and increased F (2) isoprostane (a product of cerebral oxidative damage) in both post-mortem [34] and *in vivo* [35] CSF samples.

### *BIOCHEMICAL BIOMARKERS AS MEASURES OF DISEASE PROGRESSION*

The putative diagnostic CSF biomarkers t-tau, p-tau and Aβ may also be useful in measuring disease progression. It is likely that there is a dynamic relationship between CSF markers and disease severity with tau and p-tau rising steadily from early disease, plateauing at moderate clinical disease and then falling in the most severe disease after the most rapid phase of axonal degeneration is completed in moderately severe illness. These longitudinal changes may be complicated by diluting effects in the CSF secondary to brain atrophy [13]. Natural history studies of CSF t-tau and p-tau are helping to describe if these hypothetical changes are indeed observed and can be predicted.

The natural history of changes to CSF Aβ levels are less easy to predict. It may be that in early disease Aβ levels in CSF increase from a low baseline and elevate above normal levels as the overproduction of Aβ exceeds the rate at which it can be sequestered into plaque. At a later stage, the levels of CSF Aβ may drop as APP metabolism to form Aβ diminishes and plaque sequestration increases relatively. The curves and factors associated with changes to CSF Aβ are less well-understood than those with tau and p-tau.

If these curves are well-described in normal disease progression, then an opportunity exists to measure the effect of ADMTs on these biomarkers. Considering CSF tau and p-tau, in mild disease an ADMT would be expected to reduce these levels. The relationship between an effective ADMT and CSF Aβ levels is less predictable. A drug that inhibits the metabolism of Aβ would be expected to show a reduction of Aβ in CSF, whereas a drug which prevents the aggregation of Aβ could lead to an increase in CSF Aβ. This is complicated though by the fact that drugs may also act on other parts of the metabolic process, i.e. drugs that inhibit aggregation may also promote enzymic breakdown of Aβ and hence CSF levels may remain constant or indeed fall.

The unpredictability of what to expect from an ADMT in terms of changes to biomarkers has bedevilled a consensus on what to expect from an ADMT in terms of regulatory approval. Currently, an observable effect on a biomarker in a placebo-controlled trial in the presence of conspicuous cognitive improvement would be encouraging. In fact, we will learn much about biomarkers and AD by observing the effect of drugs which interact with the pathology.

In this regard, three examples are given of potential ADMTs tested under optimal trial conditions which impacted on biomarkers. Clioquinol is a metal protein attenuating compound that interacts with zinc and copper to prevent Aβ aggregation and disaggregate plaque [36]. In a small 36-week, double-blind, randomized controlled trial, treated patients exhibited a stabilization of plasma Aβ levels which was significantly different from an observed increase in plasma Aβ levels in placebo-treated patients [37]. A recent study with simvastatin, despite pre-clinical optimism failed to show an effect on CSF Aβ [38]. However, a recent publication investigating the effect of a γ-secretase inhibitor demonstrated a decrease in plasma and CSF $A\beta_{40}$ after 6 weeks of treatment [39]. This decrease relative to placebo was a consistent direction and magnitude of change to that observed with clioquinol.

## NEUROIMAGING BIOMARKERS

Like biochemical and genetic biomarkers, neuroimaging theoretically offers the possibility of assisting diagnosis of AD and differentiating clinically defined dementias. As the disease is associated with progressive cortical atrophy, longitudinal assessment of brain volumes with neuroimaging may assist diagnosis and potentially measure the effect of ADMTs.

Neuroimaging techniques can be separated into two types: structural (using magnetic resonance imaging [MRI] or computed tomography [CT]) and functional (using positron emitting tomography [PET], functional MRI [fMRI] and single photon emission computed tomography [SPECT]).

### *STRUCTURAL IMAGING AS A DIAGNOSTIC TEST FOR AD*

Because of the modern availability of MRI and its improved resolution compared with CT, most structural imaging research uses MRI.

Despite a plethora of research to aid diagnostic accuracy in AD with MRI, only one MRI tool has shown any additional benefit of scanning over a clinical diagnosis and that is medial temporal lobe atrophy [40] which is reasonably straightforward to attain clinically [41].

### *STRUCTURAL IMAGING AS A MEASURE OF DRUG EFFICACY*

There is evidence that neuroimaging changes precede the onset of clinical symptoms by several years [42, 43] and by the time clinical AD has developed atrophy in hippocampus may have exceeded 25% [44]. Serial MRI studies have allowed for the description of not only how atrophy proceeds as disease advances but also what atrophy has preceded clinical diagnosis [45]. The observation that detectable differences occur in MRI measurements in pre-clinical disease compared with normal ageing suggests that serial MRI scanning may assist pre-clinical diagnosis of AD in an at-risk population [46].

### *FUNCTIONAL IMAGING AS A DIAGNOSTIC TEST FOR AD*

There are three main types of functional neuroimaging useful in AD research and clinically. SPECT uses γ-emitting radioisotopes attached to biologically relevant molecules which can then be mapped three-dimensionally to show, e.g. blood flow or receptor binding. As the radioisotopes have a short half-life in terms of $\gamma$-emission and can alter the pharmacological activity of drugs under study, only a limited number of ligands have been developed and this has limited the use of SPECT.

PET is a more specific test than SPECT and the source of positrons ($^{11}C$) can more easily be incorporated into biological molecules compared with the sources of $\gamma$-emissions used in SPECT ($^{123}I$ and $^{99m}Tc$). The very short half-lives of PET isotopes means that they must be created 'on site' and hence limits the availability of PET scanners.

fMRI can measure brain activity due to the differential activity of haemoglobin and deoxyhaemoglobin within the MRI field [47].

The most useful of these diagnostically for AD may be PET differentiating AD from both MCI and normal ageing [48, 49]; though this is currently the least available technique. SPECT performs less well diagnostically than PET [50], though dopamine SPECT may have particular merit in differentiating AD from Lewy body dementia (DLB) and Parkinson's disease dementia [51]. This advantage has led to dopamine SPECT or PET being included in the latest diagnostic criteria for DLB [52].

## *FUNCTIONAL IMAGING AS A MEASURE OF DRUG EFFICACY*

Functional imaging has the potential to measure both brain activity and the pathological lesions in AD.

A positive effect of donepezil on regional cortical blood flow (rCBF) has been observed after 12 months of treatment where untreated AD patients demonstrated a decrease in rCBF and treated patients had no decline [53]. Further work with donepezil demonstrated that additional improvement in frontal lobe blood flow was achieved in patients who responded to the drug with those who clinically did not [54] suggesting that treatment response may be anticipated through demonstration of an effect on frontal lobe perfusion. The localized effect on frontal lobe perfusion supported earlier work identifying this location as the area for the most significant effect of donepezil [55]. This specific effect in responders and in the frontal lobe has also been demonstrated with another acetylcholinesterase inhibitor rivastigmine [56], though there is no published evidence investigating this effect with galantamine. The other licensed symptomatic treatment for AD, namely memantine, has also not been investigated in this manner.

In terms of a direct effect on underlying AD pathology, attention has focused on labelling A$\beta$ and measuring through PET scanning the extent of amyloid burden in AD. As this is a 'diagnostic marker' of the disease it would be assumed that this would be a gold standard diagnostic test. Techniques for labelling amyloid for neuroimaging are in their infancy but progress in this area is anticipated and the implications both diagnostically and in terms of measuring ADMT efficacy are profound.

Of the tracers under testing, the most excitement currently surrounds Pittsburgh Compound-B (PIB). PIB is thought to bind to a particular site on the A$\beta$ fibril [57] with reasonable specificity though this property may also be shared by other tracers namely [11C] SB-13 [58] and aminonaphthalene (FDDNP) [59]. Radio labelling clioquinol has also been investigated with SPECT with encouraging preliminary results [60].

PIB has the most comprehensive research evidence base for its potential as a biomarker [61, 62]. Its use is also complementing investigations with other biomarkers. A recent comparative study of PIB with CSF markers demonstrated an inverse relationship between CSF $A\beta_{42}$ and intracerebral amyloid as measured with PIB, though no relationship between CSF tau, p-tau, plasma $A\beta_{40/42}$ or CSF $A\beta_{40}$ [63]. This data strongly supported the hypothesis that in early disease the amyloid plaque is acting as a sink to sequester $A\beta_{42}$ preferentially with a consequent lowering of CSF $A\beta_{42}$ levels in the CSF.

## SUMMARY

Biomarker research is important and will inevitably transfer into clinical practice to aid diagnosis. ADMTs will be developed at some point in the future, hopefully sooner rather than later. To test these drugs' disease-modifying capabilities, trial designs must employ biomarkers as outcomes whether these are imaging or biochemical or a combination of the two. The danger is that testing a novel compound with an outcome measure whose behaviour in untreated AD is uncertain could lead to a great deal of difficulty in the interpretation of results. At the moment, drug development targeting various aspects of the disease process in AD is ahead of biomarker research. Currently, the most sensible approach in trial design of ADMTs is that one uses a biomarker with the strongest most consensual evidence surrounding it. This would argue that longitudinal MRI structural imaging and CSF tau and p-tau should be included wherever possible in these trials. Other biomarkers could be included but interpretation of their changes with treatment over placebo (or lack of it) should be made with many caveats and cautions; they should certainly not constitute 'go, no-go' decisions in clinical development programs.

Consideration must also be given to the size and duration of studies as the cost of doing biomarker outcomes in large, long phase 3 trials may be prohibitive. Fundamentally a drug, whether disease-modifying or symptomatic will only be licensed if it has a beneficial impact on cognitions, behaviour and function in AD; an effect on a biomarker in the absence of a clinical effect is meaningless.

Phase 2a trials of ADMTs, where small size and short duration may preclude observation of a clinical effect, should include biomarkers. These trials represent the first opportunity to assess the impact of the new drug on AD pathology in an AD population, though 'negative' findings of a non-significant effect should not be seen as a failure of the drug due to the inherent uncertainty of biomarker behaviour and heterogeneity in assay results across a clinically defined population.

The future will witness greater diagnostic accuracy at a pre-clinical stage of disease and the prescription of combinations of symptomatic treatments for an immediate improvement in cognition and disease modifiers to halt or minimize decline. Given the high prevalence of AD and the global ageing population, the achievement of this is an absolute priority and clinical services must be in place in preparation to perform the necessary investigations and instigate the appropriate treatments.

## REFERENCES

1. Ritchie CW, Ames D, Clayton T *et al*. A meta-analysis of randomized trials for the efficacy and safety of donepezil, galantamine and rivastigmine for the treatment of Alzheimer's disease. *Am J Geriatr Psychiatry* 2004; 12:358–369.
2. McKhann G, Drachman D, Folstein M *et al*. Clinical diagnosis of Alzheimer's disease: report of the NINCDS-ADRDA Work Group under the auspices of Department of Health and Human Services Task Force on Alzheimer's disease. *Neurology* 1984; 34:939–944.
3. Saunders AM. Apolipoprotein E and Alzheimer's disease: an update on genetic and functional analyses. *J Neuropathol Exp Neurol* 2000; 59:751–758.
4. Saunders AM, Strittmatter WJ, Schmechel D *et al*. Association of apolipoprotein E allele epsilon 4 with late-onset familial and sporadic Alzheimer's disease. *Neurology* 1993; 43:1467–1472.
5. Relkin NR, Kwon YJ, Tsai J *et al*. The National Institute on Ageing/Alzheimer's Association recommendations on the application of apolipoprotein E genotyping to Alzheimer's disease. *Ann N Y Acad Sci* 1996; 802:149–176.
6. Lendon CL, Talbot CJ, Craddock NJ *et al*. Genetic association studies between dementia of the Alzheimer's type and three receptors for apolipoprotein E in a Caucasian population. *Neurosci Lett* 1997; 222:187–190.
7. Blacker D, Wilcox MA, Laird NM *et al*. Alpha-2 macroglobulin is genetically associated with Alzheimer disease. *Nat Genet* 1998; 19:357–360.

8. Risner ME, Saunders AM, Altman JFB *et al.* Efficacy of rosiglitazone in a genetically defined population with mild-to-moderate Alzheimer's disease. *Pharmacogenomics J* 2006; 1–9 [Epub ahead of print].
9. Peskind ER, Riekse R, Quinn JF *et al.* Safety and acceptability of the research lumbar puncture. *Alzheimer's Dis Assoc Disord* 2005; 19:220–225.
10. Wischik CM, Edwards PC, Lai RYK. Quantitative analysis of tau protein in paired helical filament preparations: implications for the role of tau protein phosphorylation in PHF assembly in Alzheimer's disease. *Neurobiol Ageing* 1995; 16:409–431.
11. Jensen M, Basun H, Lannfelt L. Increased cerebrospinal fluid tau in patients with Alzheimer's disease. *Neurosci Lett* 1995; 186:189–191.
12. Sjogren M, Davidsson P, Tullberg M *et al.* Both total and phosphorylated tau are increased in Alzheimer's disease. *J Neurol Neurosurg Psychiatry* 2001; 70:624–630.
13. de Leon MJ, DeSanti S, Zinkowski R *et al.* MRI and CSF studies in the early diagnosis of Alzheimer's disease. *J Intern Med* 2004; 256:205–223.
14. Lavados M, Farias G, Rothhammer F *et al.* ApoE alleles and tau markers in patients with different levels of cognitive impairment. *Arch Med Res* 2005; 36:474–479.
15. Andreasen N, Blennow K. CSF biomarkers for mild cognitive impairment and early Alzheimer's disease. *Clin Neurol Neurosurg* 2005; 107:165–173.
16. Maynard CJ, Bush AI, Masters CL *et al.* Metals and amyloid-beta in Alzheimer's disease. *Int J Exp Pathol* 2005; 86:147–159.
17. Reddy PH. Amyloid precursor protein-mediated free radicals and oxidative damage: implications for the development and progression of Alzheimer's disease. *J Neurochem* 2006; 96:1–13.
18. Atwood CS, Obrenovich ME, Liu T *et al.* Amyloid-beta: a chameleon walking in two worlds: a review of the trophic and toxic properties of amyloid-beta. *Brain Res Brain Res Rev* 2003; 43:1–16.
19. Wallin AK, Blennow K, Andreasen N *et al.* CSF biomarkers for Alzheimer's Disease: levels of beta-amyloid, tau, phosphorylated tau relate to clinical symptoms and survival. *Dement Geriatr Cogn Disord* 2006; 21:131–138.
20. Beal MF. Mitochondria take center stage in ageing and neurodegeneration. *Ann Neurol* 2005; 58:495–505.
21. Sunderland T, Mirza N, Putnam KT *et al.* Cerebrospinal fluid beta-amyloid1–42 and tau in control subjects at risk for Alzheimer's disease: the effect of APOE epsilon4 allele. *Biol Psychiatry* 2004; 56:670–676.
22. Blennow K, Vanmechelen E. Combination of the different biological markers for increasing specificity of in vivo Alzheimer's testing. *J Neural Transm* (suppl) 1998; 53:223–235.
23. Russo R, Borghi R, Markesbery W *et al.* Neprylisin decreases uniformly in Alzheimer's disease and in normal ageing. *FEBS Lett* 2005; 579:6027–6030.
24. Maruyama M, Higuchi M, Takaki Y *et al.* Cerebrospinal fluid neprilysin is reduced in prodromal Alzheimer's disease. *Ann Neurol* 2005; 57:832–842.
25. Mocchegiani E, Bertoni-Freddari C, Marcellini F *et al.* Brain, ageing and neurodegeneration: role of zinc ion availability. *Prog Neurobiol* 2005; 75:367–390.
26. Olsson A, Hoglund K, Sjogren M. Measurement of alpha- and beta-secretase cleaved amyloid precursor protein in cerebrospinal fluid from Alzheimer patients. *Exp Neurol* 2003; 183:74–80.
27. Csernansky JG, Miller JP, McKeel D *et al.* Relationships among cerebrospinal fluid biomarkers in dementia of the Alzheimer type. *Alzheimer Dis Assoc Disord* 2002; 16:144–149.
28. Blennow K, Hesse C, Fredman P. Cerebrospinal fluid apolipoprotein E is reduced in Alzheimer's disease. *Neuroreport* 1994; 5:2534–2536.
29. Yamagishi S, Nakamura K, Inoue H *et al.* Serum or cerebrospinal fluid levels of glyceraldehyde-derived advanced glycation end products (AGEs) may be a promising biomarker for early detection of Alzheimer's disease. *Med Hypotheses* 2005; 64:1205–1207.
30. Iqbal K, Grundke-Iqbal I. Elevated levels of tau and ubiquitin in brain and cerebrospinal fluid in Alzheimer's disease. *Int Psychogeriatr* 1997; 9(suppl 1):289–296.
31. Hu YY, He SS, Wang XC *et al.* Elevated levels of phosphorylated neurofilament proteins in cerebrospinal fluid of Alzheimer disease patients. *Neurosci Lett* 2002; 320:156–160.
32. Sjogren M, Minthon L, Davidsson P *et al.* CSF levels of tau, beta-amyloid(1–42) and GAP–43 in frontotemporal dementia, other types of dementia and normal ageing. *J Neural Transm* 2000; 107:563–579.
33. Regland B, Lehmann W, Abedini I *et al.* Treatment of Alzheimer's disease with clioquinol. *Dement Geriatr Cogn Disord* 2001; 12:408–414.

34. Montine TJ, Markesbery WR, Morrow JD *et al.* Cerebrospinal fluid F2-isoprostane levels are increased in Alzheimer's disease. *Ann Neurol* 1998; 44:410–413.
35. Montine TJ, Kaye JA, Montine KS. Cerebrospinal fluid abeta42, tau, and f2-isoprostane concentrations in patients with Alzheimer disease, other dementias, and in age-matched controls. *Arch Pathol Lab Med* 2001; 125:510–512.
36. Cherny RA, Atwood CS, Xilinas ME *et al.* Treatment with a copper-zinc chelator markedly and rapidly inhibits beta-amyloid accumulation in Alzheimer's disease transgenic mice. *Neuron* 2001; 30:665–676.
37. Ritchie CW, Bush AI, Mackinnon A. Metal-protein attenuation with iodochlorhydroxyquin (clioquinol) targeting Aβ amyloid deposition and toxicity in Alzheimer disease: a pilot phase 2 clinical trial. *Arch Neurol* 2003; 60:1685–1691.
38. Hoglund K, Thelen KM, Syversen S. The effect of simvastatin treatment on the amyloid precursor protein and brain cholesterol metabolism in patients with *Alzheimer's disease. Dement Geriatr Cogn Disord* 2005; 19:256–265.
39. Siemers ER, Quinn JF, Kaye J. Effects of a gamma-secretase inhibitor in a randomized study of patients with Alzheimer disease. *Neurology* 2006; 66:602–604.
40. O'Brien JT. Is hippocampal atrophy on magnetic resonance imaging a marker for Alzheimer's disease? *Int J Geriatr Psychiatry* 1995; 10:431–435.
41. Frisoni GB. Structural imaging in the clinical diagnosis of Alzheimer's disease: problems and tools. *J Neurol Neurosurg Psychiatry* 2001; 70:711–718.
42. Killiany RJ, Hyman BT, Gomez-Isla T *et al.* MRI measures of entorhinal cortex vs hippocampus in preclinical AD. *Neurology* 2002; 58:1188–1196.
43. Scahill RI, Schott JM, Stevens JM *et al.* Mapping the evolution of regional atrophy in Alzheimer's disease: unbiased analysis of fluid-registered serial MRI. *Proc Nat Acad Sci USA* 2002; 99:4703–4707.
44. Fox NC, Rossor MN. Diagnosis of early Alzheimer's disease. *Rev Neurol* 1999; 155(suppl 4):S33–S37.
45. Schott JM, Fox NC, Frost C *et al.* Assessing the onset of structural change in familial Alzheimer's disease. *Ann Neurol* 2003; 53:181–188.
46. Barber R, O'Brien J. Structural brain imaging. In: Burns A, O'Brien J, Ames D (eds). *Dementia*, 3rd edition. Hodder Arnold, London, 2005.
47. Ebmeier KP, Sutherland JK, Dougall NJ. Functional imaging. In: Burns A, Ames D, O'Brien J (eds). *Dementia*, 3rd edition. Hodder Arnold, London, 2005, pp 94–104.
48. Kawachi T, Ishii K, Sakamoto S *et al.* Comparison of the diagnostic performance of FDG-PET and VBM-MRI in very mild Alzheimer's disease. *Eur J Nucl Med Mol Imaging*. 2006; [Epub ahead of print].
49. Silverman DH, Small GW, Chang CY *et al.* Positron emission tomography in evaluation of dementia. *JAMA* 2001; 286:2120–2127.
50. Dougall NJ, Bruggink S, Ebmeier KP. Systematic review of the diagnostic accuracy of 99mTc-HMPAO-SPECT in dementia. *Am J Geriatr Psychiatry* 2004; 12:554–570.
51. Walker Z, Costa DC, Walker RW *et al.* Differentiation of dementia with Lewy bodies from Alzheimer's disease using a dopaminergic presynaptic ligand. *J Neurol Neurosurg Psychiatry* 2002; 73:134–140.
52. McKeith I, Dickson D, Emre M *et al.* Dementia with Lewy Bodies: Diagnosis and Management: Third Report of the DLB Consortium. *Neurology* 2005; 65:1863–1872.
53. Nobili F, Vitali P, Canfora M *et al.* Effects of long-term Donepezil therapy on rCBF of Alzheimer's patients. *Clin Neurophysiol* 2002; 113:1241–1248.
54. Shimizu S, Hanyu H, Iwamoto T *et al.* SPECT follow-up study of cerebral blood flow change during Donepezil therapy in patients with Alzheimer's disease. *J Neuroimaging* 2006; 16:16–23.
55. Staff RT, Gemmell HG, Shanks MF *et al.* Changes in the rCBF images of patients with Alzheimer's disease receiving Donepezil therapy. *Nucl Med Commun* 2000; 21:37–41.
56. Vennerica A, Shanks MF, Staff RT *et al.* Cerebral blood flow and cognitive responses to rivastigmine treatment in Alzheimer's disease. *Neuroreport* 2002; 13:83–87.
57. Ye L, Morgeenstern JL, Gee AD *et al.* Delineation of positron emission tomography imaging agent binding sites on beta-amyloid peptide fibrils. *J Biol Chem* 2005; 280:23599–23604.
58. Verhoeff NP, Wilson AA, Takeshita S *et al.* In-vivo imaging of Alzheimer disease beta-amyloid with [11C]SB-13 PET. *Am J Geriatr Psychiatry* 2004; 12:584–595.
59. Agdeppa ED, Kepe V, Petri A *et al.* In vitro detection of (S)-naproxen and ibuprofen binding to plaques in the Alzheimer's brain using the positron emission tomography molecular imaging probe 2(1[6[(2[(18)F] fluoroethyl)(methyl)amino]-2-naphthyl]ethylidene)malononitrile. *Neuroscience* 2003; 117:723–730.
60. Opazo C, Luza S, Villemagne VL *et al.* Radioiodinated clioquinol as a biomarker for beta-amyloid: Zn complexes in Alzheimer's disease. *Ageing Cell* 2006: 5:69–79.

61. Price JC, Klunk WE, Lopresti BJ *et al*. Kinetic modeling of amyloid binding in humans using PET imaging and Pittsburgh Compound-B. *J Cereb Blood Flow Metab* 2005; 25:1528–1547.
62. Klunk WE, Engler H, Nordberg A *et al*. Imaging brain amyloid in Alzheimer's disease with Pittsburgh Compound-B. *Ann Neurol* 2004; 55:306–319.
63. Fagan AM, Mintum MA, Mach RH *et al*. Inverse relation between in vivo amyloid imaging load and cerebrospinal fluid Abeta42 in humans. *Ann Neurol* 2006; 59:512–519.

# Section III

## Management of non-cognitive issues in dementia

# 15

# Non-pharmacological interventions for BPSD

*J. Cohen-Mansfield*

## INTRODUCTION

Non-pharmacological approaches to the care of persons with dementia differ from pharmacological treatment in that they consider the interaction between the person, caregiver, environment, and system of care in the treatment design. Such interventions generally provide more personalized care for these individuals, addressing their needs and considering their preferences. Non-pharmacological interventions have been used to address many types of behavioural and psychological symptoms of dementia (BPSD), such as depressed affect, delusions, hallucinations, sleep disturbances, and agitation, which includes restlessness, aggression, and verbal/vocal behaviour problems. This chapter presents a framework for implementing such interventions, provides examples from the literature on existing interventions, discusses the research findings regarding these interventions, and argues for increased advocacy to support their research and use.

### *WHY USE NON-PHARMACOLOGICAL APPROACHES?*

Non-pharmacological approaches to care for persons with dementia are based on a wide range of theoretical orientations and present a broad array of methodologies. Rather than viewing the patient's disease or symptoms as the problem, this perspective considers the interaction between the patient, caregiver, environment, and system of care, and ascertains treatment accordingly (Figure 15.1). While the specific goals of treatment can also differ between pharmacological and non-pharmacological approaches, both can be used for many purposes, including addressing BPSD. The exact scope of BPSD varies in the literature, and tends to include affective, perceptual and behavioural problems in dementia [1]. Non-pharmacological interventions have also been used for purposes beyond BPSD, such as improving function (activities of daily living [ADL] performance), enhancing cognition, and reinforcing a positive sense of self. In this chapter, we will focus on non-pharmacological interventions addressing BPSD. Non-pharmacological interventions have been described in the literature and summarized in many recent reviews [2–11].

A number of questions must be answered before decision makers commit to any treatment plan, including: What is the goal of treatment? Who needs to be treated? Whose problem is being treated? Whose reality is being considered? Whose needs and preferences take precedence? Answers to these questions will determine the treatment's ultimate goal, which will then dictate the selection of intervention.

**Jiska Cohen-Mansfield**, PhD, ABPP, Professor/Research Director, Research Institute on Aging, Hebrew Home of Greater Washington, Professor, Department of Health Care Services and of Prevention and Community Health, George Washington University Medical Center and School of Public Health, Washington, DC, USA

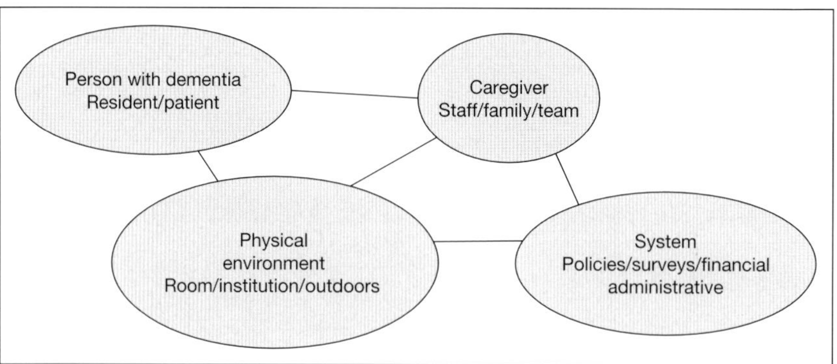


**Figure 15.1** Who needs to be treated?

The goal of treatment is especially important to identify when dealing with a conflict of interests. For example, reminding a person with dementia of an unpleasant event (e.g. that his father died) may improve his grasp of reality, but will conflict with the goal of patient comfort. Cleanliness may at times be at odds with personal autonomy, as an individual with dementia may prefer not to take a bath. (Autonomy is extremely important, but at times may need to be compromised to prevent pain and suffering due to infection.) Sometimes it is possible to accomplish both goals or to minimally compromize both, but in other instances a choice must be made. Comfort and positive life experiences are often more relevant for persons with dementia than experiencing reality that is consistent with that of caregivers. The approach underlying the discussion in this chapter assumes that a positive life experience, or at least the absence of negative experiences, is a goal that takes priority over those of improved function.

## *PRELIMINARY REQUIREMENTS FOR NON-PHARMACOLOGICAL INTERVENTIONS*

The provision of information to caregivers of persons with dementia is an essential non-pharmacological intervention. Knowledge of the disease, as well as specific symptoms and their aetiology, meaning, and management will allow caregivers to better understand the individual's behaviours rather than attributing them to resistance, difficult personality, malicious intent, craziness, or indifference. Ongoing caregiver support offering continuous opportunities to seek advice has been shown to help caregivers and postpone the institutionalization of persons with dementia [12].

A second prerequisite for non-pharmacological interventions is communication training. Although an individual's ability to communicate declines in advanced dementia, communication skills are crucial for maintaining quality of life and for understanding the perspective of the person with dementia. Caregivers must therefore be educated in communication techniques, learning to observe, listen, speak, ask questions, and offer alternatives in ways that will maximize the individual's ability to receive and transmit information. Communication training for caregivers of persons with dementia focuses on environmental aspects of communication (e.g. approaching slowly, communicating at eye level), content, phrasing, and interpreting non-verbal or confused verbal communication. Phrasing sentences in a short and clear way [13], on a level compatible with the person's understanding [14], and asking questions in a simple, yes/no format have been recommended as helpful. Others have advised using broad opening sentences, treating the person with dementia as an equal, sharing experiences and feelings, and finding topics that are meaningful [15].

Finally, caregivers must be aware that even when individuals with dementia do not speak in coherent sentences, their individual words may be meaningful, and their messages may be embedded in those words. Most essential is to not ignore, discount, or negate the verbalizations of persons with dementia, but rather to view these as insights into their perspectives, and to use them to improve their situations whenever possible [16–18].

A third condition necessary for successful implementation of non-pharmacological interventions is a positive practice style by the intervener (usually a caregiver). This practice style requires respect for the patient as a person, empathy, willingness to enhance the person's autonomy, flexibility in addressing both care and environmental issues, and compassion towards the individual. In targeting the system, caregiver, or environment for intervention, the non-pharmacological approach imparts a greater significance to the patient's point of view. Providing maximal autonomy to the person with dementia is a central guiding principle, which bestows greater importance on the person's habits or preferences than to the convenience of the caregiving system. Understanding this point of view is an important stage in the determination of treatment. For example, in this framework, a nursing home may be expected to adapt meal times to residents' habits and wishes rather than to the convenience of the kitchen staff members.

An intervention targeting specific behaviours should follow a thorough assessment, which should include a functional analysis examining the nature of the behaviours (assessment of specific symptoms), an evaluation of the interaction of symptoms with the environment (antecedents, consequences), and clarification of who is negatively affected by the symptom. Systematic observation is often useful for this assessment. In addition to information about physical and mental health, the assessment taps the topics of identity, habits and preferences, and past stress, thus guiding the understanding of the aetiology of presented symptoms as well as determining realistic goals and options for treatment. In ascertaining the aetiology of symptoms, the assessor examines a multitude of issues which may elucidate their causes, including when and where the behaviour occurred, what seemed to trigger it, whether relationships between the caregiver and recipient affected the behaviour, whether the caregiver had the resources necessary to perform his/her tasks, whether the person with dementia understood the intent of the caregiver, whether the person had sufficient activities and social contacts, etc.

Following assessment, an intervention is chosen to match the hypothesized aetiology of symptoms, the individual's prior habits and preferences, and his or her current abilities and limitations. The intervention may target a change in the environment, the behaviour of the staff member, the system of care, or the person with dementia. After the intervention is implemented, another evaluation is performed to determine whether the approach was helpful or whether it should be changed. A change may require a different intervention entirely, or may focus on a specific aspect of the intervention such as timing, dosage, presentation style, etc.

### *GENERAL FRAMEWORK*

The heterogeneity of the manifestations of dementia stems from three sources: predisposing characteristics, life events, and the individual's current condition. Each of these occurs in several domains: a genetic/biological/medical domain, a psychosocial domain, and an environmental domain [19]. These factors affect how dementia is manifested in areas of functioning such as affect and behaviour. Mapping these sources through correlation studies has proven useful in illuminating common causes for difficulties in caring for individuals with dementia.

Non-pharmacological intervention techniques used with persons with dementia can be organized along several dimensions: the function of the intervention, its underlying theory, the type of activity undertaken during the intervention, and the population subgroups for which a technique is appropriate. Interventions should be ranked by their effectiveness within a subgroup for certain goals with specific outcome criteria. This chapter will examine examples of interventions according to their purposes, namely: management of agitation/behaviour problems, treatment of depression and improvement of affect, treatment of psychotic symptoms, and addressing sleep disturbances. The list of interventions is not exhaustive, but provides examples of currently available interventions.

## BEHAVIOUR PROBLEMS/AGITATION

Agitated behaviours in the nursing home manifest as three subtypes: aggressive behaviours (e.g. hitting, kicking, pushing, scratching, tearing things, biting, spitting, cursing, or verbal aggression); physically non-aggressive behaviours (e.g. pacing, inappropriate dressing and undressing, trying to leave the nursing home, handling things inappropriately, general restlessness, repetitious mannerisms); and verbal and vocal agitated behaviours (e.g. complaining, constant requests for attention, negativism, repetitious sentences or questions, screaming) [20].

*Verbally and vocally agitated* individuals suffer from more medical conditions and higher levels of pain and depressed affect in comparison to others in the same care setting [21]. These behaviours are more likely to manifest themselves in the evening, when persons are alone, physically restrained, and/or when they are involved in ADL, especially toileting and bathing [22]. These findings support the notion that at least some verbally agitated behaviours are associated with discomfort, pain, or unmet social needs.

*Physically non-aggressive behaviours.* Persons who engage in physically non-aggressive problem behaviours have been reported to have fewer medical diagnoses and better appetites than other nursing home residents [21]. Wandering and pacing, the most common forms of physically non-aggressive agitation, occur most frequently in a corridor and near the nurses' station, where other people often spend time [23]. Wandering/pacing takes place under normal conditions of light, noise, and temperature, rather than during uncomfortable environmental conditions. Relatively healthy individuals who suffer from advanced dementia [24, 25] may manifest these behaviours as a form of stimulation, as opportunities for meaningful activities are limited by their dementia and the nursing home environment.

*Physically aggressive disruptive behaviours* are more likely to be manifested by individuals with severe cognitive impairment [24–26], particularly when individuals with advanced dementia respond to uncomfortable stimuli (while performing ADLs, or feeling cold) or perceive situations to be threatening (e.g. invasion of personal space) [27, 28]. One study found aggressive behaviours to be related to physical pain [29]. Aggressive behaviours are also more likely to be manifested by males and by persons with pre-morbid tendencies towards aggressive behaviour [30–32].

*Conditions affecting most types of inappropriate behaviours.* Most disruptive behaviours (with the exception of pacing) have been shown to be manifested more frequently under the following conditions: when physical restraints are used, when residents are inactive, when residents are alone, when staffing levels are low, or when it is cold at night. Disruptive behaviours are less likely to be demonstrated when structured activities are offered, when music is playing, or when residents are involved in social interaction [27]. These results concur with the hypothesis that agitated behaviours frequently signal discomfort and unmet needs.

Based on the findings described above, agitated behaviours are conceptualized as resulting from an interaction between lifelong habits and personality, current physical and mental conditions, and physical and psychological environmental factors [33]. More specifically, most agitated behaviours are manifestations of unmet needs. An individual with dementia is unable to independently fulfill these needs because of a combination of perceptual problems, communication difficulties, and an inability to manipulate the environment through appropriate channels. The goal of treatment should therefore focus on uncovering and addressing the unmet needs of these individuals.

The most common needs of persons with dementia are for social and physical stimulation, both of which are limited by the combination of the effects of dementia, sensory deficits, and the monotony of the nursing home environment. Other commonly unmet needs in this population are those relating to discomfort and pain.

*Non-pharmacological interventions to treat inappropriate behaviours* can be organized according to the needs they address, most of which are for social contact, engaging activities, and relief from discomfort. (Table 15.1). Many interventions address more than one of these, such as meaningful social contact which is aimed at alleviating both loneliness and boredom.

## PROVIDING SOCIAL SUPPORT AND CONTACT

At the most basic level, providing social support and contact involves talking to persons with dementia, even if the caregiver conducts the majority of the conversation. One-on-one interaction is a potent intervention that can be performed by relatives, paid caregivers, or volunteers. There are two major difficulties in providing positive social contact for persons with dementia, as these individuals may prefer socializing with loved ones rather than formal caregivers, and providing one-on-one interaction with staff members can become costly. Two successful interventions that have addressed both of these issues are videotapes of family members addressing their relative with dementia [34, 35] and simulated presence therapy [36, 37], in which a family member audiotapes his or her side of a telephone conversation, which is then played for the older person. Interventions addressing cost issues include training staff members to view all interactions with individuals in their care as opportunities for social contact (including during ADL), and interaction videos for persons with dementia. These commercially produced videotapes often incorporate memories from the past and viewers are invited to sing along to familiar music [112]. Pet therapy is another option [38], and may include visits with dogs, cats, fish, or even plush stuffed animals or robotic pets [39]. In addition to interaction with the animal, pet therapy provides a topic for interaction with other people. Dolls have also been used to simulate companions/babies, and massage may be an effective mechanism for social contact with non-verbal persons with advanced dementia when other forms of communication are hampered by the disease process.

## PROVIDING ENGAGING ACTIVITIES

Engaging persons with dementia can be accomplished by providing them with stimulation (passive engagement), providing activities (active engagement), and allowing them to self-stimulate by accommodating their inappropriate behaviours (Table 15.1). Providing stimulation includes the use of music, which should be tailored to the person's preferences [40], and other sensory stimulation such as aromatherapy [41] or touch therapy [42]. Music interventions take many forms, including listening to recorded music, playing musical games, dancing or moving to music, and singing. (Prior to initiating music therapy, hearing must be tested, and an amplifier, headphone, or hearing aid may be necessary.) One example of sensory stimulation is the 'Snoezelen' program, which was developed in Holland and includes a variety of relaxing stimuli [43].

More active engagement is usually offered in the form of structured activities, including group and individual activities. One such intervention, known as 'simple pleasures', includes a range of activities such as tetherball [44]. Activity interventions may involve manipulation (e.g. ball throwing), nurturing (e.g. watering a plant), sorting, cooking, sewing, or sensory interventions as described above, such as music or tactile stimulation with a fabric book. *Montessori-based activities* are a set of activities based on Maria Montessori's principles [45], such as task breakdown, immediate feedback and use of everyday, real world materials. Alternatively, the content of activities may be based on information regarding *'pleasant activities'*, i.e. which activities were or are reinforcing to the individual [46], or on

**Table 15.1** Non-pharmacological interventions for behavioural problems: examples of treatment by need

| ***Need general treatment approach*** | ***Social contacts*** | | | ***Engagement*** | | | | ***Discomfort*** | | |
|---|---|---|---|---|---|---|---|---|---|---|
| | ***Real human*** | ***Simulated significant others*** | ***Non-human*** | ***Provide*** | | ***Accommodate behaviour*** | | ***Pain/ discomfort*** | ***Sleep*** | ***Discomfort during ADL*** |
| | | | | ***Active*** | ***Passive*** | ***Decrease risk*** | ***Make behaviour more acceptable*** | | | |
| Interventions | One-on-one social interaction<br>Small group interaction<br>Massage | Simulated presence therapy<br>Family video-tapes | Pets<br>Dolls | Walking<br>Exercise<br>Activity programs<br>Flower arranging | Provide hearing aids and glasses to allow persons to process ongoing stimulation<br>Sensory stimulation<br>Music<br>Aromatherapy<br>Massage | Environmental design, such as: tape on floor, covering doors or exists, relocating areas | Activity apron<br>Provide materials to handle<br>Environmental design<br>Changing the visual, auditory, and olfactory stimuli on corridors, wandering garden | Pain medication<br>Repositioning<br>Removal of physical restraints | Light therapy<br>Melatonin<br>Increase exercise and decrease awakening at night | Environmental redesign of bathing process (bird pictures and sounds in baths, offering food)<br>Music during bath<br>Use of sponge bath rather than shower or bath<br>Change location of meals |
| Behaviour addressed | V-A | V-A | V-A<br>PhyNA | V-A<br>PhyNA | V-A<br>PhyNA | Exit seeking<br>Trespassing | PhyNA | V-A<br>Agg | All | Agg<br>V-A |

Agg = aggressive behaviours; PhyNA = physical non-aggressive behaviours; V-A = vocal.verbal agitation.

information about the individual's *role-identity* in the past or in the present [47–50]. Activities can involve *exercise* [51], or they may incorporate an *adaptation of ADL*, such as setting the table or cooking [52]. *Cognitive tasks* are activities that stimulate cognitive and memory skills. Group examples include '*Question Asking Readings*' in which a group reads a script accompanied by questions typed on cards that encourage participants to discuss related topics. Another group memory task is *memory bingo*, a game in which participants match beginnings and endings of popular sayings, which can also stimulate group discussion [53]. Individual *cognitive tasks* include sorting cards or objects by category, and additional examples are available elsewhere [54–57].

Interventions for accommodating pacing or wandering behaviour include outdoor walks [58] and the use of wandering areas. Outdoor walks may take place in the company of a caregiver, in which case they also involve a social component, or they may occur in secure outdoor wandering areas [59, 60]. Accommodating pacing and wandering often involves protection of others from trespassing while wandering. To prevent trespassing into another person's room cloth strips across the door connected with Velcro have been used as deterrent to entry; to prevent exit through emergency exit doors, doors and doorknobs can be camouflaged with cloth panels or murals [61], thereby disguizing the doors. Additionally, providing alternative doors, which can be controlled by the person with dementia and permit movement into another secured area, can be useful in reducing trespassing [62].

Inappropriate handling or the constant manipulation of objects can be accommodated by providing appropriate materials, such as books and pamphlets for handling [63], activity aprons (aprons that have buttons, zippers, and other articles sewn on) and other appropriate and safe items for persons to handle. Similarly, rocking chairs and gliding swings have been used to accommodate restless behaviour and provide more acceptable stimulation.

### *PROVIDING RELIEF FROM DISCOMFORT*

Interventions addressing discomfort target pain, hearing and vision problems, positioning problems, difficulties adjusting to ADLs, and unmet ADL-related needs. Although these can be considered medical and nursing care interventions rather than 'non-pharmacological' interventions, they are included here because it is the behavioural assessment that is used to reveal the underlying aetiology of negative affect or behaviour problems that allows a medical or nursing intervention to relieve the condition. Interventions such as pain management, light therapy to improve sleep, reduction of discomfort by improved seating or positioning, and removal of physical restraints have all been related to improvement in behaviour. Once needs have been identified, many of these interventions call for straightforward medical or nursing interventions, while others require more complex approaches, such as assessing pain. Many articles have described the difficulties involved in assessing pain in this population [64] and some recent findings suggest strategies for approaching these complexities [65, 66]. One small study found that pain medication reduced difficult behaviours and allowed discontinuation of psychotropic medication [67]. Improvement in eating or drinking, resulting from the use of enhanced light during meals, has been linked with a decrease in inappropriate behaviours [68], as has the use of hearing aids [69, 70]. Since physical restraints have been shown to result in increased levels of agitation [71], the removal of physical restraints may eliminate those behaviours [72, 73]. Changes in the methods and environment of providing ADLs have also been associated with reduction in inappropriate behaviours. For example, tape recordings and pictures of birds, flowing water and small animals in baths as well as offering food during bathing have been associated with a decrease of such behaviours during bathing [74]. Person-centered showering and towel baths resulted in decreased agitation in comparison with usual bathing routines [75].

Similarly, changing location of meals from central dining to dining on the unit was effective in reducing patient-to-patient assaults on an Alzheimer's and related dementias unit [76].

*Other types of interventions.* Additional categories of non-pharmacological intervention studies include: (1) staff training studies [77–80], in which staff members are trained in communication, in providing ADLs, or in techniques to handle inappropriate behaviours. Many of these programs focus on improved understanding of the older person and the impact of dementia. Changing caregiver behaviour through training is a complex and difficult challenge, and often requires ongoing instruction, modelling, monitoring, feedback, and support of the caregiver. Therefore, in institutional settings, staff training is closely tied to management. Home based caregiver training has also shown promise in decreasing behaviour problems [81]. A review of findings concerning family and staff caregivers' education regarding Alzheimer's disease can be found elsewhere [82]; (2) behavioural interventions [83] employ several techniques, including differential reinforcement (providing positive reinforcement contingent on non-agitated behaviour), time out (moving the person to a quiet area when agitated), restriction (denying the person goods, activities, etc. when agitated), or stimulus control (changing the properties of the stimuli that tend to trigger a behaviour); (3) interventions employing a combination of treatments [84].

## AFFECT

Depressed affect has been conceptualized as resulting from lack of control and a sense of helplessness [85, 86], or to insufficient reinforcing activities [87], and has also been linked to loneliness [88]. All of these models can be used to address depressed affect in persons with dementia, and affirmation of self can also improve affect in this population.

*Increasing sense of control/decreasing helplessness.* Providing opportunities for persons with dementia to exercise control, such as making decisions about meals or clothes or caring for a plant, may be used to target depression in this population [89].

*Pleasant activities.* Individualizing activities based on knowledge of what experiences are reinforcing for persons with dementia has been used to treat depressed affect in this population [46, 90].

*Self-affirming interventions* also target improving affect. These include *reminiscence therapy,* which encourages persons with dementia to talk about their pasts, and may utilise audiovisual aids such as old family photos and objects. Reminiscence can enhance individuals' sense of identity, sense of worth, or general well being [91], and may also stimulate memory processes. *Validation therapy,* in which a therapist accepts the disorientation of a person with dementia and validates his or her feelings, was developed by Naomi Feil [92]. This self-affirming intervention is based on the assumption that persons return to unfinished conflicts in their pasts, providing a background for meaningful conversations addressing their emotions.

*Social contact interventions.* Loneliness is highly correlated with depressed affect, and social interaction and contact interventions are therefore also appropriate for improving affect. The best intervention for loneliness is a positive interaction with a person who is meaningful to the elderly person [34]. Because such interventions are often not feasible, a variety of alternative social interventions have been developed, including simulated interaction and most group activities (including cognitive activities), which can be used as vehicles to promote social contacts (Table 15.1).

*Cognitive interventions* based on the work of Beck [93] and Ellis [94] have been used to treat depressed persons with mild levels of dementia [95].

*Combined interventions.* In a program that utilized a wheelchair bicycle in a recreation therapy protocol, Buettner and Fitzsimmons [96] combined small-group activity therapy and one-to-one bike rides with a staff member, resulting in a significant decrease in depression levels of long-term care residents with dementia.

## SLEEP DISTURBANCES

A number of methods have been used to improve sleep in persons with dementia [97]. Some of these studies focused on sleep as the primary target, whereas others aimed to improve sleep as a method to decrease behaviour problems. Several studies report improving sleep function in persons with dementia. One such study involved caregiver training in improving sleep hygiene, including daily walks and use of a light box, and training in behaviour management skills [98]. Another study utilized 1–2 h of individualized social activities [99]. Other interventions that have been used include bright light [100, 101], aromatherapy [102], and melatonin, though the larger studies on melatonin failed to find a significant impact on sleep [103–106].

Studies that aimed to improve sleep as well as decrease agitation, included the use of bright light therapy (BLT) [107, 108], use of melatonin [109], increased exercise [51], and a decrease in nighttime interruptions [110].

## PSYCHOTIC SYMPTOMS: HALLUCINATIONS AND DELUSIONS

When a person with dementia is considered to present psychotic symptoms, those symptoms require additional investigation as described elsewhere [9]. When addressing psychotic symptoms, the clinician must first ask several questions: Do these symptoms represent real psychosis? What are the consequences of the symptoms for the individual and his or her caregivers? What are possible reasons for the symptoms? Each of these is briefly reviewed below.

*Misinterpretation of stimuli.* At times, the diagnosed 'delusion' or 'hallucination' is triggered by an environmental stimulus. For example, a loudspeaker system may sound like voices from outside, or an image seen through a mirror may be interpreted as someone being in the room. This is facilitated by the combination of sensory deficits and cognitive limitations that occur with dementia, raising an incorrect interpretation of an initially vague or unclear stimulus. Interventions to minimize this confusion would most often remove or change the stimulus so as not to elicit the mistaken interpretation.

*Disturbing stimuli.* In a small study of BLT and its effects on patients with dementia of Alzheimer's type, one individual began hallucinating after eight days of treatment, and her eyes became markedly red. The hallucinations stopped 1 day after discontinuing BLT [111].

*Delusion as a reflection of reality.* At times, it is possible that the 'delusion' is an actual representation of reality. Examples are delusions of theft, as theft is common in many nursing homes, or the delusions of abandonment that may occur when a person enters a nursing home. Whether this feeling reflects reality from the point of view of the caregiver is irrelevant, as the move into a strange environment represents abandonment from the point of view of the person with dementia. The goal of interventions to alleviate this feeling is to re-establish trust in the relationship. Residents may eventually change their perceptions when they become comfortable with their care and when they sense consistent caring by the family. Positive frequent contact with family members, either real or simulated (e.g. videotaped family members or simulated presence therapy [35–37, 112], phone calls, and items from home, may provide a sense of love and familiarity, thus countering the feelings of abandonment and betrayal.

*Delusion as confabulation in the face of memory loss.* Many delusions are misinterpretations of actual events in the environment. When a person with dementia complains that an object has been stolen, she may be forgetting where she has placed her personal belongings and interpreting her inability to find them as theft. A number of potential solutions can be offered to residents, including marking personal belongings in clear ways so that they are easily identifiable, attaching a finder such as a KeyRinger™ to a personal belonging, or purchasing multiple inexpensive copies of personal articles so they may be easily replaced when necessary. Similarly, the delusion that a caregiver is an imposter is often the result of an individual's inability to recognize the caregiver. In that case, an intervention should work toward improving the individual's relationship with the caregiver.

*Delirium*. Delusions can also result from delirium associated with acute medical conditions that should be treated.

*Depressed affect*. Delusions have been linked to depressed affect in many studies [27, 113–119]. It is unclear whether the delusions lead to depression, or if the depression leads to delusions (e.g. through inactivity and isolation), or if both are caused by other factors. Delusions may be changed by treating the depression non-pharmacologically, such as by increasing levels of reinforcing events, by enhancing an individual's sense of control, or by other non-pharmacological psychotherapeutic methodologies (Table 15.2).

*Pleasant 'psychotic symptoms'*. At times hallucinations are pleasurable. Some people talk with deceased relatives and derive happiness from these encounters. If a person seems to enjoy such hallucinations and does not suffer any ill effects, an optimal intervention may be to explain this situation to caregivers in a manner that will make the practice acceptable to them.

*Visual and auditory problems/sensory deprivation*. Hallucinations are more likely to occur in persons with visual problems [116, 120–122], and may be linked to sensory deprivation [123, 124]. Additionally, there is evidence that in the absence of the stimulation of sensory areas by external objects, people experience hallucinations [124]. Correction of visual problems through medical intervention or through aids such as eyeglasses, enhanced contrast, larger type/object, or improved lighting, is a first step in addressing hallucinations among persons with visual impairments. To the extent that sensory deprivation may be a contributing cause of hallucinations, sensory stimulation, such as music, massage, and aromatherapy, may be beneficial.

*Cultural differences between caregivers and persons with dementia*. In some cultures, 'talking' to the dead is a fairly common practice [125–126], yet persons who speak to deceased loved ones may be diagnosed as hallucinating. In addition, someone who is heard speaking aloud in a certain way, or singing, could in fact be praying, invoking a higher power based on religious beliefs or practices, or self-stimulating in an environment that is lacking appropriate stimuli.

## EFFICACY, EFFECTIVENESS, UTILITY

The two basic questions about interventions concern their effectiveness and their costs. There is insufficient research to fully address either issue, though partial answers have been provided. Several studies [127, 128] report the benefits of validation therapy and reality orientation therapy for reducing aggressive behaviours and depressed affect while increasing scores on cognitive functioning tests in comparison to control groups. However, in a review of reality orientation, validation therapy, and reminiscence therapy, Gagnon [129] concluded that reality orientation and validation therapy do not produce sufficient change to justify their costs. Other reviews report insufficient information or limited evidence [130–132]. Cohen-Mansfield [3] reviewed 83 studies of non-pharmacological interventions for inappropriate behaviours in dementia and described the majority as reporting a positive, though not always significant impact. Many of the studies include small samples and other methodological limitations, most often resulting from limited funding for this type of research, and from the fact, that unlike pharmacological interventions, there is no financial entity that is likely to reap monetary benefits from this knowledge.

Despite the lack of conclusive evidence regarding the efficacy of non-pharmacological interventions, the research shows (even with the many difficulties associated with conducting research in this population) that a wide variety of approaches have been used successfully. Many non-pharmacological approaches resulted in a statistically and clinically meaningful improvement in the manifestation of behaviour problems, sleep disturbances, and affect according to some of the studies. However, for some areas, such as delusions and hallucinations, no studies were found regarding the efficacy of non-pharmacologic approaches.

**Table 15.2** Non-pharmacological interventions by purpose: examples

| *Sleep* | *Affect/self affirming* | *Psychotic symptoms* |
|---|---|---|
| Bright light therapy | Providing pleasurable activities<br>Meaningful activities (e.g. social wheelchair bike ride, helping others) | Remove, cover or change stimulus that is misinterpreted, such as a reflecting mirror or window |
| Caregiver training in improving sleep hygiene, including daily walks and use of a light box | Enhancing control | Delusion of theft, investigate the possibility of real theft, if the person misplaces the object, either try to teach the person to always place the object in the same place (possibly through spaced retrieval), or provide multiple copies of object, or use technology to locate the object |
| 1–2 h of individualized social activities | Provide social contacts (see Table 15.1) | For delusion of abandonment, utilize techniques to promote trust |
| Aromatherapy | Reminiscence therapy | If the person has delirium or depression, treat those conditions |
| Increased exercise | Validation therapy | If the person hallucinating has severe sensory impairment, examine options to correct the impairment or use aids to compensate for it, or otherwise provide sensory stimulation |
| Decrease nighttime interruptions | Self-identity activities/ use of objects that were meaningful in the past | If the hallucination does not bother anyone, and provides stimulation or positive affect, or if it fits with the person's cultural habits, allow it to continue |
| Melatonin (?) | Cognitive restructuring for persons with mild dementia | |

*Note*: This is not a comprehensive list, but a list that provides examples of the types of available interventions. Note that some interventions may belong to several categories.

### *BARRIERS TO PRACTICE OF NON-PHARMACOLOGICAL INTERVENTIONS IN DEMENTIA*

The actual utilization of non-pharmacological interventions in dementia falls far short of its potential. A number of systemic issues are responsible for this gap. Funding is lacking both for the practice of non-pharmacological interventions and for the acquisition of knowledge about them through systematic research. The commonly used alternative intervention of psychoactive medication is reimbursed, and the underlying structure for its delivery, such as physicians, medicine aids, pharmacy, monitoring and quality control systems, are largely in place. However, the provision of non-pharmacological interventions is generally not reimbursed, and a system for providing them is often absent. No one in the care system is currently responsible for assessing, observing, and analysing inappropriate behaviour or psychotic symptoms in order to determine their aetiology and their impact on individuals' lives. The ability of caregivers to provide non-pharmacological interventions is further limited by lack of staff member knowledge, insufficient staffing levels, and lack of support for their delivery.

As mentioned previously, there are several prerequisites to good non-pharmacological care of persons with dementia. In order to provide non-pharmacological interventions, the system of care must promote an atmosphere and practice of caring that goes beyond what is currently found in most care settings. A practice style that includes good communication skills, compassion and empathy by caregivers, as well as a high level of flexibility of direct care staff and the larger organization are needed, and are often lacking. In order to allow for alternative interventions, the system of care must promote autonomy and respect for the person with dementia and maximize flexibility in all procedures. Greater monetary resources must also be allocated for research to develop the knowledge necessary for optimizing such care. There is an urgent need to improve our ability to answer basic questions: Which interventions are efficacious for which individuals? Which aspects of an intervention are necessary for it to be efficacious? What are the active ingredients, or principles at work, in different interventions? Which personal characteristics (gender, culture, prior stress) should be considered in matching an intervention with an individual? What is the impact of the person delivering the intervention and the manner in which it is delivered? Only once these basic questions are answered can the issues of effectiveness and costs be properly addressed.

In order to increase the use of non-pharmacological interventions in dementia care, there is a need for public education and advocacy concerning the importance of such interventions and their support. Non-pharmacological interventions generally provide more personalized care for persons with dementia, addressing their needs, and thereby preventing or treating inappropriate behaviours and enhancing affect and overall quality of life.

## ACKNOWLEDGEMENTS

Funding for this work was obtained from NIH grant AG 10172 and NIMH grant MH59617. Portions of this chapter are published elsewhere [133–137] and are reproduced here with permission.

## REFERENCES

1. Zaudig M. Behavioral and psychological symptoms of dementia in the international classification of diseases (ICD)-10 and beyond (ICD-11). *Int Psychogeriatr* 2000; 12(suppl 1):29–40.
2. Opie J, Rosewarne R, O'Connor D. The efficacy of psychosocial approaches to behaviour disorders in dementia: a systematic literature review. *Aust N Z J Psychiatry* 1999; 33:789–799.
3. Cohen-Mansfield J. Nonpharmacologic interventions for inappropriate behaviors in dementia: a review, summary, and critique. *Am J Geriatr Psychiatry* 2001; 9:361–381.
4. Bates J, Boote J, Beverley C. Psychosocial interventions for people with a milder dementing illness: a systematic review. *J Adv Nurs* 2004; 45:644–658.
5. Grasel E, Wiltfang J, Kornhuber J. Non-drug therapies for dementia: an overview of the current situation with regard to proof of effectiveness. *Dement Geriatr Cogn Disord* 2003; 15:115–125.
6. Kasl-Godley J, Gatz M. Psychosocial interventions for individuals with dementia: an integration of theory, therapy, and a clinical understanding of dementia. *Clin Psychol Rev* 2000; 20:755–782.
7. Snowden M, Sato K, Roy-Byrne P. Assessment and treatment of nursing home residents with depression or behavioral symptoms associated with dementia: a review of the literature. *J Am Geriatr Soc* 2003; 51:1305–1317.
8. Cohen-Mansfield J. Cognitive and behavioral interventions for persons with dementia. In: *Encyclopedia of Applied Psychology*. Elsevier Inc, Philadelphia, 2004, p 1.
9. Cohen-Mansfield J. Nonpharmacologic interventions for psychotic symptoms in dementia. *J Geriatr Psychiatry Neurol* 2003; 16:219–224.
10. Allen-Burge R, Stevens AB, Burgio LD. Effective behavioral interventions for decreasing dementia-related challenging behavior in nursing homes. *Int J Geriatr Psychiatry* 1999; 14:213–228.

11. Siders C, Nelson A, Brown LM *et al*. Evidence for implementing nonpharmacological interventions for wandering. *Rehabil Nurs* 2004; 29:195–206.
12. Mittelman MS, Ferris SH, Steinberg G, Sulman E. An intervention that delays institutionalization of Alzheimer's disease patients: Treatment of spouse-caregivers. *Gerontologist* 1993; 33:730–740.
13. Small JA, Gutman G, Makela S, Hillhouse B. Effectiveness of communication strategies used by caregivers of persons with Alzheimer's disease during activities of daily living. *J Speech Lang Hear Res* 2003; 46:353–367.
14. Hart B, Wells D. The effects of language used by caregivers on agitation in residents with dementia. *Clin Nurse Spec* 1997; 11:20–23.
15. Tappen RM, Williams-Burgess C, Edelstein J, Touhy T, Fishman S. Communicating with individuals with Alzheimer's disease: examination of recommended strategies. *Arch Psychiatr Nurs* 1997; 11:249–256.
16. Small JA, Gutman G. Recommended and reported use of communication strategies in Alzheimer caregiving. *Alzheimer Dis Assoc Disord* 2002; 16:270–278.
17. Ripich DN, Wykle M, Niles S. Alzheimer's disease caregivers: the focused program. A communication skills training program helps nursing assistants to give better care to patients with disease. *Geriatr Nurs* 1995; 16:15–19.
18. Ripich DN. Functional communication with AD patients: a caregiver training program. *Alzheimer Dis Assoc Disord* 1994; 8:95–109.
19. Cohen-Mansfield J. Heterogeneity in dementia: challenges and opportunities. *Alzheimer Dis Assoc Disord* 2000; 14:60–63.
20. Cohen-Mansfield J, Marx MS, Rosenthal AS. A description of agitation in a nursing home. *J Gerontol* 1989; 44:M77–M84.
21. Cohen-Mansfield J, Marx MS, Werner P. Agitation in elderly persons: an integrative report of findings in a nursing home. *Int Psychogeriatr* 1992; 4(suppl 2):221–241.
22. Cohen-Mansfield J, Werner P, Marx MS. Screaming in nursing home residents. *J Am Geriatr Soc* 1990; 38:785–792.
23. Cohen-Mansfield J, Werner P, Marx MS. The social environment of the agitated nursing home resident. *Int J Geriatr Psychiatry* 1992; 7:789–798.
24. Cohen-Mansfield J, Culpepper WJ, Werner P. The relationship between cognitive function and agitation in senior day care participants. *Int J Geriatr Psychiatry* 1995; 10:585–595.
25. Cohen-Mansfield J, Marx MS, Rosenthal AS. Dementia and agitation in nursing home residents: how are they related? *Psychol Aging* 1990; 5:3–8.
26. Nasman B, Bucht G, Eriksson S , Sandman PO. Behavioral symptoms in the institutionalized elderly: relationship to dementia. *Int J Geriatr Psychiatry* 1993; 8:843–849.
27. Cohen-Mansfield J, Werner P. Environmental influences on agitation: an integrative summary of an observational study. *Am J Alzheimer's Care Relat Disord Res* 1995; 10:32–37.
28. Bridges-Parlet S, Knopman D, Thompson T. A descriptive study of physical aggressive behavior in dementia by direct observation. *J Am Geriatr Soc* 1994; 42:192–197.
29. Feldt KS, Warne MA, Ryden MB. Examining pain in aggressive cognitively impaired older adults. *J Gerontol Nurs* 1998; 24:14–22.
30. Spector WD, Jackson ME. Correlates of disruptive behaviors in nursing home, a reanalysis. *J Aging Health* 1994; 6:173–184.
31. Ryden MB. Aggressive behavior in persons with dementia who live in the community. *Alzheimer Dis Assoc Disord* 1988; 2:342–355.
32. Hamel M, Gold DP, Andres D *et al*. Predictors and consequences of aggressive behavior by community-based dementia patients. *Gerontologist* 1990; 30:206–211.
33. Cohen-Mansfield J, Deutsch L. Agitation: subtypes and their mechanisms. *Semin Clin Neuropsychiatry* 1996; 1:325–339.
34. Cohen-Mansfield J, Werner P. Management of verbally disruptive behaviors in nursing home residents. *J Gerontol A Biol Sci Med Sci* 1997; 52A:M369–M377.
35. Werner P, Cohen-Mansfield J, Fischer J, Segal G. Characterization of family-generated videotapes for the management of verbally disruptive behaviors. *J Appl Gerontol* 2000; 19:42–57.
36. Camberg L, Woods P, Ooi WL *et al*. Evaluation of simulated presence: a personalized approach to enhance well-being in persons with Alzheimer's disease [see comments]. *J Am Geriatr Soc* 1999; 47:446–452.
37. Woods P, Ashley J. Simulated presence therapy: using selected memories to manage problem behaviors in Alzheimer's disease patients. *Geriatr Nurs* 1995; 16:9–14.

38. Churchill M, Safaoui J, McCabe B, Baun M. Using a therapy dog to alleviate the agitation and desocialization of people with Alzheimer's disease. *J Psychosoc Nurs Ment Health Serv* 1999; 37:16–24.
39. Libin A, Cohen-Mansfield J. Therapeutic robocat for nursing home residents with dementia: preliminary inquiry. *Am J Alzheimers Dis Other Dement* 2004; 19:111–116.
40. Gerdner LA. Effects of individualized versus classical 'relaxation' music on the frequency of agitation in elderly persons with Alzheimer's disease and related disorders. *Int Psychogeriatr* 2000; 12:49–65.
41. Ballard CG, O'Brien JT, Reichelt K, Perry EK. Aromatherapy as a safe and effective treatment for the management of agitation in severe dementia: the results of a double-blind, placebo-controlled trial with Melissa. *J Clin Psychiatry* 2002; 63:553–558.
42. Snyder M, Egan EC, Burns KR. Interventions for decreasing agitation behaviors in persons with dementia. *J Gerontol Nurs* 1995; 21:34–40.
43. Baillon S, Van Diepen E, Prettyman R, Redman J, Rooke N, Campbell R. A comparison of the effects of Snoezelen and reminiscence therapy on the agitated behaviour of patients with dementia. *Int J Geriatr Psychiatry* 2004; 19:1047–1052.
44. Buettner LL. Simple pleasures: a multilevel sensorimotor intervention for nursing home residents with dementia. *Am J Alzheimers Dis Other Dement* 1999; 14:41–52.
45. Camp C, Cohen-Mansfield J, Capezuti E. Nonpharmacological interventions for dementia: Enhancing and maintaining mental health in long-term care residents. *Psychiatr Serv* 2002; 53:1397–1404.
46. Teri L, Logsdon RG. Identifying pleasant activities for Alzheimer's disease patients: the pleasant events schedule-AD. *Gerontologist* 1991; 31:124–127.
47. Cohen-Mansfield J, Golander H, Arnheim G. Self-identity in older persons suffering from dementia: preliminary results. *Soc Sci Med* 2000; 51:381–394.
48. Cohen-Mansfield J, Parpura-Gill A, Golander H. Utilization of self-identity roles for designing interventions for persons with dementia. *J Gerontol B Psychol Sci Soc Sci* (in press).
49. Cohen-Mansfield J, Parpura-Gill. A, Golander H. Salience of self-identity roles in persons with dementia: differences in perceptions among patients themselves, family members and caregivers. *Soc Sci Med* 2006; 62:745–757.
50. Parpura-Gill A, Cohen-Mansfield J. Utilization of self-identity roles in individualized activities designed to enhance well-being in persons with dementia. In: Hyer L, Intrieri RC (Eds.) Clinical Applied Gerontological Interventions in Long-Term Care, Chapter 7; 157–184.
51. Zisselman MH, Rovner BW, Shmuely Y, Ferrie P. A pet therapy intervention with geriatric psychiatry inpatients. *Am J Occup Ther* 1996; 50:47–51.
52. Marsden JP, Meehan RA, Calkins MP. Therapeutic kitchens for residents with dementia. *Am J Alzheimers Dis Other Dement* 2001; 16:303–311.
53. Camp CJ, Foss JW, O'Hanlon AM, Stevens AB. Memory interventions for persons with dementia. *Appl Cogn Psychol* 1996; 10:193–210.
54. Bowlby C. *Therapeutic Activities with Persons Disabled by Alzheimer's Disease and Related Disorders*. Aspen Publishers, Gaithersberg, MD, 1993.
55. Hellen C. *Alzheimer's Disease: Activity Focused Care*. Butterworth-Heinemann, Woburn, MA, 1998, p 1.
56. Zgola JML. *Doing things: a Guide to Programming Activities for Persons with Alzheimer's Disease and Related Disorders*. The Johns Hopkins University Press, Baltimore, MD, 1987.
57. Russen-Rondinone T, DesRoberts AM. Success through individual recreation: working with the low-functioning resident with dementia or Alzheimer's disease. *Am J Alzheimers Dis Other Dement* 1996; 11:32–35.
58. Cohen-Mansfield J, Werner P. Visits to an outdoor garden: impact on behavior and mood of nursing home residents who pace. In: Vellas B, Fitten J, Frisoni G (eds). *Research and Practice in Alzheimer's Disease*. Serdi, Paris, France, 1998, pp 419–436.
59. Namazi KH, Johnson BD. Pertinent autonomy for residents with dementias: modification of the physical environment to enhance independence. *Am J Alzheimer's Care Relat Disord Res* 1992; 7:16–21.
60. Cohen-Mansfield J, Werner P. Outdoor wandering parks for persons with dementia: a survey of characteristics and use [In Process Citation]. *Alzheimer Dis Assoc Disord* 1999; 13:109–117.
61. Kincaid C, Peacock JR. The effect of a wall mural on decreasing four types of door-testing behaviors. *J Appl Gerontol* 2003; 22:76–88.
62. Namazi KH, Rosner TT, Calkins MP. Visual barriers to prevent ambulatory Alzheimer's patients from exiting through an emergency door. *Gerontologist* 1989; 29:699–702.
63. Cohen-Mansfield J, Werner P. The effects of an enhanced environment on nursing home residents who pace. *Gerontologist* 1998; 38:199–208.

64. Cohen-Mansfield J, Lipson S. Pain in cognitively impaired nursing home residents: how well are physicians diagnosing it? *J Am Geriatr Soc* 2002; 50:1039–1044.
65. Feldt KS. Improving assessment and treatment of pain in cognitively impaired nursing home residents. *Ann Long Term Care* 2000; 8:36–42.
66. Huffman JC, Kunik ME. Assessment and understanding of pain in patients with dementia. *Gerontologist* 2000; 40:574–581.
67. Douzjian M, Wilson C, Shultz M *et al*. A program to use pain control medication to reduce psychotropic drug use in residents with difficult behavior. *Ann Long Term Care* 1998; 6:174–179.
68. Koss E, Gilmore GC. Environmental interventions and functional ability of AD patients. In: Vellas B, Fritten J, Frisoni G (eds). *Research and Practice in Alzheimer's Disease*. Serdi, Paris, France, 1998, pp 185–192.
69. Palmer CV, Adams SW, Bourgeois M, Durrant J, Rossi M. Reduction in caregiver-identified problem behavior in patients with Alzheimer Disease post hearing-aid fitting. *J Speech Lang Hear Res* 1999; 42:312–328.
70. Leverett M. Approaches to problem behaviors in dementia. *Phys Occup Ther Geriatr* 1991; 9:93–105.
71. Werner P, Cohen-Mansfield J, Braun J, Marx MS. Physical restraints and agitation in nursing home residents. *J Am Geriatr Soc* 1989; 37:1122–1126.
72. Yeh SH, Lin LW, Wang SY, Wu SZ, Lin JH, Tsai FM. The outcomes of restraint reduction program in nursing homes [Abstract, article in Chinese]. *Hu Li Yan Jiu* 9:183–193.
73. Werner P, Cohen-Mansfield J, Koroknay V, Braun J. Reducing restraints: Impact on staff attitudes. *J Gerontol Nurs* 1994; 20:19–24.
74. Whall A, Black M, Groh C, Yankou D, Kupferschmid B, Foster N. The effect of natural environments upon agitation and aggression in late stage dementia patients. *Am J Alzheimers Dis Other Dement* 1997; 216–220.
75. Sloane PD, Hoeffer B, Mitchell CM *et al*. Effect of person-centered showering and the towel bath on bathing-associated aggression, agitation, and discomfort in nursing home residents with dementia: a randomized, controlled trial. *J Am Geriatr Soc* 2004; 52:1795–1804.
76. Negley EN, Manley JT. Environmental interventions in assaultive behavior. *J Gerontol Nurs* 1990; 16:29–33.
77. Mentes JC, Ferrario J. Calming aggressive reactions: a preventive program. *J Gerontol Nurs* 1989; 15:22–27.
78. Williams DP, Wood EC, Moorleghen F. An in-service workshop for nursing personnel on the management of catastrophic reactions in dementia victims. *Clin Gerontol* 1994; 14:47–53.
79. McCallion P, Toseland RW, Lacey D, Banks S. Educating nursing assistants to communicate more effectively with nursing home residents with dementia. *Gerontologist* 1999; 39:546–558.
80. Savage T, Crawford I, Nashed Y. Decreasing assault occurrence on a psychogeriatric ward: an agitation management model. *J Gerontol Nurs* 2004; 30:30–37.
81. Huang HL, Shyu YI, Chen MC, Chen ST, Lin LC. A pilot study on a home-based caregiver training program for improving caregiver self-efficacy and decreasing the behavioral problems of elders with dementia in Taiwan. *Int J Geriatr Psychiatry* 2003; 18:337–345.
82. Bower FL, McCullough CS, Pille BL. Synthesis of research findings regarding the care of people with Alzheimer's disease – Part II. *Online J Knowl Synth Nurs* 2002; 29:4.
83. Doyle C, Zapparoni T, O'Connor D, Runci S. Efficacy of psychosocial treatments for noisemaking in severe dementia. *Int Psychogeriatr* 1997; 9:405–422.
84. Rovner BW, Steele CD, Shmuely Y, Folstein MF. A randomized trial of dementia care in nursing homes. *J Am Geriatr Soc* 1996; 44:7–13.
85. Seligman MEP. Depression and learned helplessness. In: *The Psychology of Depression: Contemporary Theory and Research*. Winston-Wiley, Washington, DC, 1974.
86. Seligman MEP. *Helplessness: On Depression, Development, and Death*. W.H. Freeman, San Francisco, CA, 1975.
87. Lewinsohn PM, Youngren MA. The symptoms of depression. *Compr Ther* 1976; 2:62–69.
88. Cohen-Mansfield J, Parpura-Gill A. Loneliness in elderly persons: a theoretical model and empirical findings. *Int Psychogeriatr* (in press).
89. Langer EJ, Rodin J. Effects of choice and enhanced personal responsibility for the aged: a field experiment in an institutional setting. *J Pers Soc Psychol* 1976; 34:191–198.
90. Teri L, Logsdon RG, Uomoto J, McCurry SM. Behavioral treatment of depression in dementia patients: a controlled clinical trial. *J Gerontol B Psychol Sci Soc Sci* 1997; 52B:P159–P166.
91. Brooker D, Duce L. Wellbeing and activity in dementia: a comparison of group reminiscence therapy, structured goal-directed group activity and unstructured time. *Aging Ment Health* 2000; 4:354–358.

92. Feil N. *Validation: The Feil Method*. Feil Productions, Cleveland, Ohio, 1982.
93. Beck A. The past and future of cognitive therapy. *J Psychother Pract Res* 1997; 6:276–284.
94. Ellis A. *Reason and Emotion in Psychotherapy*. Lyle Stuart, New York, 1962.
95. Scholey KA, Woods BT. A series of brief cognitive therapy interventions with people experiencing both dementia and depression: a description of techniques and common themes. *Clin Psychol Psychother* 2003; 10:175–185.
96. Buettner LL, Fitzsimmons S. AD-venture program: therapeutic biking for the treatment of depression in long-term care residents with dementia. *Am J Alzheimers Dis Other Dement* 2002; 17:121–127.
97. McCurry SM, Reynolds CF, Ancoli-Israel S, Teri L, Vitiello MV. Treatment of sleep disturbance in Alzheimer's disease. *Sleep Med Rev* 2000; 4:603–628.
98. McCurry SM, Gibbons LE, Logsdon RG, Vitiello MV, Teri L. Nighttime insomnia treatment and education for Alzheimer's disease: a randomized, controlled trial. *J Am Geriatr Soc* 2005; 53:793–802.
99. Richards KC, Beck C, O'Sullivan PS, Shue VM. Effect of individualized social activity on sleep in nursing home residents with dementia. *J Am Geriatr Soc* 2005; 53:1510–1517.
100. Kim S, Song HH, Yoo SJ. The effect of bright light on sleep and behavior in dementia: an analytic review. *Geriatr Nurs* 2003; 24:239–243.
101. Fetveit A, Skjerve A, Bjorvatn B. Bright light treatment improves sleep in institutionalized elderly – an open trial. *Int J Geriatr Psychiatry* 2003; 18:520–526.
102. Wolfe N, Herzberg J. Can aromatherapy oils promote sleep in severely demented patients? *Int J Geriatr Psychiatry* 1996; 11:926–927.
103. Singer C, Tractenberg RE, Kaye J *et al*. Alzheimer's Disease Cooperative Study. A multicenter, placebo-controlled trial of melatonin for sleep disturbance in Alzheimer's disease. *Sleep* 2003; 26:893–901.
104. Mahlberg R, Kunz D, Sutej I, Kuhl KP, Hellweg R. Melatonin treatment of day–night rhythm disturbances and sundowning in Alzheimer disease: an open-label pilot study using actigraphy. *J Clin Psychopharmacol* 2004; 24:456–459.
105. Asayama K, Yamadera H, Ito T, Suzuki H, Kudo Y, Endo S. Double blind study of melatonin effects on the sleep-wake rhythm, cognitive and non-cognitive functions in Alzheimer type dementia. *J Nippon Med Sch* 2003; 70:334–341.
106. Serfaty M, Kennell-Webb S, Warner J, Blizard R, Raven P. Double blind randomized placebo controlled trial of low dose melatonin for sleep disorders in dementia. *Int J Geriatr Psychiatry* 2002; 17:1120–1127.
107. Mishima MK, Okawa M, Hishikawa Y. Morning bright light therapy for sleep and behavior disorders in elderly patients with dementia. *Acta Psychichiatr Scand* 1994; 89:1–7.
108. Okawa M, Mishima K, Hishikawa Y, Hozumi S, Hori H, Takashi K. Circadian rhythm disorders in sleep – waking and body temperature in elderly patients with dementia and their treatment. *Sleep* 1991; 14:478–485.
109. Cohen-Mansfield J, Garfinkel D, Lipson S. Melatonin for treatment of sundowning in elderly persons with dementia – a preliminary study. *Arch Gerontol Geriatr* 2000; 31:65–76.
110. Alessi CA, Yoon EJ, Schnelle JF, Al-Samarrai NR, Cruise PA. A randomized trial of a combined physical acitivity and environmental intervention in nursing home residents: do sleep and agitation improve? *J Am Geriatr Soc* 1999; 47.
111. Schindler SD, Graf A, Fischer P, Tolk A, Kasper S. Paranoid delusions and hallucinations and bright light therapy in Alzheimer's disease. *Int J Geriatr Psychiatry* 2002; 17:1071–1072.
112. Hall L, Hare J. Video respite for cognitively impaired persons in nursing homes. *Am J Alzheimers Dis Other Dement* 1997; 12:117–121.
113. Ballinger BR, Reid AH, Heather BB. Cluster analysis of symptoms in elderly demented patients. *Br J Psychiatry* 1982; 140:257–262.
114. Bassiony MM, Steinberg MS, Warren A, Rosenblatt A, Baker AS, Lyketsos CG. Delusions and hallucinations in Alzheimer's disease: prevalence and clinical correlates. *Int J Geriatr Psychiatry* 2000; 15:99–107.
115. Bassiony MM, Warren A, Rosenbaum A *et al*. The relationship between delusions and depression in Alzheimer's disease. *Int J Geriatr Psychiatry* 2002; 17:549–556.
116. Cohen-Mansfield J, Taylor L, Werner P. Delusions and hallucinations in an adult day care population: A longitudinal study. *Am J Geriatr Psychiatry* 1998; 6:104–121.
117. Cooper JK, Mungas D, Verma M, Weilers PG. Psychotic symptoms in Alzheimer's disease. *Int J Geriatr Psychiatry* 1991; 6:721–726.
118. Cummings JL, Ross W, Absher J, Gornbein J, Hadjiaghai L. Depressive symptoms in Alzheimer disease assessment and determinants. *Alzheimer Dis Assoc Disord* 1995; 9:87–93.

119. Giladi N, Treves A, Paleacu D *et al.* Risk factors for dementia, depression and psychosis in long-standing Parkinson's disease. *J Neural Transm* 2000; 107:59–71.
120. Chapman FM, Dickinson J, McKeith I, Ballard C. Association among visual hallucinations, visual acuity, and specific eye pathologies in Alzheimer's disease: treatment implications. *Am J Psychiatry* 1999; 156:1983–1985.
121. Forsell Y. Predictors for depression, anxiety and psychotic symptoms in a very elderly population: data from a 3-year follow-up study. *Soc Psychiatry Psychiatr Epidemiol* 2000; 35:259–263.
122. Holroyd S. Hallucinations and delusions in Alzheimer's disease. In: Vellas BJ, Fitten J, Frisconi G (eds). *Research and Practice in Alzheimer's Disease Intervention in Gerontology*. Serdi Publishing, Paris, France, 1998.
123. Holroyd S, Sheldon-Keller A. A study of visual hallucinations in Alzheimer's Disease. *Am J Geriatr Psychiatry* 1996; 3:198–205.
124. Zubek JP, Pushkar DSW, Gowing J. Perceptual changes after prolonged sensory isolation (darkness and silence). *Canad J Psychol* 1961; 15:83–100.
125. Howland LG. Spirit communication at the carib dugu. *Lang Commun* 1984; 4:89–103.
126. MacDonald WL. Idionecrophanies: the social construction of perceived contact with the dead. *J Sci Study Relig* 1992; 31:215–223.
127. Toseland RW, Diehl M, Freeman K *et al.* The impact of validation group therapy on nursing home residents with dementia. *J Appl Gerontol* 1997; 16:31–50.
128. Baldelli MV, Pirani A, Motta M, Abati E, Mariani E, Manzi V. Effects of reality orientation therapy on elderly patients in the community. *Arch Gerontol Geriatr* 1993; 17:211–218.
129. Gagnon DL. A review of reality orientation, validation therapy, and reminiscence therapy with the Alzheimer's client. *Phys Occup Ther Geriatr* 1996; 14:61–77.
130. Neal M, Briggs M. Validation therapy for dementia. *Cochrane Database Syst Rev* 2003; 3(CD001394).
131. Spector A, Orrell M, Davies S, Woods RT. Reminiscence therapy for dementia. *Cochrane Database Syst Rev* 2000; 4(CD001120).
132. Spector A, Davies S, Woods B, Orrell M. Reality orientation for dementia: a systematic review of the evidence of effectiveness from randomized controlled trials. *Gerontologist* 2000; 40:206–212.
133. Camp C, Cohen-Mansfield J, Capezuti E. Mental health services in nursing homes: Use of nonpharmacologic interventions among nursing home residents with dementia. *Psychiatr Serv* 2002; 53:1397–1404. *Reprinted with permission from the Psychiatric Services, Copyright (2002). American Psychiatric Association.*
134. Cohen-Mansfield J. Cognitive and behavioural interventions for persons with dementia. *Encyclopedia of Applied Psychology*, vol. 1. Elsevier Inc., 2004; 377–385. *Reprinted with permission from Elsevier Inc.*
135. Cohen-Mansfield J. Nonpharmacologic interventions for psychotic symptoms in dementia. *J Geriatr Psychiatry Neurol 2003;* 16:219–224. *Reprinted with permission from Sage Publications.*
136. Cohen-Mansfield J. Nonpharmacologic approaches to the care of dementia with Lewy Bodies. In: O'Brien J, McKeith I, Ames D, Chiu E (eds). *Dementia with Lewy Bodies*. Taylor & Francis Medical Books, London, UK, 2006; 193–207 (from the 'Hallucinations and Delusions' section of the work.) *Reprinted with permission from Thomson Publishing Services.*
137. Cohen-Mansfield, J. Non pharmacological interventions for persons with dementia. *Alzheimer's Care Q* 2005; 6:129–145. *Reprinted with permission from Lippincott Williams & Wilkins.*

# 16

# Pharmacological interventions for BPSD

*A. Shah, A. T. Lopes*

## INTRODUCTION

Non-cognitive symptoms of dementia have been described as behavioural and psychological signs and symptoms of dementia (BPSD) by the International Psychogeriatric Association [1, 2]. Burns and colleagues [3–6], in their pioneering work on Alzheimer's disease (AD), classified BPSD into four domains: disorders of behaviour (including aggression, agitation, sleep disturbance, sexual disinhibition etc.), mood (including depression, anxiety and mania), thought content (including delusions) and perception (including hallucinations and misidentifications). These BPSD categories are now applied to all types of dementia [7]. They are common [8] and can cause distress to patients, informal carers and professionals, lead to institutionalization and over-medication [9].

## PHARMACOLOGICAL STUDIES

Both non-pharmacological and pharmacological treatments are utilized in the treatment of BPSD. Pharmacological treatments include neuroleptics, cholinesterase inhibitors, antidepressants, anti-convulsants, steroids, benzodiazepines, propranolol and herbal medicines. Case-reports, open-label studies, randomized and double-blind studies, and pooled-analyses are systematically examined using a hierarchical approach. A detailed summary of all the studies identified through a literature search is illustrated in Appendix 1.

## METHODOLOGICAL ISSUES

Case-reports and open-label studies provide a useful guide, but they do not provide conclusive evidence of efficacy. Randomized, double-blind and placebo-controlled studies can provide better evidence of efficacy. However, a number of methodological issues need consideration.

Findings from different studies are difficult to compare because of differing types of dementias, sampling frames, study settings, study durations, doses, definitions of BPSD, BPSD measurement instruments and designs (e.g. parallel-group and crossover design). This raises concerns about the application of findings from individual studies with specific characteristics to patients in clinical settings with different characteristics. Can findings from studies of a mixed group of dementias be applied to specific types of dementia? Can findings from studies of AD be applied to other types of dementias? Can findings of studies in specific clinical settings (e.g. nursing home or outpatient clinic) be applied to other clinical settings? Only a few studies have precisely defined the entry criteria for BPSD, including the threshold level

**Ajit Shah**, MBChB, MRCPsych, Consultant in Old Age Psychiatry and Honorary Senior Lecturer, West London Mental Health NHS Trust, Southall, Middlesex and Imperial College School of Medicine, London, UK

**Antonio T. Lopes**, MBBS, Senior House Officer in Psychiatry, West London Mental Health NHS Trust, Southall, Middlesex, UK

of BPSD. Where the entry criteria for BPSD have been defined, the definition has amounted to a cut-off score on a BPSD measurement instrument. The relevance of this approach to clinical practice is unclear because clinicians usually treat BPSD if it results in distress or dangerousness. Moreover, clinicians may have difficulty in applying cut-off scores to individual patients. Studies using these entry criteria have erroneously assumed that BPSD are a homogeneous entity and they have lumped all the four BPSD domains and symptoms within each domain together; and, they have evaluated the efficacy of pharmacological interventions for all the BPSD domains and all the symptoms within a given domain simultaneously. Often the total score on a BPSD measurement instrument has been used as the main outcome measure and *post hoc* analyses have been conducted on the individual symptoms within one or more BPSD domain. Only a small number of studies have examined the efficacy of a pharmacological intervention with either an individual BPSD domain or a specific symptom within a given BPSD domain. Most studies do not provide an *a priori* hypothesis for efficacy in treating an individual BPSD domain or an individual symptom in a given BPSD domain. Most studies have not stratified individual BPSD domains or individual symptoms within a given BPSD domain at the randomization stage. Furthermore, studies designed to evaluate efficacy for improving cognition, have been retrospectively analysed for efficacy of anti-dementia drugs in treating BPSD. Such analysis included subjects without clinically significant BPSD because the entry criteria were based on the severity of cognitive impairment and not BPSD. Also, very few studies have provided data on power calculations for treating individual BPSD domains or individual symptoms within a BPSD domain. Some studies have not used formally evaluated instruments to measure the outcome and other studies have used instruments which have not been evaluated for use in dementia. Some studies have compared two drugs (with each other) without a placebo group, making interpretation of absolute efficacy difficult. Duration of individual studies has been variable and many studies do not provide data on the duration of treatment before efficacy was observed and the duration for which treatment should be continued. There is also a paucity of placebo-controlled studies examining two drugs from the same class, two drugs from different classes, drug combinations, and pharmacological treatments with non-pharmacological treatments.

## SUMMARY OF TREATMENT STUDIES FOR DISORDERS OF BEHAVIOUR

### *OPEN-LABEL STUDIES (APPENDIX 1)*

Risperidone, at daily doses of 0.5–1.8 mg, had efficacy for treating some individual disorders of behaviour: agitation [10–14]; sleep disturbance [10, 14]; verbal and physical aggression [10, 12–14, 15]; activity disturbance [12, 14, 15]; irritability [12]; wandering [14]; diurnal rhythm disturbance [15]; and, avolition and social withdrawal [12]. Olanzapine, at a daily dose of up to 10 mg, improved irritability, social misunderstanding and wandering [16]. Quetiapine, at a dose of 45–77 mg, improved activity disturbance, aggression and diurnal rhythm disturbance [17]. Olanzapine was superior to risperidone and haloperidol in improving aggression [18]. Tacrine, at a daily dose of 99 mg, improved disinhibition [19]. Galantamine, at a daily dose of 8–24 mg, improved apathy, agitation, apathy and aberrant motor behaviours [20]. Rivastigmine, at a daily dose of 12 mg, improved apathy, dishibition and irritability [21]. Donepezil, at a daily dose of 5–10 mg, improved irritability and disinhibition [22]. Topiramate (with or without a neuroleptic), at a daily dose of 50–75 mg, improved aggression [23]. Gabapentin, at daily dose of 980 mg, improved agitation, aggression, sleep disturbance, apathy and wandering [24].

### *RANDOMIZED AND DOUBLE-BLIND STUDIES (APPENDIX 1)*

Total scores on BPSD rating scales improved as follows: Neuropsychiatric Inventory (NPI) [25] with olanzapine [26, 27] and risperidone [27]; Behavioural Pathology in Alzheimer's

Disease Rating Scale (BEHAVE-AD) [28] with risperidone [29]; Cohen-Mansfield Agitation Inventory (CMAI) [30] with risperidone [31, 32], haloperidol [33], trazodone [33], and valproate [34]; Nurses Observation Scale for Inpatient Behaviour (NOSIE) [35] with thioridazine and diazepam [36, 37]; Brief Psychiatric Rating Scale (BPRS) [38] with carbamazepine [39] and fluvoxamine augmenting perphenazine [40]; and, Overt Aggression Scale (OAS) [41] with carbamazepine [39]. Risperidone (1–2 mg) and olanzapine (5–10 mg) as a combined group were superior to promazine in improving the total NPI score [27].

Efficacy for individual symptoms within the BPSD domain of disorders of behaviour are described here. Olanzapine, at a daily dose of 5–10 mg, improved agitation, aggression, irritability, lability and apathy [26, 42]. Risperidone, at a daily dose of 0.5–2 mg, improved aggression [29, 43, 31]. Risperidone was superior to haloperidol for treating aggression in two studies [43, 32], but there was no difference in another study [44]. Both haloperidol and trazodone improved agitation compared to baseline, but in the trazodone group improvement was predicted by depression score and improvement in the depression score with trazodone [33]. Thioridazine, compared to diazepam, improved social competence and retardation [37]. Galantamine, at a daily dose of 16–24 mg, improved aberrant motor behaviours [45]. Rivastigmine, at a mean daily dose of 99 mg, improved aberrant motor behaviours, apathy and indifference [46]. Metrifonate, at a daily dose of 50 mg, improved agitation, aggression and aberrant motor behaviours [47]. Donepezil, at a daily dose of 5–10 mg, improved apathy, indifference and irritability [48]. Trazodone, at a daily dose of 300 mg, improved irritability and agitation [49]. Combined citalopram (30 mg) and perphenazine (6.5 mg) improved agitation, lability and aggression [50]. Carbamazepine improved hostility [51] and aggression [39] at a mean daily dose of 388 and 300 mg respectively. Valproate, at a mean daily dose of 826–1000 mg, improved agitation [52, 34]. One study of oestrogen reported efficacy in treating aggression [53], but another study did not reproduce these findings [54]. Propranolol improved agitation and aggression in one study [55]. A Chinese herbal medicine, Yi-Cam San, improved agitation, aggression, irritability, lability and aberrant motor behaviours [56].

### *POOLED-ANALYSIS (APPENDIX 1)*

A pooled-analysis of three randomized and placebo-controlled studies of risperidone reported efficacy for individual symptoms within the BPSD domain of disorders of behaviour including hitting, hurting self and others, physical and verbal aggression, agitation, repeating sentences and questions, scratching, restlessness, grabbing onto people, constantly requesting attention, pacing and aimless wandering and repetitive mannerisms [57]. Another pooled-analysis of two of three studies in the last sentence reported that risperidone had efficacy for physical and verbal aggression [58]. A meta-analysis of seven studies of conventional neuroleptics reported modest efficacy for agitation [59]. A Cochrane review reported that haloperidol had efficacy for aggression [60]. A pooled-analysis of two studies of metrifonate reported efficacy for agitation, aggression, apathy and aberrant motor behaviours [61]. A pooled-analysis of two studies of memantine reported efficacy for agitation and aggression [62]. A pooled-analysis of three studies of rivastigmine reported efficacy for aggression [63]. A Cochrane review of two studies of trazodone [64] and three studies of valproate [65] concluded that there was insufficient evidence of efficacy for agitation.

## SUMMARY OF TREATMENT STUDIES FOR DISORDERS OF MOOD

### *OPEN-LABEL STUDIES (APPENDIX 1)*

Risperidone, at daily dose of 0.5–1.75 mg improved depressed mood [10, 12, 14] and affective disturbance [15]. Quetiapine, at a daily dose of 45–77 mg, improved anxiety and phobias [17]. Anxiety was improved by tacrine [19], galantamine [20] and rivastigmine [21] at daily doses of 99, 8–24 and up to 24 mg, respectively. Galantamine also improved depression [20].

### RANDOMIZED AND DOUBLE-BLIND STUDIES (APPENDIX 1)

Improvement in the total scores on BPSD rating scales is described above in the section on 'Summary of Treatment Studies for Disorders of Behaviour'.

Improvement occurred in the following individual symptoms within the BPSD domain of disorders of mood: olanzapine improved anxiety [42] and depression [26] at daily doses of 7.5 and 5–10 mg, respectively; risperidone, at a daily dose of 1.1 mg, improved affective disturbance and anxiety and phobias [31]; risperidone, at a daily dose of 0.8 mg, was superior to haloperidol in treating anxiety and phobias [32]; thioridazine, at a daily dose of 33 mg, was superior to diazepam in treating anxiety, fears and tension [36]; and, anxiety was improved by galantamine [45], rivastigmine [46] and donepezil [48] at daily doses of 16–24, 99 and 5–10 mg, respectively; and, the donepezil study also reported efficacy for depression and dysphoria [48].

Depression in dementia, measured using validated instruments, was improved by clomipramine [66], sertraline [67], moclobemide [68], citalopram [69] and trazodone [49] at daily doses of 100, 95, 400, 30 and 300 mg, respectively. None of the randomized and double-blind studies of anti-convulsants reported efficacy for depression.

### POOLED-ANALYSIS (APPENDIX 1)

Pooled-analysis of randomized and double-blind studies reported the following efficacy: risperidone improved tearfulness [57]; metrifonate improved depression and dysphoria [61]; and, for anti-depressants there was only weak evidence of efficacy [70].

## SUMMARY OF TREATMENT STUDIES FOR DISORDERS OF THOUGHT CONTENT AND DISORDERS OF PERCEPTION

### OPEN-LABEL STUDIES (APPENDIX 1)

The following efficacies were reported for individual symptoms within the BPSD domains of disorders of thought content and disorders of perception: risperidone for delusions, hallucination and undifferentiated psychotic features at a daily dose of 0.5–1.8 mg [10–15]; olanzapine for delusions and hallucinations at a daily dose of up to 10 mg [16]; quetiapine for delusions and hallucinations at a daily dose of 45–77 mg [17]; galantamine for delusions and hallucinations at a daily dose of 8–24 mg [20]; rivastigmine for delusions at a daily dose of up to 12 mg [21] and, donepezil for delusions at a daily dose of 5–10 mg [22]. One study reported olanzapine to be superior to both risperidone and haloperidol in treating delusions and hallucinations [18].

### RANDOMIZED AND PLACEBO-CONTROLLED STUDIES (APPENDIX 1)

Improvement in the total BPSD rating scale scores are described above in the section on 'Summary of treatment studies for disorders of behaviour'.

The following efficacies were reported for individual symptoms within the BPSD domains of disorders of thought content and disorders of perception: olanzapine for psychosis and delusions at a daily dose of 5–10 mg [26, 42]; risperidone for delusions and hallucinations at a daily dose of 1.1 mg [31]; rivastigmine for delusions and hallucinations at a daily dose of 9 mg [31]; metrifonate for hallucinations at a daily dose of 30–60 mg [71]; and, donepezil for delusions and hallucinations at a daily dose of 5–10 mg [48]. Thioridazine was superior to diazepam in treating positive symptoms (i.e. psychotic symptoms) [36]. A Chinese herbal medicine, Yi Gan San, improved hallucinations [56].

### *POOLED-ANALYSIS (APPENDIX 1)*

Several pooled-analyses revealed the following efficacies: risperidone improved non-paranoid delusions [57]; metrifonate improved hallucinations [61]; and, rivastigmine improved delusions [63].

## CONCLUSIONS FOR EFFICACY

Only data from randomized and double-blind studies and pooled-analysis are considered here. Several drugs, from different classes, improved total scores on several BPSD rating scales. However, these findings are difficult to translate into clinical practice because patients usually present with specific BPSD symptoms. However, these instruments can be used to monitor the progress of treatment.

Specific symptoms within the BPSD domain of disorders of mood including affective disturbance, depressed mood, anxiety and phobias improved with olanzapine, risperidone, thioridazine and galantamine. Thioridazine is not readily available in some countries because of concern over sudden deaths, and it also has a poor side-effect profile. Ideally, however, if disorders of mood are identified (as opposed to specific symptoms), then anti-depressants should be used. There is fair evidence that depression in dementia, measured by validated instruments, improves with sertraline, citalopram, moclobemide, clomipramine and trazodone. Clomipramine has potent anti-cholinergic properties and a poor side-effect profile, and it may not be the best drug to use for depression in dementia. It is difficult to ascertain the first line drug treatment because of an absence of head-to-head comparisons of efficacy and side-effects between the remaining four anti-depressants.

Symptoms of delusions and hallucinations within the BPSD domains of disorders of thought content and perception improved with risperidone, olanzapine, thioridazine, rivastigmine, donepezil and metrifonate. As noted above, thioridazine is not available in many countries. Metrifonate has been withdrawn because of serious side-effects. A head-to-head study of risperidone and olanzapine demonstrated no difference between the two drugs. It is difficult to ascertain the first line drug treatment of delusions and hallucinations due to the paucity of head-to-head studies of efficacy and side-effects between different neuroleptics and between neuroleptics and cholinesterase inhibitors.

Within the domain of disorders of behaviour the most common symptoms of agitation, aggression and aberrant motor behaviours improved with risperidone, olanzapine, galantamine, metrifonate, donepezil, trazodone, combination of citalopram and perphenazine, carbamazepine and valproate. Metrifonate has been withdrawn. It is difficult to ascertain the first line drug treatment due to a paucity of head-to-head comparisons between drugs within the same category and across different categories.

When cholinesterase inhibitors are used to treat cognitive impairment, it would not be unreasonable to withhold drugs from other categories to treat BPSD until there is evidence of poor treatment response with cholinesterase inhibitors for BPSD. The rationale for this is the reported efficacy for cholinesterase inhibitors in treating BPSD. However, this approach may be difficult to pursue due to paucity of data on the duration of treatment before the appearance of efficacy for BPSD with cholinesterase inhibitors (i.e. when should the decision be made that cholinesterase inhibitors are not effective?).

The following caveats should be fulfilled before using psychotropic drugs. First, the methodological issues described earlier should always be considered. Second, non-pharmacological interventions including treatment of intercurrent medical illness, correction of sensory deficits, evaluation of drug interactions and side-effects of prescribed drugs, identification and treatment of delirium, control of pain, support for carers, interventions directed at carers, psychological approaches in treating BPSD, aromatherapy, light therapy (although not widely available), reality orientation therapy, validation therapy, reminiscence therapy, music therapy, day care, nursing the dementia-sufferer in an appropriate environment with appropriately skilled staff (e.g. nursing home), respite care and carer training should always be considered [72]. However, despite these strategies there may be a case for prescribing psychotropic drugs.

Some authorities have suggested that pharmacological treatment should be postponed until BPSD have been present for at least 4 weeks because of a high rate of spontaneous resolution and a high placebo response rate [73].

## TIMING OF THE ONSET OF EFFICACY AND DURATION OF TREATMENTS

Accurate data on the time interval between prescribing and the onset of efficacy can only be obtained from randomized and double-blind studies. However, most studies have not reported this precise information despite serial measurements because they have simply reported efficacy at the study endpoint. Risperidone improved BEHAVE-AD total score [29, 31, 43], and CMAI total score [43] and aggression score [29, 43] by weeks 2–4 after prescription. Olanzapine improved psychotic symptoms by week 2 after prescription [26]. Thioridazine and diazepam improved agitation and affective symptoms by week 1 after prescription [36]. Thioridazine improved affective symptoms and positive symptoms by week 1 after prescription [37]. Intramuscular olanzapine and lorazepam improved agitation within 2 h and this was sustained for 24 h [74]. Depression improved after 2 weeks with clomipramine [66], 6 weeks with sertraline [67] and citalopram [69], and 10 days with moclobemide [68]. Carbamazepine improved agitation and aggression by week 3 after prescription [39].

Randomized, placebo-controlled and double-blind studies demonstrating efficacy at endpoint have been of the following duration: neuroleptics, 6–12 weeks; cholinesterase inhibitors, 21–26 weeks; anti-depressants, 17 days to 12 weeks; and, anti-convulsants, 6 weeks. A recent study suggests that psychotropic drugs can be withdrawn successfully in patients who have been free of BPSD for 3 months [75].

## RECENT CONTROVERSY WITH OLANZAPINE AND RISPERIDONE

In March 2004, the United Kingdom Committee of Safety of Medicines (CSM) informed clinicians that risperidone and olanzapine should not be used to treat BPSD because a meta-analysis of randomized placebo-controlled studies of risperidone in dementia demonstrated a 3-fold increase in strokes and a pooled-analysis of randomized placebo-controlled studies of olanzapine in dementia demonstrated a 3-fold increase in strokes and a 2-fold increase in mortality [76]. Moreover, they concluded, 'the magnitude of this risk is sufficient to outweigh likely benefits in the treatment of behavioural disturbances associated with dementia and is a cause for concern in any patient with a high baseline risk of stroke'. Similar concerns about risperidone were previously raised in Canada and the United States [77]. However, concerns about olanzapine are new. Clinicians were alarmed as these two drugs were widely used to treat BPSD because of evidence of efficacy and generally accepted better side-effect profiles than conventional neuroleptics, which show more severe and frequent adverse events like parkinsonism, tremor, dystonia, sedation, postural hypotension and anti-cholinergic effects [78].

The CSM provided the following prescribing advice:

- Both drugs should not be used to treat behavioural symptoms of dementia (essentially referring to 'disorders of behaviour' in the BPSD classification).
- Use of risperidone for the management of acute psychotic conditions in dementia should be limited to short-term use under specialist advice.

- Prescribers should consider carefully the risk of cerebrovascular events before treating any patient with a previous history of stroke or transient ischaemic attack. Furthermore, consideration should be given to other risk factors for cerebrovascular disease including hypertension, diabetes, atrial fibrillation and current smoking.

The arguments against a complete ban on these drugs can be summarized as follows [72]: (i) the risk of cerebrovascular adverse events (CVAEs) and mortality were derived from unsophisticated statistical analysis without adequately controlling for influential variables in the analysis; (ii) increased risk of CVAEs appeared to be confined to subjects with vascular dementia or mixed dementia and those with cerebrovascular risk factors; (iii) many of the studies used in the meta-analyses and pooled-analysis were not published in peer-reviewed journals and the pooled-analyses were not published after peer-review; (iv) CVAEs were not formally defined and reliable and valid methods of ascertaining CVAEs were not used; (v) studies included in pooled-analysis were not designed and powered to examine the relationship between prescription of these two drugs and the risk of CVAEs and mortality; (vi) there was no clear relationship between risk of CVAEs and mortality and the duration of exposure and the dosage of these two drugs; (vii) there was no clear evidence of a temporal relationship between prescription of these two drugs and development of CVAEs and death; and, (viii) patients with a pure dementia type were not examined except in two studies.

There is a serious risk that if the use of these two drugs is discouraged then clinicians will either use older neuroleptics (with modest efficacy, less desirable side-effect profile and poorly studied risk of CVAEs and mortality, which may be worse or comparable at best) or other newer neuroleptics (without evidence of efficacy and possibly similar problems which to date have not been studied), and patients may be exposed to unidentified side-effects with these drugs. There is a case from the evidence that these two drugs should not be used to treat BPSD in patients with vascular dementia and those with previous CVAEs and cerebrovascular risk factors. However, in patients with AD and without previous CVAEs and cerebrovascular risk factors the evidence is debatable. After exhausting non-pharmacological treatment strategies, if a decision is made to consider neuroleptics, patients and carers should be given a choice to consider these two drugs.

## A WAY FORWARD

There is evidence of efficacy in treating different BPSD domains and symptoms within specific BPSD domains for several psychotropic drugs. However, findings from different studies are difficult to interpret and compare because of various methodological issues discussed earlier. There is a need for a more robust research base to unequivocally support the use of these drugs. Future studies should be prospective, randomized, placebo-controlled (there should be a placebo group even when head-to-head comparisons are made to establish the superiority of active treatments over placebo), double-blind and have an *a priori* hypothesis. *Post hoc* analyses of studies designed for a different purpose, like those evaluating efficacy of cholinesterase inhibitors in treating cognitive impairment, should be avoided. The entry criteria for a specific BPSD domain or specific symptom within a BPSD domain should be clearly defined (and this definition should incorporate clinical criteria of distress and dangerousness that clinicians use for treating BPSD rather than just a cut-off score on BPSD measurement instrument). Studies should specifically either focus on an individual BPSD domain or individual symptoms within a BPSD domain. If several BPSD domains or specific symptoms are examined simultaneously then stratification of these parameters should occur at the randomization stage and the study should be adequately powered to examine multiple variables simultaneously. Another approach is to measure outcome using the factor structure of BPSD measurement instruments because this allows evaluation of efficacy for treating BPSD symptoms that cluster together; this method was successfully used in one study [48]. Studies should examine specific types of dementia and in specific settings. Where more than one type of dementia and/or study settings are considered, stratification of these variables should occur at the randomization stage. Only BPSD measurement instruments that have been formally evaluated for use in dementia should be used. There is a clear need for head-to-head comparisons between different drugs within the same class and across different classes, for both efficacy and side-effects, to allow clinicians to make decisions on first line treatments. There is also a need for comparisons between pharmacological treatments and non-pharmacological treatments for both efficacy and side-effects. All efficacy studies should provide data on the time interval for the onset of efficacy after prescription by using serial measurements. There is also a need for randomized and double-blind studies of discontinuation of psychotropic drugs as well as efficacy studies to ascertain the required duration of treatment.

## APPENDIX 1

### NEUROLEPTICS

#### *OPEN-LABEL STUDIES*

1. A retrospective open-label study evaluated the efficacy of risperidone in treating BPSD in 41 outpatients with a mixed group of dementias [11] using an unevaluated scale. At a mean daily dose of 1.8 mg and a mean treatment duration of 4 months, agitation (their definition included wandering, disrobing, non-violent disruptive behaviour, and physical and verbal aggression) and psychosis improved. Pre-existing extrapyramidal symptoms worsened ($n = 5$) and new extrapyramidal symptoms ($n = 6$) emerged.
2. A 6-month, open-label study evaluated the efficacy of risperidone in treating BPSD in 109 nursing home subjects with a mixed group of dementias using an unevaluated questionnaire completed by nurses [10]. Physical aggression, physical agitation, problems sleeping at night, problems sleeping during the day, verbal outbursts, anxiety, depressed mood, delusions and hallucinations improved in 74%, 70%, 85%, 67%, 62%, 65%, 64%, 75% and 73% of the subjects respectively. Most subjects received risperidone 0.25–0.5 mg twice daily. Risperidone was discontinued in 17 subjects because of oversedation, postural hypotension, agitation, sensitivity, urinary retention and exacerbation of existing extrapyramidal symptoms.
3. A 6-week, open-label study evaluated the efficacy of risperidone in treating BPSD in 938 subjects with a mixed group of dementias in primary care [14]. Significant improvement was reported for sleep disturbances, restlessness, agitation, wandering during the daytime, hostility, verbal aggression, screaming, physical aggression, depressed mood and delusions on an unevaluated questionnaire. Most patients were treated with daily dose of between 1 and 1.75 mg. Tolerance to risperidone was judged as being 'excellent' or 'satisfactory' in 99.3% of the sample with adverse events occurring in 7.4% of the sample.
4. A 4-month, open-label study of 26 subjects with a mixed group of dementias [79] reported efficacy for risperidone in treating agitation measured by the Behavioural and Emotional Activities Manifested in Dementia Scale [80]. The initial daily dose of 0.25 mg was gradually increased to a maximum of 3 mg. Five subjects developed new extrapyramidal symptoms.
5. A 12-week, open-label study evaluated the efficacy of risperidone in treating BPSD in 50 outpatients with Alzheimer's disease [12]. Significant improvement was reported in the Positive and Negative Symptoms Scale (PANSS) [81] excitement, depression and positive (equivalent to psychotic symptoms) factors, the Scale for the Assessment of Negative Symptoms in Alzheimer's Disease (SANS-AD) [82] items of avolition and social withdrawal, the Hamilton Depression Rating Scale (HDRS) [83]

scores and BEHAVE-AD subscale scores for aggressivity and activity disturbance. Risperidone related adverse events included extrapyramidal symptoms, confusion, dizziness and sedation.

6. An 8-week, open-label study of 34 inpatients and outpatients with a mixed group of dementias reported efficacy for risperidone in treating the NPI sub-items of agitation/aggression, irritability, delusions and hallucinations by week 8 [13]. The mean daily dose at endpoint was 1.1 mg. Risperidone was well tolerated with no clinically relevant changes in extrapyramidal symptoms, vital signs or weight.
7. An 8-week, open-label study evaluated the efficacy of risperidone in treating BPSD in 48 AD subjects receiving psychiatric services [15]. There was significant improvement in the total BEHAVE-AD score and BEHAVE-AD subscale scores for activity disturbance, aggressivity, diurnal rhythm disturbance, affective disturbance, delusions and hallucinations. Doses of either 0.25–0.5 or 0.75–1 mg were more efficacious than higher doses. The main adverse event was the development of extrapyramidal symptoms, and this was dose-dependent (42% of subjects receiving more than 1 mg developed extrapyramidal symptoms).
8. A 16-week, open-label study, using a complex design, evaluated the efficacy of risperidone in treating BPSD in 35 subjects with a mixed group of dementias who were refractory to an 8-week trial of haloperidol [84]. Haloperidol was substituted by risperidone, at a daily dose of 0.5 mg for 4 weeks, and then the daily dose was increased to 1 mg for a further 8 weeks. At the end of this 12-week period subjects were switched back to haloperidol for 4 weeks. Risperidone was effective in reducing the total Brief Psychiatric Rating Scale (BPRS) [38] scores and the total BEHAVE-AD scores. Vascular dementia predicted better efficacy. The incidence of side-effects was low.
9. A 12-week, open-label study of 8 subjects with dementia with Lewy bodies examined the efficacy of olanzapine using the BEHAVE-AD ($n = 4$) or the NPI ($n = 4$) as the outcome measure [85]. The dose range was 2.5–7.5 mg per day. Two subjects showed clear improvement. Three subjects could not tolerate olanzapine and in three subjects there was minimal benefit.
10. A 24-month, open-label study evaluated the efficacy of olanzapine in treating BPSD in vascular dementia, AD, frontal lobe dementia, Lewy body disease and Parkinson's dementia complex in 64 outpatients [16]. The total BEHAVE-AD score improved in the vascular dementia, frontal lobe dementia, Lewy body dementia and Parkinson's dementia complex, but not in AD. The total NPI score improved in frontal lobe dementia and Parkinson's dementia complex. In frontal lobe dementia, social misconduct, irritability, and wandering improved. In Lewy body dementia aggression and agitation improved. Delusions improved in frontal lobe dementia, Lewy body disease and Parkinson's dementia complex. Hallucinations improved in Lewy body disease and Parkinson's dementia complex. Flexible dosing of up to 10 mg was used. Olanzapine was considered safe.
11. An 8-week, open-label study evaluated the efficacy of quetiapine in treating BPSD in 16 inpatients and outpatients with AD [17]. The total CMAI score, the total BEHAVE-AD score, and BEHAVE-AD subscale scores for activity disturbance, aggressivity, diurnal rhythm disturbance, anxiety and phobias, delusions and hallucinations improved. The mean daily doses at baseline and endpoint were 45 and 77 mg, respectively. There was no difference in the baseline and the endpoint on measures of extrapyramidal symptoms.
12. A retrospective open-label study of 998 inpatients with a mixed group of dementias reported that olanzapine was more efficacious than risperidone and haloperidol in treating aggressive behaviour (active, passive and verbal), delusions and hallucinations [18] measured by the Psychogeriatric Dependency Rating Scale [86]. Olanzapine was also more efficacious than risperidone for manipulative behaviour and noisiness. Although data on side-effects were not reported, there were no differences in the rate of prescription of anti-cholinergics between the three groups.

## *RANDOMIZED, DOUBLE-BLIND STUDIES*

1. A 6-week, randomized, double-blind, placebo-controlled and parallel-group study evaluated the efficacy of olanzapine in treating BPSD in 206 institutionalized AD subjects [26]. The NPI Core

total (sum of agitation/aggression, hallucinations and delusion items), and scores on the NPI sub-items of agitation, aggression and psychosis significantly improved at daily doses of 5 and 10 mg, but not with 15 mg dose. Delusions only improved in the 5 mg group. The BPRS anxiety and depression scores significantly improved in the 5 and 10 mg groups. Improvement in the Core total score was observed from week 2. Somnolence was more common in the olanzapine group and was dose-related. Gait disturbance was more common in the 5 and 15 mg per day olanzapine groups compared to the placebo group. There were no significant differences in cognitive impairment, central anti-cholinergic effects and extrapyramidal symptoms between the olanzapine and placebo groups. A secondary analysis of 165 subjects without delusions or hallucinations at baseline was also undertaken [87]. Those without both hallucinations or delusions and those without hallucinations, at baseline, were more likely to develop these symptoms if they were on placebo. This effect was most pronounced when compared with higher doses of 10 and 15 mg. No effect was evident for the group without delusions at baseline. A *post hoc* analysis of 29 patients who had dementia with Lewy bodies [88] reported that patients on 5 mg showed significant improvement on the NPI sub-items of delusions and hallucination. Patients on 10 mg of olanzapine showed significant improvement on the NPI sub-item score for delusions. There was no effect on psychotic symptoms in the 15 mg olanzapine group. Analysis of the BPRS confirmed these findings. There was no significant exacerbation of extrapyramidal symptoms, worsening of cognitive impairment and development of anti-cholinergic toxicity.

2. A 10-week, randomized, placebo-controlled, double-blind and parallel-group study evaluated the efficacy of olanzapine at four dosages (1, 2.5, 5 and 7.5 mg per day) in treating BPSD in 652 institutionalized subjects with AD [42]. NPI sub-item scores for psychosis, delusions, agitation/aggression and irritability/lability improved significantly with only the 7.5 mg group compared to placebo. NPI sub-item scores for anxiety, euphoria/elation, irritability/lability and apathy/indifference improved in the 5 mg group compared to placebo. BPRS positive symptoms scores improved significantly in the 7.5 mg group compared to placebo. The incidence and the total number of adverse events were not significantly different between the four active treatment groups and the placebo group.
3. A 12-week, randomized, double-blind, placebo-controlled and parallel-group study of 625 institutionalized subjects with a mixed group of dementias evaluated the efficacy of risperidone in treating BPSD at three daily doses of 0.5, 1 and 2 mg [29]. A categorical reduction in total BEHAVE-AD score of more than 50% occurred significantly more frequently in the 1 and 2 mg group. There was also a significant reduction in the total BEHAVE-AD score and BEHAVE-AD subscale scores for aggressivity with all three risperidone groups. This improvement was observed at week 2 or 3 for the 1 and 2 mg groups, and at week 12 for the 0.5 mg group. This improvement was evident even after controlling for improvement in psychosis. Findings with the CMAI were similar. There was also a significant reduction in the BEHAVE-AD psychosis subscale score (mainly accounted for by delusions as hallucination at baseline were at a low frequency) at the 1 and 2 mg doses. In the 1 mg group, this improvement was evident from week 3. There was no difference in development of extrapyramidal symptoms between the placebo group and 0.5 and 1 mg risperidone groups; however, there was a higher incidence of extrapyramidal symptoms in the 2 mg risperidone group. The incidence of other adverse events was similar in the three risperidone groups and the placebo group. The most common dose-related adverse events were extrapyramidal symptoms, somnolence and peripheral oedema. A subgroup analysis of this study was conducted to examine the specific efficacy of risperidone in treating psychosis and aggression in those with psychotic symptoms [89]. In this group of patients both psychosis and aggression (measured by specially validated psychosis and aggression severity indices derived from other data in this study) improved and the improvement was dose-dependent, with the greatest efficacy with daily risperidone doses of 1–2 mg, and the improvement was sustained over 12 weeks.
4. A 12-week, randomized, double-blind, placebo-controlled and parallel-group study evaluated the efficacy of risperidone in treating BPSD among 344 institutionalized subjects with AD, vascular

dementia or mixed dementia [43]. This study also included a randomized haloperidol group with the secondary purpose of comparing the tolerability of risperidone with haloperidol. Risperidone, compared to placebo, resulted in significant reduction in the total BEHAVE-AD score, BEHAVE-AD subscale score for aggressivity, total CMAI score and CMAI subscale score for aggression. Improvement was evident by week 2. *Post hoc* analysis revealed that haloperidol also reduced BEHAVE-AD and CMAI aggression subscale scores, but risperidone was superior to haloperidol. The mean daily dose of haloperidol and risperidone at endpoint were 1.2 and 1.1 mg, respectively. There were no significant differences between the three groups for serious or severe adverse events. The severity of extrapyramidal symptoms did not differ between the risperidone and the placebo group, but was less in the risperidone group compared to the haloperidol group. Somnolence was more prevalent in both the treatment groups compared to the placebo group.

5. A 12-week, randomized, double-blind, placebo-controlled and parallel-group study evaluated the efficacy of risperidone in treating BPSD in 345 institutionalized subjects with AD, vascular dementia or mixed dementia [31]. Risperidone significantly improved the total CMAI score, CMAI total aggression score, CMAI physical and verbal aggression scores, CMAI total non-aggression score, CMAI verbal non-aggression score, total BEHAVE-AD score, and BEHAVE-AD subscale scores for aggressivity, affective disturbance, anxiety and phobias, delusions and hallucinations. The mean daily dose of risperidone was 0.95 mg. Improvement was evident by week 4 for the total BEHAVE-AD score. Somnolence and urinary tract infection were more prevalent in the risperidone group. There was no significant difference between the two groups for extrapyramidal symptoms.
6. A 12-week, randomized, double-blind and parallel-group study evaluated the efficacy of risperidone and haloperidol in treating BPSD in 58 inpatients and outpatients with AD or vascular dementia [44]. At the endpoint, in both the haloperidol and the risperidone groups compared to the baseline, a reduction in the total CMAI score and BEHAVE-AD subscale scores for aggressivity and psychosis was observed. Risperidone also resulted in significant reduction in the total BEHAVE-AD score and subscale scores for activity disturbance and diurnal rhythm disturbance. There were no differences between the two groups on the total CMAI score, total BEHAVE-AD score and all BEHAVE-AD subscale scores. The daily mean doses of haloperidol and risperidone were 0.9 and 0.85 mg, respectively. There was an excess of extrapyramidal symptoms in the haloperidol group.
7. An 18-week, double-blind, randomized and crossover design study of 120 institutionalized subjects with AD, vascular dementia and mixed dementia compared the efficacy of risperidone and haloperidol in treating BPSD [32]. Risperidone was more efficacious than haloperidol for the BEHAVE-AD subscales of aggressivity and anxiety and phobias, total CMAI score and CMAI subscale scores for aggressive behaviour, verbally agitated behaviour and physically non-aggressive behaviour. The mean daily dose of haloperidol and risperidone was 0.83 and 0.8 mg, respectively. Extrapyramidal symptoms, somnolence, insomnia and sialorrhoea were more common with haloperidol.
8. An 8-week randomized, double-blind and parallel-group study evaluated the efficacy of risperidone, olanzapine and promazine in treating BPSD in 60 patients with AD, vascular dementia and mixed dementia [27]. The combined risperidone and olanzapine groups, compared to the promazine group, produced greater reduction in the total NPI score. Data comparing risperidone and olanzapine were not provided. The daily dose range for risperidone, olanzapine and promazine were 1–2, 5–10 and 50–100 mg, respectively. The main side-effects with risperidone included hypotension, somnolence, dyspepsia and extrapyramidal symptoms. The main side-effects with olanzapine were somnolence, weight gain, dizziness, constipation, postural hypotension and akathisia. The main side-effects of promazine were constipation, hypotension, xerostomy, sinus tachycardia, cognitive impairment, extrapyramidal symptoms, confusion and somnolence.
9. An 8-week, randomized, double-blind and parallel-group study compared the efficacy of haloperidol, oxazepam and diphenhydramine in treating agitation rated by clinicians in 59 institutionalized subjects with a mixed group of dementias [90]. All three drugs modestly improved agitation on the BPRS and Alzheimer's Disease Assessment Scale [91], but there were no differences between the

three groups. The mean daily doses of haloperidol, oxazepam and diphenhydramine were 1.5, 30 and 81 mg, respectively. There were no differences between the three groups for adverse events.

10. A 14-day, double-blind, randomized and parallel-group study [92] comparing olanzapine and risperidone in 39 institutionalized subjects with dementia (mainly AD) reported that both drugs had efficacy for reducing the total NPI scores and the NPI sub-item scores for agitation, disinhibition, irritability, aberrant motor behaviours, depression/dysphoria, anxiety and the combined NPI sub-item score for delusions and hallucinations. However, there were no differences between the two drugs. The mean daily dose of olanzapine and risperidone were 6.65 and 1.47 mg, respectively. The side-effect profile of both drugs was similar.
11. A randomized, double-blind, placebo-controlled and parallel-group study evaluated the efficacy of intramuscular olanzapine (at doses of 2.5 and 5 mg per injection) and lorazepam (1 mg) for the treatment of acute agitation in inpatients and nursing home residents with a mixed group of dementia [74]. At 2 h after the first injection, both olanzapine groups and the lorazepam group showed significant improvement over placebo on the PANSS Excited Component and Agitation-Calmness Evaluation Scale (ACES) scores, and improvement on the CMAI was observed in the 5 mg olanzapine and the lorazepam groups only. At 24 h both olanzapine groups maintained superiority over placebo on the PANNS Excited Component, but lorazepam did not; improvement in the ACES score was observed in the 5 mg olanzapine and lorazepam groups only. At 24 h, however, there was no effect on CMAI in any of the treatment groups. Adverse events were not significantly different between any of the active treatment groups compared to the placebo group.
12. A 9-week, randomized, double-blind and parallel-group study compared the efficacy of haloperidol and trazodone in treating agitation in 28 inpatients with a mixed group of dementias [33]. CMAI scores improved in both treatment groups. In the haloperidol group improvement was not associated with baseline BEHAVE-AD delusions subscale score or with change in scores on this scale with treatment. In the trazodone group improvement in CMAI scores was associated with baseline score on the HDRS and with improvement in HDRS scores with treatment. The mean daily optimal doses of haloperidol and trazodone were 2.5 and 218 mg, respectively. Data on side-effects were not reported.
13. A 16-week, randomized, parallel-group, placebo-controlled and single-blind study evaluated the efficacy of haloperidol, trazodone and behaviour management technique (BMT) in treating agitation in 149 subjects with AD [93]. The mean daily doses of haloperidol and trazodone were 1.8 and 200 mg, respectively. BMT consisted of 8 weekly and 3 biweekly structured sessions that provided information about AD, strategies for decreasing agitation, and structured in-session and 'out of session' assignments. There were no significant differences in outcome between the three treatment groups and the placebo group. However, significantly fewer side-effects (including bradykinesia and parkinsonian gait) were observed in the BMT group.
14. A 6-week, pilot, randomized, double-blind, placebo-controlled and parallel-group study reported no difference in the efficacy of haloperidol and fluoxetine in treating agitation in 15 outpatients with AD. Side-effects were more prevalent in the active treatment groups [94].
15. A 4-week, randomized, double-blind and parallel-group study compared the efficacy of thioridazine and diazepam in treating behaviour disturbance in 56 hospitalized elderly patients with 'senility' using the Hamilton Anxiety Rating Scale (HARS) [95] and a modified Nurses' Observation Scale for Inpatient Behaviour (NOSIE) [35] as the main outcome measures [36]. Although senility was not formally defined, their description suggests this was likely to equate with dementia. Thioridazine improved NOSIE scores more significantly. On the HARS, thioridazine improved scores for the items of anxiety, tension, fears, and behaviours at interview, overall mental illness and global change compared to diazepam. Patients on diazepam improved scores on the items of insomnia, intellect, depressed mood and agitation. Improvement for most items was evident as early as week one. The mean daily doses of thioridazine and diazepam were 39 and 9 mg per day. The main side-effect was drowsiness.

16. A 4-week, randomized, double-blind and parallel-group study compared thioridazine and diazepam in treating BPSD in 59 non-psychotic 'senile' patients [37]. Although dementia was not formally defined, the description of senility is similar to dementia. There were no significant differences between diazepam and thioridazine on the HDRS. Within the thioridazine group agitation, fears, anxious mood and depressed mood improved significantly from baseline; no such improvement was observed in the diazepam group. Patients on thioridazine compared to those on diazepam significantly improved on NOSIE symptom clusters of social competence, retardation, depressive manifestations, total positive factors and total patient assets. The mean daily dose of thioridazine and diazepam were 33 and 7 mg, respectively. Improvement was evident by week 1. No adverse events were reported for either drug.
17. A 26-week, randomized, double-blind, parallel group and placebo-controlled study of 93 institutionalized AD patients [96] reported no difference in efficacy for both quetiapine and rivastigmine in reducing agitation measured by the CMAI. The mean daily doses of the drugs were not provided, but they had aimed for quetiapine 50 mg twice a day and rivastigmine 9 mg or more once a day between weeks 12 and 26. Quetiapine was associated with greater cognitive decline then placebo. Data on other adverse events were not provided.

### *POOLED-ANALYSIS*

1. A *post hoc* pooled-analysis of 3 double-blind, randomized, parallel-group and placebo-controlled studies [29, 31, 43] examined the efficacy of risperidone in treating individual BPSD symptoms in nursing home subjects with a mixed group of dementias [57]. On the CMAI, hitting, hurting self or others, cursing or verbal aggression, repetitive sentences or questions, scratching, general restlessness, grabbing onto people, constant requests for attention, pacing and aimless wandering and performing repetitive mannerisms improved significantly. On the BEHAVE-AD, physical threats, violence, verbal outbursts, agitation, tearfulness and non-paranoid delusions improved significantly.
2. A pooled-analysis of two studies evaluating the efficacy of risperidone in the treatment of BPSD [29, 43] demonstrated that risperidone improved BEHAVE-AD aggressivity subscale scores, and CMAI total aggression scores, physical and verbal aggression scores compared to placebo [58]. Moreover, this effect was dose-dependent.
3. A meta-analysis of 7 placebo-controlled, randomized and parallel-group studies reported that conventional neuroleptics were superior to placebo in treating agitation in dementia with a modest effect size of 0.18 [97].
4. A systematic Cochrane database review, using pooled-analysis, concluded that haloperidol was useful in controlling aggressive behaviour in dementia, but was associated with increased side-effects [60].

## CHOLINESTERASE INHIBITORS AND RELATED DRUGS

### *OPEN-LABEL STUDIES*

1. A 24-week, open-label study evaluated the efficacy of tacrine in treating BPSD in 36 outpatients with AD [19]. There was improvement in the total NPI score and sub-item scores for anxiety and disinhibition. The average maximum daily dose of tacrine was 99 mg. Although precise data on side-effects were not provided, elevation of alanine aminotransferase and intolerable gastrointestinal side-effects prevented the attainment of maximum daily dose set at 160 mg.
2. A 3-month, open-label study of 124 AD patients [20] reported efficacy for galantamine in improving the total NPI score and sub-item scores for irritability, apathy, agitation, aberrant motor behaviour, night-time behaviour, depression, anxiety and euphoria, delusions and hallucinations at endpoint. The daily dose was increased from 8 to 24 mg over an 8-week period. Adverse events were mainly gastrointestinal.

3. A 52-week, open-label study of 72 institutionalized moderate to severe AD subjects [21] reported that rivastigmine significantly reduced the total NPI score and sub-item scores for apathy/indifference, disinhibition, irritability/lability, aberrant motor behaviours, appetite/eating changes, anxiety, euphoria/elation, delusions and hallucinations by the week 52 measurement. Mean daily dose was not provided, but patients either received the maximum tolerable dose or a maximum dose of 6 mg twice a day. Between week 27 and week 52, 95% of the sample experienced at least one adverse event, but most were considered mild or moderate in severity. The most commonly occurring serious adverse events were sepsis and pneumonia.
4. A 24-week, open-label study of donepezil (daily dose of 5 mg for 4 weeks and 10 mg for the remaining 20 weeks) of 10 hospitalized AD subjects reported efficacy for improving the NPI sub-item scores for irritability/lability, disinhibition and delusions by week 24 [22]. Donepezil was well-tolerated.
5. A 6-month, open-label study of donepezil in 28 outpatients with AD [98] reported a significant reduction in the total NPI score. Donepezil was given at a daily dose of 5 mg for 4 weeks and then increased to 10 mg for the remainder of the study. Only three adverse events were reported.
6. A 4-week, open-label, parallel-group and randomized study evaluated the efficacy of donepezil (5 mg per day) and perphenazine (8 mg per day) and perphenazine (16 mg per day) alone in treating psychotic symptoms in 12 AD inpatients who were resistant to perphenazine alone (8 mg per day) [99]. Total score on the PANSS improved more significantly in the combined donepezil and perphenazine group. Combined donepezil and perphenazine did not produce serious adverse events.

## *RANDOMIZED DOUBLE-BLIND STUDIES*

1. A secondary analysis of a 28-week, randomized, double-blind, placebo-controlled and parallel-group study of memantine (20 mg per day), primarily designed to evaluate efficacy for improving cognition in moderate to severe AD among community residents, reported no significant differences between placebo and memantine on the total NPI score [100].
2. A secondary analysis of a 21-week, randomized, double-blind, parallel-group and placebo-controlled study of 978 mild to moderate AD subjects [45] reported that galantamine at daily doses of 16 and 24 mg (compared to placebo and galantamine at 8 mg per day) significantly improved the total NPI score and sub-item scores for aberrant motor behaviours and anxiety. This study was originally designed to evaluate efficacy for cognitive improvement and, therefore, subjects with and without behavioural problems at the start were separately examined. In those without behavioural symptoms at entry, galantamine had efficacy in maintaining lower scores on the NPI sub-items of aberrant motor behaviours, apathy and disinhibition. In those with behavioural symptoms at the start, galantamine had efficacy in reducing NPI sub-item scores for agitation and aggression and aberrant motor behaviours. These improvements were mainly at galantamine dosage of 16 and 24 mg per day.
3. A 23-week, randomized, double-blind, placebo-controlled and parallel-group study evaluated the efficacy of rivastigmine in treating BPSD in 120 outpatients with dementia with Lewy bodies [46]. Rivastigmine was prescribed for 20 weeks and this was followed by a 3-week rest period. The total score on the 4-item and 10-item NPI improved more significantly in the rivastigmine group compared to placebo by week 20. After discontinuation of rivastigmine these differences tended to disappear. Specific NPI symptoms that improved included apathy, indifference, aberrant motor behaviours, anxiety, delusions and hallucinations. At week 8, when the titration period ended, the mean daily dose of rivastigmine was 99.4 mg. Known adverse effects of cholinesterase inhibitors including nausea, vomiting and anorexia were more common in the rivastigmine group, but the tolerability of these drugs was judged to be acceptable.
4. A 26-week, randomized, double-blind, placebo-controlled and parallel-group study, primarily designed to evaluate efficacy in improving cognition, evaluated the efficacy of metrifonate in treating BPSD in 264 outpatients with AD [47]. At a daily dose of 50 mg, significant improvement

in the total NPI score and sub-item scores for agitation/aggression and aberrant motor behaviours were observed. Metrifonate was reported to be well tolerated with adverse events being mild.

5. A 36-week, randomized, double-blind (for 26-weeks), placebo-controlled and parallel-group study, primarily designed to evaluate efficacy for improving cognition, evaluated the efficacy of metrifonate in treating BPSD in 408 outpatients with AD [71]. The total NPI score and sub-item score for hallucinations significantly improved compared to placebo at a daily metrifonate dose of 30–60 mg compared to placebo. Metrifonate was said to be well-tolerated.
6. A sub-analysis of a 24-week randomized, double-blind, placebo-controlled and parallel-group study of donepezil, primarily designed to evaluate efficacy for improving cognition [48], also evaluated its efficacy in treating BPSD [101]. Donepezil was given at a daily dose of 5 mg for 28 days and then increased to 10 mg in 144 subjects (placebo group $n = 146$). Factor analysis revealed three factors for the NPI sub-items. There was significant improvement in the donepezil group compared to the placebo group in the factor containing NPI items of agitation/aggression, depression/dysphoria, anxiety, apathy/indifference and irritability/lability, and in the factor containing delusions, hallucinations and appetite/eating change. Donepezil was well-tolerated.

### *POOLED-ANALYSIS*

1. A *post hoc*, pooled-analysis of two [47, 71] 26-week placebo-controlled, randomized, double-blind and parallel-group studies evaluated the efficacy of metrifonate in treating BPSD in 672 subjects with AD [61]. In the metrifonate group, the total NPI score and sub-items scores for agitation/aggression, apathy, aberrant motor behaviours, depression/dysphoria and hallucinations improved significantly. Improvement was evident by week 12 and maintained until week 26.
2. A *post hoc*, pooled-analysis of two studies of memantine in mild to moderately severe AD, designed to evaluate improvement in cognition, evaluated its efficacy in treating BPSD [62]. The first study was a 24-week (monotherapy with 20 mg per day memantine) double-blind, randomized, placebo-controlled, parallel-group study in 252 subjects [100]. The second study was a 24-week, randomized, double-blind, placebo-controlled and parallel-group study of 404 subjects receiving either placebo and donepezil (5–10 mg per day) or memantine (20 mg per day) and donepezil (5–10 mg per day) [102]. In the combination study there was significant improvement in total NPI scores at the endpoint. Memantine showed improvement in both studies compared to placebo for scores on the NPI sub-items of agitation/aggression. Memantine was well-tolerated in both studies.
3. A pooled-analysis of three [103, 104, 97] 6-month randomized, double-blind, placebo-controlled studies of rivastigmine involving 1840 subjects with AD, primarily designed to evaluate efficacy in improving cognition, reported that BEHAVE-AD subscales of delusions and aggressivity improved in the rivastigmine group at a daily dose range of 6–12 mg [63]. Emergence of activity disturbance was also prevented by rivastigmine. In subjects with more advanced AD, the BEHAVE-AD hallucinations and aggressivity subscale scores significantly improved.

## ANTI-DEPRESSANTS

### *CASE-REPORTS*

1. Several case-reports describe efficacy for trazodone in treating agitation in dementia [105–107].

### *RANDOMIZED, DOUBLE-BLIND STUDIES*

1. An 8-week, randomized, double-blind, placebo-controlled and parallel-group study evaluated the efficacy of imipramine in 61 (33 without depression and 28 with depression) outpatients with AD at a daily mean dose of 82–83 mg [108]. Those with and without depression were separately randomized and analysed. There was no difference between the treatment and placebo groups for changes in the HDRS. Data on side-effects were not provided.

2. A 14-week, randomized, double-blind, placebo-controlled and crossover design study evaluated the efficacy of clomipramine in treating depression among 21 outpatients with probable AD [66]. Clomipramine was more efficacious in improving the HDRS score. This effect was evident as early as week 2. The daily dose was titrated by 25 mg per week to a maximum of 100 mg by weeks 4–6. Only one patient developed serious side-effects, but mild side-effects were frequent with clomipramine including dry mouth, dizziness, sleep problems, constipation, headaches, stomach aches, nausea and tremor.
3. A 12-week, randomized, double-blind, placebo-controlled and parallel-group study evaluated the efficacy of sertraline in treating major depression in 44 AD outpatients [67]. Sertraline significantly improved scores on the Cornell Scale for Depression in Dementia (CSDD) [109] and the HDRS, and the number of full and partial responders was significantly higher in the sertraline group. The mean daily dose was 95 mg. There were no differences in the adverse events in the two groups. Response to treatment was observed by week 6 and continued until week 12. An initial analysis of this study with 22 subjects previously reported similar findings, except that treatment response was seen at week 3 [110].
4. An 8-week, randomized, placebo-controlled, double-blind and parallel-group study evaluated the efficacy of sertraline in treating depression in 31 female nursing home residents with late-stage AD [111]. Three outcome measures were used: CSDD, the Gestault Scale for depression [112] and the CMAI. Although scores on all three scales improved in the sertraline and placebo group compared to the baseline, there were no significant differences between the two groups. The dose was titrated from 25 mg at the outset to 100 mg between weeks 5 and 8. Data on adverse events were not reported.
5. A 6-week randomized, double-blind, placebo-controlled and parallel-group study evaluated the efficacy of fluoxetine (up to 40 mg per day) in treating depression in 41 outpatients with AD [113]. There were no differences between the treatment and the placebo group for remission and improvement in HDRS and HARS.
6. A 6-week, randomized, double-blind, placebo-controlled and parallel-group study evaluated the efficacy of moclobemide in treating 511 subjects with dementia and depression and 183 subjects with depression and cognitive decline at a daily dose of 400 mg [68]. Moclobemide, compared to placebo, produced significantly greater improvement on the HDRS in both (dementia and depression, and depression with cognitive decline) groups. Cognition also improved significantly. Improvement was evident from day 10 onwards.
7. A 6-week, randomized, double-blind, placebo-controlled and parallel-group study evaluated the efficacy of citalopram in 149 inpatients and outpatients with depression with ($n$ = 29) and without dementia [69]. Citalopram compared to placebo, improved scores on the Montgomery Asberg Depression Rating Scale (MADRS) [114] and HDRS more significantly. Improvement was observed at week 6. Data on the dementia sub-group were not separately reported. The daily dose of citalopram was increased up to 30 mg. Citalopram was well-tolerated.
8. A randomized, placebo-controlled and parallel-group study evaluated the efficacy of citalopram in treating emotional disturbances in 98 dementia-sufferers (both AD and vascular dementia) using a complicated design [115]. Subjects were randomized to placebo or citalopram for the first 4 weeks (phase A). After this all subjects received citalopram for 8 weeks (phase B). Following this subjects were again randomized to placebo or citalopram (phase C) and this phase was designed to study withdrawal effects. Initial dose of citalopram was 20 mg and this was reduced or increased by 10 mg by the clinician. Although MADRS scores improved in the active treatment group for AD (but not vascular dementia) during phase A, there were no significant differences between the treatment and placebo groups. Also, it is unclear what entry criteria, in addition to dementia, were used. Side-effects were few and mild with citalopram.
9. A 12-week, randomized, placebo-controlled and crossover study of trazodone in 31 outpatients with fronto-temporal dementia reported that trazodone improved the total NPI score and sub-items scores for irritability/agitation and depression [49]. The protocol allowed daily doses of up to

300 mg, but the mean doses used were not given. Adverse events were more prevalent in the trazodone group including fatigue, dizziness, hypotension and cold extremities.

10. An 8-week, randomized, double-blind and parallel-group study compared the efficacy of paroxetine and imipramine in treating depression in 198 subjects with a mixed group of dementias [116]. There were no significant differences between the two groups on the MADRS and the CSDD. However, MADRS scores improved in both groups compared to baseline at weeks 2, 4, and 8; the CSDD scores improved at weeks 2 and 4, but not at week 8, in both groups compared to baseline. The daily doses of paroxetine and imipramine ranged from 20 to 40, and 25 to 100 mg, respectively. Anti-cholinergic and serious non-fatal adverse events were reported more frequently in the imipramine group.
11. A 17-day, randomized, double-blind, placebo-controlled and parallel-group study compared citalopram and perphenazine in treating psychosis and behaviour disturbance in 85 non-depressed hospitalized patients with AD, vascular dementia and mixed dementia [50]. Total scores improved on the Neurobehavioural Rating Scale (NBRS) [117] in both the citalopram and perphenazine groups compared to baseline. However, only citalopram was superior to placebo. Furthermore, citalopram demonstrated improvement in the NBRS subscales of agitation/aggression and lability/tension compared to placebo. There was no efficacy for treating psychotic symptoms by both the active treatments. The mean daily dose of citalopram and perphenazine were 20 and 6.5 mg, respectively. There were no differences in the side-effect profile between the two drugs and placebo.
12. A 12-week, randomized, placebo-controlled, double-blind and parallel-group study evaluated the efficacy of sertraline augmentation to donepezil in 144 (24 patients with sertraline and donepezil and 120 patients with placebo and donepezil) outpatients with AD [118]. The mean daily dose of sertraline at endpoint was 125 mg. There was no statistically significant effect for sertraline on the NPI. However, in a subgroup of patients with moderate to severe BPSD, a greater number of subjects receiving sertraline demonstrated a reduction of 50% or more on the NPI subscale of behavioural disturbance. Only diarrhoea was more common in the sertraline group.
13. A pilot, randomized, double-blind, placebo-controlled and crossover design study with a complicated design evaluated the efficacy of fluvoxamine (50 mg) augmenting perphenazine in treating psychosis in AD [40]. During the first week all 20 subjects received perphenazine 4 mg and placebo three times a day. During the second week, in one group this regime was continued and in the other group placebo was replaced by 50 mg per day of fluvoxamine. After three weeks the regimes were crossed over for a further three weeks. In the combined fluvoxamine and perphenazine group there was significant improvement in BPRS scores when compared to the placebo and perphenazine group. Fluvoxamine alone or in combination with perphenazine was well-tolerated.

### *POOLED-STUDIES*

1. A systematic Cochrane database review, using pooled-analysis of 104 dementia-sufferers from two studies [49, 93], concluded that there was insufficient evidence from randomized, placebo-controlled studies to support a recommendation for prescribing trazodone to treat agitation in dementia [64].
2. A systematic Cochrane database review, using meta-analysis of three randomized, double-blind studies [66, 108, 110], concluded that there is weak evidence of efficacy of anti-depressants in treating depression in dementia [70].

## ANTI-CONVULSANTS

### *OPEN-LABEL STUDIES*

1. An open-label study, with a mean duration of 18 days, reported that either topiramate alone, or in combination with a neuroleptic, reduced aggression measured by the CMAI in 15 inpatients with a

mixed group of dementias at the endpoint [23]. The median daily doses of topiramate when used alone and with a neuroleptic were 75 and 50 mg, respectively. Data on side-effects were not provided.

2. A retrospective case-note review reported efficacy for sodium valproate in treating (undefined) behaviour disturbance in 25 dementia patients without psychotic symptoms [119]. Formally evaluated instruments were not used to measure BPSD. The final mean daily dose of valproate was 1650 mg with a mean serum level of 64 μg/ml. Valproate was well-tolerated except for reversible sedation in 8 subjects and transient worsening of gait and confusion in one patient.

## RANDOMIZED, DOUBLE-BLIND STUDIES

1. A pilot 6-week, double-blind, randomized, parallel-group and placebo-controlled study evaluated the efficacy of carbamazepine in treating agitation resistant to treatment with neuroleptics in 21 AD outpatients [51]. The BPRS item of hostility significantly improved. The mean daily dose towards the end of the study was 388 mg and the mean serum level was 4.9 g/ml. Adverse events were mild and included diarrhoea.
2. A 6-week, double-blind, randomized, placebo-controlled and parallel-group study of 51 institutionalized subjects with a group of mixed dementias [52] reported efficacy for carbamazepine in reducing the total BPRS score, score on the BPRS factors of agitation and hostility, and the total score on the OAS. Improvement was evident by week 3. The daily modal dose at week 6 was 300 mg with a mean serum level of 5.3 μg/ml. There were more adverse events in the carbamazepine group, but they were clinically significant in two patients.
3. A 6-week, randomized, double-blind, placebo-controlled and parallel-group study evaluated the efficacy of valproate in treating agitation in 56 nursing home residents with AD, vascular dementia and mixed dementia [120]. The daily mean dose at termination was 826 mg and the mean serum level was 45 μg/ml. There was significant improvement in the BPRS agitation factor score in the valproate group compared to the placebo group at endpoint. Side-effects were more common in the valproate group and were generally rated as mild, and were similar to those generally reported for valproate. Following this double-blind study, a 6-week open-label extension study was conducted in 46 subjects [120]. The mean daily optimum dose was 851 mg with a mean serum level of 47.5 μg/ml. There was significant improvement on the total BPRS score, BPRS agitation factor score, total Overt Aggression Scale (OAS) score and the total score on the Clinical Consortium to Establish Registry for Alzheimer's Disease Behaviour Rating Scale for Dementia [121] at endpoint.
4. An 8-week, randomized, placebo-controlled, double-blind and crossover design study evaluated the efficacy of valproate in treating aggressive behaviour in 42 inpatients with a mixed group of dementias [122]. A fixed daily dose of 480 mg was used and the mean serum level at the end of the valproate phase (3 weeks) was 41 μg/ml. Treatment with valproate showed no effect for aggressive behaviour compared to placebo on the main outcome measure of Social Dysfunction and Aggression Scale-9 [123]. Side-effects were reported to be rare in both periods and were not related to serum valproate levels. This study was followed by a 12-week open-label extension in 39 subjects [124]. The mean daily dose and serum levels at endpoint were 611 mg and 45 μg/ml respectively. Aggression scores improved significantly compared to baseline scores at endpoint. Although seven subjects died, death was not associated with valproate and the only side-effect reported was drowsiness in three subjects.
5. A 6-week, randomized, double-blind, placebo-controlled and parallel-group study evaluated the efficacy of valproate in treating BPSD (and the main objective was to improve mania secondary to dementia) in 172 institutionalized subjects with a mixed group of dementias [34]. There was efficacy in improving total CMAI scores and scores on the CMAI subscale of verbally agitated behaviours; this improvement occurred by day 14. There was no efficacy for BPRS and Bech-Rafaelsen Mania Scale [125]. The median daily dose of valproate was 1000 mg at endpoint and the mean weekly serum level ranged from 55.3 to 68.9 μg/ml. Side-effects of somnolence and thrombocytopenia were more prevalent in the treatment group.

### *POOLED-ANALYSIS*

1. A systematic Cochrane database review was unable to perform meta-analysis of three studies [34, 52, 122], but concluded that there was no evidence for valproate having efficacy in treating agitation in dementia [65].

## OTHER DRUGS

### *CASE-REPORTS*

1. Two case-reports described efficacy for cyproterone acetate in treating sexual disinhibition in vascular dementia and dementia associated with Parkinson's disease without relevant side-effects at a daily dose of 10 mg [126].
2. Two case-reports described efficacy for gabapentin augmentation of donepezil in improving total NPI scores in AD [127].
3. Two case-reports described efficacy for buspirone in treating agitation in dementia [128, 129].

### *OPEN-LABEL STUDIES*

1. A 15-month, open-label study evaluated the efficacy of gabapentin, at a mean daily dose of 980 mg, in treating BPSD in 20 nursing home residents with probable AD and significant medical comorbidity [24]. The total NPI and CMAI scores improved at both 7 and 15 months evaluation. NPI sub-items of agitation, aggressiveness, anxiety and sleep disturbance improved at 7 and 15 months, and apathy and wandering improved at 15 months. No serious adverse events were reported.

### *RANDOMIZED, DOUBLE-BLIND STUDY*

1. A 4-week, randomized, parallel-group, placebo-controlled and double-blind study evaluated the efficacy of oestrogen in 15 subjects with moderate to severe dementia (undifferentiated) and reported reduction in overall aggression and physically aggressive behaviour scores on the Overt Aggression Scale [53]. The daily dose ranged from 0.625 to 2.5 mg. There were no adverse events.
2. An 8-week, randomized, placebo-controlled, double-blind and parallel-group study evaluated the efficacy of weekly oestrogen patches in treating aggressive behaviour in 27 subjects with a mixed group of dementias [54]. There were no differences in scores on the Rating Scale for Aggressive Behaviour in the Elderly [130] and the CSDD between the two groups. Patients received 100 μg oestrogen patch weekly (two received 50 μg patches). There were no differences in adverse events between the two groups.
3. A randomized, placebo-controlled, double-blind and parallel-group study evaluated the efficacy of propranolol in treating BPSD in 31 institutionalized AD patients [55]. Propranolol was titrated over 9 days and then maintained at that dose for 6 weeks (mean daily dose was 106 mg). Propranolol improved the total NPI score and NPI sub-item scores for aggression/agitation approached significance. Propranolol was well-tolerated.
4. A 4-week randomized, parallel-group (the only comparison group was without any medication) and observer-blind study evaluated the efficacy of a traditional Chinese herbal medicine Yi-Gan San in treating BPSD in 52 institutionalized subjects with a mixed group of dementias [56]. If patients showed insufficient improvement after one week then a dopamine D1 selective neuroleptic tiapride was added, and 11 subjects in the comparison group required this addition compared to none in the treatment group. The total NPI score and sub-item scores for agitation/aggression, irritability/lability, aberrant motor activity and hallucinations significantly improved in the treatment group at a dose of 2.5 g three times a day. No treatment emergent adverse events were observed in either group.

## REFERENCES


1. Finkel SI. Behavioral and psychological signs and symptoms of dementia: implications for research and treatment. *Int Psychogeriatr* 1996; 8(suppl 3):215–552.
2. Finkel SI, Burns A. Introduction to behavioral and psychological symptoms of dementia (BPSD): a clinical and research update. *Int Psychogeriatr* 2000; 12(suppl 1):9–12.
3. Burns A, Jacoby R, Levy R. Psychiatric phenomena in Alzheimer's disease. I: Disorders of thought content. *Br J Psychiatry* 1990; 15:72–76.
4. Burns A, Jacoby R, Levy R. Psychiatric phenomena in Alzheimer's disease. II: Disorders of perception. *Br J Psychiatry* 1990; 157:76–81.
5. Burns A, Jacoby R, Levy R. Psychiatric phenomena in Alzheimer's disease. III: Disorders of mood. *Br J Psychiatry* 1990; 157:81–86.
6. Burns A, Jacoby R, Levy R. Psychiatric phenomena in Alzheimer's disease. IV: Disorders of behavior. *Br J Psychiatry* 1990; 157:86–94.
7. Shah AK, Foli S, Nnatu I. Measurement of behavioral disturbance, non-cognitive symptoms and quality of life. In: O'Brien J, Ames D, Burns A (eds). *Dementia*. Arnold Hodder, London, 2005, pp 72–80.
8. Foli S, Shah A. Measurement of behavior disturbance, non-cognitive symptoms and quality of life. In: O'Brien J, Ames D, Burns A (eds). *Dementia*. Hodder Arnold, London, 2000, pp 87–100.
9. Shah AK. Aggressive behavior in the elderly. *Int J Psychiatry Clin Pract* 1999; 3:85–103.
10. Goldberg RJ, Goldberg J. Risperidone for dementia-related disturbed behavior in nursing home residents: a clinical experience. *Int Psychogeriatr* 1997; 9:65–68.
11. Irizarry MC, Ghaemi SN, Lee-Cherry ER *et al.* Risperidone treatment of behavioral disturbance in outpatients with dementia. *J Neuropsychiatry Clin Neurosci* 1999; 11:336–342.
12. Negron AE, Reichman WE. Risperidone in the treatment of patients with Alzheimer's disease with negative symptoms. *Int Psychogeriatr* 2000; 12:527–536.
13. Rainer MK, Masching AJ, Ertl M *et al.* Effect of risperidone on behavioral and psychological symptoms and cognitive function in dementia. *J Clin Psychiatry* 2001; 62:894–900.
14. Wancata J. Efficacy of risperidone for treating patients with behavioral and psychological symptoms of dementia. *Int Psychogeriatr* 2004; 16:107–115.
15. Yoon JS, Kim JM, Lee H *et al.* Risperidone use in Korean patients with Alzheimer's disease: optimal dosage and effect on behavioral and psychological symptoms, cognitive function and activities of daily living. *Hum Psychopharmacol* 2003; 18:627–633.
16. Moretti R, Torre P, Antonella RM *et al.* Olanzapine as a treatment of neuropsychiatric disorders of Alzheimer's disease and other dementias: a 24 month follow-up of 68 patients. *Am J Alzheimers Dis Other Dement* 2003; 18:205–214.
17. Fujikawa T, Takahashi T, Kinoshita A *et al.* Quetiapine treatment for behavioral and psychological symptoms in patients with senile dementia of Alzheimer's type. *Neuropsychobiol* 2004; 49:201–204.
18. Edell WS, Tunis SL. Antipsychotic treatment of behavioral and psychological symptoms of dementia in geropsychiatric inpatients. *Am J Geriatr Psychiatry* 2001; 9:289–297.
19. Kaufer DI, Cummings J, Christine D. Effect of tacrine on behavioral symptoms in Alzheimer's disease: an open label study. *J Geriatr Psychiatry Neurol* 1996; 9:1–6.
20. Monsch AU, Giannakopoulos P, on behalf of the GAL-SUI-1 Study Group. Effects of galantamine on behavioral and psychological disturbances and caregiver burden in patients with Alzheimer's disease. *Curr Med Opin Res* 2004; 20:931–938.
21. Aupperle PM, Koumaras B, Chen M *et al.* Long-term effects of rivastigmine treatment of neuropsychiatric and behavioral disturbances in nursing home residents with moderate to severe Alzheimer's disease: results of a 52-week open label study. *Curr Med Res Opin* 2004; 20:1605–1612.
22. Barak Y, Bodner E, Zemishlani H *et al.* Donepezil for the treatment of behavioral disturbances in Alzheimer's disease: a 6-month open trial. *Arch Gerontol Geriatr* 2001; 33:237–241.
23. Fhager B, Meiri I, Sjogren M *et al.* Treatment of aggressive behavior in dementia with the anticonvulsant topiramate: a retrospective pilot study. *Int Psychogeriatr* 2003; 15:307–309.
24. Moretti R, Torre P, Antonella RM *et al.* Gabapentin for the treatment of behavioral alterations in dementia. Preliminary 15-month investigation. *Drugs Aging* 2003; 20:1035–1040.
25. Cummings JL, Mega M, Gray K *et al.* The Neuropsychiatric Inventory: comprehensive assessment of psychopathology in dementia. *Neurology* 1994; 44:2308–2314.
26. Street JS, Clark S, Gannon KS *et al.* Olanzapine treatment of psychotic and behavioral symptoms in patients with Alzheimer's disease in nursing care facilities. *Arch Gen Psychiatry* 2000; 57:968–976.

27. Gareri P, Cotroneo A, Lacava R *et al.* Comparison of the efficacy of new conventional antipsychotic drugs in the treatment of behavioral and psychological symptoms of dementia (BPSD). *Arch Gerontol Geriatr* 2004; (suppl 9):207–215.
28. Reisberg B, Borensteen J, Sabb S *et al.* Behavioral symptoms in Alzheimer's disease: phenomenology and treatment. *J Clin Psychiatry* 1987; 48(suppl):9–15.
29. Katz IR, Jeste D, Mintzer JE *et al.* Comparison of risperidone and placebo for psychosis and behavioral disturbances associated with dementia: a randomized, double-blind trial. *J Clin Psychiatry* 1999; 60:107–115.
30. Cohen-Mansfield J. Agitated behavior in the elderly II. Preliminary results in the cognitively deteriorated. *J Am Geriatr Soc* 1986; 34:722–727.
31. Brodaty H, Ames D, Snowdon J *et al.* A randomized placebo-controlled trial of risperidone for the treatment of aggression, agitation and psychosis of dementia. *J Clin Psychiatry* 2003; 64:134–143.
32. Suh GK, Son HG, Ju YS *et al.* A randomized, double-blind, crossover comparison of risperidone and haloperidol in Korean dementia patients with behavioral disturbances. *Am J Geriatr Psychiatry* 2004; 12:509–516.
33. Sultzer DL, Gray KF, Gunay I *et al.* Does behavioral improvement with haloperidol or trazodone treatment depend on psychosis or mood symptoms in patients with dementia? *J Am Geriatr Soc* 2001; 49:1294–1300.
34. Tariot PN, Schneider LS, Mintzer J *et al.* Safety and tolerability of divalproex sodium in the treatment of mania in elderly patients with dementia: results of a double-blind, placebo-controlled trial. *Curr Therapeutic Res* 2001; 62:51–67.
35. Honigfeld G. NOSIE-30. A treatment sensitive ward behavior scale. *Psychol Rep* 1966; 19:180–185.
36. Kirven LE, Montero EF. Comparison of thioridazine and diazepam in the control of non-psychotic symptoms associated with senility: double blind study. *J Am Geriatr Soc* 1973; 21:546–551.
37. Covington JS. Alleviating agitation, apprehension and related symptoms in geriatric patients: a double-blind comparison of a phenothiazine and a benzodiazepine. *South Med J* 1975; 68:719–724.
38. Overall JE, Gorham DR. Introduction to the brief psychiatric rating scale (BPRS): recent developments in ascertainment and scaling. *Psychopharmacol Bull* 1988; 24:97–98.
39. Tariot PN, Erb R, Podgorski CA *et al.* Efficacy and tolerability of carbamazepine for agitation and aggression in dementia. *Am J Psychiatry* 1998; 155:54–61.
40. Levkovitz Y, Bloch Y, Kaplan D *et al.* Fluvoxamine for psychosis in Alzheimer's disease. *J Nervous Ment Disord* 2001; 189:126–129.
41. Yudofsky SC, Silver JM, Jackson W *et al.* The overt aggression scale for the objective rating of verbal and physical aggression. *Am J Psychiatry* 1986; 143:35–39.
42. De Deyn PP, Carrasco MM, Deberdt W *et al.* Olanzapine versus placebo in the treatment of psychosis with or without associated behavioral disturbances in patients with Alzheimer's disease. *Int J Geriatr Psychiatry* 2004; 19:115–126.
43. De Deyn PP, Rabheru K, Rasmussen A *et al.* A randomized trial of risperidone, placebo and haloperidol for behavioral symptoms of dementia. *Neurology* 1999; 53:946–955.
44. Chan W, Lam LC, Choy CN *et al.* A double-blind randomized comparison of risperidone and haloperidol in the treatment of behavioral and psychological symptoms in Chinese dementia patients. *Int J Geriatr Psychiatry* 2001; 16:1156–1162.
45. Cummings JL, Schneider L, Tariot P *et al.* Reduction of behavioral disturbances and caregiver distress by galantamine in patients with Alzheimer's disease. *Am J Psychiatry* 2004; 161:532–538.
46. McKeith I, Del Ser T, Spano PF *et al.* Efficacy of rivastigmine in dementia with Lewy bodies: a randomized, double-blind, placebo-controlled international study. *Lancet* 2000; 356:2031–2036.
47. Raskind MA, Cyprus PA, Ruzicka BB *et al.* The effects of metrifonate on the cognitive, behavioral, and functional performance of Alzheimer's disease patients. *J Clin Psychiatry* 1999; 60:318–325.
48. Feldman H, Gauthier S, Hecker J *et al.* A 24-week, randomized, double-blind study of donepezil in moderate to severe Alzheimer's disease. *Neurology* 2001; 57:613–620.
49. Lebert F, Stekke W, Hasenbroekx C *et al.* Frontotemporal dementia: a randomized, controlled trial with trazodone. *Dement Geriatr Cogn Disord* 2004; 17:355–359.
50. Pollock BG, Mulsant BH, Rosen J *et al.* Comparison of citalopram, perphenazine, and placebo for acute treatment of psychosis and behavioral disturbances in hospitalized, demented patients. *Am J Psychiatry* 2002; 159:460–465.
51. Olin JT, Fox LS, Pawluczyk S *et al.* A pilot randomized trial of carbamazepine for behavioral symptoms in treatment resistant outpatients with Alzheimer's disease. *Am J Geriatr Psychiatry* 2001; 9:400–405.

52. Porsteinsson AP, Tariot PN, Erb R *et al.* Placebo controlled study of divalproex sodium for agitation in dementia. *Am J Geriatr Psychiatry* 2001; 9:58–66.
53. Kyomen HH, Satlin A, Hennen J *et al.* Estrogen therapy and aggressive behavior in elderly patients with moderate-to-severe dementias: results from a short-term randomized, double-blind trial. *Am J Geriatr Psychiatry* 1999; 4:339–349.
54. Hall KA, Keks NA, O'Connor DW. Transdermal oestrogen patches for aggressive behavior in male patients with dementia: a randomized, controlled trial. *Int Psychogeriatr* 2005; 17:165–178.
55. Peskind ER, Tsuang DW, Bonner LT *et al.* Propranolol for disruptive behaviors in nursing home residents with probable and possible Alzheimer's disease. *Alzheimer Dis Assoc Disord* 2005; 19:23–28.
56. Iwasaki K, Satoh-Nakagawa T, Maruyama M *et al.* A randomized, observer-blind, controlled trial of the traditional Chinese medicine Yi-Gan San for improvement of behavioral and psychological symptoms and activities of daily living in dementia patients. *J Clin Psychiatry* 2005; 66:248–252.
57. Rabinowitz J, Katz IR, De deyn P *et al.* Behavioral and psychological symptoms in patients with dementia as a target for pharmacotherapy with risperidone. *J Clin Psychiatry* 2004; 65:1329–1334.
58. De Deyn PP, Katz IR. Control of aggression and agitation in patients with dementia: efficacy and safety of risperidone. *Int J Geriatr Psychiatry* 2000; 15:S14–S22.
59. Schneider LS, Pollock VE, Lyness SA. A meta-analysis of controlled trials of neuroleptic treatment in dementia. *J Am Geriatr Soc* 1990; 38:553–563.
60. Lonergan ET, Luxenberg J, Colford J. Haloperidol for agitation in dementia. *Cochrane Database Syst Rev* 2002; CD002852.
61. Cummings JL, Nadel A, Mastermann D *et al.* Efficacy of metrifonate in improving the psychiatric and behavioral disturbances of patients with Alzheimer's disease. *J Geriatr Psychiatry Neurol* 2001; 14:101–108.
62. Gauthier S, Wirth Y, Mobius HJ. Effects of memantine on behavioral symptoms in Alzheimer's disease: an analysis of the neuropsychiatric inventory (NPI) data of two randomized, controlled studies. *Int J Geriatr Psychiatry* 2005; 20:459–464.
63. Finkel SI. Effects of rivastigmine on behavioral and psychological symptoms of dementia in Alzheimer's disease. *Clin Ther* 2004; 26:980–990.
64. Martinon-Torres G, Fioravanti M, Grimley Evans J. Trazodone for agitation in dementia. *Cochrane Database Syst Rev* 2004; CD004990.
65. Lonergan ET, Luxenberg J. Valproate preparations for agitation in dementia. *Cochrane Database Syst Rev* 2004; CD003945.
66. Petracca G, Teson A, Chemerinski E *et al.* A double-blind placebo-controlled study of clomipramine in depressed patients with Alzheimer's disease. *J Neuropsychiatry* 1996; 8:270–275.
67. Lyketsos CG, DelCampo L, Steinberg M *et al.* Treating depression in Alzheimer's disease: efficacy and safety of sertraline therapy, and the benefits of depression reduction: The DIADS. *Arch Gen Psychiatry* 2003; 60:737–744.
68. Roth M, Mountjoy CQ, Amrien R *et al.* Moclobemide in elderly patients with cognitive decline and depression. An international double-blind, placebo-controlled trial. *Br J Psychiatry* 1996; 168:149–157.
69. Nyth AL, Godfries CG, Lyby K *et al.* A controlled multicentre clinical study of citalopram and placebo in elderly depressed patients with and without concomitant dementia. *Acta Psychiatr Scand* 1992; 86:138–145.
70. Bains J, Birks JS, Dening TR. The efficacy of antidepressant in the treatment of depression in dementia. *Cochrane Database Syst Rev* 2002; CD003944.
71. Morris JC, Cyprus PA, Orazem J *et al.* Metrifonate benefits cognitive, behavioral, and global function in patients with Alzheimer's disease. *Neurology* 1998; 50:1222–1230.
72. Shah AK, Suh GK. A case for judicious use of olanzapine and risperidone in dementia. *Int Psychogeriatr* 2005; 17:12–29.
73. Ballard C, O'Brien J. Treating behavioral and psychological signs in Alzheimer's disease. *Br Med J* 1999; 319:138–139.
74. Meehan KM, Wang H, David SR *et al.* Comparison of rapidly acting intramuscular olanzapine, lorazepam, and placebo: a double-blind, randomized study in acutely agitated patients with dementia. *Neuropsychopharmacology* 2002; 26:494–504.
75. Committee of Safety of Medicines. Atypical antipsychotic drugs and stroke. http://medicines.mhra.gov.uk/ourwork/monitorsafequalmed/messages/risperidoneclinicaltrialdata final.pdf. Date of Access: May 13, 2004.
76. Ballard C, Thomas A, Fossey J *et al.* A 3-month randomized placebo controlled neuroleptic discontinuation study in 100 people with dementia: the neuropsychiatric inventory median cut-off is a predictor of clinical outcome. *J Clin Psychiatry* 2004; 65:114–119.

77. Smith D, Beier M. Association between risperidone treatment and cerebrovascular adverse events: examining the evidence and postulating hypotheses for an underlying mechanism. *J Am Med Dir Assoc* 2004; 5:129–132.
78. Saxe T. Risperidone questioned as dementia first-line treatment. *Geriatrics* 2004; 59:11.
79. Laks J, Engelhardt E, Marinho V *et al.* Efficacy and safety of risperidone oral solution in agitation associated with dementia in the elderly. *Arq Neuropsiquiatr* 2001; 59:859–864.
80. Sinha D, Zamlan FP, Nelson S. A new scale for assessing behavioral agitation in dementia. *Psychiatr Res* 1992; 41:73–88.
81. Kay SR, Opler LA, Fizbein A. Positive and negative syndrome scale (PANSS) for schizophrenia. *Schizophr Bull* 1987; 13:261–276.
82. Reichman WE, Coyne AC, Amirneri S *et al.* Negative symptoms in Alzheimer's disease. *Am J Psychiatry* 1996; 153:424–426.
83. Hamilton M. A rating scale for depression. *J Neurol Neurosurg Psychiatry* 1960; 23:56–62.
84. Lane HY, Chang YC, Su MH *et al.* Shifting from haloperidol to risperidone for behavioral disturbances in dementia: safety, response predictors, and mood effects. *J Clin Pharmacol* 2002; 22:4–10.
85. Walker Z, Grace, J, Overshot R *et al.* Olanzapine in dementia with Lewy bodies: a clinical study. *Int J Geriatr Psychiatry* 1999; 14:459–466.
86. Wilkinson IM, Graham-White J. Psychogeriatric Dependency Rating Scale (PGDRS): a method of assessment for use by nurses. *Br J Psychiatry* 1980; 137:558–565.
87. Clark WS, Street JS, Feldman PD *et al.* The effect of olanzapine in reducing the emergence of psychosis among nursing home patients with Alzheimer's disease. *J Clin Psychiatry* 2001; 62:34–40.
88. Cummings JL, Street J, Masterman D *et al.* Efficacy of olanzapine in the treatment of psychosis in dementia with Lewy bodies. *Dement Cogn Disord* 2002; 13:67–73.
89. Schneider LS, Katz IR, Park S *et al.* Psychosis of Alzheimer's disease. Validity of the construct and response to risperidone. *Am J Geriatr Psychiatry* 2003; 11:414–425.
90. Coccaro E, Kramer E, Zemishlany Z *et al.* Pharmacologic treatment of noncognitive behavioral disturbance in elderly demented patients. *Am J Psychiatry* 1990; 147:1640–1645.
91. Rosen WG, Mohs RC, Davis KL. A new rating scale for Alzheimer's disease. *Am J Psychiatry* 1984; 141:1356–1364.
92. Fontaine CS, Hynan LS, Koch K *et al.* A double-blind comparison of olanzapine versus risperidone in the acute treatment of dementia-related behavioral disturbances in extended care facilities. *J Clin Psychiatry* 2003; 64:726–730.
93. Teri L, Logsdon RG, Peskind E *et al.* Treatment of agitation in AD: a randomized, placebo-controlled clinical trial. *Neurology* 2000; 55:1271–1278.
94. Auchus AP, Bissey-Black C. Pilot study of haloperidol, fluoxetine, and placebo for agitation in Alzheimer's disease. *J Neuropsychiatry* 1997; 9:591–593.
95. Hamilton M. The assessment of anxiety states by rating. *Br J Med Psychology* 1959; 32:50–53.
96. Ballard C, Margallo-Lana M, Juszczak E *et al.* Quetiapine and rivastigmine and cognitive decline in Alzheimer's disease: randomized double-blind placebo controlled trial. *Br Med J* 2005; 330:874–877.
97. Schneider LS, Anand R, Farlow M. Systematic review of the efficacy of rivastigmine in patients with Alzheimer's disease. *Int J Geriatr Psychopharmacol* 1998; (suppl 1):26–34.
98. Paleacu D, Mazeh D, Mirecki I *et al.* Donepezil for the treatment of behavioral symptoms in patients with Alzheimer's disease. *Clin Neuropharmacol* 2002; 6:313–317.
99. Bergman J, Brettholz I, Shneidman M *et al.* Donepezil as add-on treatment of psychotic symptoms in patients with dementia of Alzheimer's type. *Clin Neuropharmacol* 2003; 26:88–92.
100. Reisberg B, Doody R, Stoffler A *et al.* Memantine in moderate-to-severe Alzheimer's disease. *N Engl J Med* 2003; 348:1333–1341.
101. Gauthier S, Feldman H, Hecker J *et al.* Efficacy of donepezil on behavioral symptoms in patients with moderate to severe Alzheimer's disease. *Int Psychogeriatr* 2002; 14:389–404.
102. Tariot PN, Farlow MR, Grossberg GT *et al.* Memantine treatment in patients with moderate to severe Alzheimer's disease already receiving donepezil: a randomized controlled trial. *J Am Med Assoc* 2004; 291:317–324.
103. Corey-Bloom JF, Anand R, Veach J, for the ENA 713 B352 Study Group. A randomized trial evaluating the efficacy and safety of ENA 713 (rivastigmine tartrate), a new acetylcholinesterase inhibitor, in patients with mild to moderately severe Alzheimer's disease. *Int J Geriatr Psychopharmacol* 1998; 1:55–65.
104. R Sler M, Anand R, Cicin-Sain A *et al.* Efficacy and safety of rivastigmine in patients with Alzheimer's disease: International randomized controlled trial. *Br Med J* 1999; 318:633–638.

105. Greenwald BS, Marin DB, Silverman SM. Serotoninergic treatment of screaming and banging in dementia. *Lancet* 1986; ii:1464–1465.
106. O'Neil M, Page N, Adkins WN *et al.* Tryptophan-trazodone treatment of aggressive behavior. *Lancet* 1986; ii:859–860.
107. Simpson DN, Foster D. Improvement in organically disturbed behavior with trazodone treatment. *Gen Clin Psychiatry* 1986; 47:192–193.
108. Reifler B, Teri L, Raskind M *et al.* Double-blind trial of imipramine in Alzheimer's disease patients with and without depression. *Am J Psychiatry* 1989; 146:45–49.
109. Alexopoulos GS, Abrahams RC, Young RC *et al.* Cornell Scale for depression in dementia. *Biol Psychiatry* 1988; 23:271–284.
110. Lyketsos CG, Sheppard JM, Steele CD *et al.* Randomized, placebo-controlled, double-blind clinical trial of sertraline in the treatment of depression complicating Alzheimer's disease: initial results from depression in Alzheimer's disease study (DIADS). *Am J Psychiatry* 2000; 157:1686–1689.
111. Magai C, Kennedy G, Cohen CI *et al.* A controlled clinical trial of sertraline in the treatment of depression in nursing home patients with late-stage Alzheimer's disease. *Am J Geriatr Psychiatry* 2000; 8:66–74.
112. Abrahams RC, Alexopoulos GS. Assessment of depression in dementia. *Alzheimer's Dis Relat Disord* 1994; 8:S227–S229.
113. Petracca GM, Chemerinski E, Starkstein SE. A double-blind, placebo-controlled study of fluoxetine in depressed patients with Alzheimer's disease. *Int Psychogeriatr* 2001; 13:233–240.
114. Montgomerie SA, Asberg M. A new depression rating scale designed to be sensitive to change. *Br J Psychiatry* 1979; 134:382–389.
115. Nyth AL, Gottfries CG. The clinical efficacy of citalopram in treatment of emotional disturbances in dementia disorders. A Nordic Multicentre Study. *Br J Psychiatry* 1990; 157:894–901.
116. Katona C, Hunter BN, Bray J. A double-blind comparison of the efficacy and safety of paroxetine and imipramine in the treatment of depression in dementia. *Int J Geriatr Psychiatry* 1998; 13:100–108.
117. Levin HS, High WM, Goethe KE *et al.* The neurobehavioral rating scale: assessment of the behavioral sequalae of head injury by the clinician. *Neurol Neurosurg Psychiatry* 1987; 50:183–193.
118. Finkel S, Mintzer J, Dysken M *et al.* A randomized, placebo-controlled study of the efficacy and safety of sertraline in the treatment of behavioral manifestations of Alzheimer's disease in outpatients treated with donepezil. *Int J Geriatr Psychiatry* 2004; 19:9–18.
119. Narayan M, Nelson JC. Treatment of dementia with behavioral disturbance using divalproex or a combination of divalproex and a neuroleptic. *J Clin Psychiatry* 1997; 58:351–354.
120. Porsteinsson AP, Tariot PN, Jakimovich LJ *et al.* Valproate therapy for agitation in dementia. *Am J Geriatr Psychiatry* 2003; 11:434–440.
121. Tariot PN, Mack JL, Patterson MB *et al.* The behavior rating scale for dementia of the consortium to establish a registry for Alzheimer's disease. *Am J Psychiatry* 1995; 152:1349–1357.
122. Sival RC, Haffmans PMJ, Jansen PAF *et al.* Sodium valproate in the treatment of aggressive behavior in patients with dementia – a randomized placebo controlled clinical trial. *Int J Geriatr Psychiatry* 2002; 17:579–585.
123. Wistedt B, Rasmussen A, Pederson L *et al.* The development of an observer-scale for measuring social dysfunction and aggression. *Pharmacopsychiatry* 1990; 23:249–252.
124. Sival RC, Duivenvoorden HJ, Jansen PAF *et al.* Sodium valproate in aggressive behavior in dementia: a twelve-week open label follow-up study. *Int J Geriatr Psychiatry* 2004; 19:305–312.
125. Bech P, Rafaelsen OJ, Kramp P *et al.* The mania rating scale: scale construction and interobserver agreement. *Neuropharmacology* 1978; 17:430–431.
126. Haussermann P, Goecker D, Beier K *et al.* Low-dose cyproterone acetate treatment of sexual acting out in men with dementia. *Int Psychogeriatr* 2003; 15:181–186.
127. Dallocchio C, Buffa C, Ligure N *et al.* Combination of donepezil and gabapentin for behavioral disorders in Alzheimer's disease. *J Clin Psychiatry* 2000; 61:64.
128. Colenda CC. Buspirone in treatment of agitated demented patients. *Lancet* 1988; i:1169.
129. Tiller JWG, Dakis JA, Shaw JM. Short-term buspirone treatments in disinhibition with dementia. *Lancet* 1988; ii:510.
130. Patel V, Hope RA. A rating scale for aggressive behavior in the elderly – the RAGE. *Psychol Med* 1992; 22:211–221.

# 17

# Management of affective disorders in dementia

*A. Thomas*

## INTRODUCTION

Non-cognitive symptoms occur in the great majority of people with dementia and affective disturbances are among the most common of these symptoms. These are dominantly depression with or without associated anxiety and agitation, although mania does occur. In a community study in England depression was identified in 24% of those with Alzheimer's disease (AD), whereas mania occurred in 'only' 3.5% [1]. In the Cache County study, the Neuropsychiatric Inventory was used to rate the presence of psychiatric symptoms in people with dementia and it was reported that 23.7% had depression, 17% anxiety, but only 0.9% had elation [2]. Since depression is so much more frequent in dementia than elation and most research has focused on this, the management of depression in dementia will be the main consideration here.

## DEPRESSION IN DEMENTIA

Depression and dementia have a complex inter-relationship. It is now recognized that people with depression have cognitive impairments, characteristically frontal-subcortical in pattern [3], and these are probably more severe in those whose depression begins in late life [4]. It is also now clear that depression is itself an independent risk factor for dementia [5]. In many cases in which the onset of dementia occurs a year or two after the depression it is likely that the depression was in a fact a harbinger of the dementia, since the risk of dementia in such people is substantially increased [6]. In these cases depression may be a prodrome to the cognitive decline, and some of these cases may have been diagnosed as 'depressive pseudodementia' [7]. However, even when such cases are excluded, depression is a risk factor for subsequent dementia when it occurs many years before the dementia diagnosis is made [5]. Here the focus is on the development of depression in people with a pre-existing dementia.

### *DEPRESSION IN PRE-EXISTING DEMENTIA*

#### *What do we mean by depression in dementia?*

The term depression is a slippery one, being used for a symptom (low mood), a vague group of related symptoms (low mood, anergia, anhedonia etc), or a more clearly defined syndrome (e.g. DSM major depressive episode). Knowing which kind of meaning is being used is clearly important because it affects the interpretation of each study in the field. This

**Alan Thomas**, BSc, MBChB, MRCPsych, PhD, Senior Lecturer and Honorary Consultant in Old Age Psychiatry, Newcastle University and Gateshead Health NHS Foundation Trust, Newcastle upon Tyne, UK

question merges into that of whether we conceive of depression as a continuum, in practice leaving the clinician to decide when the number and severity of symptoms is sufficient to merit intervention, or as a discrete illness, with the clinician needing to satisfy himself that diagnostic criteria are met. In clinical practice such a difference in approach probably is less important in terms of deciding whom to treat than other issues specific to depression in dementia. For in the context of dementia, the additional problem arises as to whether we consider the symptoms of depression as being separate and potentially distinguishable from the same symptoms occurring outside depression in dementia (an additional syndrome, albeit one which is likely to be due to the same underlying disease process), or whether symptoms consistent with depression are taken to be indicative of a potentially treatable depression regardless of whether they appear the same as in many other people with dementia. Whilst obviating the diagnostic difficulties of the former approach, taking this latter approach will lead to high rates of 'depression', and by implication large numbers of people needing intervention for depression. Given that, as shown below, many apparent depressive episodes are transient in dementia, that evidence for the efficacy of current treatments is modest and that pharmacological treatments are associated with adverse effects, it appears prudent to take the former approach. This is the approach encapsulated in the provisional diagnostic criteria for depression of AD recently published by a group of North American investigators [8]. They aimed to capture those people whose affective disturbance in dementia was likely to be a significant depression and so, as in DSM-IV criteria for major depression, these criteria include the 2 week rule for persistence of symptoms and symptoms are to be associated with clinically significant distress or disruption in functioning. The details of the symptoms differ from those 'standard' depression criteria, as shown in Table 17.1, and clinicians are encouraged to try to distinguish symptoms due to depression from those due to dementia. Also two depression items (irritability and social withdrawal) are added and the total number required in the 2-week period to meet the diagnosis is 3 or more (compared with 5 or more for major depression in DSM-IV).

#### *How common is depression in dementia?*

Reported prevalence figures vary enormously, due in part to the differences discussed above in how depression is defined as well as to other issues such as variation in the assessment methods employed and the population sampled. For example in the Cache County study the prevalence of depression (as a symptom on the Neuropsychiatric Inventory [9]) was 24% in those with dementia compared with 7% in those without [2]. In a prospective study over 5 years, 59% AD patients were rated as having depressed mood at some time, whereas 'only' 28% had depressed mood associated with vegetative signs [10]. These findings are consistent with earlier reports that isolated symptoms were much more common than depressive syndromes [11] and this 28% figure is also within the usual prevalence range for depression syndromes of 20–40%, e.g. 25% with major depression and 27% with minor depression in a hospital sample [12].

Although most research has focused on depression in AD, evidence suggests that depression is more frequent in the other two main causes of dementia in late-life. Depression is more frequent in vascular dementia than in AD in both community (32% vs. 20% [2]) and clinic (19% vs. 8% [13]) samples. In dementia with Lewy bodies (DLB) depression is reported in 48% compared with 18% of AD subjects [14] and this high prevalence has led to it being added as a supportive diagnostic feature [15]. These findings imply that even more careful attention should be paid to detecting depression in these patient groups. Another important feature of depression in dementia is that it appears to fluctuate [11] and to be less persistent than in primary depression. In an important prospective study it was found that depressed mood with vegetative signs, approximating to a depression syndrome, rarely persisted [10].

**Table 17.1** Provisional diagnostic criteria for depression of AD [35]

A. Three (or more of the following symptoms have been present during the same 2-week period and represent a change from previous functioning: at least one of the symptoms is either (1) depressed mood or (2) decreased positive affect or pleasure

**Note:** Do not include symptoms that, in your judgement, are clearly due to a medical condition other than AD, or are a direct result of non-mood-related dementia symptoms (e.g. loss of weight due to difficulties with food intake)

1. Clinically significant depressed mood (e.g. depressed, sad, hopeless, discouraged, tearful)
2. Decreased positive affect or pleasure in response to social contacts and usual activities
3. Social isolation or withdrawal
4. Disruption in appetite
5. Disruption in sleep
6. Psychomotor changes (e.g. agitation or retardation)
7. Irritability
8. Fatigue or loss of energy
9. Feelings of worthlessness, hopelessness, or excessive or inappropriate guilt
10. Recurrent thoughts of death, suicidal ideation, plan or attempt

B. All criteria are met for dementia of the Alzheimer type (DSM-IV-TR)
C. The symptoms cause clinically significant distress or disruption in functioning
D. The symptoms do not occur exclusively during the course of a delirium
E. The symptoms are not due to the direct physiological effects of a substance (e.g. a drug of abuse or a medication)
F. The symptoms are not better accounted for by other conditions such as major depressive disorder, bipolar disorder, bereavement, schizophrenia, schizoaffective disorder, psychosis of AD, anxiety disorders, or substance-related disorder

*Specify if*:

**Co-occurring onset:** if onset antedates or co-occurs with the AD symptoms
**Post-AD onset:** if onset occurs after AD symptoms

*Specify*:

**With psychosis of AD**
**With other significant behavioural signs or symptoms**
**With past history of mood disorder**

### *The adverse impact of depression in dementia*

When depression occurs in dementia it adds considerably to the overall morbidity, further impairing activities of daily living [16], increasing agitation, wandering and aggression [16, 17] and worsening quality of life [18]. Consequently it is associated with a more rapid decline [19], earlier placement in nursing care [20] and a higher mortality [21]. If depression in dementia can be successfully treated then these adverse effects of the illness might also be reduced.

## *RECOGNITION AND DIAGNOSIS*

Concerns about failure to recognize depression in old people with and without dementia continue, although the increasing numbers of prescriptions for depression for the aged suggests this may be a diminishing problem. Starting from the point where someone has recognized that the person with dementia may now also have depression, we come to the problems touched on earlier of diagnosing depression in someone with dementia. We can slightly simplistically separate these difficulties into the conceptual and practical.

#### *Conceptual difficulties*

Approaching the problem of diagnosing depression in people with dementia on the theoretical level one can immediately see major difficulties. A good history remains the most important element in diagnosis in medicine and yet this is not going to be available from the majority of people with dementia. The patient is also unable accurately to describe their current psychopathology during the mental state assessment and, as mentioned above, most of the symptoms needed to diagnose the depression syndrome (such as sleep disturbance, appetite and weight loss, anergia, psychomotor symptoms) occur frequently in people with dementia who show no evidence of mood disturbance. A detailed assessment of these features may enable the clinician to disentangle depression, rather than the dementia, as a 'cause' of them, although in practice such fine distinctions are very difficult to make (see 'Practical difficulties' below). In fact it may be argued that only low mood and the so-called cognitive symptoms of depression, such as guilt, pessimism and suicidal ideation, do not occur frequently in people who have dementia without depression. Yet in individuals who have moderate-severe dementia, it is difficult in most cases to elicit convincing evidence of negative ideation. Thus we can see why the clinician asked to assess for the presence of depression in someone with dementia often finds himself reduced to trying to discern if the patient is sad and wondering if there are any other reliable symptoms to support such an impression.

#### *Practical difficulties*

The solution to the absence of valid information from the patient for a history is to speak with an informant. Yet in practice many of those referred are living alone, when only the account of a neighbour or friend may be available, or are in residential care when the clinician can only obtain a report from a formal carer. In both of these situations, the report is usually very difficult to weigh up (how often does she see her? How well does he know her?) and on some occasions is clearly erroneous. Whilst thus far the difficulty of trying to recognize depression in dementia has focused on the confounding effects of the dementia itself, in clinical practice the presence of other illnesses frequently further complicates the situation. It is not uncommon for the onset of depression symptoms, such as a reduction in physical activity and social withdrawal, to be due to the development of an infection or the worsening of pain due to long-standing arthritis.

#### *What is helpful in diagnosing depression in dementia?*

These practical difficulties are minimized in those with milder dementia, although even here the amnesia is likely to reduce the volume and quality of reliable history. If historical information is available from the patient or an informant, then a previous history of depressive illness or a strong family history will increase the likelihood that this is a depressive episode. Of more importance is the development of new symptoms consistent with a depression; i.e. these symptoms are not long-standing and unchanged aspects of the patient's dementia. An account of recent withdrawal from previous activities or social situations is suggestive of depression, although other explanations clearly need to be excluded and the onset of a cluster of characteristic symptoms over a period of several weeks or a few months is strongly indicative of a depressive episode. For each symptom a search for a non-depressive cause should be made, e.g. confirming that a loss of appetite is not due to dysphagia or social withdrawal due to worsening physical impairment, and an attempt should be made to determine the severity of the symptom. As studies have shown [10, 22] that depressive symptoms and episodes are often transient in dementia, then detailing the duration of the symptoms is important. As mentioned above, any clear evidence from the history or at interview of recurrent pessimistic ideation or persistent suicidal thinking strongly suggests depression. Psychomotor features may be present at assessment and if so it will again be important to ascertain whether these are a new development. A low and unreactive mood at interview and/or reports of recent tearfulness suggest a depression may have developed. Finally, a physical assessment with investigations to exclude an acute illness is needed to help exclude confounding illnesses which will need to be dealt with in their own right.

## *NEUROPATHOLOGICAL AND NEUROCHEMICAL STUDIES OF DEPRESSION IN DEMENTIA*

The few post-mortem investigations of depression in dementia have, unsurprisingly, generally focused on aminergic nuclei in the brainstem in AD. These have shown marked neurodegenerative changes, with earlier studies reporting an increase in depressed compared with non-depressed subjects with dementia [23], but more recent investigations have not confirmed these findings in AD [24, 25] or DLB [26]. Neurochemistry studies in depression in dementia have also had mixed results, with marked reductions in 5-HT-2 receptors in frontal, temporal and cingulate cortices but only moderate decreases or no change in 5-HT1 receptors [27], and studies of the 5-HT transporter have shown no change [27] or a reduction in both frontal and temporal cortices [28].

These varied findings may merely reflect an underlying heterogeneity in the population of dementia subjects, but they might also represent real differences in the chemistry and pathology underpinning depression in dementia compared with primary depression. For example, neurotransmitters involved in the frontal-subcortical circuits (γ-aminobutyrinic acid [GABA], glutamate, acetylcholine and dopamine) may be important since reductions in cholinergic innervation of cortical regions is a consistent finding in dementia [29, 30] and dopaminergic neuronal loss occurs in DLB [31]. Also the focus of potential treatment for late-life primary depression has recently widened to include the D3 receptor [32] as well as GABA and glutamate transmission [33]. It may prove to be that one reason for the modest efficacy of current anti-depressants in depression in dementia, is that the wrong transmitter systems are being targeted.

## *EFFICACY OF TREATMENT OF DEPRESSION IN DEMENTIA*

Anti-depressants have established efficacy in primary late-life depression [34] but, although depression in people with dementia is recognized to be a common and serious issue, there have been few empirical studies investigating any treatment approaches and very few randomized trials in this group [35]. Furthermore, the studies that have been reported use different criteria for depression, vary in whether dementia, AD or broad cognitive impairment is the other diagnosis and usually include small numbers of subjects in inadequately designed trials.

### *Efficacy of anti-depressants in dementia*

There appear to be only 8 randomized placebo-controlled studies (one has been reported at two stages) investigating standard anti-depressants in people with depression in dementia. However, the limitations in several of these studies resulted in the systematic review from the Cochrane collaboration [36] including only three of them [37–39] in its final analysis and concluding the evidence for the benefit of anti-depressants in depression in dementia is weak. However, it should be noted that the most recent update of this meta-analysis does not include two of the 'larger' studies [40, 41]. These studies are summarized in Table 17.2. All were parallel group studies except one which was a randomized crossover trial [38]. Consistent with only three being included in the Cochrane review the quality of several of these studies is poor, making firm conclusions difficult to draw. The two reports of tricyclic anti-depressants (TCAs) are both small and conflicting, with one [37] reporting no benefits from imipramine and the other modest benefits from clomipramine [38]. Both included patients with mild–moderate levels of depression and it may be significant that the negative

**Table 17.2** Randomized controlled trials of anti-depressants vs. placebo in depression in dementia

| *Study* | *n* | *Age* | *Setting* | *Dementia criteria* | *Depression criteria* | *Instruments* | *Comparisons* | *Duration (weeks)* | *Outcome* |
|---|---|---|---|---|---|---|---|---|---|
| Reifler et al. [37] | 28 | ~73 | Outpatients | DSM-III<br>MMSE ≤ 25 | DSM-III<br>HDRS ≥ 15 | HDRS | Imipramine vs. placebo | 8 | No difference |
| Nyth and Gottfries [42] | 89 | ~78 | Unclear | DSM-III<br>AD or VaD | None<br>Mean baseline MADRS of ~8 | MADRS, GBS | Citalopram vs. placebo | 4 | Citalopram > placebo in AD<br>No difference in VaD |
| Nyth *et al.* [43] | 29 | ~77 | Inpatients and outpatients | GBS | HDRS ≥ 14 | HDRS, MADRS, GBS | Citalopram vs. placebo | 6 | Not reported for HDRS or MADRS<br>Citalopram > placebo on GBS |
| Petracca *et al.* [38] | 21 | ~72 | Outpatients | McKhann<br>Probable AD<br>11MMSE ≥ 10 | DSM-IIIR<br>MDD or Dysthymia<br>HDRS > 10 | HDRS | Clomipramine vs. placebo | 6 | Clomipramine > placebo |
| Roth *et al.* [56] | 51<br>1 | ~74 | Inpatients and outpatients | 476 = DSM-III<br>35 = cog decline<br>MMSE > 11 | GDS ≥ 5<br>HDRS ≥ 14 | HDRS | Moclobemide vs. placebo | 6 | Moclobemide > placebo |
| Lyketsos *et al.* [39] | 22 | 77 | Outpatients | McKhann<br>Probable AD<br>MMSE ≥ 10 | DSM-IV<br>MDD | CSDD<br>HDRS | Sertraline vs. placebo | 12 | Sertraline > placebo |
| Magai *et al.* [44] | 31 | 89 | Women in nursing home | McKhann<br>Probable or possible AD | CSDD ≥ 3<br>GS ≥ 1 | CSDD<br>Knit-brow | Sertraline vs. placebo | 8 | No difference |
| Petracca *et al.* [40] | 41 | ~71 | Outpatients | McKhann<br>Probable AD<br>MMSE ≥ 10 | DSM-IV<br>MDD or MinDep<br>HDRS ≥ 14 | HDRS | Fluoxetine vs. placebo | 6 | No difference |
| Lyketsos *et al.* [41] | 44 | ~77 | Outpatients | McKhann<br>Probable AD<br>MMSE ≥ 10 | DSM-IV<br>MDD | CSDD<br>HDRS | Sertraline vs. placebo | 12 | Sertraline > placebo |

study had a low mean imipramine dose of 83 mg. The largest study reported to date investigated the reversible monoamine oxidase type A (MAO-A) inhibitor moclobemide in a mixed group of subjects drawn from inpatient (about 80% of subjects) and outpatient units. They reported a significant benefit from moclobemide over only 6 weeks (about 13 point reduction on the Hamilton Depression Rating Scale [HDRS]) in those with dementia with depressive symptoms. In common with other studies there was a large placebo response so that the drug–placebo difference was much less impressive at about 4 points. Unfortunately the exact make-up of this 'dementia with depressive symptoms' group is difficult to determine, making interpretation problematic. The remaining five studies investigated selective serotonin reuptake inhibitors (SSRIs). Three of these (two using citalopram [42, 43] and one using sertraline [44]) did not apply clear diagnostic criteria and examined the benefits of SSRIs in people with low levels of depressive symptoms and varying levels of dementia severity. Overall they do not provide evidence of any clear benefit of using SSRIs in such patients. In contrast the other two SSRI studies (fluoxetine [40] and sertraline [41]), which are the most recent, investigated similar numbers of outpatients with clearly defined mild–moderate AD who met DSM-IV depression criteria. Fluoxetine was not found to be superior to placebo, although this study determined efficacy at only 6 weeks (5 weeks on 20 mg) and included minor and major depression, and thus the overall mean Hamilton score was only about 16 at baseline. The authors also observed that a large placebo effect might have affected their findings. Probably the best designed study so far reported is the DIADS (Depression in AD Study), which provisionally reported in 2000 (with 22 subjects) [44] and finally reported in 2003 [41] (with 44 subjects). After a 1-week placebo run-in (to exclude transient depressive symptoms) subjects were randomized and were rated with the Cornell Scale for Depression in Dementia (CSDD) and the HDRS with final efficacy at 12 weeks. Independent raters used their change scores on these scales to rate subjects as responders, partial responders and non-responders. A full response occurred in 38% on sertraline compared with 20% on placebo and any response occurred in 84% compared with 35%, corresponding to substantial effect sizes of 0.85 and 1.4. Also twice as many patients dropped out in the placebo group (25%) compared with the sertraline group. Whilst this study provides good evidence for the efficacy of sertraline in depression in AD, it is important to note that the subjects were all community residents, with most living with either their spouse or another relative, and a reasonable proportion had a previous history (about 16%) or family history (about 27%) of depressive illness. Thus it may be argued the generalizability of these findings is limited to people with persistent diagnosable depression in dementia who are living 'at home' and enjoying good family and community support.

In addition to these placebo-controlled trials there have been two investigations of head-to-head comparisons of TCAs and SSRIs. Both used recognized diagnostic criteria for dementia and depression. The first report compared fluoxetine and amitriptyline over 45 days in outpatients meeting standard criteria for probable AD [45] and major depression [46] and found no difference in efficacy, but that fluoxetine was better tolerated, with 58% dropping out on amitriptyline compared with 22% on fluoxetine [47]. The second study, of paroxetine and imipramine, investigated dementia patients with Research Diagnostic Criteria [48] defined major or minor depression. The high cut-off for entry on the Montgomery Asberg Depression Rating Scale (MADRS) of 20 meant this was also a moderate-severe depressed group and there were substantial improvements on both drugs with no difference between them other than some suggestions that paroxetine was better tolerated [49].

Overall, further large well-designed randomized trials are clearly needed and it is worth noting that no randomized trials have been reported using the commonly prescribed anti-depressants mirtazapine and venlafaxine. There is little to suggest that anti-depressants benefit people with dementia who have only depressive symptoms, but some evidence that they may help those with defined depression syndromes of at least moderate severity.

## TOLERABILITY, ADVERSE EFFECTS AND SAFETY OF ANTI-DEPRESSANTS

Given the modest evidence base for the efficacy of anti-depressants in depression in dementia it is especially important to consider how well-tolerated such treatments are in dementia patients. The two comparator trials [47, 49] are perhaps most important for confirming most clinicians' practice that SSRIs are to be preferred to TCAs in this patient group. This view is well supported by evidence from other patient groups. A Cochrane review of the tolerability of SSRIs and TCAs using data from 136 trials in adults of all ages demonstrated about 20% more subjects dropping out of treatment due to adverse effects when taking TCAs compared with those taking SSRIs [50]. Old people, and especially those with dementia who frequently have other comorbidities as well, are much more vulnerable to adverse effects from psychotropic medication [51]. They are especially likely to suffer orthostatic hypotension and falls due to adrenergic effects, worsening of confusion and the development of delirium from anti-cholinergic effects and excess sedation from the histaminergic properties of tricyclic agents. Furthermore, TCAs are cardiotoxic and prolongation of the QT interval, with the associated risk of arrhythmias and sudden death, has been shown to occur far more frequently in people taking TCAs and in old people [52]. In contrast, SSRIs are safe in cardiac disease [53, 54] and consequently for this reason alone should be the choice for old people with primary depression [55]. As there is no evidence of increased efficacy from TCAs in depression in dementia it is difficult to justify using these agents in this patient population, and SSRIs should be the first choice in these patients as well.

Less is known about other classes of anti-depressant. In the largest study to date investigating anti-depressants in depression in dementia, moclobemide was well-tolerated, with no increase in adverse effects compared with placebo, and, importantly, it was not associated with any worsening of cognition [56]. There is little other research on this agent which appears to remain underused, probably because of concerns about dietary restriction. An open-label trial of mirtazapine in 119 nursing home residents with depression and Mini-mental State Examination (MMSE) scores of $\geq$10 reported significant improvements in depression, but also that this drug was well-tolerated [57]. As this patient group was similar in age and comorbidity to those with depression and dementia, this study suggests mirtazapine is a reasonable option too, although of course randomized evidence is lacking. In contrast, a randomized trial comparing sertraline and venlafaxine in a similar population of 52 frail nursing home residents with depression found that, whilst both were equally efficacious in improving depression, serious adverse effects and dropouts were more frequent in those on venlafaxine [58]. Other concerns about venlafaxine led the National Institute for Clinical Excellence in the UK to caution against its use by non-specialists, and advise blood pressure and ECG monitoring for those taking it [59]. Such concerns clearly are particularly relevant to the treatment of depression in dementia. Thus, if an SSRI is not tolerated or produces no significant response, the limited evidence available suggests either mirtazapine or moclobemide as the next treatment of choice, with the former having the advantage of a pharmacological profile that combines well and safely with SSRIs, and the latter evidence of efficacy in this group of patients.

An alternative class of medication sometimes proposed for the treatment of depression in dementia is the cholinesterase inhibitors. These have been shown to produce improvements in global measures of behavioural and psychological symptoms of dementia (BPSD) in AD [60, 61] and DLB [62]. However, randomized trials of donepezil in AD [61, 63] and DLB [62] and galantamine in AD [60] have failed to demonstrate any specific benefit on depression symptoms. Whilst it is possible these drugs might be of benefit in depression as a syndrome in dementia there is no evidence to support their use at the current time.

## HOW LONG SHOULD TREATMENT CONTINUE?

As shown in Table 17.2 all the randomized trials of anti-depressants have been of short duration, typically only 6 or 8 weeks, with the longest being 12 weeks. In old non-demented adults with depression there is also very little research on continuation and maintenance treatment but the trials that have been reported are consistent with the findings in younger adults, demonstrating that continuing treatment over 2 years [64] and 3 years [65] leads to significantly fewer episodes of relapse and recurrence. However, since depressive episodes in dementia appear to often be short-lived and may be different from primary depression it is not clear whether these findings can be extrapolated to this patient group.

### *EFFICACY OF NON-PHARMACOLOGICAL APPROACHES FOR DEPRESSION IN DEMENTIA*

Investigation of the benefits of treatments other than medication in this patient group is rare. Electroconvulsive therapy (ECT) is of proven benefit in depression at all ages [66] and is at least as efficacious in late-life depression as in depression occurring earlier in life [67, 68]. A concern in using this treatment in old adults, especially in those with dementia, is that it may worsen cognitive impairment and precipitate delirium. A retrospective chart review study [69] of 31 patients with moderate-severe (mean MADRS 27.5) treatment-resistant depression (all had failed to respond to at least two anti-depressants) investigating the utility of ECT in this patient group found that 49% developed a delirium at some point, although they added that in all cases this delirium was short-lived, lasting only 2 or 3 days and was not associated with any fatalities. There were in addition some other serious transient complications, e.g. development of cardiac arrhythmias and prolonged seizures. Positively, treatment led to marked improvements in depression (a mean MADRS reduction of 12.3 points) and associated improvements in cognition (MMSE scores increased by a mean of 1.6 points). Thus, as in those with pure depression, although ECT does cause increases in cognitive impairment in some people, and not surprisingly more so in this group, it leads to overall improvements in cognition as the depression remits. It appears that ECT should be considered in patients with dementia whose depression is moderate to severe and does not respond to standard anti-depressant treatment although close medical supervision is especially necessary in these frail individuals.

Evidence for the benefit of specific psychotherapies in late-life depression is mixed with the few randomized trials showing no benefits compared with placebo [70, 71] or that anti-depressants are more efficacious [72–74]. The best evidence currently is for interpersonal therapy in combination with medication as a maintenance treatment [65]. These findings do not suggest psychotherapeutic treatments are likely to be of benefit in depression in dementia even if they could be applied. Given the difficulties of applying them in cognitively impaired individuals it is not surprising they have not been investigated in depression in people with dementia. However, one group has investigated behavioural treatment approaches in this patient group [75]. They compared pleasant event focused behaviour therapy ($n = 23$), problem solving focused behaviour therapy ($n = 19$), usual care ($n = 10$) and waiting list controls ($n = 20$) in moderately severely impaired people with probable AD [45] (mean MMSE 16.5) who also had mild-moderate DSM-IIIR major or minor depression (mean HDRS 15.4). After 9 weeks of treatment they found significant improvements in the two treatment groups (both 4–5 point reductions on the HDRS) but no change in the two comparison groups. They also reported benefits in depression for the carers who were administering the therapy to the patients. Whilst suggesting that such behavioural approaches may be beneficial it should be noted that no comparison with anti-depressants was made and the outcome measures were not blind to treatment assignment.

Although the evidence to support specific psychotherapies in late-life depression is weak, there is now robust evidence from randomized controlled trials supporting 'multifaceted approaches'. Although the details of the elements involved varied they included such components as psychoeducation, adherence therapy, increasing physical activity, enhancing social engagement and frequent supportive visits from experienced mental health professionals [76–80]. These trials all showed significant benefits for those in the intervention groups and since they included patients drawn from different settings (at home, outpatients, inpatients, nursing home) they appear to be applicable in a wide variety of settings. Furthermore, most of the components in these interventions appear relevant and applicable to people with depression in association with dementia. This is especially the case if carers are involved in those parts requiring some ability to retain information and remember activity programmes; carers were involved in similar ways in the behavioural treatments referred to above [75]. However, a randomized controlled trial using different care models for managing depression in dementia in nursing homes cautions against such optimism [81]. They randomized 66 subjects with DSM-IV dementia and clinically significant depressive symptoms to one of three groups (a case management model with several components applied by experienced professionals, a consultation model with advice given to nurses and general practitioners and standard care). After 12 weeks similar improvements in depression were found in all groups. The authors speculated that 'leakage' of the treatment techniques may have occurred to subjects in the other two groups as subjects were randomized individually and not by nursing home. Whilst further investigation is warranted this study does not provide support for using such packages of care in this patient group, although they may be relevant to people with depression and dementia in other settings.

### *SUMMARY OF THE MANAGEMENT OF DEPRESSION IN DEMENTIA*

In conclusion, current evidence suggests that when conducting an assessment of depression in someone with a dementia the clinician should aim to detect 'a depression syndrome' which has persisted rather than the presence of one or a few depression symptoms, and also endeavour to confirm that these symptoms are not part of the established pattern of the dementia. Any physical causes likely to be contributing to the depression, e.g. infections or thyroid disease, should be identified and treated. Isolated symptoms are much more common but there is little to suggest they will respond to intervention. If a depression syndrome appears to be present which has not persisted for more than a few weeks and is not associated with significant patient distress or increased dysfunction, the fluctuating nature of depression in dementia suggests it may be wiser to re-assess rather than immediately commence anti-depressant treatment. A period of such 'watchful waiting' will often see improvement and if not then treatment can begin.

An SSRI should be the first line treatment and one with a short half-life and few drug–drug interactions such as citalopram is especially appropriate in this group of patients. Commencing at a low dose, e.g. citalopram 10 mg daily, and slowly increasing the dose with regular review is needed to monitor for adverse effects. Involvement of an experienced nurse or other health professional to provide more frequent review and to help address issues such as inactivity and loneliness in the patient and issues of stigma and misunderstanding in carers should be considered. Treatment should continue for at least 8 weeks before a change of treatment is considered and for 12 weeks if there appears to be some response. In those who do not adequately respond to an SSRI, a review of the diagnosis is appropriate, giving special attention to comorbid physical illness and environmental factors which may be perpetuating the depression. The little evidence available suggests that switching to moclobemide or mirtazapine is the next step and if there has been a partial response to the SSRI then augmentation with mirtazapine is the preferred option because its pharmacological properties complement those of SSRIs and there may be concerns about using moclobemide with an SSRI. If these treatments remain ineffective then further combination treatments, e.g. using lithium or anti-psychotics, which are employed in treatment-resistant primary depression will be needed. ECT is the other main option either for such treatment resistance or at any time if the depression is severe and associated with poor intake of food and/or fluids or a high suicide risk.

## MANIA IN DEMENTIA

As noted in the introduction, elevated mood and manic states occur in dementia at a much lower frequency than depression and depressive episodes [1, 2]. When they do occur it is important to exclude delirium, as this can present in a similar way to mania, with elation and manic symptoms such as overactivity and disinhibition, and full medical assessment to exclude medical causes such as endocrine disturbance and medication should be carried out. If increased motor activity and behavioural disturbance including aggression are present then, paradoxically, an agitated depressive pattern should also be considered. In some subjects such a manic presentation will occur in someone with a history of bipolar disorder and in such cases it is appropriate to use the same treatments as in previous episodes, although lower doses may be needed.

For those with no history of mania or other causes of their manic disturbance then a watchful waiting policy is prudent initially as such episodes are frequently short-lived, although in many cases the degree of disturbance may not make this a viable option. Unfortunately the low frequency of such states means there are no available clinical trials to guide clinicians and there are also no randomized double-blind treatment studies in late-life mania occurring in people with no dementia [82]. Open studies and clinical experience suggest that similar treatment approaches used in younger bipolar subjects (lithium, carbamazepine, sodium valproate, atypical anti-psychotics) are efficacious in late-life mania and it appears reasonable to use such medication in mania occurring in dementia [83, 84].

## REFERENCES

1. Burns A, Jacoby R, Levy R. Psychiatric phenomena in Alzheimer's disease. III: Disorders of mood. *Br J Psychiatry* 1990; 157:81–86,92–94.
2. Lyketsos CG, Steinberg M, Tschanz JT, Norton MC, Steffens DC, Breitner JC. Mental and behavioral disturbances in dementia: findings from the Cache County Study on Memory in Aging. *Am J Psychiatry* 2000; 157:708–714.
3. Austin MP, Mitchell P, Goodwin GM. Cognitive deficits in depression: possible implications for functional neuropathology. *Br J Psychiatry* 2001; 178:200–206.
4. Salloway S, Malloy P, Kohn R *et al.* MRI and neuropsychological differences in early- and late-life-onset geriatric depression. *Neurology* 1996; 46:1567–1574.
5. Jorm AF. History of depression as a risk factor for dementia: an updated review. *Aust N Z J Psychiatry* 2001; 35:776–781.
6. Alexopoulos GS, Meyers BS, Young RC, Mattis S, Kakuma T. The course of geriatric depression with 'reversible dementia': a controlled study. *Am J Psychiatry* 1993; 150:1693–1699.
7. Baldwin R. Depressive illness. In: Jacoby R, Oppenheimer C (eds). *Psychiatry in the Elderly*. Oxford University Press, Oxford, 2002.
8. Olin JT, Schneider LS, Katz IR *et al.* Provisional diagnostic criteria for depression of Alzheimer disease. *Am J Geriatr Psychiatry* 2002; 10:125–128.
9. Cummings JL, Mega M, Gray K, Rosenberg-Thompson S, Carusi DA, Gornbein J. The Neuropsychiatric Inventory: comprehensive assessment of psychopathology in dementia. *Neurology* 1994; 44:2308–2314.
10. Devanand DP, Jacobs DM, Tang MX *et al.* The course of psychopathologic features in mild to moderate Alzheimer disease. *Arch Gen Psychiatry* 1997; 54:257–263.
11. Wragg RE, Jeste DV. Overview of depression and psychosis in Alzheimer's disease. *Am J Psychiatry* 1989; 146:577–587.
12. Ballard C, Bannister C, Solis M, Oyebode F, Wilcock G. The prevalence, associations and symptoms of depression amongst dementia sufferers. *J Affect Disord* 1996; 36:135–144.

13. Ballard C, Neill D, O'Brien J, McKeith IG, Ince P, Perry R. Anxiety, depression and psychosis in vascular dementia: prevalence and associations. *J Affect Disord* 2000; 59:97–106.
14. Ballard C, Holmes C, McKeith I *et al.* Psychiatric morbidity in dementia with Lewy bodies: a prospective clinical and neuropathological comparative study with Alzheimer's disease. *Am J Psychiatry* 1999; 156:1039–1045.
15. McKeith IG, Galasko D, Kosaka K *et al.* Consensus guidelines for the clinical and pathologic diagnosis of dementia with Lewy bodies (DLB): report of the consortium on DLB international workshop. *Neurology* 1996; 47:1113–1124.
16. Lyketsos CG, Steele C, Baker L *et al.* Major and minor depression in Alzheimer's disease: prevalence and impact. *J Neuropsychiatry Clin Neurosci* 1997; 9:556–561.
17. Lyketsos CG, Steele C, Galik E *et al.* Physical aggression in dementia patients and its relationship to depression. *Am J Psychiatry* 1999; 156:66–71.
18. Gonzalez-Salvador T, Lyketsos CG, Baker A *et al.* Quality of life in dementia patients in long-term care. *Int J Geriatr Psychiatry* 2000; 15:181–189.
19. Ritchie K, Touchon J, Ledesert B. Progressive disability in senile dementia is accelerated in the presence of depression. *Int J Geriatr Psychiatry* 1998; 13:459–461.
20. Steele C, Rovner B, Chase GA, Folstein M. Psychiatric symptoms and nursing home placement of patients with Alzheimer's disease. *Am J Psychiatry* 1990; 147:1049–1051.
21. Burns A, Lewis G, Jacoby R, Levy R. Factors affecting survival in Alzheimer's disease. *Psychol Med* 1991; 21:363–370.
22. Ballard CG, Patel A, Solis M, Lowe K, Wilcock G. A one-year follow-up study of depression in dementia sufferers. *Br J Psychiatry* 1996; 168:287–291.
23. Forstl H, Levy R, Burns A, Luthert P, Cairns N. Disproportionate loss of noradrenergic and cholinergic neurons as cause of depression in Alzheimer's disease – a hypothesis. *Pharmacopsychiatry* 1994; 27:11–15.
24. Hoogendijk WJ, Sommer IE, Pool CW *et al.* Lack of association between depression and loss of neurons in the locus coeruleus in Alzheimer disease. *Arch Gen Psychiatry* 1999; 56:45–51.
25. Hendricksen M, Thomas AJ, Ferrier IN, Ince P, O'Brien JT. Neuropathological study of the dorsal raphe nuclei in late-life depression and Alzheimer's disease with and without depression. *Am J Psychiatry* 2004; 161:1096–1102.
26. Ballard C, Johnson M, Piggott M *et al.* A positive association between 5HT re-uptake binding sites and depression in dementia with Lewy bodies. *J Affect Disord* 2002; 69:210–223.
27. Leake A, Moore PB, Leitch M *et al.* The Serotonergic System in Alzheimer's Disease and normal neocortical post-mortem brain: neurochemical and clinical correlates. *Neurol Psychiatr Brain Res* 1993; 2:53–59.
28. Palmer AM, Wilcock GK, Esiri MM, Francis PT, Bowen DM. Monoaminergic innervation of the frontal and temporal lobes in Alzheimer's disease. *Brain Res* 1987; 401:231–238.
29. Perry EK, Gibson PH, Blessed G, Perry RH, Tomlinson BE. Neurotransmitter enzyme abnormalities in senile dementia: choline acetyltransferase and glutamate acid decarboxylase activities in necropsy brain tissue. *J Neurol Sci* 1977; 34:247–265.
30. Gottfries CG, Blennow K, Karlsson I, Wallin A. The neurochemistry of vascular dementia. *Dementia* 1994; 5:163–167.
31. Piggott MA, Marshall EF, Thomas N *et al.* Striatal dopaminergic markers in dementia with Lewy bodies, Alzheimer's and Parkinson's diseases: rostrocaudal distribution. *Brain* 1999; 122:1449–1468.
32. Alexopoulos GS. The depression-executive dysfunction syndrome of late life: a specific target for D3 agonists? *Am J Geriatr Psychiatry* 2001; 9:22–29.
33. Krystal JH, Sanacora G, Blumberg H *et al.* Glutamate and GABA systems as targets for novel antidepressant and mood-stabilizing treatments. *Mol Psychiatry* 2002; 7:S71–S80.
34. Wilson K, Mottram P, Sivanranthan A, Nightingale A. Antidepressants versus placebo for the depressed elderly. *Cochrane Database Syst Rev* 2005; 3.
35. Olin JT, Katz IR, Meyers BS, Schneider LS, Lebowitz BD. Provisional diagnostic criteria for depression of Alzheimer disease: rationale and background. *Am J Geriatr Psychiatry* 2002; 10:129–141.
36. Bains J, Birks JS, Dening TR. Antidepressants for treating depression in dementia. *Cochane Database Syst Rev* 2006; 1.
37. Reifler BV, Teri L, Raskind M *et al.* Double-blind trial of imipramine in Alzheimer's disease patients with and without depression. *Am J Psychiatry* 1989; 146:45–49.

38. Petracca G, Teson A, Chemerinski E, Leiguarda R, Starkstein SE. A double-blind placebo-controlled study of clomipramine in depressed patients with Alzheimer's disease. *J Neuropsychiatry Clin Neurosci* 1996; 8:270–275.
39. Lyketsos CG, Sheppard JM, Steele CD *et al.* Randomized, placebo-controlled, double-blind clinical trial of sertraline in the treatment of depression complicating Alzheimer's disease: initial results from the Depression in Alzheimer's Disease study. *Am J Psychiatry* 2000; 157:1686–1689.
40. Petracca GM, Chemerinski E, Starkstein SE. A double-blind, placebo-controlled study of fluoxetine in depressed patients with Alzheimer's disease. *Int Psychogeriatr* 2001; 13:233–240.
41. Lyketsos CG, DelCampo L, Steinberg M *et al.* Treating depression in Alzheimer disease: efficacy and safety of sertraline therapy, and the benefits of depression reduction: the DIADS. *Arch Gen Psychiatry* 2003; 60:737–746.
42. Nyth AL, Gottfries CG. The clinical efficacy of citalopram in treatment of emotional disturbances in dementia disorders. A Nordic multicentre study. *Br J Psychiatry* 1990; 157:894–901.
43. Nyth AL, Gottfries CG, Lyby K *et al.* A controlled multicenter clinical study of citalopram and placebo in elderly depressed patients with and without concomitant dementia. *Acta Psychiatrica Scand* 1992; 86:138–145.
44. Magai C, Kennedy G, Cohen CI, Gomberg D. A controlled clinical trial of sertraline in the treatment of depression in nursing home patients with late-stage Alzheimer's disease. *Am J Geriatr Psychiatry* 2000; 8:66–74.
45. McKhann G, Drachman D, Folstein M, Katzman R, Price D, Stadlan EM. Clinical diagnosis of Alzheimer's disease: report of the NINCDS-ADRDA Work Group under the auspices of Department of Health and Human Services Task Force on Alzheimer's Disease. *Neurology* 1984; 34:939–944.
46. American Psychiatric Association. *Diagnostic and Statistical Manual of Mental Disorders*, 3rd edition revised. APA, Washington, DC, 1987.
47. Taragano FE, Lyketsos CG, Mangone CA, Allegri RF, Comesana-Diaz E. A double-blind, randomized, fixed-dose trial of fluoxetine vs. amitriptyline in the treatment of major depression complicating Alzheimer's disease. *Psychosomatics* 1997; 38:246–252.
48. Spitzer RL, Endicott J, Robins E. Research diagnostic criteria, rationale and reliability. *Arch Gen Psychiatry* 1978; 35:78–82.
49. Katona CL, Hunter BN, Bray J. A double-blind comparison of the efficacy and safely of paroxetine and imipramine in the treatment of depression with dementia. *Int J Geriatr Psychiatry* 1998; 13:100–108.
50. Barbui C, Hotopf M, Freemantle N *et al.* Selective serotonin reuptake inhibitors versus tricyclic and heterocyclic antidepressants: comparison of drug adherence. *Cochrane Database Syst Rev* 2000; CD002791.
51. Pollock BG. Adverse reactions of antidepressants in elderly patients. *J Clin Psychiatry* 1999; 60 (suppl 20):4–8.
52. Reilly JG, Ayis SA, Ferrier IN, Jones SJ, Thomas SH. QTc-interval abnormalities and psychotropic drug therapy in psychiatric patients. *Lancet* 2000; 355:1048–1052.
53. Glassman AH, O'Connor CM, Califf RM *et al.* Sertraline treatment of major depression in patients with acute MI or unstable angina. *JAMA* 2002; 288:701–709.
54. Sauer WH, Berlin JA, Kimmel SE. Selective serotonin reuptake inhibitors and myocardial infarction. *Circulation* 2001; 104:1894–1898.
55. Skerritt U, Evans R, Montgomery SA. Selective serotonin reuptake inhibitors in old patients. A tolerability perspective. *Drugs Aging* 1997; 10:209–218.
56. Roth M, Mountjoy CQ, Amrein R. Moclobemide in elderly patients with cognitive decline and depression: an international double-blind, placebo-controlled trial. *Br J Psychiatry* 1996; 168:149–157.
57. Roose SP, Nelson JC, Salzman C, Hollander SB, Rodrigues H, Mirtazapine in the Nursing Home Study G. Open-label study of mirtazapine orally disintegrating tablets in depressed patients in the nursing home. *Curr Med Res Opin* 2003; 19:737–746.
58. Oslin DW, Ten Have TR, Streim JE *et al.* Probing the safety of medications in the frail elderly: evidence from a randomized clinical trial of sertraline and venlafaxine in depressed nursing home residents. *J Clin Psychiatry* 2003; 64:875–882.
59. NICE. *Depression: Management of Depression in Primary and Secondary Care*. 2004.
60. Cummings JL, Schneider L, Tariot PN, Kershaw PR, Yuan W. Reduction of behavioral disturbances and caregiver distress by galantamine in patients with Alzheimer's disease. *Am J Psychiatry* 2004; 161:532–538.

61. Holmes C, Wilkinson D, Dean C *et al.* The efficacy of donepezil in the treatment of neuropsychiatric symptoms in Alzheimer disease. *Neurology* 2004; 63:214–219.
62. McKeith I, Del Ser T, Spano P *et al.* Efficacy of rivastigmine in dementia with Lewy bodies: a randomized, double-blind, placebo-controlled international study. *Lancet* 2000; 356:2031–2036.
63. Tariot PN, Cummings JL, Katz IR *et al.* A randomized, double-blind, placebo-controlled study of the efficacy and safety of donepezil in patients with Alzheimer's disease in the nursing home setting [see comment]. *J Am Geriatr Soc* 2001; 49:1590–1599.
64. OADIG. How long should the elderly take antidepressants? A double blind placebo-controlled study of continuation/prophylaxis therapy with dothiepin. *Br J Psychiatry* 1993; 162:175–182.
65. Reynolds CF 3rd, Frank E, Perel JM *et al.* Nortriptyline and interpersonal psychotherapy as maintenance therapies for recurrent major depression: a randomized controlled trial in patients older than 59 years. *JAMA* 1999; 281:39–45.
66. Group UER. Efficacy and safety of electroconvulsive therapy in depressive disorders: a systematic review and meta-analysis. *Lancet* 2003; 361:799–808.
67. Tew JD Jr, Mulsant BH, Haskett RF *et al.* Acute efficacy of ECT in the treatment of major depression in the old-old. *Am J Psychiatry* 1999; 156:1865–1870.
68. O'Connor MK, Knapp R, Husain M *et al.* The influence of age on the response of major depression to electroconvulsive therapy: a C.O.R.E. Report. *Am J Geriatr Psychiatry* 2001; 9:382–390.
69. Rao V, Lyketsos CG. The benefits and risks of ECT for patients with primary dementia who also suffer from depression. *Int J Geriatr Psychiatry* 2000; 15:729–735.
70. Beutler B, Cerami A. The history, properties, and biological effects of cachectin. *Biochemistry* 1988; 27:7575–7582.
71. Thompson LW, Coon DW, Gallagher-Thompson D, Sommer BR, Koin D. Comparison of desipramine and cognitive/behavioral therapy in the treatment of elderly outpatients with mild-to-moderate depression. *Am J Geriatr Psychiatry* 2001; 9:225–240.
72. Jarvik LF, Mintz J, Steuer J, Gerner R. Treating geriatric depression: a 26-week interim analysis. *J Am Geriatr Soc* 1982; 30:713–717.
73. Reynolds CF 3rd, Miller MD, Pasternak RE *et al.* Treatment of bereavement-related major depressive episodes in later life: a controlled study of acute and continuation treatment with nortriptyline and interpersonal psychotherapy. *Am J Psychiatry* 1999; 156:202–208.
74. Williams JW Jr, Barrett J, Oxman T *et al.* Treatment of dysthymia and minor depression in primary care: A randomized controlled trial in old adults. *JAMA* 2000; 284:1519–1526.
75. Teri L, Logsdon RG, Uomoto J, McCurry SM. Behavioral treatment of depression in dementia patients: a controlled clinical trial. *J Gerontol B Psychol Sci Soc Sci* 1997; 52:P159–P166.
76. Banerjee S, Shamash K, Macdonald AJ, Mann AH. Randomized controlled trial of effect of intervention by psychogeriatric team on depression in frail elderly people at home. *BMJ* 1996; 313:1058–1061.
77. Llewellyn-Jones RH, Baikie KA, Smithers H, Cohen J, Snowdon J, Tennant CC. Multifaceted shared care intervention for late life depression in residential care: randomized controlled trial. *BMJ* 1999; 319:676–682.
78. Ciechanowski P, Wagner E, Schmaling K *et al.* Community-integrated home-based depression treatment in old adults: a randomized controlled trial. *JAMA* 2004; 291:1569–1577.
79. Unutzer J, Katon W, Callahan CM *et al.* Collaborative care management of late-life depression in the primary care setting: a randomized controlled trial. *JAMA* 2002; 288:2836–2845.
80. Sirey JA, Bruce ML, Alexopoulos GS. The Treatment Initiation Program: an intervention to improve depression outcomes in old adults. *Am J Psychiatry* 2005; 162:184–186.
81. Brodaty H, Draper BM, Millar J *et al.* Randomized controlled trial of different models of care for nursing home residents with dementia complicated by depression or psychosis. *J Clin Psychiatry* 2003; 64:63–72.
82. Young RC. Bipolar disorder in old persons. *Am J Geriatr Psychiatry* 2005; 13:265–267.
83. Sajatovic M, Gyulai L, Calabrese JR *et al.* Maintenance treatment outcomes in old patients with bipolar I disorder. *Am J Geriatr Psychiatry* 2005; 13:305–311.
84. Gildengers A, Mulsant BH, Begley AE *et al.* A Pilot Study of standardized treatment in geriatric bipolar disorder. *Am J Geriatr Psychiatry* 2005; 13:319–323.

# 18

# Management of vascular and other risks

*R. Stewart*

## INTRODUCTION

The primary objective of research into risk factors for any disorder is to identify ways in which that disorder might be prevented. For a gradually progressive disorder such as dementia, risk factors that influence its development may also influence its subsequent progression. Over the last 10–15 years there has been a rapid increase in epidemiological studies of risk factors for dementia. The purpose of this chapter is to review the current state of knowledge for the most established risk factors, considering the potential for intervention, and to review the much more limited evidence for the efficacy of given interventions. It is beyond the scope of this chapter to discuss the numerous causes of 'secondary' dementia or dementia-like syndromes which are obvious candidates for intervention, where interventions exist.

## IMPORTANT ISSUES IN DEMENTIA RISK FACTOR RESEARCH

### *THE LONG PRODROMAL PHASE*

The over-riding issue for all attempts to draw conclusions in this field is the long period over which dementia develops. Alzheimer's disease (AD), for example, may take 10 or 20 years to develop as a clinical syndrome from the first pathological changes. Risk factors may operate at any point during this period, but may not operate at all stages. They may even be influenced themselves by neurodegenerative changes. For example high blood pressure appears to be a risk factor for dementia, but neurodegenerative changes may act to lower blood pressure closer to the development of the disorder and obscure earlier associations. Dementia may be prevented at a variety of stages – through preventing the onset of earliest pathological changes, through preventing or slowing progression of these changes and early cognitive decline, or through preventing transition to dementia from a state of mild cognitive impairment where neurodegeneration may already be advanced. Finally, a given risk factor might continue to influence the progression of dementia after it has become manifest – although an identified risk factor cannot be assumed to be also a prognostic factor.

### *INTERVENING MORTALITY*

It is not currently known whether dementia is an inevitable consequence of brain ageing, and there is disagreement on whether prevalence rates accelerate or decelerate at extreme

**Robert Stewart**, MD, MSc, MRCPsych, Clinical Senior Lecturer, King's College London (Institute of Psychiatry), London, UK

old age. A clinical examination of the oldest living person in 1993 (at age 118 years) showed no evidence of substantial cognitive impairment [1]. However most people will die several decades earlier and the objective of any preventative intervention is not to reduce dementia prevalence at extreme old age, but that an increased proportion of the population will die without having been troubled by dementia beforehand. The concept of 'prevention' in dementia may therefore be synonymous with delayed onset. In this context, even delaying the onset of dementia by 2–3 years may have a substantial effect on risk at a population level: large numbers of people who in theory were 'destined' to develop dementia will die of another cause before this develops, and a further proportion will die during early stages where a clinical diagnosis might be made, but where quality of life is relatively unimpaired or can be maintained by appropriate formal and informal support.

### *MULTIPLE RISK FACTORS AND ENVIRONMENTAL INFLUENCES*

As with any other disorder manifesting in late life, it is misleading to assume that the majority of cases of dementia have a single underlying cause. Several risk factors and causal processes may have been operating over the long prodromal period before clinical manifestation. Not all of these will be directly linked to the underlying neurodegenerative process itself. For example, a person may manifest the clinical syndrome of dementia at an earlier stage if cognitive function was relatively low before the development of neurodegenerative processes – either because of limited 'development' of cognitive function in early life or because of intervening adverse events, health states or behaviours. Furthermore, at a later stage, the extent to which a given degree of cognitive impairment results in clinical dementia (i.e. more globally impaired function) will depend on a variety of unrelated factors: both individual (level of physical health and functional impairment caused by other factors), environmental (level of family and other societal support) and ecological (social expectations of 'function' in an older person). The focus for preventative interventions therefore need not be on the neurodegenerative process itself, but may instead work with equal efficiency if they alter other factors contributing to the dementia syndrome. Similarly 'prognosis' in dementia encompasses many factors besides cognitive decline itself.

## METHODOLOGICAL CHALLENGES

The factors listed above present important challenges for research in this area, and inevitably limit the conclusions which can be drawn from individual studies. The long prodromal period for dementia means that it is very difficult, in observational studies, to know whether a factor predicting dementia is a cause or effect of the condition – even for cohort studies with relatively long follow-up periods. Furthermore, these studies rely on the concept of 'incidence' which is difficult to apply to dementia because of its gradual emergence and its definition as a clinical syndrome rather than a discrete disorder. The transition of most clinical interest, that between 'mild cognitive impairment' and dementia, is particularly problematic. Cognitive impairment is present by definition in both states and there are no criteria for distinguishing the two according to performance on a given test. Instead, cognitive impairment in dementia should have reached a stage where it is causing difficulties with activities of daily living. In practice it may be very difficult to distinguish whether someone's functional impairment at follow-up, which was not present when they were last examined, has occurred because of cognitive decline or an unrelated occurrence such as physical illness or changes in available social support. This has important implications for studies which seek to identify factors which may protect against such an occurrence since these cannot be assumed to be modifying the underlying neurodegenerative disease or its effects. A further limitation in dementia prevention research is that many candidate interventions are already known to be effective in the prevention or treatment of other disorders. Evidence for their effectiveness in preventing dementia may be limited because it is not ethically possible to carry out randomized controlled trials (at least those which would involve denying the intervention to a comparison group).

## 'NON-PREVENTABLE' RISK FACTORS – AGE, GENDER AND GENES

For this group of risk factors, the risk factor itself cannot be prevented or changed. However, this does not imply that there is no scope for modifying its actual effects on dementia risk. For example, the strongest risk factor for dementia is increased age. Whilst chronological age cannot be modified, the relationships remain uncertain between chronological age, 'biological ageing' and dementia syndromes. This is illustrated by research investigating incidence rates in extreme old age. If dementia is explained simply by a brain ageing process, then incidence rates would be expected to rise until the disorder became inevitable at a certain age. However, if dementia is related to other risk factors which are associated with old age but not inevitable, then a slowing or reduction of incidence rates might be expected as a proportion of the population lives beyond the point where these factors have their impact. Currently, the trajectory of incidence rates at extreme old age is controversial because of obvious methodological difficulties, with some studies suggesting a continued acceleration [2] and others a plateau [3]. If dementia is related to a physiological ageing process then this could conceivably be modified, although no agents have been developed to date, which achieve this despite vigorous research activity. Other risk factors which become more common with age, and which may partly explain chronological age as a risk factor, may also be modifiable, as will be discussed later.

Gender also modifies risk of some dementia subtypes, although to a less strong extent than age. For example, most studies find a higher risk of AD in women [4]. As with age this cannot be changed, although the basis for gender differences, if clarified, might reveal modifiable causal pathways.

Research into genetic factors underlying AD and other causes of dementia may also identify opportunities for disease modification, although this is likely to be a distant prospect given that treatments for disorders with a better understood genetic basis such as cystic fibrosis and Huntingdon's chorea remain elusive. With rapidly advancing research, it may be possible in future to modify directly the expression of risk factor alleles such as ApoE-ε4 and, in effect, change a person's genotype. However, genes such as ApoE may have a variety of physiological roles giving rise to unforeseen consequences of such global modification, so that progress is more likely through modification of more specific allele effects.

## PARTLY PREVENTABLE RISK FACTORS – THE EARLY LIFE ENVIRONMENT

It has long been recognized that factors arising or acting early in life may influence risk of dementia. The association which has received most research attention is level of education with the majority of studies finding associations between low education and dementia as a whole or AD specifically [5, 6]. The reasons for this have not been fully clarified. One possibility is that higher levels of education delay the onset of the clinical dementia syndrome at a given stage of neurodegeneration through increased 'cognitive reserve'. Supporting this, there is some evidence that people with higher education, once they develop dementia, have more severe underlying brain changes [7] and increased subsequent cognitive decline [8]. However, other research suggests that low educational attainment may be a marker of brain development in early life which itself determines risk of subsequent dementia. This is supported by stronger associations with dementia for pre-morbid intelligence than education [9], and by the associations between early linguistic ability and Alzheimer pathology reported from the Nun Study [10]. There is also some research evidence to suggest that education may modify vulnerability to risk factors occurring later in life such as hypertension and diabetes [11, 12].

Other early life risk factors have received less attention but suggest that a more generally adverse environment may influence risk of dementia. These have included area of residence [13], parental occupation, and household size [14]. Dementia has been found to be associated with shorter leg length [15], which is a potential marker of nutritional status in early life [16] and several studies have found associations between dementia and smaller intracranial volume [17], which is likely to be a risk factor determined in early life. Low birth weight is associated with later cognitive impairment [18] and is therefore also a potential risk factor.

An adverse environment in early life may therefore be an important determinant of risk for later dementia through a variety of mediating pathways. Although these risk factors could in theory be modified at source, they clearly are not high priority targets for preventative interventions. However, there may be some reason for optimism that previously improving child health for generations entering the risk period for dementia might result in lower than expected incidence rates. Like age, gender and genetic factors, the effect of childhood factors on risk for dementia is potentially amenable to modification. However, the likely effectiveness of any intervention depends on the causal pathway responsible. 'Cognitive reserve' might be influenced by later intellectual activity or 'brain exercise' – this will be discussed later – but any benefits accrued through delaying (and therefore preventing in some instances) the onset of clinical dementia may be partly outweighed by more rapid cognitive decline once this has developed. Factors which are markers of underlying vulnerability to neurodegeneration are less easily modifiable. Part of the effect, however may be mediated through other disorders, such as cardiovascular disease, occurring later in life which itself may be modifiable as discussed below. Effects of education or other early-life factors in modifying the impact of other risk factors may have relevance for preventative interventions since groups with higher vulnerability may require specific targeting to ensure that they have access to a given programme.

## VASCULAR RISK FACTORS AND DEMENTIA

Rapid progress has been made over the last decade in clarifying the role of vascular risk factors in the aetiology of dementia. 'Vascular risk factors' in this context are the collection of well-recognized risk factors for cardiovascular disease and stroke: high blood pressure, diabetes, dyslipidaemia, obesity and smoking. Several large prospective studies have found that raised mid-life blood pressure is a risk factor for later cognitive impairment, dementia or AD [19–21]. Several other studies have found increased incidence rates of dementia and AD associated with diabetes [22, 23], as well as associations with insulin resistance and the 'metabolic syndrome' [24–26]. Smoking has also been found to be a risk factor for dementia in several studies [27, 28]. Although mid-life obesity has been identified as a risk factor in some studies [26, 29], the role of lipid levels is more uncertain. Raised total cholesterol was found to be a risk factor in one study [21], but a protective factor in another [30]. Furthermore, a large neuropathological series from another cohort study found associations between Alzheimer pathology and increased rather than decreased HDL-cholesterol [31].

The particular importance of vascular factors in dementia is that they are potential targets for intervention and, because they have high prevalence rates in older populations, any intervention could have substantial population-level effects on risk of dementia or, potentially, on its prognosis. The difficulty is that many of these factors may exert their actions at particular stages in the development of dementia and their influence may have changed by the time this develops. For example, studies which have found that high blood pressure is a risk factor for dementia have generally involved follow-up periods of 10–20 years. By the time dementia has developed, blood pressure is lower than that in controls [32]. Therefore, studies with shorter follow-up periods frequently find no association between the risk factor and outcome [33]. The same may be true for total cholesterol levels where studies with less than 10-year follow-up periods more often find associations with low rather than high levels [34]. Dementia is a catabolic condition and is accompanied by profound metabolic changes, particularly at advanced stages. However, a growing body of research suggests that these changes may begin at relatively early stages, and certainly before the clinical syndrome develops. These include weight loss [35] and falling blood pressure [36]. The likelihood is that these changes are secondary to neurodegenerative processes and there is no evidence that they are brought about by medication. However, they have important implications for the likely detectable effect of interventions – since the lag period from effective intervention to reduced outcome is likely to be considerably longer than the usual follow-up period for a clinical trial.

## OPPORTUNITIES TO PREVENT DEMENTIA THROUGH MODIFYING VASCULAR RISK

### *LOWERING BLOOD PRESSURE*

Early observational studies suggested that the association between raised mid-life blood pressure and cognitive impairment was strongest in those who had not received anti-hypertensive agents [19], suggesting that dementia might be prevented through treating high blood pressure. However, evidence from randomized controlled trials has been much less conclusive. The UK Medical Research Council (MRC) placebo-controlled trial of a diuretic and/or β-blocker in hypertensive people aged 65–74 years found no effect of either treatment on cognitive decline over a 54-month period [37]. The more recent SCOPE and HOPE trials also found no effect of an $\alpha_2$ antagonist or an angiotensin-converting enzyme (ACE) inhibitor/diuretic respectively on cognitive decline [38, 39]. The SHEP trial of diuretic, β-blocker and reserpine found no effect of any treatment on cognitive impairment over a 4.5 year follow-up, although secondary analyses suggested that protective effects might have been missed due to differential attrition [40]. The PROGRESS trial of an ACE-inhibitor with or without a diuretic, the largest of these trials so far, did not find any effect on dementia or cognitive decline over a 3.9 year follow-up period in a sample of people with cerebrovascular disease. However, both these outcomes were reduced in the treatment group for the subsample with recurrent strokes during the follow-up period [41]. Furthermore, a subsequent substudy has recently reported a significant effect of treatment in reducing white matter lesion progression [42], suggesting at least some potentially beneficial effect. Of all the trials to date, only the Syst-Eur study of a calcium antagonist (with or without a β-blocker or diuretic) for people with isolated systolic hypertension has found any evidence of substantial reduction in dementia risk [43]. Although numbers of people with dementia were very small in this study, further open-label follow-up suggested continued risk reduction in the originally treated group [44]. The problem with this, as in other trials, is that benefits in the primary endpoint (incident stroke) were identified before sufficient numbers of dementia cases were accumulated, and the trial could not ethically continue to allow this. Although the positive findings from the Syst-Eur study are widely cited as supporting anti-hypertensive treatment as a preventative intervention, the largely negative findings from other large trials are hard to ignore. Since the Syst-Eur study is the only trial so far to evaluate a calcium antagonist, the stronger protective effect found might reflect other properties of the agent used rather than the effect of blood pressure lowering *per se*. However, the long lag period between the emergence of hypertension and that of dementia should be borne in mind since it may obscure any effect of treatment over what are relatively short periods.

### *DIABETES CONTROL*

The association between diabetes and dementia is beginning to be recognized although it has received less research as a risk factor. If diabetes is acting directly as a risk factor, it would be expected that there would be a higher risk in people with worse control and that interventions to improve glycaemic control would prevent cognitive decline. To date, this question has received little or no investigation either in observational or interventional research. Some studies have found the association to be strongest in people receiving insulin (compared to other anti-diabetic agents) which might be a proxy indicator of poor control [22]. Findings of associations between insulin resistance and risk of dementia also suggest that interventions to improve insulin sensitivity might also be effective in reducing risk, but to date there has been little evaluation of this.

### *IMPROVING LIPID PROFILE*

The role of cholesterol-lowering therapy is discussed in detail in a previous chapter. As described earlier, the association between raised cholesterol and dementia is substantially less clear than that for raised blood pressure as a risk factor. This may partly arise from the fact that total cholesterol levels are markers of more than one process, particularly in later life. For example, in older people, low rather than high cholesterol predicts mortality [45]. A fall in cholesterol levels is associated with poor health and frailty, and may be secondary specifically to poor nutritional status or chronic inflammatory processes [46], both of which are implicated in dementia. Furthermore, the role of cholesterol in AD is potentially complex and the effect of circulating levels on the vasculature may only be one factor underlying any association. Although some observational studies had suggested that people with dementia were less likely to be taking statins (3-hydroxy-3-methyl-glutaryl coenzyme A reductase inhibitors), suggesting a possible protective effect, prospective research has failed to demonstrate a negative association between the two [47], and there were no demonstrable effects on cognitive function in three randomized controlled trials of lovastatin, simvastatin or pravastatin [48–50]. On the other hand, one recent trial found a beneficial effect of atorvastatin on progression of AD [51]. Since all these agents have been shown to lower circulating cholesterol levels but only one has been found to have any effect on cognition, it is not certain whether effects on cholesterol levels as a 'vascular risk factor' have any role in treatment effects.

### *ASPIRIN*

Given the length of time that vascular disease has been recognized as a risk factor for dementia, and that aspirin has been recognized as a protective factor for cerebrovascular disease, it is surprising that it has received so little research attention as a potential protective factor for dementia. One of the difficulties encountered is that people who take aspirin have a higher than average level of vascular risk, so that any protective effects may be obscured in observational research. Despite this, there is some evidence that aspirin use is positively, although weakly, correlated with cognitive function [52]. Furthermore, there is evidence from one randomized trial that aspirin, possibly to a greater extent than warfarin, has a beneficial effect on cognitive function in men at risk of cardiovascular disease [53].

### *CHANGES IN LIFESTYLE – DIET, SMOKING AND OBESITY*

Diet, smoking and obesity are all important factors in cardiovascular disease and improvement in any of these may have an impact on risk of dementia. For smoking, it is possible that cessation may have a relatively rapid effect on risk, since only current smokers were at increased risk of developing dementia over a 2-year follow-up in one study, with no increased risk in former smokers [54]. Former smokers also had substantially reduced risk of incident dementia compared to current smokers in the Rotterdam Study [27]. However, it is possible that smoking cessation is accompanied by other beneficial lifestyle changes in those who achieve it and differences in risk between current and former smokers may be overestimated in observational studies. Obesity as a risk factor is less well-established and is complicated by the weight loss that occurs early on in dementia [35]. Given that low rather than high body mass index (BMI) emerges as a risk factor for morbidity/mortality in late life, it is likely that the avoidance of obesity in mid-life will be more protective than the management of obesity once this has developed. The role of diet in the aetiology of dementia has received a large amount of attention recently and it is beyond the scope of this chapter to provide a comprehensive review. The field is understandably complex because of the difficulties involved in accurately measuring diet, because of the multitude of factors which could be measured, and because of close correlations between different dietary factors and the difficulty of dealing with confounding. In general, however, there is growing evidence from observational studies that a diet which would be expected to lower cardiovascular risk is also a potential protective factor for dementia [55–57]. Because people's diet measured at a single time-point is likely to reflect a long period of exposure, it is difficult to conclude from observational findings whether modification at a late stage will alter dementia risk.

### *PROLONGED SURVIVAL AND RISK OF DEMENTIA*

There is reasonable evidence from observational studies that vascular risk in middle age is also an important determinant of risk for dementia in those who survive into old age. While it is still uncertain whether modification of risk in later life will prevent dementia, it is reasonable to suppose that a general improvement in mid-life health at a population level might be an important means of reducing the prevalence of dementia 10–20 years later. What is less certain is whether this would be reflected in reduced lifetime risk – because improved health will also increase life-expectancy and hence will reduce the likelihood of someone dying of another cause (principally cardiovascular disease) prior to dementia 'onset'. It is possible that cohorts who would once have died in their eighth decade will soon be surviving well into their ninth with levels of vascular disease which are not sufficiently severe to be life-threatening but which are sufficiently severe to accelerate neurodegenerative processes or precipitate dementia. To date, predictions of dementia prevalence have been predominantly based on population age and gender structures. With increasing knowledge of risk factor–outcome relationships, it is likely that future modelling will need to become more complex and to consider also changes in population health status.

## OTHER RISK MARKERS AND THE OPPORTUNITY FOR DEMENTIA PREVENTION – PHYSICAL, SOCIAL AND COGNITIVE ACTIVITY

There has been growing evidence from observational research that risk of cognitive decline and dementia may be influenced by other aspects of individuals' lifestyles, besides those which directly influence risk of vascular disease. Evidence is emerging that a socially and cognitively stimulating environment may be associated with decreased risk of dementia. In one study, people who lived alone and/or lacked close social ties were at increased risk of developing dementia over a 3-year period [58]. In another, participation in cognitively stimulating activities was strongly negatively associated with risk of later dementia, partly explaining associations with education and occupation as exposures [59]. Another study with a long follow-up period from birth to middle age found that cognitive function in childhood predicted later cognitive decline – but also suggested that protective effects could be acquired in adulthood [60]. These last two studies suggest that the impact of low educational attainment on risk of dementia may be substantially modifiable later on in life.

Physical activity may also be a protective factor. Several studies have found a lower risk of dementia in people who are more physically active [61–63]. In general, the levels of activity involved were relatively mild and easily achievable. Protective effects of exercise may be mediated through effects on cardiovascular disease or on vascular risk factors such as obesity and hyperinsulinaemia. However, there are a variety of other pathways which may be important, such as effects on growth factors and hormone metabolism [61]. One randomized controlled trial found aerobic exercise improved cognitive function in sedentary men to a greater extent than anaerobic exercise, with only a small gain in physical fitness required [64].

Whether it is physical activity or social/cognitive activity which is most important in determining risk of dementia has not been fully established. However, the changes in lifestyle involved are likely to be easily achievable and the potential for other benefits (e.g. on mood and general health) are such that large-scale controlled intervention studies specific for dementia or cognitive function as outcomes may be difficult to achieve or justify.

## SUMMARY OF DEMENTIA PREVENTION RESEARCH

There is a growing body of evidence that risk factors for dementia operate across the life course, some of which may be amenable to intervention. However, the periods between the action of the risk factor and the manifestation of the outcome are likely to be too long in many instances for traditional randomized controlled trials to be applicable. Furthermore, many of the potential risk factors have well-recognized associations with other disorders, such as heart disease and stroke, where incidence rates are substantially higher than those for dementia and beneficial effects more demonstrable in trials. Placebo-controlled trials with incident dementia as an outcome may therefore be unethical as well as infeasible. Cognitive decline is an alternative outcome but limited by the large number of tests to choose from, the poor psychometric properties of many of these, and the lack of predictive validity for dementia (since a large proportion of people with cognitive decline will not develop dementia). Therefore, for many risk factors it is likely that recommendations for primary prevention will have to rely on findings from observational rather than interventional research, with all the potential difficulties of deducing cause and effect. Fortunately, to date, the risk factors identified have been those where interventions can be justified on numerous other grounds besides the impact on dementia.

## TREATMENT OF DEMENTIA THROUGH CONTROLLING RISK FACTORS

While there have been considerable advances in understanding factors which influence risk of dementia occurring, substantially less is known about those which influence its progression. The progression of most dementia syndromes is unpredictable: cognitive decline in AD, for example, shows very wide inter-individual variation with a significant proportion of clinically confirmed cases showing no appreciable change over at least 4 years in one study [65]. Because of the very long prodromal periods for most types of dementia, and the different contributing causal pathways, it is not appropriate to assume that a risk factor which influences risk of dementia will continue to influence its progression. The ApoE-ε4 allele, e.g. is a well-recognized risk factor for AD, but several studies have failed to find any substantial influence on disease progression [66–68].

### *INFLUENCES OF CAUSAL PATHWAYS*

Taking vascular risk factors as an example, it is now accepted that they predict the occurrence of AD (at least as clinically defined) as well as 'vascular' dementia (i.e. dementia with clinical evidence of cerebrovascular disease). However, there are various ways in which cerebrovascular and Alzheimer pathology may interact and which have different implications for how responsive the disorder may be to modifying vascular risk factors after its clinical onset [69]. There are some theoretical pathways by which vascular damage may actually accelerate AD pathological changes and neurodegeneration, for example through inflammatory changes secondary to ischaemia or through disruption of the blood–brain barrier. These suggest that ischaemia or infarction may continue to influence the progression of AD throughout its course and both before and after the diagnosis. However, it is also possible that vascular damage may act to diminish 'reserve' – so that AD manifests as a clinical syndrome at earlier pathological stages. This causal pathway predicts no further influence on decline once the clinical syndrome has developed.

### *EVIDENCE FOR CAUSAL PATHWAYS BETWEEN VASCULAR FACTORS AND ALZHEIMER'S DISEASE*

The nature of the relationship between vascular and AD pathology is therefore important in predicting the extent to which AD can be treated through modifying vascular risk factors. Evidence to date still remains preliminary and tentative but, if anything, supports the second pathway. Although most neuropathological studies are small and carried out in select clinical samples, there is little evidence to suggest a direct link between the two pathological processes, since this would predict worse AD pathology in the presence of cerebrovascular disease. Instead, evidence from the Nuns study suggests an interaction in clinical manifestations as described above [70], supported by similar results from the OPTIMA study [71]. Furthermore, there is no evidence from the limited research in this area that co-occurring cerebrovascular disease predicts more rapid decline in AD. One autopsy study found no associations between the presence of infarcts and previous cognitive decline [72]. Another clinical study found that cerebrovascular disease was associated with faster cognitive decline in people with dementia aged 80 years or above and with slower decline in those younger than 80, suggesting that any differences may be explained by the extent of AD pathology at the time of presentation rather than cerebrovascular disease [73].

Currently, there is therefore little evidence from observational research to suggest that improving vascular risk factors at least will have a substantial impact on cognitive decline in AD, once the stage of clinical dementia has been reached. Whether the same is true for 'vascular dementia' is less certain. The difficulty with vascular dementia as a construct is that it is a very heterogeneous disorder with a substantial degree of overlap with AD [74]. Trial evidence is lacking in this area with only one very tentative finding from a pilot study suggesting that aspirin might have a protective effect [75], which is still awaiting replication. A recent trial of one cholesterol-lowering agent (atorvastatin) indicated potential benefits in people with AD [51]. However, it is not yet clear whether this is mediated through improvements in lipid profile and reduced vascular risk, or through more specific actions of this particular agent.

## A POSSIBLE ROLE OF INTER-CURRENT INFECTIONS IN DEMENTIA

Inflammatory pathways have long been implicated in AD from neuropathological research [76]. Several more recent epidemiological studies have found that raised circulating levels of inflammatory markers, particularly cytokines, are associated with an increased risk of cognitive decline or dementia [77–80]. While these may simply be markers of more severe vascular disease, it is also possible that disorders associated with acute or chronic inflammatory responses may influence some of the pathological processes underlying dementia. It is a common clinical observation that people with gradually progressive dementia often experience a more rapid deterioration associated with a systemic infection, or that they experience an episode of delirium after which they do not regain their previous level of function. A small prospective study addressing this issue found that raised cytokine levels were associated with increased cognitive decline in people with AD, and also that cognitive impairment in this group persisted at least two months after the resolution of a systemic infection [81]. Reducing the risk of infections, or possibly interventions at the time of an infection, might present opportunities both to delay the manifestation of dementia and to improve prognosis. However, this requires further evaluation before conclusions can be drawn.

## STROKE PREVENTION IN DEMENTIA

While there may be substantial potential for preventing dementia through modifying certain risk factors such as mid-life vascular factors, it is controversial whether modification of these risk factors will affect cognitive decline once dementia has developed. However, it is important to take a more broad view of what risk factor modification represents. The purpose of clinical care in dementia is not only to reduce cognitive decline if possible but also to improve quality of life, or at least to prevent its deterioration. As discussed earlier, most of the risk factors for dementia are risk factors for other disorders as well. Stroke is an important cause of morbidity and disability, whether a person has dementia or not and it is important that factors which might increase the risk of stroke are identified and appropriate actions taken in someone with dementia, just as rigorously as would be expected in someone else of the same age.

## SUMMARY

A growing body of evidence is accumulating on risk factors for dementia, principally for AD and vascular dementia. Many of these are potentially modifiable, particular vascular factors. However, the long period of time which elapses between the emergence of the risk factor and the manifestation of dementia means that it will be difficult, if not impossible, to demonstrate the efficacy of many of these potentially preventative interventions through randomized controlled trials. There is also a large degree of uncertainty over whether risk factor modification will make any difference to the clinical course of dementia, once this has become manifest. However, this may be the wrong question to be asking if these interventions can improve quality of life (or prevent its deterioration) in other respects.

## REFERENCES

1. Ritchie K. Mental status examination of an exceptional case of longevity: J.C. aged 118 years. *Br J Psychiatry* 1995; 166:229–235.
2. Kawas C, Gray S, Brookmeyer R *et al*. Age-specific incidence rates of Alzheimer's disease: The Baltimore Longitudinal Study of Aging. *Neurology* 2000; 54:2072–2077.
3. Miech RA, Breitner JCS, Zandi PP *et al*. Incidence of AD may decline in the early 90s for men, later for women: The Cache County study. *Neurology* 2002; 58:209–218.
4. van Duijn CM, Stijnen T, Hofman A. Risk factors for Alzheimer's disease: overview of the EURODEM collaborative re-analysis of case-control studies. *Int J Epidemiol* 1991; 20(suppl 2):S1–S73.
5. Canadian Study of Health and Aging. Risk factors for Alzheimer's disease in Canada. *Neurology* 1994; 44:2073–2080.
6. Stern Y, Gurland B, Tatemichi TK *et al*. Influence of education and occupation on the incidence of Alzheimer's disease. *JAMA* 1994; 271:1004–1010.
7. Stern Y, Alexander GE, Prohovnik I *et al*. Inverse relationship between education and parietotemporal perfusion deficit in Alzheimer's disease. *Ann Neurol* 1992; 32:371–375.
8. Stern Y, Albert S, Tang M-X *et al*. Rate of memory decline in AD is related to education and occupation. *Neurology* 1999; 53:1942–1947.
9. Schmand B, Smit JH, Geerlings MI *et al*. The effects of intelligence and education on the development of dementia. A test of the brain reserve hypothesis. *Psychol Med* 1997; 27:1337–1344.
10. Snowdon DA, Kemper SJ, Mortimer JA *et al*. Linguistic ability in early life and cognitive function and Alzheimer's disease in late life. *JAMA* 1996; 275:528–532.
11. Stewart R, Richards M, Brayne C *et al*. Vascular risk and cognitive impairment in an older, British, African-Caribbean population. *J Am Geriatr Soc* 2001; 49:263–269.

12. Stewart R, Kim J-M, Shin I-S *et al.* Education and the association between vascular risk factors and cognitive function. A cross-sectional study in older Koreans with cognitive impairment. *Int Psychogeriatr* 2003; 15:27–36.
13. Moceri VM, Kukull WA, Emanuel I *et al.* Early-life risk factors and the development of Alzheimer's disease. *Neurology* 2000; 54:415–420.
14. Moceri VM, Kukull WA, Emanuel I *et al.* Using census data and birth certificates to reconstruct the early-life socioeconomic environment and the relation to the development of Alzheimer's disease. *Epidemiology* 2001; 12:383–389.
15. Kim J-M, Stewart R, Shin I-S *et al.* Limb length and dementia in an older Korean population. *J Neurol Neurosurg Psychiatry* 2003; 74:427–432.
16. Wadsworth MEJ, Hardy RJ, Paul AA *et al.* Leg and trunk length at 43 years in relation to childhood health, diet and family circumstances; evidence from the 1946 national birth cohort. *Int J Epidemiol* 2002; 31:383–390.
17. Graves AB, Mortimer JA, Bowen JD *et al.* Head circumference and incident Alzheimer's disease. Modification by apolipoprotein E. *Neurology* 2001; 57:1453–1460.
18. Richards M, Hardy R, Kuh D *et al.* Birthweight, postnatal growth and cognitive function in a national UK birth cohort. *Int J Epidemiol* 2002; 31:342–348.
19. Elias MF, Wolf PA, D'Agostino RB *et al.* Untreated blood pressure level is inversely related to cognitive functioning: The Framingham study. *Am J Epidemiol* 1993; 138:353–364.
20. Launer LJ, Masaki K, Petrovitch H *et al.* The association between midlife blood pressure levels and late-life cognitive function. *JAMA* 1995; 274:1846–1851.
21. Kivipelto M, Helkala E-L, Laakso MP *et al.* Midlife vascular risk factors and Alzheimer's disease in later life: longitudinal, population based study. *Br Med J* 2001; 322:1447–1451.
22. Ott A, Stolk RP, van Harskamp F *et al.* Diabetes mellitus and the risk of dementia. *Neurology* 1999; 53:1937–1942.
23. Arvanitakis Z, Wilson RS, Bienias JL *et al.* Diabetes mellitus and risk of Alzheimer disease and decline in cognitive function. *Arch Neurol* 2004; 61:661–666.
24. Kuusisto J, Koivisto K, Mykkänen L *et al.* Association between features of the insulin resistance syndrome and Alzheimer's disease independently of apolipoprotein E4 phenotype: cross sectional population based study. *Br Med J* 1997; 315:1045–1049.
25. Luchsinger JA, Tang M-X, Shea S *et al.* Hyperinsulinemia and risk of Alzheimer disease. *Neurology* 2004; 63:1187–1192.
26. Kivipelto M, Nganda T, Fratiglioni L *et al.* Obesity and vascular risk factors at midlife and the risk of dementia and Alzheimer's disease. *Arch Neurol* 2005; 62:1556–1560.
27. Ott A, Slooter AJC, Hofman A *et al.* Smoking and the risk of dementia and Alzheimer's disease in a population-based cohort study: The Rotterdam Study. *Lancet* 1998; 351:1840–1843.
28. Launer LJ, Andersen K, Dewey ME *et al.* Rates and risk factors for dementia and Alzheimer's disease. *Neurology* 1999; 52:78–84.
29. Gustafson D, Rothenberg E, Blennow K *et al.* An 18-year follow-up of overweight and risk of Alzheimer disease. *Arch Intern Med* 2003; 163:1524–1528.
30. Mielke MM, Zandi PP, Sjögren M *et al.* High total cholesterol levels in late life associated with a reduced risk of dementia. *Neurology* 2005; 64:1689–1695.
31. Launer LJ, White LR, Petrovitch H *et al.* Cholesterol and neuropathologic markers of AD. A population-based autopsy study. *Neurology* 2001; 57:1447–1452.
32. Skoog I, Lernfelt B, Landahl S *et al.* 15-year longitudinal study of blood pressure and dementia. *Lancet* 1996; 347:1141–1145.
33. Posner HB, Tang M-X, Luchsinger J *et al.* The relationship of hypertension in the elderly to AD, vascular dementia, and cognitive function. *Neurology* 2002; 58:1175–1181.
34. Reitz C, Tang M-X, Luchsinger J *et al.* Relation of plasma lipids to Alzheimer disease and vascular dementia. *Arch Neurol* 2004; 61:705–714.
35. Stewart R, Masaki K, Xue Q-L *et al.* A 32-year prospective study of change in body weight and incident dementia: the Honolulu-Asia Aging Study. *Arch Neurol* 2005; 62:55–60.
36. Qiu C, von Strauss E, Winblad B *et al.* Decline in blood pressure over time and risk of dementia: a longitudinal study from the Kungsholmen Project. *Stroke* 2004; 35:1810–1815.
37. Prince MJ, Bird AS, Blizard RA *et al.* Is the cognitive function of older patients affected by antihypertensive treatment? Results from 54 months of the Medical Research Council's treatment trial of hypertension in older adults. *Br Med J* 1996; 312:801–804.

38. Starr JM, Whalley LJ, Deary IJ. The effects of antihypertensive treatment on cognitive function: results from the HOPE study. *J Am Geriatr Soc* 1996; 44:411–415.
39. Lithell H, Hansson L, Skoog I *et al*. The Study on Cognition and Prognosis in the Elderly (SCOPE): principal results of a randomized double-blind intervention trial. *J Hypertension* 2003; 21:875–886.
40. Di Bari M, Pahor M, Franse LV *et al*. Dementia and disability outcomes in large hypertension trials: lessons learned from the systolic hypertension in the elderly program (SHEP) trial. *Am J Epidemiol* 2001; 153:72–78.
41. Tzourio C, Anderson C, Chapman N *et al*. Effects of blood pressure lowering with perindopril and indapamide therapy on dementia and cognitive decline in patients with cerebrovascular disease. *Arch Intern Med* 2003; 163:1069–1075.
42. Dufouil C, Chalmers J, Coskun O *et al*. Effects of blood pressure lowering on cerebral white matter hyperintensities in patients with stroke: the PROGRESS (Perindopril Protection Against Recurrent Stroke Study) Magnetic Resonance Imaging Substudy. *Circulation* 2005; 112:1644–1650.
43. Forette F, Seux M-L, Staessen JA *et al*. Prevention of dementia in randomized double-blind placebo-controlled Systolic Hypertension in Europe (Syst-Eur) trial. *Lancet* 1998; 352:1347–1351.
44. Forette F, Seux M-L, Staessen JA *et al*. The prevention of dementia with antihypertensive treatment. New evidence from the Systolic Hypertension in Europe (Syst-Eur) study. *Arch Intern Med* 2002; 162:2046–2052.
45. Corti M-C, Guralnik JM, Salive ME *et al*. Clarifying the direct relation between total cholesterol levels and death from coronary heart disease in older persons. *Ann Intern Med* 1997; 126:753–760.
46. Hu P, Seeman TE, Harris TB *et al*. Does inflammation or undernutrition explain the low cholesterol-mortality association in high-functioning older persons? MacArthur Studies of Successful Aging. *J Am Geriatr Soc* 2003; 51:80–84.
47. Zandi PP, Sparks DL, Khachaturian AS *et al*. Do statins reduce risk of incident dementia and Alzheimer's disease? The Cache County Study. *Arch Gen Psychiatry* 2005; 62:217–224.
48. Santanello NC, Barber BL, Applegate WB *et al*. Effect of pharmacologic lipid lowering on health-related quality of life in older persons: results from the Cholesterol Reduction in Seniors Program (CRISP) Pilot Study. *J Am Geriatr Soc* 1997; 45:8–14.
49. Heart Protection Study Collaborative Group MRC/BHF Heart Protection Study of cholesterol lowering with simvastatin in 20,536 high-risk individuals: a randomized placebo-controlled trial. *Lancet* 2002; 360:7–22.
50. Shepherd J, Blauw GJ, Murphy MB *et al*. Pravastatin in elderly individuals at risk of vascular disease (PROSPER): a randomized controlled trial. *Lancet* 2002; 360:1623–1630.
51. Sparks DL, Sabbagh MN, Connor DJ *et al*. Atorvastatin for the treatment of mild to moderate Alzheimer Disease. *Arch Neurol* 2005; 62:753–757.
52. Peacock JM, Folsom AR, Knopman DS *et al*. Association of nonsteroidal anti-inflammatory drugs and aspirin with cognitive performance in middle-aged adults. *Neuroepidemiology* 1999; 18:134–143.
53. Richards M, Meade TW, Peart S *et al*. Is there any evidence for a protective effect of antithrombotic medication on cognitive function in men at risk of cardiovascular disease? Some preliminary findings. *J Neurol Neurosurg Psychiatry* 1997; 62:269–272.
54. Merchant C, Tang M-X, Albert M *et al*. The influence of smoking on the risk of Alzheimer's disease. *Neurology* 1999; 52:1408–1412.
55. Luchsinger JA, Tang M-X, Shea S *et al*. Caloric intake and the risk of Alzheimer disease. *Arch Neurol* 2002; 59:1258–1263.
56. Morris MC, Evans DA, Bienias JL *et al*. Consumption of fish and n-3 fatty acids and risk of incident Alzheimer disease. *Arch Neurol* 2003; 60:940–946.
57. Laurin D, Masaki KH, Foley DJ *et al*. Midlife dietary intake of antioxidants and risk of late-life incident dementia. *Am J Epidemiol* 2004; 159:959–967.
58. Fratiglioni L, Wang H-X, Ericsson K *et al*. Influence of social network on occurrence of dementia: a community-based longitudinal study. *Lancet* 2000; 355:1315–1319.
59. Wilson RS, Mendes de Leon CF, Barnes LL *et al*. Participation in cognitively stimulating activities and risk of incident Alzheimer disease. *JAMA* 2002; 287:742–748.
60. Richards M, Shipley B, Fuhrer R *et al*. Cognitive ability in childhood and cognitive decline in mid-life: longitudinal birth cohort study. *Br Med J* 2004; 328:552–554.
61. Laurin D, Verreault R, Lindsay J *et al*. Physical activity and risk of cognitive impairment and dementia in elderly persons. *Arch Neurol* 2001; 58:498–504.

62. Abbott RD, White LR, Ross GW *et al*. Walking and dementia in physically capable elderly men. *JAMA* 2004; 292:1447–1453.
63. Rovio S, Kareholt I, Helkala E-L *et al*. Leisure-time physical activity at midlife and the risk of dementia and Alzheimer's disease. *Lancet Neurol* 2005; 4:705–711.
64. Kramer AF, Hahn S, Cohen NJ *et al*. Ageing, fitness and neurocognitive function. *Nature* 1999; 400:418–419.
65. Galasko D, Fillenbaum GG, Morris JC *et al*. Variability in annual Mini-Mental State Examination score in patients with probable Alzheimer disease. *Arch Neurol* 1999; 56:862.
66. Growdon JH, Locascio JJ, Corkin S *et al*. Apolipoprotein E genotype does not influence rates of cognitive decline in Alzheimer's disease. *Neurology* 1996; 47:444–448.
67. Holmes C, Levy R, McLoughlin DM *et al*. Apolipoprotein E: non-cognitive symptoms and cognitive decline in late onset Alzheimer's disease. *J Neurol Neurosurg Psychiatry* 1996; 61:580–583.
68. Kurz A, Egensperger R, Haupt M *et al*. Apolipoprotein E e4 allele, cognitive decline, and deterioration of everyday performance in Alzheimer's disease. *Neurology* 1996; 47:440–443.
69. Stewart R. Cardiovascular factors in Alzheimer's disease. *J Neurol Neurosurg Psychiatry* 1998; 65:143–147.
70. Snowdon DA, Greiner LH, Mortimer JA *et al*. Brain infarction and the clinical expression of Alzheimer disease. *JAMA* 1997; 277:813–817.
71. Esiri MM, Nagy Z, Smith MZ *et al*. Cerebrovascular disease and threshold for dementia in the early stages of Alzheimer's disease. *Lancet* 1999; 354:919–920.
72. Lee J-H, Olichney JM, Hansen LA *et al*. Small concomitant vascular lesions do not influence rates of cognitive decline in patients with Alzheimer disease. *Arch Neurol* 2000; 57:1474–1479.
73. Mungas D, Reed BR, Ellis WG *et al*. The effects of age on rate of progression of Alzheimer disease and dementia with associated cerebrovascular disease. *Arch Neurol* 2001; 58:1243–1247.
74. Stewart R. Vascular dementia: a diagnosis running out of time. *Br J Psychiatry* 2002; 180:152–156.
75. Meyer JS, Rogers RL, McClintic K *et al*. Randomized clinical trial of daily aspirin therapy in multi-infarct dementia. *J Am Geriatr Soc* 1989; 37:549–555.
76. Breitner JCS. Inflammatory processes and antiinflammatory drugs in Alzheimer's disease: a current appraisal. *Neurobiol Aging* 1996; 17:789–794.
77. Schmidt R, Schmidt H, Curb JD *et al*. Early inflammation and dementia: a 25-year follow-up of the Honolulu-Asia Aging Study. *Ann Neurol* 2002; 52:168–174.
78. Weaver JD, Huang MH, Albert M *et al*. Interleukin-6 and risk of cognitive decline: MacArthur studies of successful aging. *Neurology* 2002; 59:371–378.
79. Yaffe K, Lindquist MS, Penninx BW *et al*. Inflammatory markers and cognition in well-functioning African-American and white elders. *Neurology* 2003; 61:76–80.
80. Engelhart MJ, Geerlings MI, Meijer J *et al*. Inflammatory proteins in plasma and the risk of dementia. *Arch Neurol* 2004; 61:668–672.
81. Holmes C, El-Okl M, Williams AL *et al*. Systemic infection, interleukin 1β, and cognitive decline in Alzheimer's disease. *J Neurol Neurosurg Psychiatry* 2003; 74:788–789.

# 19

# Social management of dementia for patients and carers

*H. Brodaty, K. Berman*

## INTRODUCTION

In the USA, 70% of the four million people with Alzheimer's disease are cared for at home [1] and in Europe 66–80% of the 16 million people with dementia are cared for at home [2]; clearly there are huge numbers of caregivers worldwide. The caregiving career is highly dynamic and evolving, and the kinship relationship between patient and caregiver is extremely important. Family caregivers perform an important service for their relatives and for society, but do so at great cost to themselves. Decline in cognitive abilities, loss of functional capacity, dwindling companionship and the increasing demands of physical care along with possible behavioural changes in patients with a dementing illness, all impose escalating stresses on family caregivers [3].

Management of persons with dementia (also called patients here) and their caregivers aims to maximize the quality of life of the patient and that of the caregiver [4]. This requires a long-term view and the establishment of partnerships between patients, families and clinicians.

## WHO BECOMES A CAREGIVER?

As the dementing illness progresses, usually one person in the family comes forward as caregiver. This is generally a spouse or partner if the patient is married or in a relationship (the physical health of a spouse being an important predictor in beginning and in continuing to care for a patient [5]) or a child (more commonly a daughter or daughter-in-law) if the patient is single. About 75% of caregivers are women, whom society traditionally views as responsible for nursing sick family members [3, 6, 7]. Up to 64% of these women work outside the home (50% work full-time) as well as acting as caregivers [1]. Husbands handle the caregiving role very differently from wives, demonstrating significant changes in household responsibilities, social integration, marital relationship and well-being [8]. In a study of 818 community dwelling elderly people, people more likely to become caregivers tended to be older and to have lower incomes, lower senses of self-mastery and higher levels of health risk behaviours, before becoming caregivers [9].

Caregivers of patients with dementia tend to be older people, with all the concomitant problems of ageing. Caregiving often starts as a part-time function, but then grows and expands to full-time over months if not years [10]. Typically, caregivers offer their services for emotional and economic reasons, not because they are proficient at, or feel comfortable

**Henry Brodaty**, MBBS, MD, FRACP, FRANZCP, Professor of Psychogeriatrics, Academic Department for Old Age Psychiatry, School of Psychiatry, University of New South Wales, Sydney, Australia

**Karen Berman**, MB BCh, Academic Department for Old Age Psychiatry, School of Psychiatry, Prince of Wales Hospital, Randwick, NSW, Australia

with, the type of care required. Primary caregivers spend an average of 60 h per week caring for the patient [11]. In many families, caregiving is shared with other family members taking on a secondary caregiving role and providing periodic caregiving [12]. Families tend to keep the caregiving role within the family, but may hire outside help [13]. A hierarchical pattern of caregiver preference exists, with older people turning first to a spouse, then to an adult child, then to another relative and finally to a friend for care [14–16]. The mix of formal and informal help varies from country to country [11] as do patterns of caring for elderly dementing patients and attitudes to respite care and nursing home placement [17]. Most caregiving is done 'behind closed doors' and unless help is actively sought by the caregiver, friends and neighbours may remain unaware of the family's needs.

## DEFINITION OF CAREGIVER/FAMILY TERMINOLOGY

Many terms are used for those who provide care for people with dementia. In essence:

(a) Carers = caregivers = caretaker = informal carers = family and friends = unpaid.
(b) Formal caregivers = paid caregivers.
(c) Care co-ordinators = case managers = supervise the (paid) caregivers, but do not necessarily have a role in hands-on care. May live some distance from the patient.
(d) Family = almost any relative, whether related by blood or marriage.
(e) Full-time caregivers = provide more than 40 h of care per week.

## WHAT CAREGIVERS DO

One in four caregivers assist patients with three or more activities of daily living (ADLs), while four in five caregivers assist with instrumental activities of daily living (IADLs). Caregivers must thus be multi-skilled and be prepared to take on tasks performed by physiotherapists, nurses, financial and business managers, housekeepers and cooks [1].

## EFFECTS OF CAREGIVING ON CAREGIVERS

The caregiver is often regarded as the 'second' or 'hidden' patient. The combination of loss, prolonged distress and the physical demands of caregiving in older caregivers increases their risk of physical health problems [18]. Vehadra [19] reported caregivers as having high cortisol levels and a poor antibody response to the influenza vaccine, and concluded that these caregivers may be more vulnerable to infectious diseases than a non-caregiving population of similar age. Rates of wound healing are slowed [20], and levels of mild hypertension are increased [21], as is the tendency to develop serious illness [22]. As well, over one-third of caregivers suffer high levels of distress, objective and subjective burden and depression [5, 23–25], have higher relapse rates of depression [8], higher levels of anger [26] and take more prescription medication than non-caregivers of a similar age [27]. Live-in caregivers are more likely to be depressed than non-live-in caregivers [28] and spousal caregivers are more likely to be depressed than non-spousal caregivers [29] (i.e. the closer the bond, the greater the strain for the caregiver) although this was not noted in Waite's study [30]. Male caregivers may show their stress differently, turning to substance abuse or physical violence [1]. Many of the negative symptoms listed above tend to become worse over time [9].

Caregivers providing more care have simultaneously shown more satisfaction with their lives and more burden [31–33]. Frustration has been reported in 81% and grief in 73% of carers [34]. Hostility and anxiety are also reported [35]. Some caregivers care for the patient willingly and cheerfully while others do so grudgingly and become more distressed [36].

### *Positive aspects of caregiving*

Caregivers may be able to adapt to the stress of caregiving, and may draw on previously unused strengths and resources [37]. Cohen found that over 70% of caregivers reported that they were happy or positive about the caregiving role [32]. Positive aspects included companionship, fulfilment, a rewarding feeling and pride in one's ability to handle problems [38–40]. Contacts made with other people in the caregiving world are regarded as a positive part of the caregiving experience by many caregivers [1]. Caregivers who reported more positive feelings were less likely to report burden, depression or poor health [41] and had a decreased risk of patient institutionalization [42]. This was not, however, a consistent finding [43]. Caregivers who cannot identify any positive aspects of caring may be at risk for depression and poor health outcomes as well as earlier institutionalization of their care recipients [32].

#### *Caregiver burden*

This is defined as 'the negative phenomena associated with caring for an elderly, chronically ill or disabled family member or other person' [44]. This may be further divided into objective and subjective burden.

*Objective burden*: The burden or load borne by a person who cares for an elderly, chronically ill or disabled family member or other person is a multidimensional response to physical, psychological, emotional, social and financial stressors associated with the caregiving experience and is greatly influenced by the amount of time spent with the patient [45]. Behaviour disturbance is the most consistent predictor of caregiver burden [46]. Physical and social burden are good predictors of likelihood of institutionalization. Financial burden is a more variable predictor of likelihood to institutionalize [44, 47].

*Subjective burden (sometimes called strain)*: Subjective burden is defined as the caregiver's perception of the objective burden, and includes emotional reactions such as resentment, worry, frustration, anxiety and fatigue. Feelings of 'being trapped' and 'being manipulated' are common, as is lack of privacy [10].

## INTERVENTIONS FOR CAREGIVERS

### *INTRODUCTION*

The ability of a patient to remain in the community depends largely on the caregivers and their levels of stress. Some caregiver interventions can reduce caregiver psychological morbidity and help people with dementia to stay at home longer [48–51]. Interventions are many and varied and some are more effective than others [52], though none can alter the course of the disease [53]. While most programs are targeted at one member of the dyad (i.e. either the caregiver or patient), both are affected by the intervention and the benefits to one may be outweighed by potential distress to the other [53]. As well, the whole support system should be taken into account including other family members, community services etc. [53]. Except in the early stages of the disease, patients cannot actively participate in treatment, so most treatments are generally aimed at caregivers [53]. Caregivers may benefit from support, education and training for the duration of their time as caregivers, which may be several years.

The benefits of specific interventions include decreased caregiver stress [54], improved caregiver coping skills [52], reduced caregiver psychological morbidity [54–59], decreased or delayed nursing home placements [52, 59, 60], improved survival [61] and improved knowledge of dementia [54]. Educational and emotional support *per se* appear to be only modestly effective [62], emotional support being slightly more effective, and the combination being more effective than either support alone [58]. Education alone is unlikely to produce any improvement in caregiver well-being [63]. Pinquart and Sorensen [43] suggest that as behavioural problems cause the most stress in caregivers, caregivers should be educated about coping with these as a priority. They also suggest that spouses may benefit more than other caregivers from interventions that reduce objective burden [43]. The results of interventions have been mixed [64] and these will be discussed below.

## TYPES OF INTERVENTION

A full continuum of intervention or training exists, from provision of simple information to use of specialized behavioural and psychological techniques.

### Education and information

Caregivers require the knowledge and skills pertinent to the care of the patient. Almost half of all caregivers are ill-informed of the patient's diagnosis and the disease in general [65]. The next step for caregivers after the diagnosis is education regarding the illness, medication use and ways of enhancing the care that they are providing. Once caregivers accept the diagnosis and understand that the disease is chronic and without a cure, they can participate more effectively in an intervention program [53]. Educating caregivers about the disease helps reduce caregiver negative affect [66] (although caregivers may become depressed short-term [53]) and improves communication with the patient. Information about resources, services and training is helpful, as is discussion regarding forward planning, and the use of advance directives and respite care. Even though caregivers are reluctant to use respite care [67] a better understanding of the respite care process may encourage caregivers to use and to benefit from this service [53]. While information is clearly important, information alone does not decrease caregiver burden or impact significantly on the patient [68].

### Teaching behavioural strategies

Traditionally, behaviour modification has examined ways in which the social and physical environment influences behaviour. The environment can be modified to achieve the required behaviour on the part of patients. Teri *et al.* [69] found that pleasurable event planning and the use of problem-solving techniques improved depression levels in both patients and caregivers. In another study, they demonstrated that an exercise training program for patients with Alzheimer's disease combined with teaching caregivers behavioural management techniques, decreased frailty and improved behavioural problems in patients [70]. Group and individual behaviour management therapies have been trialled with some success, as discussed below in the 'Outcomes' section.

### Counselling

This involves a therapeutic relationship between caregivers and a trained professionals. Counselling needs are different at each stage as caregiving requirements change, including comfort for the family that is mourning the slow loss of parts of the person with dementia [71]. Caring for dementia patients is very different from caring for other patients and far more demanding, changing constantly as the disease progresses. In the early stages of the illness, the caregiver is involved in minor day-to-day help, e.g. cooking, cleaning and banking. Later, personal care is needed as well. Later still, round-the-clock care may be required. Caregivers of dementia patients need to deal with the patients' lack of insight and behavioural problems in addition to their physical needs. Patient resentment, anger and communication difficulties all add to the burden of care. Counselling gives caregivers 'permission' to seek assistance and offers validation [72], helps to normalize their feelings and reassures them. The therapist may teach self-monitoring behaviour, challenge negative thoughts and help caregivers develop problem-solving skills. Counselling can offer fresh insight, introduce caregivers to alternatives, offer support, change caregiver responses to behavioural disturbances, and offer a good opportunity to include other family members in the care of the patient and so distribute the burden more equally between family members [71].

Practical legal and financial advice may be of benefit to caregivers, as is the reminder to direct attention to the caregivers' physical health. Caregivers may well benefit from discussions regarding use of formal/respite care.

***Anger management***

Anger is a common negative emotion experienced by caregivers [35]. Coon *et al.* developed an intervention project aimed at 169 female caregivers (aged 50 years and over, and with normal cognition) who were the primary caregivers of dementing patients in the community. Caregivers were randomly assigned to one of three groups: anger management, depression management and a group with no intervention (waitlisted controls, who were offered the opportunity to participate in one of the classes at a later date). Interventions were psychoeducational and skills training, enabling caregivers to master self-management skills. Skills training led to reduced symptoms of anger, hostility and depression, as well as increased self-sufficiency in manageing behaviour problems and controlling upsetting thoughts [73].

***Caregiver training programs***

Training programs that include all the above, often in conjunction with local Alzheimer's Associations, may reduce caregiver distress and delay nursing home admission [48, 49]. A program designed to teach caregivers for elderly disabled patients caregiving skills and techniques was highly valued by participants [74]. The program also enhanced the caregivers' sense of competency and reduced the risk of physical strain [74]. Caregivers can be taught to avoid triggering aggressive behaviour, new ways of dealing with aggressive behaviour and ways of lessening the severity of inappropriate behaviours when they do occur [75].

A successful program trialled in six centres in Sweden [76] trained family caregivers and volunteers together. The volunteers later relieved the caregivers by providing in-home help. Both caregivers and volunteers expressed satisfaction with this training program.

***Support groups***

Support groups for caregivers have been well received since their introduction in the late 1970s [68, 77]. They can reduce caregiver stress and improve caregiver and patient quality of life [71, 77], but are less effective than highly structured individual interventions [68, 78]. A Dutch study [79] found support groups to be particularly effective for caregivers who were dissatisfied with their caregiving role and who had no job. The groups were also more effective when the patients were more apathetic and lived in nursing homes.

Groups may be large national associations, self-help groups or telephone or computer support services. Importantly, caregivers and other family members who attend these groups are not regarded as 'patients' but as people who have an increased risk of becoming overburdened by the caregiving role. This is an important difference between a support group and a psychotherapy group [79]. Support groups teach the carers that they are not alone in their daily struggle, decrease caregivers' sense of isolation and are educational. Anecdotally, their regular newsletters are invaluable to members.

Professionally led support groups are more formally structured [80] and appear to produce greater improvement in caregivers' psychological functioning, whereas peer-led groups have been found to produce the greater increase in informal support networks and the extent to which carers feel able to handle the care-giving role [81, 82]. Facilitators of peer-led groups usually are, or have been, caregivers themselves. Support groups should appeal to the local community as far as cultural and ethnic values are concerned [80]. In some countries there is a wide choice of support groups based on gender, age, setting of care and stage of disease [83]. Computer support networks have also been found to be an effective tool in decreasing strain for some caregivers [84, 85] and are a boon for younger caregivers and those living in remote areas [85].

Alzheimer's Associations or societies exist in over 75 countries worldwide (www.alz.co.uk). They provide education, support, counselling, telephone help-lines, advocacy, and, in many places, direct services such as day centres and even nursing homes. The more developed associations fund research directly and are very effective in lobbying government (e.g. Australia = www.alzheimers.org.au; USA = www.alz.org; UK = www.alzheimers.org.uk). At the heart of the associations are the support groups. Customarily these groups are held monthly and offer local caregivers the chance to ventilate, to learn from others and to socialize. Empirical data regarding the efficacy of self-help groups are lacking but anecdotal accounts are positive [80]. Not all caregivers will join an association or even obtain information from one, e.g. caregivers with large informal networks are less likely to be members. The commonest reason for caregivers not contacting their local association is lack of awareness [80].

#### *Telemedicine services*

The CANDID (Counselling and Diagnosis in Dementia) telemedicine service was set up in the UK to provide medical advice and intervention from a distance for the patient, the caregiver, and the general practitioner or other health professional involved in dementia care (http://dementia.ion.ucl.ac.uk/). The service is promoted for (caregivers and) patients whose dementia began before the age of 65, and has been used by a broad range of caregivers and professionals, although medical professionals have made less use of the service than was anticipated [86].

'Computerlink' is an electronic network, based in the USA, designed to provide social support to caregivers of patients with Alzheimer's disease [87]. Internet support has been conducted with some success for some caregivers [84, 85]. The Dementia Adovacy and Support Network International (DASNI) is a virtual support group for people with dementia (http://www.dasninternational.org/).

#### *Home modification advice*

Adjustments in the home environment are usually necessary to create a safe living environment, e.g. protection from hot surfaces, temperature regulators on hot water systems, unlit gas stoves or sharp objects and perimeter locks to secure wandering patients [71].

#### *Formal care*

Formal care services include meals-on-wheels, home-care, day-care, in-home respite care (sitting), residential respite care and permanent care. Designed to give the primary caregiver respite from caregiving duties, these services are needed by caregivers at different stages of the caregiving process, though it is more usual in the middle-to-later stages of the dementia [88]. As well as giving the caregiver a much-needed break, residential respite can be an opportunity for a professional re-assessment of the patient's condition and care needs.

Forms of respite care are:

- Day-care – where the person with dementia attends an activity centre for a few hours.
- Night-care – where someone stays overnight to allow the caregiver a restful night.
- In-home respite – where a professional caregiver comes into the person's home to spend time with the person with dementia.
- Residential respite – where the person with dementia is admitted for a period, usually days to weeks. This may be offered as:
  - an emergency, e.g. if the caregiver becomes ill, or
  - planned respite, e.g. so that the caregiver can have treatment for themselves or take a holiday.

Other innovative forms of respite have been devised, such as taking a group of people with dementia on a holiday or a weekend camp, with or without their caregivers.

Overwhelmingly, respite care has been described as useful and necessary for family caregivers [89, 90]. Respite care may be provided by trained or untrained staff or by volunteers [91]. Ideally patients and caregivers should be able to choose the amount and the timing of the respite, but in fact this does not often occur as caregivers are limited by type and availability of respite care in their area [91]. The amount of services offered differs by country and within countries, as does the cost of using the services. Respite is often used in emergency situations, e.g. when a caregiver is unexpectedly hospitalized and here again choice of respite may be limited. The Family Survival Project [92] developed the concept of minimal required hours of respite care. It concluded that 8 h per week is the minimum number of hours necessary to achieve relief from caregiving work. Many respite programs offer fewer hours than this, and may not be meeting the respite requirements of caregivers and are thus not effective.

The use of formal support services is much higher in caregivers of dementia patients than caregivers of other elderly patients [93], particularly the use of home help, day-care and district nursing. However, even when offered residential respite care, only slightly over half of caregivers avail themselves of this service [90]. Barriers to accepting respite care often derive from the caregivers themselves [94]. They may not accept care if e.g. they feel guilty or they may see the acceptance of respite care as an admission of 'weakness' or of 'failure' [95]. Financial barriers, cultural attitudes and lack of information about respite may also impede caregivers' use of this service [94]. Overall, caregivers of people with dementia are less satisfied with formal services than caregivers of people with non-dementing illnesses and have more unmet needs [23].

In a small study by Gonyea *et al.*, the female caregivers (of male veterans) who provided more assistance to the patients and had a greater sense of objective burden or were in poorer physical health, were more likely to express an interest in hospital-based respite care. These caregivers were less accepting of using respite care for reasons relating to subjective rather than to objective burden. Care recipients were less likely to accept respite care than the caregivers [95]. This study did not measure actual use of respite care, but only an 'interest' in using respite care.

*Benefits of formal care*: There is little evidence to suggest that residential respite care provides long-term benefits to patients or to caregivers or even that it improves outcome, [91, 96] but day-care programmes are cost-effective alternatives to nursing home care and they delay institutionalization of patients who cannot be managed at home on a full-time basis [71]. Zarit *et al.* [97] found that caregivers of relatives with dementia who used adult day-care services for at least twice each week for a minimum period of 3 months, experienced lower levels of caregiver related stress and better psychological well-being than a control group not using this service. Short-term (3 months) and long-term (12 months) benefits were found, however, the caregivers' feelings of 'role-captivity' were not improved [97].

Zarit *et al.*'s [98] survey of a variety of intervention programs found that benefits from in-home respite care included improved mood, reduced distress and decreased time spent caring for the patient. Problems with in-home respite care included poorly trained home-helpers and different helpers each time [98].

Adult day-care provides supervized activities for patients during the day and allows caregivers free time. Patients may attend day-care from one to several days each week and generally for 5–6 h each day. Day-care has not been shown to be effective in delaying nursing home admission [99], but has been shown to be effective for three outcomes: caregiver burden, caregiver depression and caregiver well-being [100]. Caregivers have generally expressed satisfaction with day-care [98].

There are few data on other forms of respite care. A small study by Vernooij-Dassen *et al.* [101] showed significantly fewer nursing home or retirement home admissions among a group using in-home services than among a control group. Similarly Mohide *et al.*'s [102] small study also showed fewer nursing home admissions in the treated group, but the numbers were small and the attrition rate high.

## OUTCOMES OF INTERVENTIONS

### Introduction

Outcomes are difficult to compare as the types of measures used in studies vary widely. There is great variability in characteristics of caregivers who are very heterogeneous, in the components of intervention which are often used in combination, in the amounts or 'doses' of intervention, in the duration of time over which the intervention is administered and in the length of follow-up (or in some cases the lack of follow-up). Studies without a delayed follow-up may miss impacts of treatment, which, in some studies, may manifest after a delay and may be maintained for some time [63]. Some studies had control groups and others not. Despite all the above, some interventions can make a difference to the caregiver. Although Cooke *et al.* [63] reported that approximately 66% of interventions targeting dementia caregivers do not produce the desired outcome, it is rare for any deterioration to be recorded in outcome measures.

Several reviews or meta-analyses have been published. In the meta-analyses reported by Sorenson *et al.* [100] and Charlesworth [103] adult child caregivers benefited more from interventions than did spouse caregivers, and women benefited more than did men. Also, the majority of the benefits persisted an average of seven months post-intervention [100]. The most consistent positive effects of caregiver interventions were found for psychotherapy and psycho-educational interventions, which produced improvements across almost all outcome measures [100]. However, in their review, Pusey and Richards [104] found that individualized interventions utilizing problem-solving and behaviour management were the most effective forms of intervention.

Professionally led support groups appear to produce the greatest improvement in caregivers' psychological functioning, whereas peer-led groups have been found to produce the greatest increase in informal support networks and the extent to which caregivers feel able to handle the care-giving role [81].

Unsuccessful interventions are short educational programs, support groups alone, single interviews and brief interventions or courses that are not supplemented with long-term contact [52, 105]. Social and health services other than respite care seem to have no consistent impact on caregiver distress [88]. According to Zarit [106], spouse caregivers, caregivers with less formal education and caregivers who feel 'trapped' do not benefit from day-care. In Yates' study [107], the use of formal services did not alleviate either caregiver load or caregiver depression.

### Psychological outcomes

Brodaty *et al.*'s [105] meta-analysis reported that caregiver interventions reduced caregiver stress (effect size [ES] 0.31; 95% confidence interval [CI] 0.13–0.50), enhanced caregiver knowledge (ES 0.51; CI 0.05–0.98), delayed nursing home admission and improved patients' psychological well-being. In addition, caregivers were satisfied with the interventions, had improved coping skills and improved relationships with the care recipients [105]. Sorensen *et al.*'s [100] meta-analysis (not restricted to dementia caregivers) had similar findings, showing a significant reduction in caregiver depression. In Cooke *et al.*'s [63] review of psychosocial interventions, 60% of caregivers improved on measures of psychological well-being.

### Outcome of burden

Th evidence for reduction of burden is mixed, possibly because of differences in how burden is conceptualized and measured. While burden was not reduced by interventions in Brodaty *et al.*'s meta-analysis, with only one in twenty studies showing a significant positive effect on burden [105], Cooke *et al.* [63] reported that 47% of studies showed reduced levels of caregiver burden. However, one study in this meta-analysis found levels of burden had increased after intervention [108]. Sorensen *et al.*'s meta-analysis [109] also reported a significant decrease in burden (of 0.14–0.41 standard deviation units on average) following caregiver interventions.

#### *Outcomes of education*

All three reviews reported significant improvement in caregiver knowledge following educational intervention [63, 105, 109]. Increased knowledge however, did not necessarily lead to improved caregiver well-being or decreased caregiver burden. Indeed only 27% of studies showing improved knowledge also showed improved well-being or burden. Caregiver education can have an impact on improving patient behaviours. In a controlled trial of fifty caregivers of Alzheimer's disease patients, the provision of verbal and videotaped material, behavioural problems and lists of possible interventions led to (non-significant) improvements in patients' behavioural scores. Scores in the control group increased slightly. Despite the non-significant result, 75% of caregivers rated the interventions as 'frequently' or 'always' effective [110].

#### *Outcomes of counselling*

Whitlatch *et al.* [111] found that caregivers in individual and family counselling were more likely to have successful outcomes on all dependent measures (the Brief Symptom Inventory, personal strain and role strain) than those not receiving counselling. Li and Seltzer [112] showed that social participation improved depressive symptoms in daughter caregivers, and emotional support buffered the stress emanating from behavioural problems and functional limitations in the parent.

#### *Outcomes of patient progress*

Sorensen *et al.*'s [109] meta-analysis showed that psychotherapy specifically targeting caregivers had a positive effect on patients' behavioural symptoms. Teri's [113] study suggested that behavioural training, when part of a larger program, can have a significant positive effect on patient behaviour.

#### *Time to institutionalization*

In the review by Brodaty *et al.* [105], four of seven intervention studies demonstrated delayed nursing home admission. Behavioural training, as part of a larger program, can delay institutionalization [113]. Caregivers have reported that nursing home placement is the most difficult decision that they have ever had to make [114]. They need support through this difficult transition time [115] and some interventions for both staff and caregivers have been shown to decrease difficulties [116].

### *PREDICTORS OF SUCCESSFUL INTERVENTIONS*

Programs that involve both patients and families and that are more intensive and modified to the caregivers' needs may be more successful [105]. Statistically, the involvement of the patient in addition to the caregiver produced better outcomes [105]. Despite the modest results of caregiver interventions overall, caregivers were frequently satisfied or very satisfied with their interventions.

Psycho-educational and psychotherapeutic interventions, or a combination of the two, showed the most consistent short term effects on outcome measures in Sorensen *et al.*'s meta-analysis [109]. The 'dose' or length of the intervention is important, e.g. 7–9 sessions would be adequate to increase knowledge, but may be inadequate to improve depression [105, 109]. Spousal caregivers, who have increased risk factors for distress, benefited less than adult children. Individual interventions were better at improving caregiver well-being, whereas group interventions were better at improving patient symptoms [100].

The use of a social component, or the combination of social and cognitive components, proved to be relatively effective in improving psychological morbidity [63]. Charlesworth's [103] editorial agreed with this, adding that for interventions to be effective, they should be targeted specifically to the individual needs of both patient and caregiver. Pusey and Richards [104] observed that individualized interventions using problem-solving and behaviour management techniques were most effective. Post-intervention follow-up is important as long-term effects may be missed if the follow-up period is too short [63].

## NURSING HOME ADMISSION

### *CAREGIVER FACTORS LEADING TO NURSING HOME ADMISSION*

The ability of a person with dementia to remain in the community as the disease progresses depends largely on the caregivers and their levels of stress [117]. Some caregiver interventions can reduce caregiver psychological morbidity and help people with dementia to stay at home longer [48–51].

Caregivers who are physically healthy are more likely to continue to care for persons with dementia, while caregivers in declining physical health are more likely to stop providing care [5]. This however does not apply to mental health of caregivers, as even those with declining mental health will continue to care for persons with dementia [5]. Daughters are less likely to continue giving care than are wives [5, 118] and husbands are less likely to continue giving care than are wives [40]. In Yaffe *et al.*'s [119] study, caregiver characteristics associated with nursing home placement were higher age and higher scores on the Zarit Burden Scale. Ongoing caregiving was not associated with the number of hours of care required per week [5].

### *PATIENT FACTORS PRECIPITATING NURSING HOME ADMISSION*

Behavioural problems are the most common precipitants for a move to a nursing home. Lim *et al.* [117] found that two behavioural abnormalities (repetition and agitation) and one functional impairment (urinary incontinence) predicted the likelihood of admission to a nursing home. O'Donnell *et al.* [120] found that increased severity of dementia, disruptive behaviours and incontinence increased the probability of nursing home admission, with the best predictors of admission being paranoia, aggressive behaviour and incontinence. Cohen *et al.* [42] reported that seven variables (use of services, enjoyment of caregiving, caregiver burden and health, caregiver rating and reaction to patient behaviour and memory problems, and presence of troublesome behaviours) predicted the decision to institutionalize, and six (caregiver health and burden, use of services, patient cognitive function and troublesome behaviours and caregiver reaction to these behaviours) predicted actual institutionalization at 18 months. Yaffe's large study of 5788 ethnically diverse patients with dementia found that patient characteristics associated with nursing home placement were: black ethnicity, Hispanic ethnicity, (both inversely associated with placement), living alone, one or more dependencies in ADL, greater cognitive impairment with Mini-mental State Examination score under 20, and one or more difficult behaviours [119].

## SUMMARY

The role of the caregiver in supporting family members with dementia is vital. While demanding and stressful, the role often delivers satisfaction to caregivers. There are many adverse effects on family caregivers – psychological, physical, social and financial. Interventions can be effective but should be tailored to the needs of the caregiver and those of the patient. Predictors of negative consequences can be identified and it may be more effective to target interventions at vulnerable caregivers. General measures such as increased community awareness of dementia, reduction of stigma, referrals to Alzheimer's associations and enhancing caregiver knowledge appear useful but are more difficult to be proven to be empirically efficacious.

## REFERENCES


1. Giorgianni S (ed). *A Profile of Caregiving in America*, 2nd edition. Impact Communications, New York, 2005.
2. European Institute of Womens' Health. Remind Project: Dementia Care. Challenges for an Aging Europe. 2005.
3. Brodaty H, Hadzi-Pavlovic D. Psychosocial effects on carers of living with persons with dementia. *Aust NZ J Psychiatry* 1990; 24:351–361.
4. Brodaty H, Green A, Low L-F. Vascular dementia: consequences for family carer and implications for management. In: O'Brien J, Ames D, Gustafson L, Folstein M, Chiu E (eds). *Cerebrovascular Disease and Dementia: Pathology, Neuropsychiatry and Management*, 2nd edition. Martin Dunitz, London, 2004, pp 363–378.
5. McCann JJ, Hebert LE, Bienias JL, Morris MC, Evans DA. Predictors of beginning and ending caregiving during a 3-year period in a biracial community population of older adults. *Am J Public Health* 2004; 94:1800–1806.
6. Anonymous. Canadian study of health and aging: study methods and prevalence of dementia. *CMAJ* 1994; 150:899–913.
7. Yee JL, Schulz R. Gender differences in psychiatric morbidity among family caregivers: a review and analysis. *Gerontologist* 2000; 40:147–164.
8. Russo J, Vitaliano PP, Brewer DD, Katon W, Becker J. Psychiatric disorders in spouse caregivers of care recipients with Alzheimer's disease and matched controls: a diathesis-stress model of psychopathology. *J Abnorm Psychol* 1995; 104:197–204.
9. Burton LC, Zdaniuk B, Schulz R, Jackson S, Hirsch C. Transitions in spousal caregiving. *Gerontologist* 2003; 43:230–241.
10. Schur D, Whitlatch CJ, Clark PA. Beyond the chi-square: caregivers are more than just faceless statistics. *Lippincotts Case Manag* 2005; 10:65–71.
11. Max W, Webber P, Fox P. Alzheimer's disease. The unpaid burden of caring. *J Aging Health* 1995; 7:179–199.
12. Stone R, Cafferata GL, Sangl J. Caregivers of the frail elderly: a national profile. *Gerontologist* 1987; 27:616–626.
13. Brody EM. Parent care as normative stress. *Gerontologist* 1985; 25:19–29.
14. Himes CL, Reidy EB. The role of friends in caregiving. *Res Aging* 2000; 22:315–336.
15. Antonucci TC, Hiroko A. Convoys of social support: generational issues. *Marriage Fam Rev* 1991; 16:103–119.
16. Cantor MH. Neighbours and friends: an overlooked resource in the informal support system. *Res Aging* 1979; 1:434–463.
17. Prince M, Acosta D, Chiu H, Sczufca M, Shaji K. Cross-cultural issues for care. 10/66 program. In: *Alzheimer's Association International Conference*. Washington DC, USA, 2005.
18. Vitaliano PP, Zhang J, Scanlan JM. Is caregiving hazardous to one's physical health? A meta-analysis. *Psychol Bull* 2003; 129:946–972.
19. Vedhara K, Cox NK, Wilcock GK *et al*. Chronic stress in elderly carers of dementia patients and antibody response to influenza vaccination. *Lancet* 1999; 353:627–631.
20. Kiecolt-Glaser JK, Marucha PT, Malarkey WB, Mercado AM, Glaser R. Slowing of wound healing by psychological stress. *Lancet* 1995; 346:1194–1196.
21. Shaw WS, Patterson TL, Ziegler MG, Dimsdale JE, Semple SJ, Grant I. Accelerated risk of hypertensive blood pressure recordings among Alzheimer caregivers. *J Psychosom Res* 1999; 46:215–227.
22. Shaw WS, Patterson TL, Semple SJ *et al*. Longitudinal analysis of multiple indicators of health decline among spousal caregivers. *Ann Behav Med* 1997; 19:101–109.
23. Bedford S, Melzer D, Dening T, Lawton C. What becomes of people with dementia referred to community psychogeriatric teams? *Int J Geriatr Psychiatry* 1996; 11:1051–1056.
24. Haley WE, Levine EG, Brown SL, Berry JW, Hughes GH. Psychological, social, and health consequences of caring for a relative with senile dementia. *J Am Geriatr Soc* 1987; 35:405–411.

25. Brodaty H. The Sydney Dementia Carers Training Program. In: Copeland J, Abou-Saleh MT, Blazer DG (eds). *Principles and Practice of Geriatric Psychiatry*. John Wiley and Sons Ltd, 2002.
26. Gallagher D, Wrabetz A, Lovett S, Del Maestro S, Rose J. Depression and other negative affects in family caregivers. In: Light E, Lebowitz B (eds). *Alzheimer's Disease Treatment and Family Stress: Future Directions of Research*. Government Printing Office, Washington DC, USA, 1989, pp 218–244.
27. Oyebode J. Assessment of carer's psychological needs. *Adv Psychiatr Treat* 2003; 9:45–53.
28. Whitlatch C, Noelker L. Caregiving and Caring. *Encyclopaedia Gerontol* 1996; 1:253–268.
29. Donaldson C, Tarrier N, Burns A. Determinants of carer stress in Alzheimer's disease. *Int J Geriatr Psychiatry* 1998; 13:248–256.
30. Waite A, Bebbington P, Skelton-Robinson M, Orrell M. Social factors and depression in carers of people with dementia. *Int J Geriatr Psychiatry* 2004; 19:582–587.
31. Lawton MP, Rajagopal D, Brody E, Kleban MH. The dynamics of caregiving for a demented elder among black and white families. *J Gerontol* 1992; 47:S156–S164.
32. Cohen CA, Colantonio A, Vernich L. Positive aspects of caregiving: rounding out the caregiver experience. *Int J Geriatr Psychiatry* 2002; 17:184–188.
33. Beach SR, Schulz R, Yee JL, Jackson S. Negative and positive health effects of caring for a disabled spouse: longitudinal findings from the caregiver health effects study. *Psychol Aging* 2000; 15:259–271.
34. Luscombe G, Brodaty H, Freeth S. Younger people with dementia: diagnostic issues, effects on carers and use of services. *Int J Geriatr Psychiatry* 1998; 13:323–330.
35. Anthony-Bergstone CR, Zarit SH, Gatz M. Symptoms of psychological distress among caregivers of dementia patients. *Psychol Aging* 1988; 3:245–248.
36. Brodaty H. Dementia and the family. In: Bloch S, Hafner J, Harari E, Szmukler GI (eds). *The Family in Clinical Psychiatry*. Oxford University Press, Oxford, 1994, pp 224–246.
37. Stephens MA, Zarit SH. Family caregiving to dependent older adults: stress, appraisal, and coping. *Psychol Aging* 1989; 4:387–388.
38. Grant G, Ramcharan P, McGrath M, Nolan M, Keady J. Rewards and gratifications among family caregivers: towards a refined model of caring and coping. *J Intellect Disabil Res* 1998; 42:58–71.
39. Brodaty H, Low L. Involvement of carers, consumers and the broader community. In: Draper B, Melding P, Brodaty H (eds). *Psychogeriatric Service Delivery. An International Perspective*. Oxford University Press, Oxford, 2005, pp 293–307.
40. Kramer BJ. Husbands caring for wives with dementia: a longitudinal study of continuity and change. *Health Soc Work* 2000; 25:97–107.
41. Schulz R, Beach SR. Caregiving as a risk factor for mortality: the Caregiver Health Effects Study. *JAMA* 1999; 282:2215–2219.
42. Cohen CA, Gold DP, Shulman K, Tracey J, McDonald G, Wargon M. Factors determining the decision to institutionalize dementing individuals: a prospective study. *Gerontologist* 1993; 33:714–720.
43. Pinquart M, Sorensen S. Associations of caregiver stressors and uplifts with subjective well-being and depressive mood: a meta-analytic comparison. *Aging Ment Health* 2004; 8:438–449.
44. Stuckey JC, Neundorfer MM, Smyth KA. Burden and well-being: the same coin or related currency?... an earlier version of this article was presented in November, 1994 at the 47th Annual Meeting of the Gerontological Society of America in Atlanta, Georgia. *Gerontologist* 1996; 36:686–693.
45. Bullock R. The needs of the caregiver in the long-term treatment of Alzheimer disease. *Alzheimer Dis Assoc Disord* 2004; 18(suppl 1):S17–S23.
46. Coen RF, O'Boyle C, Oakley D, Lawlor BA. Dementia carer education and patient behaviour disturbance. *Int J Geriatr Psychiatry* 1999; 14:302–306.
47. Stull DE, Kosloski K, Kercher K. Caregiver burden and generic well-being: opposite sides of the same coin? *Gerontologist* 1994; 34:88–94.
48. Mittelman MS, Ferris SH, Shulman E, Steinberg G, Levin B. A family intervention to delay nursing home placement of patients with Alzheimer disease. A randomized controlled trial. *JAMA* 1996; 276:1725–1731.
49. Brodaty H, Gresham M, Luscombe G. The Prince Henry Hospital dementia caregivers' training programme. *Int J Geriatr Psychiatry* 1997; 12:183–192.
50. Eloniemi-Sulvaka U, Sivenius J. Support programs for demented patients and their carers: the role of dementia family co-ordinator is crucial. In: Iqbal K, Swaab D, Winblad B (eds). *Alzheimers Disease and Related Disorders*. John Wiley and Sons, West Sussex, 1999, pp 795–802.
51. Riordan J, Bennett A. An evaluation of an augmented domiciliary service to older people with dementia and their carers. *Aging Ment Health* 1998; 2:137–143.

52. Brodaty H, Gresham M. Effect of a training programme to reduce stress in carers of patients with dementia. *BMJ* 1989; 299:1375–1379.
53. Zarit SH, Leitsch SA. Developing and evaluating community based intervention programs for Alzheimer's patients and their caregivers. *Aging Ment Health* 2001; 5(suppl 1):S84–S98.
54. Kahan J, Kemp B, Staples FR, Brummel-Smith K. Decreasing the burden in families caring for a relative with a dementing illness. A controlled study. *J Am Geriatr Soc* 1985; 33:664–670.
55. Brodaty H, Gresham M. Effect of a training programme to reduce stress in carers of patients with dementia. *BMJ* 1989; 299:1375–1379.
56. Mittelman MS, Ferris SH, Shulman E, Steinberg G, Levin B. A family intervention to delay nursing home placement of patients with Alzheimer disease. A randomized controlled trial. *JAMA* 1996; 276:1725–1731.
57. Brodaty H, Gresham M, Luscombe G. The Prince Henry Hospital dementia caregivers' training programme. *Int J Geriatr Psychiatry* 1997; 12:183–192.
58. Rabins PV. The caregiver's role in Alzheimer's disease. *Dement Geriatr Cogn Disord* 1998; 3:25–28.
59. Mittelman MS, Ferris SH, Steinberg G *et al*. An intervention that delays institutionalization of Alzheimer's disease patients: treatment of spouse-caregivers. *Gerontologist* 1993; 33:730–740.
60. Ferris SH, Steinberg G, Shulman E, Kahn R, Reisberg B. Institutionalization of Alzheimer's disease patients: reducing precipitating factors through family counseling. *Home Health Care Serv Q* 1987; 8:23–51.
61. Brodaty H, McGilchrist C, Harris L, Peters KE. Time until institutionalization and death in patients with dementia. Role of caregiver training and risk factors. *Arch Neurol* 1993; 50:643–650.
62. Gitlin LN, Belle SH, Burgio LD *et al*. Effect of multicomponent interventions on caregiver burden and depression: the REACH multisite initiative at 6-month follow-up. *Psychol Aging* 2003; 18:361–374.
63. Cooke DD, McNally L, Mulligan KT, Harrison MJ, Newman SP. Psychosocial interventions for caregivers of people with dementia: a systematic review [see comment]. *Aging Ment Health* 2001; 5:120–135.
64. Brodaty H, Green A. Caregiver interventions. In: Qizibash N, Schneider L, Chui H, Tariot P, Brodaty H, Kaye J (eds). *Evidence Based Dementia Practice: A Practical Guide to Diagnosis and Management*. Blackwell Science, Oxford, 2002, pp 764–794.
65. Thomas P, Chantoin-Merlet S, Hazif-Thomas C *et al*. Complaints of informal caregivers providing home care for dementia patients: the Pixel study. *Int J Geriatr Psychiatry* 2002; 17:1034–1047.
66. Chiverton P, Caine ED. Education to assist spouses in coping with Alzheimer's disease. A controlled trial. *J Am Geriatr Soc* 1989; 37:593–598.
67. Brodaty H, Gresham M. Prescribing residential respite care for dementia – effects, side-effects, indications and dosage. *Int J Geriatr Psychiatry* 1992; 7:357–362.
68. Marriott A, Donaldson C, Tarrier N, Burns A. Effectiveness of cognitive-behavioural family intervention in reducing the burden of care in carers of patients with Alzheimer's disease. *Br J Psychiatry* 2000; 176:557–562.
69. Teri L, Gibbons LE, McCurry SM *et al*. Exercise plus behavioral management in patients with Alzheimer disease: a randomized controlled trial. *JAMA* 2003; 290:2015–2022.
70. Teri L, Logsdon RG, Uomoto J, McCurry SM. Behavioral treatment of depression in dementia patients: a controlled clinical trial. *J Gerontol B Psychol Sci Soc Sci* 1997; 52:159–166.
71. Mendez MF, Cummings JL. *Dementia. A Clinical Approach*, 3rd edition. Butterworth Heinemann, Philadelphia, 2003, pp 583–603.
72. Kasuya RT, Polgar-Bailey P, Takeuchi R. Caregiver burden and burnout. A guide for primary care physicians. *Postgrad Med* 2000; 108:119–123.
73. Coon DW, Thompson L, Steffen A, Sorocco K, Gallagher-Thompson D. Anger and depression management: psychoeducational skill training interventions for women caregivers of a relative with dementia. *Gerontologist* 2003; 43:678–689.
74. Mahoney DF, Shippee-Rice R. Training family caregivers of older adults: a program model for community nurses. *J Community Health Nurs* 1994; 11:71–78.
75. Brodaty H. Caregivers and behavioral disturbances: effects and interventions. *Int Psychogeriatr* 1996; 3:455–458.
76. Jansson W, Almberg B, Grafstrom M, Winblad B. The Circle Model – support for relatives of people with dementia. *Int J Geriatr Psychiatry* 1998; 13:674–681.
77. Fuller J, Ward E, Evans A, Massam K, Gardner A. Dementia: supportive groups for relatives. *Br Med J* 1979; 1:1684–1685.

78. Gallagher-Thompson D, DeVries HM. 'Coping with frustration' classes: development and preliminary outcomes with women who care for relatives with dementia. *Gerontologist* 1994; 34:548–552.
79. Cuijpers P, Hosman CM, Munnichs JM. Change mechanisms of support groups for caregivers of dementia patients. *Int Psychogeriatr* 1996; 8:575–587.
80. Brodaty H, Green A, Graham N. Alzheimer's (disease and related disorders) associations and societies: supporting family carers. In: O'Brien J, Ames D, Burns A (eds). *Dementia* 2nd edition. Arnold, London, 2000, pp 361–367.
81. Toseland RW, Rossiter CM, Labrecque MS. The effectiveness of peer-led and professionally led groups to support family caregivers. *Gerontologist* 1989; 29:465–471.
82. Zarit SH, Femia EE, Watson J, Rice-Oeschger L, Kakos B. Memory Club: a group intervention for people with early-stage dementia and their care partners. *Gerontologist* 2004; 44:262–269.
83. Gwyther LP. Social issues of the Alzheimer's patient and family. *Am J Med* 1998; 104:27.
84. Bass DM, McClendon MJ, Brennan PF, McCarthy C. The buffering effect of a computer support network on caregiver strain. *J Aging Health* 1998; 10:20–43.
85. Brennan PF, Moore SM, Smyth KA. The effects of a special computer network on caregivers of persons with Alzheimer's disease. *Nurs Res* 1995; 44:166–172.
86. Harvey R, Roques PK, Fox NC, Rossor MN. CANDID – Counselling and Diagnosis in Dementia: a national telemedicine service supporting the care of younger patients with dementia. *Int J Geriatr Psychiatry* 1998; 13:381–388.
87. Brennan PF, Moore SM, Smyth KA. Alzheimer's disease caregivers' uses of a computer network. *West J Nurs Res* 1992; 14:662–673.
88. Knight BG, Lutzky SM, Macofsky-Urban F. A meta-analytic review of interventions for caregiver distress: recommendations for future research. *Gerontologist* 1993; 33:240–248.
89. Brodaty H, Gresham M. Effect of a training programme to reduce stress in carers of patients with dementia. *BMJ* 1992; 299:1375–1379.
90. Lawton MP, Brody EM, Saperstein AR. A controlled study of respite service for caregivers of Alzheimer's patients. *Gerontologist* 1989; 29:8–16.
91. Lee H, Cameron M. Respite care for people with dementia and their carers. *Cochrane Database Syst Rev* 2004; 2.
92. Family Survival Project. *Annual Reports: Family Survival Program Pilot Project*. San Francisco, Family Survival Project, 1984.
93. Philp I, McKee KJ, Meldrum P *et al*. Community care for demented and non-demented elderly people: a comparison study of financial burden, service use, and unmet needs in family supporters. *BMJ* 1995; 310:1503–1506.
94. Lawton MP, Brody EM, Saperstein AR. *Respite for Caregivers of Alzheimer Patients: Research and Practice*. Springer Publishing Co, 1991, p 164.
95. Gonyea JG, Seltzer GB, Gerstein C, Young M. Acceptance of hospital-based respite care by families and elders. *Health Soc Work* 1988; 13:201–208.
96. Montgomery R, Borgatta E. The effects of alternative support strategies on family caregiving. *Gerontologist* 1989; 29:457–464.
97. Zarit SH, Stephens MA, Townsend A, Greene R. Stress reduction for family caregivers: effects of adult day care use. *J Gerontol Ser B Psychol Sci Soc Sci* 1998; 53:S267–S278.
98. Zarit SH, Gaugler JE, Jarrott SE. Useful services for families: research findings and directions. *Int J Geriatr Psychiatry* 1999; 14:165–177.
99. Ballinger BR. The effects of opening a geriatric psychiatry day hospital. *Acta Psychiatr Scand* 1984; 70:400–403.
100. Sorensen S, Pinquart M, Duberstein P. How effective are interventions with caregivers? An updated meta-analysis. *Gerontologist* 2002; 42:356–372.
101. Vernooij-Dassen M, Huygen F, Felling A, Persoon J. Home care for dementia patients. *J Am Geriatr Soc* 1995; 43:456–457.
102. Mohide EA, Pringle DM, Streiner DL, Gilbert JR, Muir G, Tew M. A randomized trial of family caregiver support in the home management of dementia. *J Am Geriatr Soc* 1990; 38:446–454.
103. Charlesworth GM. Reviewing psychosocial interventions for family carers of people with dementia. *Aging Ment Health* 2001; 5:104–106.
104. Pusey H, Richards D. A systematic review of the effectiveness of psychosocial interventions for carers of people with dementia. *Aging Ment Health* 2001; 5:107–119.

105. Brodaty H, Green A, Koschera A. Meta-analysis of psychosocial interventions for caregivers of people with dementia. *J Am Geriatr Soc* 2003; 51:657–664.
106. Zarit SH. Interventions for family caregivers: do they work and why. In: *Powerpoint Presentation*. 2005.
107. Yates ME, Tennstedt S, Chang BH. Contributors to and mediators of psychological well-being for informal caregivers. *J Gerontol B Psychol Sci Soc Sci* 1999; 54:12–22.
108. Goodman C, Pynoos J. A model telephone and information support program for caregivers of Alzheimer's patients. *Gerontologist* 1990; 30:399–405.
109. Sorensen S, Pinquart M, Duberstein P. How effective are interventions with caregivers? An updated meta-analysis. *Gerontologist* 2002; 42:356–372.
110. Burgener SC, Bakas T, Murray C, Dunahee J, Tossey S. Effective caregiving approaches for patients with Alzheimer's disease. *Geriatr Nurs* 1998; 19:121–126.
111. Whitlatch CJ, Zarit SH, von Eye A. Efficacy of interventions with caregivers: a reanalysis. *Gerontologist* 1991; 31:9–14.
112. Li LW, Seltzer MM, Greenberg JS. Social support and depressive symptoms: differential patterns in wife and daughter caregivers. *J Gerontol B Psychol Sci Soc Sci* 1997; 52:S200–S211.
113. Teri L. Training families to provide care: effects on people with dementia. *Int J Geriatr Psychiatry* 1999; 14:110–116.
114. Fink SV, Picot SF. Nursing home placement decisions and post-placement experiences of African-American and European-American caregivers. *J Gerontol Nurs* 1995; 21:35–42.
115. Ryan AA, Scullion HF. Family and staff perceptions of the role of families in nursing homes. *J Adv Nurs* 2000; 32:626–634.
116. Maas ML, Reed D, Park M *et al*. Outcomes of family involvement in care intervention for caregivers of individuals with dementia. *Nurs Res* 2004; 53:76–86.
117. Lim PP, Sahadevan S, Choo GK, Anthony P. Burden of caregiving in mild to moderate dementia: an Asian experience. *Int Psychogeriatr* 1999; 11:411–420.
118. Seltzer MM, Li LW. The dynamics of caregiving: transitions during a three-year prospective study. *Gerontologist* 2000; 40:165–178.
119. Yaffe K, Fox P, Newcomer R *et al*. Patient and caregiver characteristics and nursing home placement in patients with dementia. *JAMA* 2002; 287:2090–2097.
120. O'Donnell BF, Drachman DA, Barnes HJ, Peterson KE, Swearer JM, Lew RA. Incontinence and troublesome behaviors predict institutionalization in dementia. *J Geriatr Psychiatry Neurol* 1992; 5:45–52.

# Section IV

## Treatment of non-Alzheimer's disease cognitive impairment

# 20

## Vascular dementia

*S. Gauthier, T. Erkinjuntti, K. Rockwood*

### INTRODUCTION

Cerebrovascular disease (CVD), as well as ischaemic brain injury secondary to cardiovascular disease, are common causes of dementia in elderly people. Importantly, CVD frequently contributes to cognitive loss in patients with Alzheimer's disease (AD). Progress in understanding the pathogenesis of vascular dementia (VaD) has resulted in promising symptomatic and preventive treatments of these conditions. Of note, cholinergic deficits can be demonstrated even in 'pure' VaD and are due to ischaemia of cholinergic pathways and can be treated with the use of the cholinesterase inhibitor agents. Controlled clinical trials with donepezil, galantamine, and rivastigmine in VaD, as well as galantamine in patients with AD with CVD, have demonstrated improvement in cognition, behaviour and activities of daily living (ADL). The use of the *N*-methyl-D-aspartate (NMDA) receptor antagonist, memantine, has also demonstrated symptomatic benefit in VaD in comparison to placebo. Primary and secondary prevention of stroke, in particular with control of hypertension and hyperlipidaemia, can also result in decreased incidence of VaD. From the public health viewpoint, recognition of the risk state towards VaD after transient ischaemic attacks (TIA) or stroke before the development of dementia, and correction of vascular risk factors could lead to a global decrease of incident dementia in the elderly. This chapter will review available evidence, already summarized by Erkinjuntti *et al.* [1], and will argue that the treatment of global risk as suggested by Elkind [2] will be more effective than treating individual risk factors.

### EPIDEMIOLOGY OF STROKE AND DEMENTIA

Stroke and dementia increase exponentially with population ageing [3]. Less well-known is the fact of the important interplay between these two conditions, so that stroke can result in VaD, but also brain ischaemia can worsen the cognitive effects of AD pathology [4]. Post-stroke dementia occurs in up to one-third of patients with clinically manifest ischaemic stroke after age 65 [5]. Moreover, magnetic resonance imaging (MRI)-documented silent brain infarcts more than double the risk of developing dementia in elderly people [6]. In addition, in these age groups vascular cognitive impairment (VCI) short of dementia, is also common [7–9]. Current projections indicate that with increasing longevity of the oldest age groups and the damaging effects of CVD and heart disease on cognition, VaD will become one of the main causes of dementia in the elderly [10].

**Serge Gauthier**, MD, FRCPC, Director, Alzheimer's Disease & Related Disorders Research Unit, McGill Center for Studies in Aging, Douglas Hospital, Montreal, Canada

**Timo Erkinjuntti**, MD, PhD, Professor in Applied Neurology, Department of Neurology, University of Helsinki, Helsinki, Finland

**Kenneth Rockwood**, MPA, BSc, MD, FRCPC, Consultant Geriatrician (Geriatrics & Neurology), Department of Medicine, Dalhousie University Centre for Health Care of the Elderly, Halifax, Nova Scotia, Canada

## VASCULAR DEMENTIA – TERMINOLOGY AND CRITERIA

Dementia is a syndrome of acquired intellectual deficit that results in significant impairment of social or occupational functioning [11]. AD is the most common cause of dementia and this has influenced our understanding of the dementia syndrome. Indeed, all diagnostic criteria for 'dementia' require a core amnestic disorder and a progressive, irreversible decline, despite the fact that VaD may present with relatively mild memory impairment and a more 'subcortical' pattern of presentation in which impaired executive function is particularly prominent. Historically, VaD has been the second most common cause of dementia. Until recently, the term used was 'multi-infarct dementia' (MID), which was thought to arise from the additive effect of sequential cerebral infarcts [12]. MID and post-stroke VaD can be defined clinically by sudden onset, stepwise deterioration, and presence of focal (usually motor) neurological features. The Hachinski Ischaemia Score [13] is useful in the clinical diagnosis of MID. It is now apparent, however, not all cases of VaD are represented by MID. More common than MID are cases of subcortical ischaemic VaD (SIVD; [14]), manifested clinically as a subcortical form of dementia with prominent involvement of prefrontal executive functions, apathy, slowing of psychomotor functions, and gait abnormalities; SIVD may result from lacunar strokes and incomplete white matter ischaemia.

By analogy to the concept of amnestic mild cognitive impairment (MCI), which is considered the earliest manifestation of AD, it has been proposed that the notion of VaD should be broadened to encompass early forms of cognitive loss due to CVD. The nosology of this has been confusing, as it is variously called VCI and VCI no-dementia, abbreviated as either vascular CIND or VCI-ND, [8, 15–17]. VCI is also the term introduced to capture the full range of VCI no-dementia, VaD and AD with CVD.

## VASCULAR DEMENTIA CRITERIA

All of the available clinical criteria for VaD identify with varying specificity a common group of patients. Therefore, any and all of them are useful to diagnose VaD in a clinical setting [18–20]. However, for controlled clinical trials, or for other research purposes where false-positive cases must be excluded, only those criteria that have high specificity are used. Specificity is usually obtained at the cost of decreased sensitivity, first, by using strict requirements for the diagnosis of dementia, and second, by requiring that brain imaging identify cerebrovascular pathology. In the early 1990s, two influential sets of diagnostic criteria were developed for the identification of VaD for research purposes. The criteria of the California Alzheimer's Disease Diagnostic and Treatment Centres (CAD-DTC; [21]) were developed for the diagnosis of VaD caused exclusively by ischaemic cerebrovascular lesions. The criteria of the National Institute of Neurological Disorders and Stroke and the Association Internationale pour la Recherche et l'Enseignement en Neurosciences (NINDS-AIREN; [22]) recognize that VaD may result from a variety of cerebrovascular disorders including complete or incomplete brain ischaemia, cerebral haemorrhage, and other vascular or circulatory brain injuries. Perhaps unavoidable at the time of inception was the use in both sets of criteria of dementia definitions modelled on the dementia of AD. Although both criteria went beyond the MID concept, they still operationalized VaD in a way that was heavily influenced by the notion of 'strokes large and small'. Nonetheless, the important role of single strategic infarcts was recognized by both sets of criteria.

In keeping with the emphasis on cerebrovascular injury arising from demonstrable infarction, both sets of VaD criteria rely on neuroimaging for confirmation of cerebrovascular lesions. These lesions include both large vessel and small vessel ischaemia. Large vessel injuries are either multiple cortical or cortico-subcortical infarcts, or single, strategically placed infarcts that occur in areas that are crucial for cognition or behaviour (e.g. angular gyrus, basal forebrain, thalamus, anterior or posterior cerebral artery strokes). Small-vessel injury is manifested as multiple basal ganglia and white-matter lacunae or as extensive white-matter lesions, or combinations thereof. Patients can have evidence of either large- or small-vessel disease, or both.

The diagnosis of 'probable' VaD by the NINDS-AIREN criteria [22] identifies the best-defined clinical phenotype of VaD; i.e. post-stroke VaD, where the relationship between the CVD and the dementia has a temporal basis. In these patients, onset of dementia occurs within 3 months of a stroke. By excluding cases with prodromal and progressive amnestic disorder prior to the stroke, these criteria effectively exclude patients with 'mixed' dementia, i.e. AD with CVD.

## CLINICAL FEATURES OF VASCULAR DEMENTIA AND ITS SUBTYPES

The following descriptions of cardinal clinical subtypes of VaD outline subgroups that form the probable VaD spectrum within the current generation of VaD studies [23].

*Post-stroke VaD* (also called multi-infarct dementia, or MID when present after multiple strokes). Classic clinical features of post-stroke VaD include abrupt, onset of focal neurological symptoms and signs, and presence of cortical cognitive impairments such as aphasia, apraxia, or agnosia. True MID is relatively uncommon nowadays, given appropriate secondary stroke prevention. MID remains relatively stable or evolves in association with silent infarction without classical stroke signs. Classically, the progression of MID is stepwise, with long plateaux between events and day-to-day fluctuations in severity. Correlation between infarction and impairment is imprecise, and patients may progress or remain stable despite similar neuroimaging profiles. Therefore, the MID concept misses other important types of VaD, such as the slowly progressive forms associated with diffuse white-matter changes and subcortical infarction. In the absence of clinically eloquent stroke and MID, these definitions of VaD have led to the conclusion that, in the early stages, cognitive impairment can be missed easily. Most patients have some evidence of the dysexecutive syndrome, exhibiting difficulties with higher functions such as goal formulation, initiation, planning and organizing. Abstract thought is also affected.

*Single 'strategic' infarct dementia.* It was originally felt that VaD could not occur without less than 100 cc of infarcted brain tissue [24]. Over the years, however, it was finally recognized that small but strategically located infarcts affecting structures such as thalamus, basal forebrain, and caudate, could also produce a dementia syndrome [11]. The clinical features of strategic infarct VaD vary considerably with the precise location of the lesions, which can be either cortical or subcortical. Severe memory impairment is often apparent and there may be confusion and fluctuating levels of consciousness. Behavioural changes may include apathy, lack of spontaneity, and perseveration [25].

*Subcortical VaD.* In the last several years, there has been considerable focus on the 'SIVD' phenotype [14]. This has been driven in part by the recognition that, in addition to forming a recognizable clinical entity, patients with SIVD may respond differently to drug therapy than those with MID. Diagnostic criteria for SIVD have been proposed [26]. Cerebrovascular lesions in subcortical VaD tend to be located in specific areas in the prefrontal subcortical circuits. Clinically, the most prominent cognitive feature is loss of executive function [27–28]. Memory deficits tend to be less severe than in AD. Recognition and cuing effects remain relatively intact. Mood changes with depression, personality changes and emotional lability are common. Onset is usually slow and often very subtle. Acute stroke-like episodes are usually missing. There are often admixed upper motor neurone signs, gait disorder, urinary urgency, and psychomotor slowing.

*Mixed AD with CVD.* AD and VaD have much in common and frequently coexist as 'mixed' dementia. They share risk factors, clinical features, and pathogenic mechanisms [29]. It is likely that CVD has an important role in determining clinical symptoms in AD [30]. The presence of lacunar cerebral infarcts was reported to raise the risk of dementia by as much as 20-fold in patients who had pathology confirmed AD lesions [31]. Moreover, neuropathological studies suggest that concurrent AD and CVD lesions are a frequent occurrence, particularly in the oldest patients [32].

## CLINICAL COURSE

The cognitive outcome of patients with VaD may be as severe as in AD but their morbidity and mortality are usually worse. In a review, Chui and Gonthier [33] showed shorter survival in VaD than in AD; also, those VaD survivors had a more variable course. Survival variability may produce a length bias whereby patients whose disease progresses too rapidly are usually excluded in prevalence surveys [34].

Although natural history studies have found poor cognitive outcome in patients with VaD, this has not been the case in clinical trials of VaD. In such trials, patients in the placebo groups have had little progression of impairment – the so-called 'stable placebo response' [35]. The most likely explanation is the degree of exclusion of cases with mixed AD + CVD, since these mixed patients usually have a progression midway between AD and VaD cases. Other explanations have been proposed, including: (i) selection bias since patients enrolled in trials are generally more fit than patients studied in natural history settings; (ii) expectation bias or placebo effects; (iii) co-intervention, resulting in better control of vascular risk factors that might also explain both less disease progression and lower mortality rates. Finally, outcome measures used in these trials and adopted from AD trials may be relatively unresponsive to decline.

## PRIMARY AND SECONDARY PREVENTION

*Primary prevention* aims to reduce incident disease by eliminating its cause or main risk factors [36]. In primary prevention, the target is the person with a 'brain at risk' from CVD before stroke or VCI occur. The intent is to treat putative risk factors and to promote protection. Risk factors include those related to CVD, stroke, VCI, VaD, as well as AD. Such vascular risk factors include arterial hypertension, lipid abnormalities, atrial fibrillation, myocardial infarction, coronary heart disease, diabetes, atherosclerosis, smoking, and hyperhomocysteinaemia [37]. Possible protective factors include anti-inflammatory drugs, and lipid-lowering agents.

The effect of primary prevention in populations free of cognitive impairment remains unknown. Unfortunately, most cardiovascular and cerebrovascular studies on primary prevention have missed the opportunity to study cognition as an endpoint. The Syst-Eur Study demonstrated that the treatment of isolated systolic hypertension in the elderly with a calcium-channel agent decreased significantly the incidence of dementia [38]. Other inferences about the positive effects of primary prevention are based on cumulative experience with the treatment of vascular risk factors in the primary prevention of stroke.

*Secondary prevention* aims to prevent disease progression by means of early detection and appropriate treatment. In secondary prevention, the target is CVD in the brain at risk of VCI and VaD. The basis of secondary prevention therefore includes: (i) diagnosis and treatment of acute stroke in order to limit the extent of ischaemic brain changes and to promote recovery; (ii) prevention of recurrence of stroke, according to the type of CVD; (iii) slowing the progression of brain changes associated with VaD e.g. ischaemic white-matter lesions; (iv) management of risk factors of incident dementia, as well as (v) intensifying treatment of risk factors individually or as a group [2].

There have been significant advances in acute stroke therapy, particularly in regard to anti-platelet agents, thrombolysis, and acute stroke care [39] although neuroprotection has been disappointing [40]. Treatments for recurrent stroke prevention are also well-defined [41]. Selection of treatment is guided by the aetiology of CVD, such as large-artery disease (e.g. anti-platelet agents, carotid endarterectomy), cardiac embolic events (e.g. anti-coagulation), small-vessel disease (e.g. aspirin), and haemodynamic mechanisms (e.g. control of hypotension and cardiac arrhythmias). Hypoxic ischaemic events (cardiac arrhythmias, congestive heart failure, myocardial infarction, seizures, pneumonia) are important risk factors for incident dementia in patients with stroke [42]. There is a paucity of knowledge on the effects of secondary prevention of VaD. Most trials on acute stroke and secondary prevention of stroke have again missed the opportunity to study cognition as an endpoint.

Given that HMG Co-A reductase inhibitors (statins) are important in the secondary prevention of stroke [43] there are incentives to undertake trials in patients with mild VaD. Not all statins cross the blood–brain barrier but the relevance of this to reducing the risk of dementia is still unclear [44]. In an animal model, simvastatin inhibited β-secretase metabolism of the amyloid precursor protein [45]. In addition, lovastatin and simvastatin inhibit human butyrylcholinesterase [46]. Clearly, further studies and targeted clinical trials will be needed to understand the role of statins in the prevention and treatment of dementia.

Perindopril, an angiotensin-converting enzyme inhibitor used in a trial of secondary prevention of stroke [47] showed a strikingly beneficial effect (usually coupled with the diuretic indapamide) in patients who had had a previous stroke. Lowering of blood pressure was associated with reduction in the risk of dementia and severe cognitive impairment among patients who experienced recurrent stroke.

## TREATMENT TARGETS AND TRIAL METHODS

Disease expression in VaD is heterogeneous and provides several potential targets for treatment, including: (i) symptomatic improvement of the core symptoms (cognition, function and behaviour); (ii) slowing of progression; and (iii) treatment of secondary manifestations that affect cognition (e.g. depression, anxiety, agitation) [48].

Current VaD trials have closely used the instruments from AD trials as recommended by the United States Food and Drug Administration (FDA) regulatory specifications [49]. The instruments adopted as primary outcome measures for the current generation of clinical trials include the cognitive portion of the Alzheimer's Disease Assessment Scale (ADAS-Cog), the Clinician's Interview-Based Impression of change plus caregiver input (CIBIC+), or the Clinical Global Impression of Change (CGIC) [50]. The European Commission for Medicinal and Pharmaceutical Compounds (CPMC), mostly requires positive impact on ADL and a responder analysis. To the extent that ADAS-Cog and CIBIC+ measures have proved to be sensitive in cholinergic AD trials, and since the cholinergic hypothesis is being endorsed in VaD, it is not unreasonable to use the same measures in both patient populations. On the other hand, the CIBIC+ might be particularly difficult to apply in VaD, a condition with unclear rates of decline and greater variability of disease course. Quinn *et al.* [51] showed that physicians have most difficulty with CIBIC+ ratings in AD in the face of clinical improvement. The cause is not entirely clear, but physicians lack a good model of successful disease treatment beyond reversal of the untreated natural history of progression. This is likely to be an even greater problem in VaD as illustrated in a recently reported clinical trial of memantine in VaD: the ADAS-Cog, the primary cognitive outcome measure, was strongly positive whereas the CIBIC+ rating did not reach significance [52].

Moreover, the current tests are relatively insensitive to frontal/subcortical dysfunction, which is likely to be a key cognitive domain, particularly in VaD [28, 53]. This has given rise to proposals to incorporate such testing in future clinical trials, and to the development of the vascular equivalent of the ADAS-Cog, the VADAS-Cog [50]. One of the shortcomings of these trials was the absence of formal measurement of executive function; however, ADLs have been considered a proxy evaluation of executive function. Pohjasvaara *et al.* [54] confirmed that executive dysfunction was the main determinant of abnormalities in both basic ADLs and instrumental ADLs (IADLs) in patients with post-stroke VaD. Executive function tests, including IADLs, may be sensitive tools for the diagnosis of VaD and could accurately measure the effects of potential therapies.

The role of mood and behavioural symptoms on functional abilities in VaD studies remain to be clarified in order to define their utility as outcome measures in VaD trials [55, 56]. Their rates of emergence and patterns of symptomatic involvement across the continuum of VaD are unclear. Their current use requires assumptions of uncertain validity and in consequence it is only appropriate to use them as secondary outcome measures. The heterogeneity of subtypes of VaD and functional rates of decline are not well characterized making their use as a primary outcome measure premature. Functional decline related directly to the sequelae of stroke has a different significance than functional decline evolving out of cognitive impairment. The current ADL scales do not allow this distinction to be clearly made.

## HISTORY OF PHARMACOTHERAPY IN VaD

Published data on interventions for patients with dementia believed to have a vascular component go back several decades. The American physician Arthur C. Walsh published on an 'anti-coagulant-psychotherapy' intervention for a broadly constructed 'senility' in which he claimed notable success [57]. A vascular aetiology, or at least pathogenesis, also underlay the use of several compounds purported to be useful in the symptomatic treatment of VaD. These included anti-thrombotics, ergot alkaloids, nootropics, TRH-analogue, Ginkgo biloba extracts, plasma viscosity drugs, hyperbaric oxygen, anti-oxidants, serotonin and histamine receptor antagonists, vasoactive agents, xanthine derivates, and calcium antagonists [12, 48, 58]. These studies have mostly had negative results, were based on small numbers, short treatment periods, variations in diagnostic criteria and tools, often included mixed populations, and have had variations in the application of clinical endpoints. Currently, there is not a widely accepted standard symptomatic treatment of VaD.

Many agents have been studied carefully in VaD but none has reached regulatory approval: propentofylline, nimodipine, memantine and the cholinesterase inhibitors donepezil and galantamine. The latter two are discussed in a separate section considering the importance of the cholinergic dysfunction in VaD.

*Propentofylline*, a glial modulator, is no longer under development despite observed beneficial effect on learning and memory in European and Canadian double-blind, placebo-controlled, randomized, parallel group trials [35, 59] in patients with mild-to-moderate VaD according to NINDS-AIREN criteria. Significant improvement and long-term efficacy using the ADAS-Cog and the CIBIC+ were noted up to 48 weeks compared to placebo. In addition, sustained treatment effects for at least 12 weeks after withdrawal were present suggesting an effect on disease progression.

*Nimodipine*, a dihydropyridine calcium-antagonist was primarily tested in subcortical VaD. Nimodipine has effects on autoregulation of cerebral blood flow, causing vasodilatation without a steal effect, and blocks L-type calcium receptors, potentially providing a neuroprotective effect. Nimodipine has specific effects on small vessels. Encouraging results from an open-label trial [60] led to a larger double-blind, placebo-controlled study known as the Scandinavian Multi-Infarct Dementia trial [61, 62]. Patients were divided between MID and subcortical VaD groups, according to computed tomography (CT) findings and were blindly assessed. Nimodipine had a beneficial effect on attention and psychomotor performances in the subcortical group, although no clear advantage was seen in the combined sample. These preliminary results are currently being tested in an international, multicentre, randomized, double-blind trial enrolling patients with subcortical VaD, defined on a clinical–radiological basis [63]. For the moment, the Cochrane Collaboration review concluded that there is no convincing evidence that nimodipine is a useful treatment for the symptoms of VaD [64].

*Memantine* is a moderate-affinity, voltage-dependent, uncompetitive NMDA receptor antagonist with fast receptor kinetics. Initial data from a double-blind, placebo-controlled nursing home trial in severe dementia of mixed aetiology (51% of patients had VaD), showed that memantine (10 mg/day) was well-tolerated, improved function, and reduced care dependency in treated patients with severe dementia, compared to patients on placebo [65]. Based on the hypothesis of glutamate-induced neurotoxicity in cerebral ischaemia, two randomized, placebo-controlled 6-month trials have studied memantine (20 mg/day) in patients with mild to moderate probable VaD by NINDS-AIREN criteria.

In the MMM 300 study 147 patients were randomized to memantine and 141 to placebo [52]. After 28 weeks, the mean ADAS-Cog scores were significantly improved relative to placebo: the memantine group mean score had gained an average of 0.4 points, whereas the placebo group mean score declined by 1.6, i.e. a difference of 2.0 points ($P = 0.0016$). The response rate for CIBIC+, defined as improved or stable, was 60% with memantine compared with 52% with placebo ($P = 0.227$). The Gottfries–Bråne–Steen (GBS) Scale and the Nurses' Observation Scale for Geriatric Patients (NOSGER) total scores at week 28 did not differ significantly between the two groups. However, the GBS Scale intellectual function subscore and the NOSGER disturbing behaviour dimension also showed a difference favouring memantine ($P = 0.04$ and 0.07, respectively).

In the MMM 500 study, 277 patients were randomized to memantine and 271 to placebo [66]. At 28 weeks the active group had gained 0.53 points and the placebo declined by 2.28 points in ADAS-Cog, a significant difference of 1.75 ADAS-Cog points between the groups ($P < 0.05$). The global assessment CGIC, the Mini-mental State Examination (MMSE), GBS or NOSGER did not reveal differences between the groups. Memantine was well-tolerated in the two studies. In a *post hoc* pooled subgroup analysis of these two studies by baseline severity as assessed by MMSE, the more advanced patients obtained a larger cognitive benefit than mildly affected patients. The subgroup with an MMSE score <15 at baseline showed an ADAS-Cog improvement of 3.2 points over placebo [67]. Subgroup analyses by radiological findings at baseline showed that the cognitive treatment effect for memantine was more pronounced in the small-vessel type group without cortical infarctions by CT or MRI. In addition, the placebo decline in this group was clearly more pronounced than in patients with (cortical) large-vessel type VaD.

## CHOLINERGIC DYSFUNCTION IN VASCULAR DEMENTIA

As noted previously in this chapter, cholinergic deficits exist in VaD, independently of any concomitant AD pathology. Cholinergic structures are vulnerable to ischaemic damage. For instance, hippocampal CA1 neurones are particularly susceptible to experimental ischaemia, and hippocampal atrophy is common in patients with VaD in the absence of AD [68, 69]. Selden *et al.* [70] described two highly organized and discrete bundles of cholinergic fibres in human brains that extend from the nucleus basalis to the cerebral cortex and amygdala. Both pathways travel in the white matter, and together carry widespread cholinergic input to the neocortex. Localized strokes may interrupt these cholinergic bundles [71]. Mesulam *et al.* [72] demonstrated cholinergic denervation from pathway lesions, in the absence of AD, in a young patient with CADASIL, a pure genetic form of VaD.

In experimental rodent models, such as the spontaneously hypertensive stroke prone rat, there is a significant reduction in cholinergic markers including acetylcholine (ACh) in the neocortex, hippocampus and cerebrospinal fluid (CSF) [73]. In human disease there is a reported loss of cholinergic neurones in 70% of AD cases and in 40% of VaD patients examined neuropathologically, and also reduced ACh activity in the cortex, hippocampus, striatum, and CSF [74].

Two cholinesterase inhibitors have been studied in VaD in placebo-controlled studies: donepezil and galantamine, and the dual inhibitor rivastigmine has been tested in an open-label study.

*Donepezil*. The safety and efficacy of donepezil has been studied in the largest clinical trial of pure VaD to date [75]. A total of 1219 subjects were recruited for a 24-week, randomized, placebo-controlled, multicentre, multinational study divided into two identical trials [76, 77]. The patients were randomized to one of three groups: placebo, donepezil at a dosage of 5 mg/day or donepezil 10 mg/day. The group receiving 10 mg/day initially received 5 mg/day for four weeks; the dosage was then titrated up to 10 mg/day. Patients with a diagnosis of either possible or probable VaD according to the NINDS-AIREN criteria were eligible for inclusion in the study. All patients had brain imaging prior to the study (CT or MRI) with demonstration of relevant cerebrovascular lesions. Patients with pre-existing AD were excluded, as were AD with CVD patients. Although patients with concomitant AD may not be totally excluded, the NINDS-AIREN criteria are able to classify patients into probable or possible VaD categories.

Probable VaD was present in 73% of the patients in the two studies. Probable VaD was diagnosed by the presence of mild to moderate dementia, clinical and brain imaging evidence of relevant CVD, and a clear temporal relationship between stroke and cognitive decline, with onset of dementia within 3 months of a clinically eloquent stroke or a stepwise course. Possible VaD was diagnosed in cases with indolent onset of the cognitive decline, and accounted for 27% of the cases. Possible VaD also included patients with silent stroke, extensive white-matter disease or an atypical clinical course. There were no differences in trial results between these two subgroups.

The endpoints included cognition measured with the ADAS-Cog and the MMSE, global function as measured with the CIBIC+ and the Sum of Boxes of the Clinical Dementia Rating (CDR-SB) and ADL as measured with Alzheimer's Disease Functional Assessment and Change Scale (ADFACS).

In one trial, the donepezil treatment group showed statistically significant improvement in cognitive functioning measured with the ADAS-Cog; the mean changes from baseline score were: donepezil 5 mg/day, −1.90 ($P = 0.001$); donepezil 10 mg/day, −2.33 ($P < 0.001$). The MMSE also showed statistically significant improvement vs. placebo. The treated group also showed significant improvement in global function on the CIBIC+ in the 5 mg/day group ($P = 0.014$), which did not reach significance in the 10 mg/day group ($P = 0.27$). CDR-SB showed non-significant benefit in the 5 mg/day group, but was significant in the 10 mg/day group ($P = 0.022$). The ADLs showed significant benefits in donepezil-treated patients over placebo using the ADFACS in both treatment groups ($P > 0.05$).

In the second trial, the donepezil treatment group showed statistically significant improvement in cognitive functioning measured with the ADAS-Cog; the mean changes from baseline score were: donepezil 5 mg/day, −1.65 ($P = 0.003$); donepezil 10 mg/day, −2.09 ($P = 0.0002$). The MMSE also showed statistically significant improvement vs. placebo. The treated group also showed significant improvement in global function on the CIBIC+ in the 5 mg/day group ($P = 0.004$), which did not reach significance in the 10 mg/day group ($P = 0.047$). CDR-SB showed non-significant benefit in the 5 mg/day group, but was significant in the 10 mg/day group ($P = 0.03$). The ADLs showed superiority in the donepezil-treated patients over placebo using the ADFACS in both treatment groups, which, however, did not reach significance at the end of the study, compared to placebo.

Of interest, cognitive decline in untreated patients with VaD in these trials was less severe than in placebo-treated patients with AD during 24 weeks of study, using similar instruments. These differences were also notable for their global impact, measured by the CIBIC+ version; and, in contrast with AD, patients with VaD showed improvements in global function. In contrast with AD trials, these VaD studies enrolled more men than women (58% vs. 38%), their mean age was older (74.5 ± 0.2 vs. 72 ± 0.2 years), their HIS score more elevated (6.6 ± 0.2 vs. <4), with higher percentages of subjects with hypertension, cardiovascular disease, diabetes, smoking, hypercholesterolaemia, previous stroke and TIA, suggesting that the two populations are clearly different.

Donepezil was generally well-tolerated, although more adverse effects were reported in the 10-mg group than in the 5-mg or placebo groups. The adverse effects were assessed as mild to moderate and transient, and were typically diarrhoea, nausea, arthralgia, leg cramps, anorexia, and headache. The incidence of bradycardia and syncope was not significantly different from the placebo group. The discontinuation rates for the groups were 15% for placebo, 18% for 5 mg, and 28% for the 10-mg group. There was no significant interaction with the numerous cardiovascular medications and anti-thrombotic agents used by this patient population.

*Galantamine* is a cholinesterase inhibitor that also modulates central nicotinic receptors to increase cholinergic neurotransmission. A randomized, double-blind, controlled clinical trial studied patients diagnosed with probable VaD, or with AD combined with CVD, who received galantamine 24 mg/day ($n = 396$) or placebo ($n = 196$) over 6 months [78]. Eligible patients met the clinical criteria of probable VaD by NINDS-AIREN criteria or of possible AD according to the NINCDS-ADRDA criteria. They also showed significant radiological (CT/MRI) evidence of CVD (i.e. AD + CVD). Evidence of CVD on a recent (within 12 months) scan included multiple large-vessel infarcts or a single, strategically placed infarct (angular gyrus, thalamus, basal forebrain, territory of the posterior or anterior cerebral artery), or at least two basal ganglia and white-matter lacunae, or white-matter changes involving at least 25% of the total white matter. The MMSE score was 10–25 and 12 or more in the ADAS-Cog/11; age ranged from 40 and 90 years.

Primary endpoints were cognition, as measured using the ADAS-Cog/11, and global functioning as measured using the CIBIC+. Secondary endpoints included assessments of ADL, using the Disability Assessment in Dementia (DAD; [79]), and behavioural symptoms, using the Neuropsychiatric Inventory (NPI; [80]).

In analyses of both groups as a whole, galantamine demonstrated efficacy on all outcome measures. Galantamine showed greater efficacy than placebo on ADAS-Cog (2.7 points; $P \leq 0.001$) and CIBIC+ (74% vs. 59% of patients remained stable or improved; $P \leq 0.001$). ADL and behavioural symptoms were also significantly improved compared with placebo (both $P < 0.05$). In an open-label extension the original galantamine group with probable VaD or AD with CVD showed similar sustained benefits in terms of maintenance of or improvement in cognition (ADS-Cog), functional ability (DAD), and behaviour (NPI) after 12 months [81].

Probable VaD was diagnosed in 81 (41%) of the placebo patients and in 171 (43%) of those on galantamine. In the probable VaD group, ADAS-Cog scores improved significantly (mean change from baseline, 2.4 points; $P < 0.0001$) in patients treated with galantamine for 6 months, but not with placebo (mean change from baseline, 0.4; treatment difference vs. galantamine 1.9; $P = 0.06$). More patients treated with galantamine than with placebo maintained or improved global function (CIBIC+, 31% vs. 23%); however, it was not statistically significant. In these patients, the cognitive benefits of galantamine were maintained at least up to 12 months, demonstrating a mean change of –2.1 in the ADAS-Cog score compared to baseline, and the active group was still close to baseline at 24 months.

*Rivastigmine* is an acetylcholinesterase and butyrylcholinesterase inhibitor. The effects of rivastigmine in the treatment of cognitive impairment associated with VaD remain to be established. In a small open-label study of patients with subcortical VaD, rivastigmine improved cognition (clock-drawing test), reduced caregiver stress and improved behaviour [82–84]. AD patients with vascular risk factors showed a relatively larger effect size in cognitive response (ADAS Cog) than those without vascular risk factors.

## SUMMARY

Rigorous control of vascular risk factors is important in primary and secondary prevention of VaD, and might be important in ameliorating disease expression in those with mild VaD.

A number of controlled clinical trials on VaD using donepezil, galantamine and memantine are available. However, at the end of 2005 none has obtained approved indication by the FDA or the CPMC. More effective therapies are needed, perhaps with combinations of memantine + AChEIs, or using other nootropic and neuroprotective agents.

## REFERENCES


1. Erkinjuntti T, Romän G, Gauthier S, Feldman H, Rockwood K. Emerging therapies for vascular dementia and vascular cognitive impairment. *Stroke* 2004; 35:1010–1017.
2. Elkind MSV. Implications of stroke prevention trials. Treatment of global risk. *Neurology* 2005; 65:17–21.
3. Launer LJ, Hofman A. Frequency and impact of neurologic diseases in the elderly of Europe: a collaborative study of population-based cohorts. *Neurology* 2000; 54(suppl 5):S1–S3.
4. Snowdon DA, Greimer LH, Mortimer JA *et al.* Brain infarction and the clinical expression of Alzheimer disease: the Nun study. *JAMA* 1997; 277:813–817.
5. Esiri MM, Nagy Z, Smith MZ, Barnetson L, Smith AD. Cerebrovascular disease and threshold for dementia in the early stages of Alzheimer's disease. *Lancet* 1999; 354:919–920.
6. Vermeer SE, Hollander M, van Dijk EJ *et al.* Silent brain infarcts and white matter lesions increase stroke risk in the general population: the Rotterdam Scan Study. *Stroke* 2003; 34:1126–1129.
7. Rockwood K, Howard K, MacKnight C, Darvesh S. Spectrum of disease in vascular cognitive impairment. *Neuroepidemiology* 1999; 18:248–254.
8. Wentzel C, Rockwood K, MacKnight C. Progression of impairment in patients with vascular cognitive impairment without dementia. *Neurology* 2001; 57:714–716.
9. Rockwood K, Davis H, MacKnight C *et al.* The consortium to investigate vascular impairment of cognition: methods and first findings. *Can J Neurol Sci* 2003; 30:237–243.
10. Román GC. Stroke, cognitive decline and vascular dementia: the silent epidemic of the 21st century. *Neuroepidemiology* 2003; 22:161–164.
11. Erkinjuntti T, Hachinski VC. Rethinking vascular dementia. *Cerebrovasc Dis* 1993; 3:3–23.
12. Erkinjuntti T. Cerebrovascular dementia. Pathophysiology, diagnosis and treatment. *CNS Drugs* 1999; 12:35–48.
13. Hachinski VC, Iliff LD, Zilhka E *et al.* Cerebral blood flow in dementia. *Arch Neurol* 1975; 32:632–637.
14. Román GC, Erkinjuntti T, Wallin A, Pantoni L, Chui HC. Subcortical ischaemic vascular dementia. *Lancet Neurol* 2002; 1:426–436.
15. Bowler JV, Steenhuis R, Hachinski V. Conceptual background of vascular cognitive impairment. *Alzheimer Dis Assoc Disord* 1999; 13:S30–S37.
16. Rockwood K, Wenzel C, Hachinski V. Prevalence and outcomes of vascular cognitive impairment. *Neurology* 2000; 54:447–451.
17. O'Brien JT, Erkinjuntti T, Reisberg B *et al.* Vascular cognitive impairment. *Lancet Neurol* 2003; 2:89–98.
18. Chui HC, Mack W, Jackson JE *et al.* Clinical criteria for the diagnosis of vascular dementia. *Arch Neurol* 2000; 57:191–196.
19. Pohjasvaara T, Mäntylä R, Ylikoski R *et al.* Comparison of different clinical criteria for the vascular cause of vascular dementia (ADDTC, DSM-III, DSM-IV, ICD-10, NINDS-AIREN). *Stroke* 2000; 31:2952–2957.
20. Gold G, Bouras C, Canuto A *et al.* Clinicopathological validation study of four sets of clinical criteria for vascular dementia. *Am J Psychiatry* 2002; 159:82–87.
21. Chui HC, Victoroff JI, Margolin D *et al.* Criteria for the diagnosis of ischemic vascular dementia proposed by the State of California Alzheimer's Disease Diagnostic and Treatment Centers. *Neurology* 1992; 42:473–480.
22. Román GC, Tatemichi TK, Erkinjuntti T *et al.* Vascular dementia: diagnostic criteria for reserach studies. Report of the NINDS-AIREN International Work Group. *Neurology* 1993; 43:250–260.
23. Erkinjuntti T, Rockwood K. Vascular cognitive impairment. *Psychogeriatrics* 2001; 1:27–38.
24. Blessed G, Tomlinson BE, Roth M. The association between quantitative measures of dementia and of senile change in the cerebral grey matter of elderly subjects. *Br J Psychiatry* 1968; 114:797–811.
25. Ballard C, McKeith I, O'Brien J *et al.* Neuropathological substrates of dementia and depression in vascular dementia, with a particular focus on cases with small infarct volumes. *Dement Geriatr Cogn Disord* 2000; 11:59–65.
26. Erkinjuntti T, Inzitari D, Pantoni L *et al.* Research criteria for subcortical vascular dementia in clinical trials. *J Neural Transm* 2000; 59:23–30.

27. Desmond DW, Erkinjuntti T, Sano M *et al.* The cognitive syndrome of vascular dementia: implications for clinical trials. *Alzheimer Dis Assoc Disord* 1999; 13:S21–S29.
28. Román GC, Royall DR. Executive control function: a rational basis for the diagnosis of vascular dementia. *Alzheimer Dis Assoc Disord* 1999; 13:69–80.
29. Kalaria RN, Ballard C. Overlap between pathology of Alzheimer disease and vascular dementia. *Alzheimer Dis Assoc Disord* 1999; 13:S115–S123.
30. Zekry D, Hauw JJ, Gold G. Mixed dementia: epidemiology, diagnosis, and treatment. *J Am Geriatr Soc* 2002; 50:1431–1438.
31. Zekry D, Duyckaerts C, Belmin J *et al.* Alzheimer's disease and brain infarcts in the elderly: agreement with neuropathology. *J Neurol* 2002; 249:1529–1534.
32. Royall DR, Palmer R, Mulroy A *et al.* Pathological determinants of clinical dementia in Alzheimer's disease. *Exp Aging Res* 2002; 28:143–162.
33. Chui HC, Gonthier R. Natural history of vascular dementia. *Alzheimer Dis Assoc Disord* 1999; 13:S124–S130.
34. Wolfson C, Wolfson DB, Asgharian M *et al.* A reevaluation of the duration of survival after the onset of dementia. *N Engl J Med* 2001; 344:1111–1116.
35. Kittner B, Rossner M, Rother M. Clinical trials in dementia with propentofylline. *Ann NY Acad Sci* 1997; 826:307–316.
36. Skoog I. Risk factors for vascular dementia: a review. *Dementia* 1994; 5:137–144.
37. Smith AD. Homocysteine, vitamins and cognitive deficit in the elderly. *Am J Clin Nutr* 2002; 75:785–786.
38. Forette F, Seux ML, Staessen JA *et al.* The prevention of dementia with antihypertensive treatment. New evidence from the systolic hypertension in Europe (Sys-Eur) study. *Arch Intern Med* 2002; 162:2046–2052.
39. Klijn CJ, Hankey GJ, American Stroke Association, European Stroke Initiative. Management of acute ischemic stroke: new guidelines from the American Stroke Association and the European Stroke Initiative. *Lancet Neurol* 2003; 2:698–701.
40. Gorelick PB. Neuroprotection in acute ischaemic stroke: a tale of for whom the bell tolls? *J Am Geriatr Soc* 2000; 355:1925–1926.
41. Gorelick PB. Stroke prevention therapy beyond antithrombotics: unifying mechanisms in ischaemic stroke pathogenesis and implications for therapy. *Stroke* 2002; 33:862–875.
42. Moroney JT, Bagiella E, Desmond DR *et al.* Cerebral hypoxia and ischemia in the pathogenesis of dementia after stroke. *Ann NY Acad Sci* 1997; 826:433–436.
43. Callahan A. Cerebrovascular disease and statins: a potential addition to the therapeutic armamentarium for stroke prevention. *Am J Cardiol* 2001; 88:33J–37J.
44. Rockwood K, Darvesh S. The risk of dementia in relation to statins and other lipid lowering agents. *Neurol Res* 2003; 25:601–604.
45. Fassbender K, Simons M, Bergmann C *et al.* Simvastatin strongly reduces levels of Alzheimer's disease beta-amyloid peptides Aβ42 and Aβ40 in vitro and in vivo. *Proc Natl Acad Sci USA* 2001; 98:5856–5861.
46. Darvesh S, Martin E, Walsh R, Rockwood K. Differential effects of lipid-lowering agents on human cholinesterases. *Clin Biochem* 2004; 37:42–49.
47. The PROGRESS Collaborative Group. Effects of blood pressure lowering with perindopril and indapime therapy on dementia and cognitive decline in patients with cerebrovascular disease. *Arch Intern Med* 2003; 163:1069–1075.
48. Rockwood K, Gauthier S, Erkinjuntti T. Prevention and treatment of vascular dementia. In: Erkinjuntti T, Gauthier S (eds). *Vascular Cognitive Impairment.* Martin Dunitz Ltd., London, 2002, pp 587–595.
49. Sawada T, Whitehouse PJ. Regulatory guidelines for antidementia drugs. In: Erkinjuntti T, Gauthier S (eds). *Vascular Cognitive Impairment.* Martin Dunitz Ltd., London, 2002, pp 619–627.
50. Ferris S, Gauthier S. Cognitive outcome measures in vascular dementia. In: Erkinjuntti T, Gauthier S (eds). *Vascular Cognitive Impairment.* Martin Dunitz Ltd., London, 2002, pp 395–400.
51. Quinn J, Moore M, Benson DF *et al.* A videotaped CIBIC. For dementia patients: validity and reliability in a simulated clinical trial. *Neurology* 2003; 58:433–437.
52. Orgogozo J-M, Rigaud A-S, Stöffler A, Möbius H-J, Forette F. Efficacy and safety of Memantine in patients with mild to moderate vascular dementia. A randomized, placebo-controlled trial (MMM 300). *Stroke* 2002; 33:1834–1839.
53. Royall DR. Executive cognitive impairment: a novel perspective on dementia. *Neuroepidemiology* 2000; 19:293–299.

54. Pohjasvaara T, Leskelä M, Vataja R *et al.* Post-stroke depression, executive dysfunction and functional outcome. *Eur J Neurol* 2002; 9:269–275.
55. Chui E, Yastrubetskaya O, Williams M. Pharmacotherapy of mood and behavior symptoms. In: Erkinjuntti T, Gauthier S (eds). *Vascular Cognitive Impairment.* Martin Dunitz Ltd., London, 2002, pp 597–605.
56. Gauthier S, Gélinas I. Evaluation of daily activities in vascular cognitive impairment. In: Erkinjuntti T, Gauthier S (eds). *Vascular Cognitive Impairment.* Martin Dunitz Ltd., London, 2002, pp 411–416.
57. Walsh AC, Walsh BH, Melaney C. Senile-presenile dementia: follow-up data on an effective psychotherapy-anticoagulant regimen. *J Am Geriatr Soc* 1978; 26:467–470.
58. Román GC. Perspectives in the treatment of vascular dementia. *Drugs Today* 2000; 36:641–653.
59. Mielke R, Möller H-J, Erkinjuntti T, Rosenkranz B, Rother M, Kittner B. Propentofylline in the treatment of vascular dementia and Alzheimer-type dementia: overview of phase I and phase II clinical trials. *Alzheimer Dis Assoc Disord* 1998; 12:29–35.
60. Pantoni L, Carosi M, Amigoni S, Mascalchi M, Inzitari D. A preliminary open trial with nomodipine in patients with cognitive impairment and leukoaraiosis. *Clin Neuropharmacol* 1996; 19:497–506.
61. Pantoni L, Rossi R, Inzitari D *et al.* Efficacy and safety of nimodipine in subcortical vascular dementia: a subgroup analysis of the Scandinavian multi-infarct dementia trial. *J Neurol Sci* 2000; 175:124–134.
62. Pantoni L, Bianchi C, Beneke M *et al.* The Scandinavian multi-infarct dementia trial: a double-blind, placebo-controlled trial on nimodipine in multi-infarct dementia. *J Neurol Sci* 2000; 175:116–123.
63. Pantoni L, del Ser T, Soglian A *et al.* Efficacy and safety of nimodipine in subcortical vascular dementia: a randomized placebo-controlled trial. *Stroke* 2205; 36:619–624.
64. Lopez-Arieta BJ. Nimodipine for primary degenerative, mixed and vascular dementia. *Cochrane Database Syst Rev* 2001; 1:CD000147.
65. Winblad B, Porotis N. Memantine in severe dementia: results of the 9M-Best Study. *Int J Geriatr Psychiatry* 1999; 14:135–146.
66. Wilcock G, Möbius HJ, Stöffler A, on behalf of the MMM 500 group. A double-blind, placebo-controlled multicentre study of memantine in mild to moderate vascular dementia (MMM 500). *Int Clin Psychopharmacol* 2002; 17:297–305.
67. Möbius HJ, Stöffler A. New approaches to clinical trials in vascular dementia: memantine in small vessel disease. *Cerebrovasc Dis* 2002; 13:61–66.
68. Gottfries CG, Blennow K, Karlsson I, Wallin A. The neurochemistry of vascular dementia. *Dementia* 1994; 5:163–167.
69. Vinters HV, Ellis WG, Zarow C *et al.* Neuropathologic substrates of ischemic vascular dementia. *J Neuropathol Exp Neurol* 2000; 60:658–659.
70. Selden NR, Gitelman DR, Salamon-Murayama N, Parrish TB, Mesulam MM. Trajectories of cholinergic pathways within the cerebral hemispheres of the human brain. *Brain* 1998; 121:2249–2257.
71. Swartz RH, Sahlas DJ, Black SE *et al.* Strategic involvement of cholinergic pathways and executive dysfunction: does location of white matter signal hyperdensities matter? *J Stroke Cerebrovasc Dis* 2003; 12:29–36.
72. Mesulam M, Siddique T, Cohen B. Cholinergic denervation in a pure multi-infarct state: observations on CADASIL. *Neurology* 2003; 60:1183–1185.
73. Togashi H, Matsumoto K, Yoshida M. Neurochemical profiles in cerebrospinal fluid of stroke-prone spontaneously hypertensive rat. *Neurosci Lett* 1994; 166:117–120.
74. Court JA, Perry EK, Kalaria RN. Neurotransmitter control of the cerebral vasculature and abnormalities in vascular dementia. In: Erkinjuntti T, Gauthier S (eds). *Vascular Cognitive Impairment.* Martin Dunitz Ltd., London, 2002, pp 167–185.
75. Roman GC, Wilkinson DG, Doody RS *et al.* Donepezil in vascular dementia: combined analysis of two large-scale clinical trials. *Dement Geriatr Cogn Disord* 2005; 20:338–344.
76. Black S, Román GC, Geldmacher DS *et al.* Efficacy and tolerability of Donepezil in vascular dementia. Positive results of a 24-week, multicenter, international, randomized, placebo-controlled clinical trial. *Stroke* 2003; 34:2323–2332.
77. Wilkinson D, Doody R, Helme R *et al.* Donepezil in vascular dementia. A randomized, placebo-controlled study. *Neurology* 2003; 61:479–486.
78. Erkinjuntti T, Kurz A, Gauthier S, Bullock R, Lilienfeld S, Damaraju CV. Efficacy of galantamine in probable vascular dementia and Alzheimer's disease combined with cerebrovascular disease: a randomized trial. *Lancet* 2002; 359:1283–1290.
79. Gélinas I, Gauthier L, McIntyre M, Gauthier S. Development of a functional measure for persons with Alzheimer's disease: the Disability Assessment for Dementia. *Am J Occup Ther* 1999; 53:471–481.

80. Cummings JL, Mega M, Gray K *et al.* The Neuropsychiatric Inventory: comprehensive assessment of psychopathology in dementia. *Neurology* 1994; 44:2308–2314.
81. Erkinjuntti T, Kurz A, Small GW *et al.* An open-label extension trial of galantamine in patients with probable vascular dementia and mixed dementia. *Clin Ther* 2003; 25:1765–1782.
82. Moretti R, Torre P, Antonello RM, Cazzato G. Rivastigmine in subcortical vascular dementia: a comparison trial on efficacy and tolerability for 12 months follow-up. *Eur J Neurol* 2001; 8:361–362.
83. Moretti R, Torre P, Antonello RM, Cazzato G, Bava A. Rivastigmine in subcortical vascular dementia: an open 22-month study. *J Neurol Sci* 2002; 203:141–146.
84. Erkinjuntti T, Skoog I, Lane R, Andrews C. Rivastigmine in patients with Alzheimer's disease and concurrent hypertension. *Int J Clin Pract* 2002; 56:791–796.

# 21

# Fronto-temporal dementia

*M. Ikeda*

## INTRODUCTION

As dementia progresses, recognition skills become impaired in combination with delusions, agitation, feelings of worry, and depression, leading to a wide range of neuropsychiatric manifestations and disturbed behaviour (now frequently called behavioural and psychological symptoms of dementia [BPSD]) [1]. In recent years, there has been considerable progress in expanding the differential diagnosis of Alzheimer's disease (AD) with clinical characterization of fronto-temporal dementia (FTD), dementia with Lewy bodies (DLB) and so on. These developments emphasize the need for disease-specific management. Each dementia has its own characteristic behavioural profile. For example, patients with AD have higher rates of delusions than FTD patients. In DLB, visual hallucinations are prominent, whereas in FTD inappropriate eating behaviour and aggression are more pronounced. These BPSD are highly prevalent in patients with dementia and are a major source of difficulty and distress for caregivers. BPSD are one of the main reasons for hospital or nursing home placement of patients, and thus contribute greatly to the cost of caring for dementia patients. While a number of intervention studies have aimed to reduce the burden of caring for patients with dementia through family support and counselling of caregivers, few studies have focused on using pharmacotherapy or non-pharmacologic management to alleviate specific BPSD and reduce the care burden [2]. Although the aetiology of these neurodegenerative diseases is still unknown, treatment should be directed toward disease-specific symptomatic improvement.

FTD is now included more in the comprehensive construct, fronto-temporal lobar degeneration (FTLD) [3], that comprises frontal type dementia, with other subtypes such as semantic dementia (SD) and progressive non-fluent aphasia (PA). In spite of the possibility that FTLD has been under-recognized clinically, it is thought to account for up to 20% of presenile dementia. The Cambridge group recently examined the prevalence of early-onset dementia in a community-based study [4]. Of 108 cases identified, FTLD accounted for 17 patients (15.7%) and AD for 25%. The FTLD group included 13 FTD and two each with SD and PA. Almost one-third of cases with FTLD (29%) had a positive family history. In our consecutive series of 330 outpatients with dementia (hospital setting without age limitation), 42 (12.7%) had FTLD and 215 (65.1%) had AD; the FTLD group comprised 22 FTD, 15 SD and 5 PA [5]. In summary, these epidemiological studies, both in community-based and hospital-based samples, demonstrate that FTD is a more common cause of early-onset dementia than was previously recognized.

**Manabu Ikeda**, MD, PhD, Associate Professor, Department of Neuropsychiatry, Neuroscience, Ehime University Graduate School of Medicine, Ehime, Japan

**Table 21.1** Behavioural features of FTD

| Behavioural features |
|---|
| Loss of social awareness and insight |
| Personal neglect |
| Disinhibition, impulsivity, restlessness ('going my way' behaviour) |
| Distractibility and impersistence |
| Inertia, aspontaneity, loss of volition |
| Mental rigidity and inflexibility |
| Sterotypies, compulsivity |
| Stimulus-bound behaviour |
| Hyperorality and dietary changes |

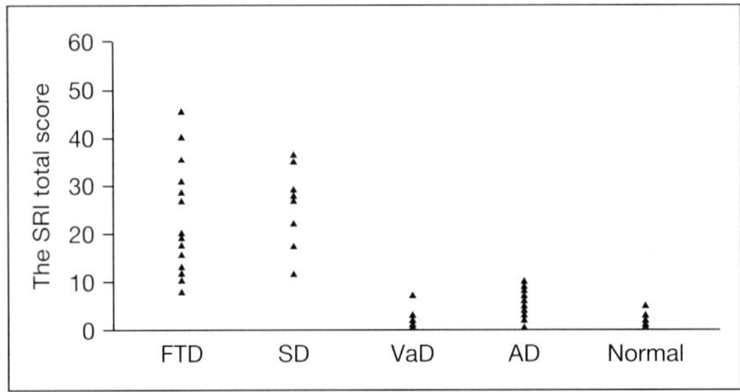


**Figure 21.1** The SRI total score of FTD, SD, VaD, AD and normal control subjects (revised from reference [8]). The SRI provides scores for 5 domains' subscales (eating and cooking behaviours, roaming, speaking, movements, and daily rhythm). Each is scored for frequency and severity, and the total subscale score can be calculated by multiplying these two factors. The SRI total score is the sum of the 5 total subscores. Total score on the SRI of FTD and SD patient groups were higher than that of VaD patients, AD patients, and normal controls with very little overlap ($P < 0.0001$) [8].

Distinctive unusual behaviours of FTD, such as disinhibition, loss of social awareness, overeating, perseverative and stereotyped behaviour, and impulsivity, are serious obstacles to managing and caring for patients with FTD [6]. The main behavioural features of FTD are listed in Table 21.1. Patients with subtypes of FTLD, especially FTD and SD, exhibit very similar profiles of abnormal behaviour. Among these peculiar behavioural disturbances, stereotypic and eating behaviours are significantly more frequent in FTLD than in other types of dementia [7–9]. These behaviours are so characteristic of FTLD that they are important symptoms for discriminating between FTLD and AD (Figures 21.1 and 21.2).

There is no known treatment to delay the progression of FTD although non-pharmacological and pharmacological interventions may potentially help considerably with behavioural management [10, 11]. Thus far there have been no systematic efforts to manage or treat patients with FTD [12].

## PRINCIPLES OF TREATMENT AND MANAGEMENT FOR CHALLENGING BEHAVIOURS

### *INSTRUCTION FOR CAREGIVERS*

Education programs should be offered to families and caregivers to improve caregiver satisfaction and reduce the caregiver's burden. Lack of knowledge can contribute to caregiver

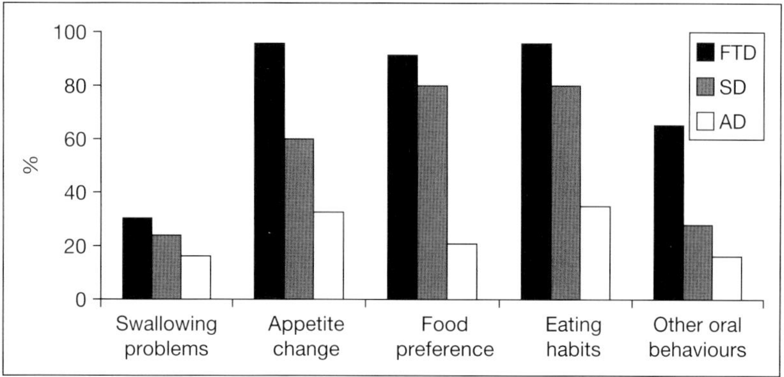


**Figure 21.2** Frequency of each symptom domain in FTD, SD, and AD groups (revised from [9]). The frequencies of all domains except swallowing problems were higher in FTD than in AD ($P < 0.001$). Patients with SD had more frequent changes in food preference and eating habits than patients with AD ($P < 0.01$) [9].

stress, particularly in a condition such as FTD where the diagnosis may be delayed [13]. In contrast to AD and vascular dementia (VaD), educational material for caregivers of FTD is usually scarce. Education should provide information regarding the diagnosis, prognosis, and the meaning and cause of specific behaviours. Once caregivers have a greater understanding of dementia, many of their anxieties and concerns are diminished [14]. For example, wandering and pacing are significant problems in AD while wandering (called roaming) in FTD is not a distressing behaviour for caregivers at least in early stages of the disease. Patients with FTD embark on long walks, usually involving the same route without getting lost owing to their relatively preserved memory and visuospatial abilities such as orientation in familiar surroundings. Sometimes caregivers will change the patient's environment based on their knowledge of specific behaviours. Some caregivers may find the use of day-care with bathing services is helpful from an early stage. This is based on information that undressing and bathing frequently become serious obstacles at home in advanced FTD and putting them into a strict daily timetable from an early stage can help avoid this issue. Education is necessary prior to commencement of any intervention and in addition to advice from the treating physician, input from a clinical psychologist, occupational therapist or specialist nurse can be a very useful resource for caregivers.

### *FOCUSING ON TARGET BEHAVIOURS AND SPECIFIC NEUROCHEMICAL ABNORMALITIES*

It is important to perform a detailed evaluation of the quality and severity of BPSD in FTD at the earliest possible time, so that the burden of caring can be reduced through tailored intervention. There is a wide range of BPSD in FTD such as disinhibition, impulsivity, aspontaneity, stereotypes, utilization behaviours, and abnormal eating behaviour, and it is essential to determine the specific target symptoms for intervention in each patient. Patients may be overactive, restless, distractible, and disinhibited at the first medical referral. Those same patients may show little spontaneous activity when left to their own devices. Moreover, overactive patients may show increasing inertia [15].

Target symptoms might also vary in different disease stages. Target symptoms might be challenging behaviours which are often antisocial, a risk for patients and/or cause profound distress for caregivers. These can result in the institutionalization of the sufferer. When overeating and hyperorality are present, dietary restrictions may be necessary to prevent excessive weight gain or eating non-edible foodstuffs [9]. Pharmacologic agents are indicated for challenging behaviours where non-pharmachological interventions – such as environmental changes – are insufficient to alleviate the behavioural disturbance.

BPSD are thought to arise from complex changes in central neurotransmitter levels, with particular categories of symptoms linked to certain neurotransmitter abnormalities [16], though more research is needed as these relationships are largely based on speculation rather than empirical evidence in FTD at present. Aggression may be associated with raised levels of noradrenaline and reduced levels of serotonin, depression with low serotonin, psychosis with low acetylcholine and elevated dopamine, stereotypy and compulsivity with low serotonin, and apathy with low acetylcholine. Many features of FTD such as stereotypic behaviour, overeating, and impulsivity are thought to be compatible with serotonergic dysfunction. Thus, the choice of treatment should be based on the neurochemical target for each BPSD. Understanding the behavioural symptomatology of different dementias provides a rational strategy for the development of novel pharmacological treatments which target specific neurochemical abnormalities.

### *USING WELL-VALIDATED AND CAREFULLY SELECTED OUTCOME MEASURES*

Objective assessment of any patient intervention – whether pharmacological, psychological, or environmental – is essential. Given the peculiar behavioural disturbances in patients with FTD, it is necessary to select an appropriate range of outcome measures that are sensitive to the effects of interventions on behaviour. Widely used behavioural assessment instruments, such as the Neuropsychiatric Inventory (NPI) [17] and BEHAVE-AD [18], may not be sufficiently sensitive to reliably detect improvement in challenging behaviours following an intervention, although they can distinguish FTD from AD to some degree [19, 20]. The NPI is a clinical rating instrument designed specifically to provide a comprehensive evaluation of neuropsychiatric symptomatology in demented patients and has been demonstrated to be sensitive to drug treatment effects in AD [21, 22]. However, this instrument does not adequately cover the range of compulsive, repetitive and bizarre stereotypic behaviours seen in FTD [23].

The Stereotypy Rating Inventory (SRI) (that can be used in conjunction with the NPI) is a validated instrument that efficiently and comprehensively assesses the stereotypic behavioural aspects of FTD [8]. The SRI assesses five distinctive stereotypic behavioural disturbances (eating and cooking behaviours, roaming, speaking, movements, daily rhythms) often seen in patients with FTD (Table 21.2).

The swallowing/appetite/eating habits questionnaire assesses the following five domains: swallowing problems, appetite change, food preference (including sweet food preference and food fads), eating habits (including stereotypic eating behaviours and decline in table manners), and other oral behaviours (including food cramming and indiscriminate eating) [9] (Table 21.3).

In summary, one is able to make a more comprehensive evaluation of the extent of psychopathological changes with the passage of time in patients with FTD by combining the NPI and these specific scales for FTD.

## NON-PHARMACOLOGIC MANAGEMENT

Behaviour modification and environmental manipulation should be considered in the care of FTD before any pharmacologic treatment. Care of patients with FTD, without memory, apraxic or visuospatial disturbances, is potentially easier than care of AD patients, if stimulus-bound behaviours and stereotypies can be appropriately utilized in a positive sense [6].

### *EXPLOITING PRESERVED MEMORY FUNCTION*

Using relatively preserved episodic and procedural memory is an important strategy in caring for patients with FTD. Fixing a specific nurse or occupational therapist for each FTD

**Table 21.2** The Stereotypy Rating Inventory [8]

*Daily rhythm*

Does the patient live with a strictly fixed daily rhythm that looks like a timetable? Or does he/she do the same thing at a certain time every day? Does he/she prefer to live with the fixed daily rhythm and dislike being disturbed from his/her daily rhythm?

No (If no, proceed to next screening question)
Yes (If yes, proceed to subquestions)

1. Is the patient concerned with going to bed and getting up at a certain time?
2. Is the patient concerned with watching TV at a certain time?
3. Is the patient concerned with taking a walk at a certain time?
4. Is the patient concerned with taking his/her meal at a certain time?
5. Is the patient concerned with doing other things at a certain time?

If the screening question is confirmed, determine the frequency and severity of the daily rhythm.

Frequency:
1. Often – about once per week
2. Moderately frequent – several times per week but less than every day
3. Frequent – every day (less than 5 times per day)
4. Extremely frequent – every day (more than 5 times per day or almost all the time)

Severity:
1. Mild – stereotypic behaviours are notable but produce little interference with daily routines
2. Moderate – stereotypic behaviours are very evident; can be overcome by the caregiver
3. Marked – stereotypic behaviours are very evident, they usually fail to respond to any intervention by the caregiver, and they are a major source of distress

**Table 21.3** Swallowing/appetite/eating habits questionnaire [9]

*Food preference*

| | Frequency | Severity |
|---|---|---|
| 1. Does he/she prefer sweet foods more than before? | 0 1 2 3 4 | 1 2 3 |
| 2. Does he/she drink more soft drinks? | 0 1 2 3 4 | 1 2 3 |
| 3. Does he/she drink more tea/coffee? | 0 1 2 3 4 | 1 2 3 |
| 4. Has his/her 'taste' in food changed in another way (e.g. eats more meat, curries, fried foods) | 0 1 2 3 4 | 1 2 3 |
| Any comments ______ | | |
| 5. Does he/she add more seasoning to their food (e.g. adds more salt)? | 0 1 2 3 4 | 1 2 3 |
| 6. Has he/she developed other food fads? | 0 1 2 3 4 | 1 2 3 |
| Any comments ______ | | |
| 7. Does he/she hoard sweets or other food? | 0 1 2 3 4 | 1 2 3 |
| 8. Does he/she drink more alcohol? | 0 1 2 3 4 | 1 2 3 |

If you have answered yes to any of these, when did the symptoms begin? ______

Frequency:
0. Never
1. Occasionally – less than once per week
2. Often – about once per week
3. Frequently – several times per week but less than every day
4. Very frequently – once or more per day or continuously

Severity:
1. Mild – changes in food preference or alcohol intake are present but easily controlled
2. Moderate – changes in food preference or alcohol intake are present, difficult to control and cause some problems in the family
3. Marked – obvious changes in food preference or alcohol intake causing considerable conflict, embarrassment, or other difficulties (e.g. drunkenness)

patient in a day-care unit or nursing home is effective to adjust them to programme routines. Preserved episodic memory means that patients with FTD can easily identify their key-worker although they may seem indifferent to other staff members. This one-to-one approach is especially useful in the beginning of institutional care.

It can often be useful to program the daily activity for FTD patients in residential or day-care based on each patient's premorbid hobbies or career. Knitting a muffler for a former housewife, even measuring blood pressures of staff members for a former physician, can be very effective to reduce their irritability and maladapted stereotypical behaviours [10, 24].

***[Case] A 65-year-old right-handed retired office worker [10]***

At 63 years old, he was referred for evaluation of inappropriate behaviour that had started 4 years earlier. He ate large amounts of sweet food, ate by stealth, and stole money from his family. Disinhibition and indifference were most conspicuous, and he was euphoric. In contrast to these behavioural changes there was scarce historical evidence of a primary impairment of language, perception, visuospatial skills or memory. Head computed tomography (CT) revealed striking circumscribed bilateral fronto-temporal atrophy. In the ward, he frequently urinated or defaecated in nearby beds of other patients. As a result, he was assaulted frequently. Based on information from his wife about his premorbid hobbies, he was offered a microphone for 'karaoke' in the ward recreation room. Being a music academy graduate, he sang several popular songs very well. After this intervention, he began to participate in recreational activities and always requested to sing. He became a popular person in the ward and troubles with other patients strikingly decreased.

## POSITIVE USE OF STIMULUS-BOUND BEHAVIOUR AND STEREOTYPIC BEHAVIOUR

The stimulus-bound behaviour appears in various forms such as tracing figures, echo symptoms (echolalia, echopraxia, or echoreading), imitation behaviour, utilization behaviour and the environmental dependency syndrome. This behaviour is thought to result from an imbalance between frontal and parietal lobe activity. Specifically, frontal lobe damage results in a loss of the normal negative feedback on parietal lobe activity, rendering the patient unable to inhibit motor responses to any stimuli from the external environment [6, 25]. In patients who exhibit stimulus-bound behaviour, this phenomenon can be channelled to promote less disruptive daily activities. For instance, by conspicuously laying out items at the entrance to the rehabilitation room (knitting needles and wool, a jigsaw puzzle etc.), such stimuli can elicit the motor actions appropriate to those objects with an attendant reduction of less desirable behaviours.

Stereotypic behaviours range from simple to complex repeated actions. Simple stereotypies are defined as iterative actions such as palilalia, paligraphia and palikinesia (e.g. repetitive knee-rubbing) – also referred to as clonic perseveration. More complex stereotypic behaviours form part of the daily repertoire, such as roaming (strolling through precisely the same route each day) and clock-watching or adherence to a strict daily timetable [15]. These behaviours are thought to be due to an imbalance between the activity of the frontal cortex and the basal ganglia [6]. Patients become increasingly inflexible and often adopt a fixed daily routine. These fixed stereotypic behaviours may become incompatible with the patient's home environment, in which case short-term hospitalization and/or SSRIs may be necessary.

***[Case] A 71-year-old right-handed housewife [26]***

At the age of 68 years, this lady began to show alterations in her personality and behaviour. She became increasingly restless and displayed flattening of affect. Her everyday routines were repeated on a regular time schedule. At 69 years old, she was referred for evaluation because of her disinhibition, distractibility, and profound palilalia. Magnetic resonance imaging (MRI) revealed marked right fronto-temporal atrophy with left orbitofrontal atrophy. She ate large amounts of food and her weight had become a serious problem. At 71 years old, she was referred for hospital admission. In the dementia ward, she wandered into other patients' rooms in fixed order, stole meals from other patients, and ate non-edible things on the floor. However, it was known that knitting had been a favourite former hobby. The occupational therapist, therefore, left a ball of yarn and knitting needles ready beforehand on the table in the dayroom. Challenging behaviours disappeared during her periods of persistent knitting. It is considered that her tendency to respond easily to external stimuli (a ball of yarn and knitting needles) and her compulsive or repetitive tendency were successfully utilized.

### *SHORT-TERM HOSPITALIZATION*

The benefits of short-term hospitalization into a special care unit are: (i) close observation and analysis of patients' behaviour in order to develop strategies for behavioural therapy; (ii) provision of adequate instruction to caregivers on coping strategies for challenging behaviours that will reduce their burden; (iii) breaking antisocial daily routines and reconstructing more adaptive stereotypical behaviours; (iv) prompting by nurses or occupational therapists for improvement of aspontaneity and indifference; (v) to familiarize patients with the hospital environment and group activities thus enabling them to maintain regular visits to the hospital and utilize day-care resources [27].

#### *[Case] A 67-year-old right-handed housewife*

At 63 years of age, she began to show profound alterations in her personality and behaviour. She was restless and would rapidly abandon activities that she had just commenced. She became incontinent of urine for which she showed no concern. Two years after onset of symptoms she began to embark on long walks, involving the same route. She strictly adhered to a practice of extinguishing her cigarettes on the floor of her own home – on one occasion causing a fire to break out. At the age of 67, while roaming her habitual route, she was caught stealing tomatoes from a nearby farm, causing the farmer to lodge a complaint. When her husband tried to interrupt her roaming, irritability or aggression was provoked which in turn exacerbated his distress. Thus an impasse had been reached in which she was unable to continue in her home environment and consequently, she was referred for admission to our dementia ward. Head CT revealed striking circumscribed atrophy of fronto-temporal lobes and amygdala. In the ward, she was unable to adhere to her destructive habits of smoking and stealing tomatoes. Her manner was disinhibited, restless, distractible, and puerile, however, 2 weeks after her admission an occupational therapist introduced her to the day-care unit. While it took her more than 2 weeks to adapt to the day-care program, she was ultimately able to adapt to the strict daily timetable. Following discharge, she adhered to participation in the day-care program 7 days per week. Her husband was relieved of both full-time caregiving responsibilities and of her antisocial stereotypical behaviours.

#### *[Case] A 68-year-old, right-handed housewife [28]*

At the age of 53 years, this lady lost interest in her surroundings. Her behaviour became stereotyped, in that she cooked the same meal day after day without variation. Her everyday routines were repeated on a regular time schedule. At 57 years old, she was referred for evaluation because of her lack of initiation, difficulty in planning, and compulsive behaviour. MRI images revealed striking circumscribed atrophy of bilateral frontal lobes. We introduced education programmes about preserved and deteriorating behaviours in FTD to her husband and occupational therapies such as stringing beads for a necklace to her once a week. With her husband's help and initiative, her functioning in the household was restored to almost the same level as it had been premorbidly. With disease progression, her loss of volition dominated the clinical picture. By the age of 59 years, she was spending 2 hours in the preparation of each meal in spite of her husband's aid. A further short-term hospitalization was arranged during which her daily activities were improved by nurses and occupational therapists through one-to-one encouragement of the initiation of actions. This intervention led to her taking only 30 minutes to prepare each meal with her husband's encouragement. She remains at home and is fundamentally self-caring.

## PHARMACOTHERAPY OF FTD

While several drugs, such as the cholinesterase inhibitors, have been shown to be effective for treatment of AD [29], few drugs have been evaluated for the treatment for FTD. Behavioural symptoms found in FTD have been associated with serotonin abnormalities [30, 31]. Data from PET imaging studies have also indicated abnormalities in serotonin metabolism [32]. Following the finding that serotonin receptor binding is decreased in the brain of FTD patients [33], it was suggested that selective serotonin reuptake inhibitors (SSRIs) might improve the behavioural symptoms of FTD patients [11]. In an open study, the use of sertraline, fluoxetine, or paroxetine improved behavioural symptoms in FTD although the outcomes of the treatments were not objectively measured. Given the abundant literature demonstrating the efficacy of SSRIs in such diverse conditions as obsessive-compulsive disorder and related disorders [34, 35], depression [36], and eating disorders [37, 38], it is not surprising that treatment with SSRIs has been proposed as a candidate therapy for a wide range of psychiatric and behavioural symptoms in FTD patients, without causing any cognitive change. Unfortunately, after this early work, there have been only four systematic studies of SSRIs and related compounds. All these studies involve the symptomatic treatment of FTD.

At this moment, there is a general lack of evidence-based therapy and even when a randomized, double-blind, placebo-controlled trial was done, the numbers were very small, making it hard to draw firm conclusions. It is difficult to do well-powered clinical trials for subjects with FTD. As indicated by the inclusiveness of diagnoses into the syndrome of FTD and/or FTLD, most clinical trials will have heterogeneous study samples. The wide range of neuropathological findings within FTD raises the possibility that including all subjects with FTD in one clinical drug trial could mask a subpopulation of FTD patients who respond to the study drug. Given these problems, it would be preferable for future drug trials in FTD to be designed on multicentre protocols [39].

### *SELECTIVE SEROTONIN REUPTAKE INHIBITORS*

#### *Fluvoxamine maleate*

Fluvoxamine is a monocyclic, specific serotonin reuptake inhibitor. There is one published study of fluvoxamine in the treatment of FTD and SD [40] (Table 21.4). Sixteen FTLD patients were treated with a fluvoxamine in an open-label, 12-week trial. Treatment responses for stereotyped behaviour and other neurobehavioural symptoms were evaluated by the SRI and the NPI. The behavioural symptoms, especially stereotyped behaviours of FTLD, significantly improved after treatment. The Mini-mental State Examination (MMSE) was not modified.

#### *Trazodone*

Trazodone is an atypical serotonergic agent that has moderate serotonin reuptake inhibition and a serotonergic antagonist effect with an active metabolite meta-chlorophenyl-piperazine (m-CPP). There is one randomized, double-blind, placebo-controlled, crossover trial in FTD [41] (Table 21.5). Thirty-one FTD patients were included and treatment responses for neurobehavioural symptoms were evaluated by the NPI. Behavioural symptoms, especially

**Table 21.4** Fluvoxamine trial for FTD [40]

| | |
|---|---|
| Design | Open, dose-finding |
| Subjects | Number = 16 (11 FTD, 5 SD)<br>Mean age = 70.0<br>M/F ratio = 6/10 |
| Entry criteria | FTD and SD groups fulfilled the consensus clinical criteria for FTLD |
| Duration | 12 weeks |
| Treatment | Started at 50 mg/day. Dose was adjusted during the first regimen 8 weeks in increments of 50 mg/day |
| Main outcome | Primary: NPI, SRI. Secondary: MMSE |

**Table 21.5** Trazodone trial for FTD [41]

| | |
|---|---|
| Design | Randomized, double-blind, placebo-controlled, crossover |
| Subjects | Number = 31<br>Mean age = 61.7<br>M/F ratio = 15/16 |
| Entry criteria | Lund and Manchester criteria for FTD<br>Frontal Behavioural Dysfunction Scale >3<br>NPI total scale >8 and a score >4 for one of subscale |
| Duration | 6-week double-blind, then 6-week double-blind crossover |
| Treatment regimen | Started at 50–100 mg/day of tradozone or placebo for a week, regimen 150 mg/day for 3 weeks, 300 mg/day for 3 weeks if patients had no side-effects |
| Maim outcome | Primary: NPI. Secondary: CGI-I, MMSE |

**Table 21.6** Paroxetine trial for FTD (1) [43]

| | |
|---|---|
| Design | Open, randomized, uncontrolled |
| Subjects | Number = 16<br>Mean age = 64.6<br>M/F ratio = 6/10 |
| Entry criteria | Lund and Manchester criteria for FTD, criteria of DSM-IV for dementia |
| Duration | 14 months |
| Treatment regimen | Paroxetine 20 mg/day or piracetam 1200 mg/day<br>Paroxetine was started at 10 mg/day and was titrated to the dose of 20 mg/day |
| Main outcome | NPI, the Clinical Insight Rating Scale (CIR), the Cornell Scale for Depression, BEHAVE-AD, MMSE, The Ten Point Clock Test, the Proverb Interpretation Tasks, the Stroop Test |

eating disorders, agitation, irritability, and depression/dysphoria of FTD, significantly improved on active treatment. There was a mild to moderate improvement in clinical severity after the tradozone period, assessed by the CGI-I scale [42]. The MMSE was not modified.

***Paroxetine***

Paroxetine is a selective and potent inhibitor of 5-HT reuptake into serotoninergic neurones. There are two trials to evaluate the effects of paroxetine in FTD patients. The first was an open-label, randomized, uncontrolled study, with no crossover [43] (Table 21.6). Patients were randomized to receive paroxetine up to 20 mg/day ($n = 8$) or piracetam up to 1200 mg/day ($n = 8$). At 14 months, the patients treated with paroxetine showed significant improvements in behavioural symptoms such as personal behaviour and social conduct,

**Table 21.7** Paroxetine trial for FTD (2) [44]

| | |
|---|---|
| Design | Randomized, double-blind, placebo-controlled, crossover |
| Subjects | Number = 10<br>Mean age = 66.3<br>M/F ratio = 7/3 |
| Entry criteria | FTD fulfilled the consensus clinical criteria for FTLD |
| Duration | 6-week double-blind, then 6-week double-blind crossover |
| Treatment regimen | Started at 20 mg/day of paroxetine or placebo for a week, 30 mg/day for a week, 40 mg/day for a month, reduced by 10 mg/day each week |
| Main outcome | NPI, Cambridge Behavioural Inventory, CANTAB, Paired association learning, Decision-making |

reflected by a reduction of caregiver stress. The second trial was a randomized, double-blind, placebo-controlled, crossover trial [44] (Table 21.7). Doses of paroxetine were progressively increased to 40 mg daily ($n = 10$). The same regimen was used for placebo capsules ($n = 10$). Treatment responses for neurobehavioural symptoms were evaluated by the NPI and Cambridge Behavioural Inventory. Cognitive function was evaluated by a broad range of neuropsychological tests. On contrast to the results from the open-label trial, paroxetine did not significantly improve scores on behavioural assessments. Paroxetine therapy selectively impaired paired associates' learning, reversal learning and delayed pattern recognition. This pattern of deficits closely resembles that seen after tryptophan depletion. The discrepancy between these two trials could be due to the procedural differences (open vs. double-blind with placebo-controlled) and/or paroxetine doses (20 mg vs. 40 mg). Forty milligram paroxetine/day is a relatively high dose. Whether low-dose paroxetine (20 mg/day) could give the optimal balance between therapeutic and side-effects awaits evaluation in a blinded, placebo-controlled trial.

### *OTHER AGENTS*

Small doses of major tranquilizers such as risperidone or olanzapine might be indicated for disinhibition, aggressiveness, or stereotypic behaviours where the above-mentioned non-pharmacological interventions or SSRIs are not effective for these challenging behaviours. However, all anti-psychotic drugs can be associated with increased drowsiness and falls. Multicentre trials of memantine for FTD are in progress, with the rationale that the neuroprotective effect of an *N*-methyle-D-aspartate (MMDA) antagonist could benefit patients with non-Alzheimer's neurodegenerative processes [39]. One randomized, double-blind, placebo-controlled, crossover trial in FTD demonstrated the effectiveness of methylphenidate on the task of risk-taking behaviour, with the rationale that methylphenidate would ameliorate reward-based deficits in FTD by stimulating dopaminergic transmission in the orbitofrontal fronto-striatal circuit [45]. The amelioration of risk-taking behaviour carries important implications for rehabilitative approaches to disinhibition and impulsivity in patients with FTD. There is no evidence of benefits from acetylcholinesterase inhibitors such as donepezil, rivastigmine, or galantamine [14].

## SUMMARY

Neurodegenerative dementia is a chronic illness that is progressive and is associated with a range of behavioural and cognitive disturbance. For these patients there are still no drugs that can cure or retard the primary pathological process. Hence, the primary aim of treatment at present is to evaluate BPSD correctly, and at the earliest possible time, so that the burden of care can be minimized through appropriate behavioural therapy or symptomatic drug treatment. This reduction is critical for the continuation of satisfactory home care and could also benefit health economics. This is particularly relevant for FTD in that patients typically manifest marked behavioural disturbance in the absence of major global cognitive deficits in the initial stages [46].

In addition to the above-mentioned BPSD, the early onset seen in FTD (often <65 years) can add to the burden and distress experienced by family members. Relative youth means patients are often employed and may have adolescent children at home. The young age of these patients is also problematic because many services designed for people with dementia are built around AD patients, who are usually much older. Many community dementia services are reluctant to accept young, physically healthy persons in their programs, particularly if that patient is male and is exhibiting challenging behaviours [47].

Not only physicians but other healthcare professionals and also caregivers need to be aware of the features of FTD to provide appropriate and specific care and social support for this early onset dementia with striking BPSD.

## ACKNOWLEDGEMENT

I thank Dr. Peter J. Nestor (Department of Neurology, University of Cambridge) for his valuable comments.

## REFERENCES

1. Finkel SI, Costa e Silva J, Cohen G *et al.* Behavioural and psychological signs and symptoms of dementia; A consensus statement on current knowledge and implications for research and treatment. *Int Psychogeriatr* 1996; 8(suppl 3):497–500.
2. Ikeda M, Tanabe H. Reducing the burden of care in dementia through the amelioration of BPSD by drug therapy. *Expert Rev Neurotherapeutics* 2004; 4:921–922.
3. Neary D, Snowden JS, Gustafson L *et al.* Frontotemporal lobar degeneration: a consensus on clinical diagnostic criteria. *Neurology* 1998; 51:1546–1554.
4. Ratnavalli E, Brayne C, Dawson K, Hodges JR. The prevalence of frontotemporal dementia. *Neurology* 2002; 58:1615–1621.
5. Ikeda M, Ishikawa T, Tanabe H. Epidemiology of frototemporal lobar degeneration. *Dement Geriatr Cogn Disord* 1999; 10:50–54.
6. Tanabe H, Ikeda M, Komori K. Behavioural symptomatology and care of patients with frontotemporal lobe degeneration: based on the aspects of the phylogenetic and ontogenetic processes. *Dement Geriatr Cogn Disord* 1999; 10(suppl 1):50–54.
7. Bozeat S, Gregory CA, Ralph MA, Hodges JR. Which neuropsychiatric and behavioural features distinguish frontal and temporal variants of frontotemporal dementia from Alzheimer's disease? *J Neurol Neurosurg Psychiatry* 2000; 69:178–186.
8. Shigenobu K, Ikeda M, Fukuhara R *et al.* The stereotypy rating inventory for frontotemporal lobar degeneration. *Psychiatry Res* 2002; 110:175–187.
9. Ikeda M, Brown J, Holland AJ *et al.* Changes in appetite, food preference, and eating habits in frontotemporal dementia and Alzheimer's disease. *J Neurol Neurosurg Psychiatry* 2002; 73:371–376.
10. Ikeda M, Tanabe H, Horino T *et al.* Care for patients with Pick's disease by using their preserved procedural memory. *Seishin Shinkeigaku Zasshi* 1995; 97:179–192 (Abstract in English).
11. Swartz JR, Miller BL, Lesser IM, Darby AL. Frontotemporal dementia: treatment response to serotonin selective reuptake inhibitors. *J Clin Psychiatry* 1997; 58:212–216.
12. Litvan I. Therapy and management of frontal lobe dementia patients. *Neurology* 2001; 56(suppl 4): S41–S45.
13. LoGiudice D, Hassett A. Uncommon dementia and carer's perspective. *Int Psychogeriatr* 2005; 17:S223–S231.
14. Mendez MF, Cummings JL. Nonpharmacologic management of dementia. In: *Dementia: A Clinical Approach*, 3rd edition. Butterworth Heinemann, Philadelphia, 2003, pp 583–603.
15. Snowden J, Neary D, Mann DMA. *Fronto-Temporal Lobar Degeneration: Fronto-Temporal Dementia, Progressive Aphasia, Semantic Dementia.* Churchill Livingstone, London, 1996.

16. Torsa R, Badino E, Scalabrino A. Therapeutic strategies for behavioural and psychological symptoms (BPSD) in dementia patients. *Arch Gerontol Geriatr Suppl* 2004; 9:443–454.
17. Cummings JL, Mega M, Gray K *et al.* The Neuropsychiatric Inventory: comprehensive assessment of psychopathology in dementia. *Neurology* 1994; 44:2308–2314.
18. Reisberg B, Borenstein J, Salob SP *et al.* Behavioural symptoms in Alzheimer's disease: phenomenology and treatment. *J Clin Psychiatry* 1987; 48(suppl):9–15.
19. Levy ML, Miller BL, Cummings JL *et al.* Alzheimer disease and frontotemporal dementias: behavioural distinctions. *Arch Neurol* 1996; 53:687–690.
20. Mendez MF, Perryman KM, Miller BL *et al.* Behavioural differences between frontotemporal dementia and Alzheimer's disease: a comparison on the BEHAVE-AD rating scale. *Int Psychogeriatr* 1998; 10:155–162.
21. Kaufer DI, Cummings JL, Christine D. Effect of tacrine on behavioural symptoms in Alzheimer's disease: An open-label study. *J Geriatr Psychiatry Neurol* 1996; 9:1–6.
22. Shigenobu K, Ikeda M, Fukuhara R *et al.* Reducing the burden of care for Alzheimer's disease through the amelioration of 'delusions of theft' by drug therapy. *Int J Geriatr Psychiatry* 2002; 17:211–217.
23. Ames D, Cummings JL, Wirshing WC *et al.* Repetitive and compulsive behaviour in frontal lobe degenerations. *J Neuropsychiatry Clin Neurosci* 1994; 6:100–113.
24. Gregory CA, Lough S. Practical issues in the management of early onset dementia. In: Hodges JR (ed). *Early-Onset Dementia: A Multidisciplinary Approach*. Oxford University Press, Oxford, 2001, pp 449–468.
25. Lhermitte F. Human autonomy and the frontal lobes. II. Patient behaviour in complex and social situations: The 'environmental dependency syndrome'. *Ann Neurol* 1986; 19:335–343.
26. Ikeda M, Tanabe H. Two forms of palilalia: a clinicoanatomical study. *Behav Neurol* 1992; 5:241–246.
27. Ikeda M, Imamura T, Ikejiri Y *et al.* The efficacy of short-term hospitalizations in family care for patients with Pick's disease. *Seishin Shinkeigaku Zasshi* 1996; 98:822–829 (Abstract in English).
28. Ikeda M, Komori K, Shimomura T *et al.* A patient with frontotemporal dementia presenting palilalias in association with intention to act. *Jpn J Neuropsychol* 1997; 13:57–63 (Abstract in English).
29. Cummings JL. Cholinesterase inhibitors: a new class of psychotropic compounds. *Am J Psychiatry* 2000; 157:4–15.
30. Miller BL, Darby A, Benson DF *et al.* Aggressive, socially disruptive and antisocial behaviour associated with fronto-temporal dementia. *Br J Pharmacol* 1997; 170:150–155.
31. Procter AW, Qurne M, Francis PT. Neurochemical features of frontotemporal dementia. *Dement Geriatr Cogn Disord* 1999; 10(suppl 1):80–84.
32 Franceschi M, Anchisi D, Pelati O *et al.* Glucose metabolism and serotonin receptors in frontotemporal lobe degeneration. *Ann Neurol* 2005; 57:216–225.
33. Sparks DL, Markesbery WR. Altered serotonergic and cholinergic markers in Pick's disease. *Arch Neurol* 1991; 48:796–799.
34. Goodman WK, Price LH, Rasmussen SA *et al.* Efficacy of fluvoxamine in obsessive-compulsive disorder: a double blind comparison with pracebo. *Arch Gen Psychiatry* 1989; 46:36–44.
35. Hollander E: Treatment of obsessive-compulsive spectrum disorders with SSRIs. *Br J Psychiatry* 1998; 173(suppl 35):7–12.
36. Janicak PG, Davis JM, Preskorn SH, Ayd FJ Jr. *Principles and Practice of Psychopharmacotherapy*. Williams and Wilkins, Baltimore, 1993.
37. Anderson IM, Tomenson BM. The efficacy of selective serotonin reuptake inhibitors in depression: a meta-analysis of studies against tricyclic antidepressants. *J Psychopharmacol* 1994; 8:238–249.
38. Fluoxetine Bulimia Nervosa Study Group. Fluoxetine in the treatment of bulimia nervosa. A multicenter, placebo-controlled, double-blind trial. *Arch Gen Psychiatry* 1992; 49:139–147.
39. Fichter MM, Kruger G, Rief W *et al.* Fluvoxamine in prevention of relapse in bulimia nervosa: effects on eating-specific psychopathology. *J Clin Psychopharmacol* 1996; 16:9–18.
40. Chow TW. Treatment approaches to symptoms associated with frontotemporal degeneration. *Curr Psychiatry Rep* 2005; 7:376–380.
41. Ikeda M, Shigenobu K, Fukuhara R *et al.* Efficacy of fluvoxamine as a treatment for behavioural symptoms in FTLD patients. *Dement Geriatr Cogn Disord* 2004; 17:117–121.
42. Lebert F, Stekke W, Hasenbroekx C *et al.* Frontotemporal dementia: a randomized, controlled trial with trazodone. *Dement Geriatr Cogn Disord* 2004; 17:355–359.
43. Mattis S. Mental status examination for organic mental syndrome in the elderly patients. In: Bellak L, Karasu TB (ed). *Geriatric Psychiatry*. Grune & Stratton, New York, 1986, pp 77–121.

44. Moretti R, Torre P, Antonello RM *et al.* Frontotemporal dementia: paroxetine as a possible treatment of behaviour symptoms. A randomized, controlled, open 14-month study. *Eur Neurol* 2003; 49:13–19.
45. Deakin JB, Rahman S, Nestor PJ *et al.* Paroxetine does not improve symptoms and impairs cognition in frontotemporal dementia: a double-blind randomized controlled trial. *Psychopharmachology* 2004; 172:400–408.
46. Rahman S, Robbins TW, Hodges JR *et al.* Methylphenidate ('Ritalin') can ameliorate abnormal risk-taking behaviour in the frontal variant of frontotemporal dementia. *Neuropsychopharmacology* 2006; 31:651–658.
47. Shinagawa S, Ikeda M, Fukuhara R *et al.* Initial symptoms in frontotemporal dementia and semantic dementia compared with Alzheimer's disease 2006; 21:74–80.
48. Yeaworth RC, Burke WJ. Frontotemporal dementia: A different kind of dementia. *Arch Psychiatr Nursing* 2000; 14:249–253.

# 22

# Lewy body disease

*R. Barber, F. Boddy*

## INTRODUCTION

Lewy body disease (LBD) is a clinico-pathological description that links a characteristic clinical phenotype to the formation of Lewy type pathology – Lewy bodies (LB) and Lewy neuritis (LN). LBs and LNs are pathological aggregations of a protein, α-synuclein, within neurones.

The core clinical features of LBD are the motor symptoms of parkinsonism, cognitive impairment and psychiatric dysfunction. The extent of these symptoms varies within individuals over time as the disease progresses and between groups of individuals with different variants of LBD. For example, individuals with dementia with Lewy bodies (DLB) develop cognitive impairment but not always the motor features of Parkinson's disease (PD), and conversely patients with established PD may never develop dementia, or do so only after many years of illness (Parkinson's disease and dementia [PDD]). Table 22.1 summarizes the main clinical and pathological features of LBD.

Detailed discussion of the pathological relationship between DLB and PDD is beyond the scope of this chapter, but given the overlap in the pathophysiology and symptoms between these 'parkinsonian-dementia syndromes' they could be viewed as part of a unitary disease process related to α-synucleinopathy.

The primary focus of this chapter is the management of the non-motor symptoms of DLB and PDD. The first part of the chapter will summarize the main neuropsychiatric complications associated with DLB and PDD. The second part will review non-pharmacological and pharmacological treatments. The management of DLB and PDD will mainly be discussed together as the principles and practice of management are similar. Indeed, evidence to date suggests that outcome to psychopharmacological agents are similar.

Two themes will run through this chapter. First, the relative scarcity of good quality evidence to inform clinical practice. Second, the underlying pathophysiology of LBD renders patients prone to experience both multiple symptoms as well as multiple side-effects to pharmacological agents.

## CLINICAL AND NEUROPSYCHIATRIC FEATURES OF DEMENTIA WITH LEWY BODIES AND PARKINSON'S DISEASE WITH DEMENTIA

### *DEMENTIA WITH LEWY BODIES*

DLB is the second commonest cause of degenerative dementia in late life after Alzheimer's disease (AD) accounting for about 15–20% of all causes of dementia.

**Robert Barber,** MDc, MD, MRCPsych, Consultant Old Age Psychiatrist and Honorary Clinical Senior Lecturer, Institute for Ageing and Health, Newcastle General Hospital, Newcastle upon Tyne, UK

**Frauke Boddy**, MRCPsych, Senior Registrar in Old Age Psychiatry, Institute for Ageing and Health, Newcastle General Hospital, Newcastle upon Tyne, UK

**Table 22.1** Common clinical and pathological features of Lewy body disease (DLB and PDD)

| *Common clinical features* | *Pathological*[1,2] |
|---|---|
| *Motor*<br>parkinsonism: rigidity, tremor, bradykinesia, postural instability<br>*Non-motor*<br>cognition: impairment and fluctuations<br>psychiatric: visual hallucinations, delusions, depression, apathy<br>sleep: REM sleep behaviour disorder, insomnia<br>*Autonomic*<br>syncope, orthostatic hypotension, urinary dysfunction<br>*Severe sensitivity to neuroleptic (anti-psychotic) medication*<br>avoid neuroleptic medication | $\alpha$-synuclein positive, neuronal inclusion Lewy bodies, Lewy neurites are found in the neocortex, limbic cortex, sub-cortical nuclei and brainstem<br>deficits in dopamine neurotransmission – notably in the nigrostriatal dopamine pathway (D2 receptor loss in DLB > PD)<br>deficits in acetylcholinergic neurotransmission (with relative preservation of post-synaptic receptors)<br>neuronal loss in striatum and substantia nigra (PD > DLB) with overall mild atrophy |

DLB = dementia with Lewy bodies; PD = Parkinson's disease; PDD = Parkinson's disease and dementia; REM = rapid eye movement.
[1]A proportion of patients will have varying degrees of 'mixed' pathologies including Alzheimer-type (tangle and neuritic plaque formation) as well as vascular disease.
[2]There are a number of other primary neurodegenerative 'parkinsonian dementia syndromes' which have overlapping clinico-pathological features with DLB and PDD. These include the parkinsonism tauopathies, progressive supranuclear palsy (PSP) and corticobasal degeneration (CBD); PD, DLB and multiple systems atrophy are synucleinopathies [70].

It is characterized by progressive cognitive impairment (usually the presenting feature), fluctuations (in up to 75% of patients), spontaneous parkinsonism (up to 75%) and recurrent visual hallucinations (up to 80%). The hallucinations are usually of animals and children and rich in detail and colour. Other psychotic experiences such as auditory hallucinations (20%) and secondary paranoid delusions (65%) may also feature, as can depression (30%).

Using consensus clinical criteria DLB can be accurately diagnosed (good specificity) though cases can be missed (lower sensitivity). The criteria have recently been revised [1], as summarized in more detail in Table 22.2. Rapid eye-movement (REM) sleep behaviour disorder, severe neuroleptic sensitivity and reduced striatal dopamine transporter activity on functional neuro-imaging have been given greater diagnostic weight as features suggestive of a DLB.

## *PARKINSON'S DISEASE WITH DEMENTIA*

Approximately 20–40% of patients with PD will develop dementia. This is not usually a feature of early PD, more often occurring after 8–10 years of illness. However, individuals with mild disease can exhibit changes consistent with frontal lobe dysfunction, such as impairment of planning and sequencing. In the main, patients with DLB and PDD will have a similar profile of cognitive impairment characterized by deficits in attention, visuospatial processing and executive function.

In a similar way to DLB, patients with PD also experience neuropsychiatric complications as well as change to sleep pattern. Psychotic symptoms such as visual hallucinations are more common in elderly patients with longer illness, more advanced disability and cognitive impairment. The main non-cognitive psychiatric complications of PD (along with possible interventions) are summarized in Table 22.3. In addition, behavioural changes can

**Table 22.2** Revised criteria for the clinical diagnosis of dementia with Lewy bodies (DLB). (With permission [1])

1. Central feature *(essential for a diagnosis of possible or probable DLB)*
   Dementia defined as progressive cognitive decline of sufficient magnitude to interfere with normal social or occupational function. Prominent or persistent memory impairment may not necessarily occur in the early stages but is usually evident with progression. Deficits on tests of attention, executive function and visuo-spatial ability may be especially prominent
2. Core features *(two core features are sufficient for a diagnosis of probable DLB, one for possible DLB)*
   Fluctuating cognition with pronounced variations in attention and alertness
   Recurrent visual hallucinations that are typically well formed and detailed
   Spontaneous features of parkinsonism
3. Suggestive features *(if one or more of these is present in the presence of one or more core features, a diagnosis of probable DLB can be made. In the absence of any core features, one or more suggestive features is sufficient for possible DLB. Probable DLB should not be diagnosed on the basis of suggestive features alone)*
   REM sleep behaviour disorder
   Severe neuroleptic sensitivity
   Low dopamine transporter uptake in basal ganglia demonstrated by SPECT or PET imaging
4. Supportive features *(commonly present but not proven to have diagnostic specificity)*
   Repeated falls and syncope
   Transient, unexplained loss of consciousness
   Severe autonomic dysfunction e.g. orthostatic hypotension, urinary incontinence
   Hallucinations in other modalities
   Systematized delusions
   Depression
   Relative preservation of medial temporal lobe structures on CT/MRI scan
   Generalized low uptake on SPECT/PET perfusion scan with reduced occipital activity
   Abnormal (low uptake) MIBG myocardial scintigraphy
   Prominent slow wave activity on EEG with temporal lobe transient sharp waves
5. A diagnosis of DLB is less likely
   In the presence of cerebrovascular disease evident as focal neurological signs or on brain imaging
   In the presence of any other physical illness or brain disorder sufficient to account in part or in total for the clinical picture
   If parkinsonism only appears for the first time at a stage of severe dementia
6. Temporal sequence of symptoms
   DLB should be diagnosed when dementia occurs before or concurrently with parkinsonism (if it is present). The term Parkinson's disease dementia (PDD) should be used to describe dementia that occurs in the context of well-established Parkinson's disease. In a practice setting the term that is most appropriate to the clinical situation should be used and generic terms such as LB disease are often helpful. In research studies in which distinction needs to be made between DLB and PDD, the existing one-year rule between the onset of dementia and parkinsonism DLB continues to be recommended

occur, such as apathy, hypo- or hypersexuality, and changes consistent with abnormal impulse control, such as excessive gambling.

The severity of extrapyramidal motor features in PD, PDD and DLB is similar, though a resting tremor is less prominent in DLB.

### *IMPLICATIONS FOR MANAGEMENT*

The interplay between the cognitive, psychiatric and motor symptoms of LBD makes the management of these symptoms complex and challenging. In particular, the pharmacological management of LBD is complicated by the risk of adverse reactions to medication. Treatments for the motor symptoms of PD can either directly precipitate psychiatric symptoms

**Table 22.3** Psychiatric complications of Parkinson's disease

| *Symptoms* | *Frequency* | *Possible interventions* |
|---|---|---|
| Cognitive impairment/ dementia | 20–40% | Treat any comorbid conditions that could further hinder cognition. Consider CHI<br>Multi-professional involvement to fully assess and manage needs |
| Major depression | 5–10% | Consider SSRI<br>Address any exacerbating factors, e.g. optimize control of motor symptoms |
| Minor depression | 10–30% | Supportive interventions and monitoring |
| Anxiety (including generalized anxiety, panic and social phobia) | 20–40% | Treat any comorbid depression<br>Consider SSRI (possible lower dose)<br>Optimize psychological interventions (relaxation therapy, problem solving, education, cognitive therapy, sleep hygiene)<br>Optimize control of motor symptoms |
| Psychosis | 10–40% (up to 70% if dementia also present) | Review medication – rationalize where possible to lowest effective dose (or withdrawal if appropriate)<br>Recognition and treatment of additional medical conditions (comorbid physical and psychiatric conditions and sleep disturbances)<br>Consider non-pharmacological interventions including social support<br>If medication required consider CHI (or if not tolerated/effective trial of low dose quetiapine) |
| Sleep disorders | Insomnia 60–70%<br>RBD 15–50% | Optimizing night-time management of PD<br>Treat comorbid medical and psychiatric conditions<br>Treat specific sleep disorders:<br>RBD: consider low-dose clonazepam (0.5–1 mg)<br>Insomnia: address any environmental issues, consider psychological intervention for insomnia ± medication (e.g. low-dose trazodone 25–100 mg) |

CHI = cholinesterase inhibitor; PD = Parkinson's disease; RBD = rapid eye movement behaviour disorder; SSRI = selective serotonin reuptake inhibitor.

and/or interact with co-prescribed psychotropic medications, and *vice versa*. This makes it difficult to find the best balance: treatment introduced for one set of symptoms may lead to deterioration in other symptoms – the 'motion–emotion' conundrum [2].

Table 22.4 summarizes some of the key potential neuropsychiatric adverse effects and drug interactions of medication used for the motor symptoms of PD.

With respect to psychotropic drugs, it is well-recognized that anti-psychotic medication can precipitate or exacerbate parkinsonism. The onset of these side-effects tends to be acute or subacute, but may persist for several months after cessation. The sensitivity to neuroleptics appears to be similar in DLB and PDD [3]. Importantly, patients with LBD can be exquisitely sensitive to anti-psychotic (neuroleptic) medication and can develop life-threatening sensitivity reactions akin to neuroleptic malignant syndrome. This reaction is recognized by the onset of sedation, increased confusion, immobility, rigidity, postural instability, and

**Table 22.4** Psychiatric consequences of medications for the motor symptoms of Parkinsonism

| *Medication* | *Potential adverse effect* | *Potential interactions with psychotropic medications* | *Potential benefits* |
|---|---|---|---|
| Levodopa | Vivid dreams, insomnia, psychosis, delirium, affective symptoms, nightmares, behavioural disturbance, agitation | MAO-I A, St John's wort, antagonize anti-psychotics | May improve some aspects of executive function |
| DA agonists | Hallucinations, confusion, drowsiness, hypersexuality, pathological gambling, repetitive, purposeless motor acts – punding | – | Pramipexole – possible anti-depressant effect |
| Selegiline | Hallucinations, confusion, sleep disorders | Caution with SSRI (and tricyclic anti-depressants) – risk of serotonergic syndromes | Possible anti-depressant effect |
| Amantadine | Hallucinations, confusion | – | – |
| Anti-cholinergic | Cognitive impairment, hallucinations, agitation, insomnia | Increase risk of anti-muscarinic effects when given with MAOIs or tricyclic anti-depressants | – |
| Catechol-O-methyl transferase (COMT) inhibitors | – | Entacapone – caution in patients with a history of neuroleptic malignant syndrome and when co-prescribed with venlafaxine – increased adrenergic side-effects theoretically possible | – |

MAO-I A = monoamine oxidase type A inhibitor.

falls. Outcome is poor with a 2–3-fold increased mortality. To manage these risks, and oversee the frequent need for multidisciplinary care, it is advisable that patients should be referred to a specialist(s) for further assessment and management.

## OVERVIEW OF MANAGEMENT OF DLB AND PDD

An important first step is to try to identify and manage any modifiable factors which could be exacerbating symptoms, such as comorbid medical and psychiatric illness or concurrent medications. The intended goals and outcome to any interventions also need to be defined. There will undoubtedly be times when possible interventions are avoided or deferred because the predicted risks are greater than the anticipated gains. For example, this could be relevant when deciding not to pursue drug management for a patient with psychotic symptoms who is not distressed or unduly disabled by these experiences.

As part of a comprehensive approach, multiple interventions are often required. These interventions will need to be managed and adjusted over time as the illness progresses and the needs of patients and their families change. Drug, behavioural and environmental approaches are not mutually exclusive and ultimately the aim is to tailor a range of interventions to try and best address the individual needs of patients and carers.

Steps to consider in the assessment and management of LBD include the following [4]:

**Step 1:** Initial medical diagnosis and the exclusion/management of comorbid illness or other causes of dementia/parkinsonism.
**Step 2:** Provide information and advice to patients and their families/caregivers.
**Step 3:** Establish the key issues for assessment and management.
**Step 4:** Introduce additional supports focusing on non-pharmacological, multi-professional interventions.
**Step 5:** Refer to specialist for further advice on diagnosis and pharmacological therapies and involvement of specialist services.

## NON-PHARMACOLOGICAL APPROACHES

In broad terms, non-pharmacological interventions approach management from a 'systems' perspective. Rather than the behaviour of individual patients being the focus of the 'problem', efforts are made to try and address any breakdown in the interaction between the patient, caregiver, environment and the prevailing system of care [5]. Within this framework, and depending on the formulation of a specific situation, the 'target' of any intervention(s) may not necessarily involve the patient directly but other people and factors involved in their care.

There has been no systematic evaluation of psychosocial interventions in LBD, so it is not possible to say they are any more or less effective than drug interventions. Nevertheless, given concerns and uncertainties about the safety and effectiveness of medications, and the high levels of associated psychological burden, the provision of educational, practical and emotional support for patients and carers will form the backbone of clinical management.

In common with other causes of dementia, the clinician will also need to work with other professionals, such as community psychiatric nurses, occupational therapists, social workers/care managers, physiotherapists, and specialist PD nurses. Consideration will need to be given to a range of issues including level of psychiatric symptoms, activities of daily living, safety, risks, mobility, medication compliance, driving, as well as physical health, environmental, social, personal and nutritional needs. Expectations and wishes of the patient and their family need to be clarified, as do the coping strategies and capacities of the care network. In some patients, symptoms such as visual hallucinations may improve with increased stimulation and novelty. Interventions for cognitive difficulties include prompts for orientation and memory. Exercise may also be beneficial in dementia [6].

## PHARMACOLOGICAL MANAGEMENT

There are no disease-modifying therapies. Instead treatments are focused on symptom relief. Whilst dopaminergic deficiency primarily determines the akinetic-rigid symptoms of PDD and DLB, cholinergic dysfunction is thought to underpin many of the cognitive impairments and psychotic features [7].

In general, drug treatments for neuropsychiatric symptoms are likely to be most appropriate when there are specifically identified symptoms, which are severe and associated significant risks to the patients and/or others. Ideally, dosing should follow the adage 'start low, go slow' and where possible the use of medication should be time-limited. They will be best used after a full discussion with patients and their family about the likely benefits and risks, and when prescribed as part of a 'bio-psycho-social' approach to management.

The main pharmacological agents will be discussed under the relevant target symptoms.

### DEPRESSION

Depressive symptoms are relatively common in LBD. However, there is insufficient evidence (due largely to a lack of well-designed trials) regarding the efficacy and safety of anti-depressants to be able to draw any definitive conclusions or recommendations [8–10].

In clinical practice, therefore, it will be a question of adapting generic guidelines on the management of depression in a way that best fits with the particular needs and issues of individuals. If symptoms are mild then they can usually be managed without the need for medication – advice, support and monitoring can be sufficient. If the symptoms are more severe and cause distress and impairment then a trial of treatment with an anti-depressant needs to be considered. Overall, selective serotonin reuptake inhibitors (SSRIs) are considered to be safer and better tolerated than tricyclic anti-depressants (TCA). Although there are case reports of SSRIs having a deleterious effect on the motor symptoms of PD, this effect is not thought to be clinically important, and they avoid the more common problem of anti-cholinergic side-effects associated with TCAs [11]. Also the dosing regimes are usually more straightforward, favouring better concordance. If an SSRI is not tolerated, an alternative is mirtazapine, which can improve sleep pattern and appetite. In severe depression, if indicated, electroconvulsive therapy may also improve the severity of the parkinsonism [12].

### SLEEP DISTURBANCE

Sleep disturbance is common. For patients, protracted sleep difficulties may cause irritability and excessive daytime tiredness which in turn can increase the risk of falling. For carers, it can be a major source of stress.

There are many potential causes. It may relate to the motor complications of parkinsonism, such as cramps, akinesia, dystonia and difficulty turning in bed [13]. Treatment of any other medical and/or psychiatric conditions, such as pain, nocturia and depression, needs to be considered. The psychiatric symptoms of LBD, such as hallucinations, may cause disruption to normal sleep, as can vivid dreams. In terms of specific sleep disorders, insomnia, REM sleep behaviour disorder (RBD) and restless legs syndrome are the commonest.

For insomnia, non-pharmacological approaches, including advice, education, daily exercise and activities, and sleep hygiene measures offer the safest first line interventions, possibly with a better outcome than drug treatments [14]. If a trial of medication is indicated, consider using low-dose trazodone (25–100 mg), mirtazapine (7.5–15 mg) or a short-acting benzodiazepine. Aim to limit the duration of treatment and be alert to the risk of falls, injury and confusion, especially with benzodiazepines. Low-dose quetiapine (6.25–50 mg) has also been used to treat insomnia in dementia [15], but is probably best reserved for patients with insomnia complicated by psychosis or vivid dreaming (which may herald the onset of daytime psychosis). In a small open-label study, rivastigmine improved sleep in DLB [16], but there was no change in sleep pattern in a larger placebo-controlled study [17].

In RBD individuals act their dreams in ways that can be both dramatic and dangerous. Due to a failure of normal muscle atonia, individuals may shout, push, punch, thrash or kick out as if, for example, they are being chased or swimming. Treatment with low doses of the long-acting benzodiazepine clonazepam (0.5–1 mg) can be helpful [18]. Melatonin may also be effective [19].

Abnormalities in REM sleep could be a risk factor for hallucinations [20], but further trials are required to know whether treating REM sleep abnormalities also improves visual hallucinations.

## PSYCHOTIC SYMPTOMS

Where possible anti-PD medication(s) should be simplified and reduced, although this does not always lead to a reduction in non-motor symptoms or indeed a worsening in the motor symptoms – suggesting an important role for non-dopaminergic mechanisms [21]. Empirically, agents could be gradually reduced/withdrawn in order of anti-cholinergics, amantadine, selegeline, dopamine agonists and levodopa [22]. Even though the dose of levodopa is not necessarily greater in those with or without psychosis, if levodopa is prescribed it is advisable to aim for the lowest acceptable dose [7].

### Anti-psychotics

The use of neuroleptic medication in LBD needs very careful consideration of the likely balance of risks vs. benefits. Where possible they are usually best avoided, but if used then this will require close supervision and monitoring.

In terms of risk, as mentioned, patients can be exquisitely sensitive to anti-psychotic agents. The anti-dopaminergic effect of neuroleptic agents can precipitate and/or exacerbate parkinsonism. High-potency typical anti-psychotics, such as haloperidol, which block D2 receptors have the greatest propensity. Atypical anti-psychotics (such as risperidone, olanzapine, clozapine, quetiapine, and aripiprazole) which have less D2 receptor antagonism (and greater 5-HT2 receptor antagonism) are less likely to cause extrapyramidal symptoms and somnolence, but this can occur, even at low doses. Atypical anti-psychotics can however cause weight gain and metabolic changes, including hyperlipidaemia and disruption of blood glucose control. Agents such as clozapine and olanzapine also have anti-muscarinic effects. There are concerns that neuroleptic medication may accelerate cognitive decline in patients with dementia.

Furthermore, meta-analyses of pooled data from published and unpublished randomized controlled trials (RCTs) indicate that use of atypical anti-psychotics in older individuals with dementia (AD, VaD or mixed dementia) is associated with an increased risk of cardiovascular disease (placebo vs. drug, – 1.1% vs. 3.3%) and mortality (2.3% vs. 3.5%) [23, 24]. This appears to be a class rather than individual drug effect [24, 25] and the risks of cerebrovascular events with typical anti-psychotics are probably similar, though the evidence is limited. Although these studies do not include subjects with DLB or PDD, as a precautionary stance, warnings about the safety of atypicals are extended to all causes of dementia [23] and all atypicals [25]. Cerebrovascular adverse events included a spectrum of events from non-specific dizziness through to transient ischaemic attacks and frank infarction/stroke. Deaths were mainly caused by heart related events (e.g. heart failure, sudden death) or infections (mostly pneumonia).

These safety concerns need to be set against the wider debate about the overall efficacy of anti-psychotics in the treatment of the behavioural and psychological symptoms in dementia [26].

*Clozapine.* Clozapine has been regarded as the 'gold standard' of anti-psychotics agents in PD. The safety and efficacy of clozapine in PD has been studied in over 30 open-label trials and two multicentre, placebo-controlled, double-blind trials. However, there have been very few studies in patients with established dementia (DLB or PDD). Studies to date have consistently demonstrated that (at lower doses and in the short term) clozapine is effective in treating 'drug-induced psychosis' in PD without adversely affecting motor symptoms – indeed tremor and dyskinesias can improve in some individuals [27–29]. The mean dose of clozapine in these trials was approximately 25–35 mg daily (range 6.25–50 mg) and the risk of side-effects was reduced with a slower dose titration. However, patients from one study were followed up for 26 months and the overall prognosis was poor whether or not psychosis persisted: 69% had persistent psychosis; 25% were dead, 42% were admitted to a nursing home, and 68% developed dementia [30]. Add to this, the prevalence of hallucinations at follow-up did not differ between patients receiving anti-psychotics vs. those on no treatment. Overall, it is not clear whether the continued use of clozapine improves the long-term prognosis of parkinsonian patients with psychosis [31].

Also, the role of clozapine in the management of LBD associated with dementia is less clear. As patients with Mini-mental State Examination (MMSE) scores below 20 were excluded from one of two RCTs, it is difficult to know whether treating 'drug-induced psychosis' in PD in the short term is clinically equivalent to managing psychosis in patients with DLB who will have more advanced dementia, recurrent, often long-standing psychotic symptoms, and may not be receiving anti-PD medication. Furthermore, approximately 1% of patients receiving clozapine develop agranulocytosis, and therefore regular and long-term blood cell counts are mandatory. This can place practical limits on the use of clozapine. There are other important side-effects including sedation, orthostatic hypotension, sialorrhoea/drooling, and seizures. Indeed the limited available evidence would suggest that clozapine has a less favourable risk–benefit outcome in more frail and cognitive impaired patients with DLB, probably because of the increased sensitivity to anti-cholinergic effects [7, 32].

*Risperidone and olanzapine.* Risperidone, even in very low doses, can be poorly tolerated in patients with parkinsonism, with reports of worsening parkinsonism, somnolence, sialorrhoea, dizziness, palpitations, constipation, delirium, fatigue, leg cramps, depression, urinary incontinence and hypotension [33]. Olanzapine has been studied in greater detail in subjects with psychosis and PD, and despite some positive findings [34], RCTs have failed to demonstrate a consistent benefit. In one study clozapine was superior to olanzapine [35] and in another (the combined results from two placebo-controlled, double-blind studies) outcome was similar to placebo [36]. Both publications report increased motor symptoms with olanzapine: indeed the trial by Goetz *et al.* [35] was aborted after 15 patients had completed the study as safety stopping rules were invoked because of exacerbated parkinsonism in olanzapine-treated subjects. Added to these concerns are reports of increased mortality and cerebrovascular adverse events in patients with dementia treated with risperidone or olanzapine as noted above.

*Quetiapine.* Low-dose quetiapine (12.5–25 mg) is an alternative to low-dose clozapine but again evidence is very limited. Uncontrolled studies suggest it can reduce psychotic symptoms in PD and is generally well-tolerated (mean dose 40 mg/day) [37]. A larger extension of this study found the outcome was similar for patients with PD and DLB [38]: around 90% of subjects in both groups had a partial to complete resolution of psychosis using quetiapine but around 30% experienced some worsening in motor function. In a later study [39] response rates were lower (around 80%) and patients with dementia were more likely to be non-responders and develop motor worsening. Quetiapine, unlike clozapine, is not associated with agranulocytosis so is a more practical option with the caveat that there are scant trial data on its efficacy.

*Aripiprazole.* Aripiprazole is a new atypical anti-psychotic which is a partial agonist at the D2 and 5-HT1a receptors and an antagonist at 5-HT2a receptors. It may have a low propensity to cause extrapyramidal side-effects because it also has a high 5-HT2/D2 ratio. However, there is inconclusive evidence regarding its safety and efficacy in dementia generally and in LBD [40, 41].

#### *Cholinesterase inhibitors*

The theoretical rationale for the use of cholinesterase inhibitors (CHIs) is based on the fact that substantial cholinergic deficits have been found both in DLB and PDD. Indeed these deficits can be more pronounced than in AD. Though the cholinergic loss in DLB affects both brain stem and basal forebrain pre-synaptic nuclei, in contrast to AD, the post-synaptic cortical muscarinic and nicotinic receptors are more functionally intact. This could mean subjects with LBD would have at least as good if not better response to CHIs than observed in AD.

Cholinergic loss in LBD has been associated with deficits in attention and cognition, but also with hallucinations, delusions and REM sleep behaviour disorder. As mentioned, there are dilemmas when making treatment decisions in patients suffering from DLB or PDD. By using CHIs it is possible to treat a number of different cognitive and neuropsychiatric symptoms with only one agent. This would help to avoid polypharmacy and minimize unwanted adverse effects on this vulnerable patient group. Indeed, as of 2006, rivastigmine is the first and so far only medicine licensed for the treatment of mild to moderately severe PDD in the European Union.

Case studies of CHIs in LBD have consistently shown improvements in psychotic symptoms and behaviour. These include improvements in visual hallucinations with donepezil [42], rivastigmine [16, 43, 44], and galantamine [45] as well as improvements in overall behaviour with donepezil in DLB [46, 47]. Open-label studies have also shown benefits. A 24-week multicentre open-label study of galantamine in DLB showed improvements in overall Neuropsychiatric Inventory (NPI) score but also the abridged NPI-4 (composite of delusions, hallucinations, apathy and depression) [48]. DLB and PDD show similar treatment response in NPI scores to CHIs [49].

There have been five randomized placebo-controlled trials (RCTs) of CHIs in PDD (×4) and DLB (×1) to date. The main results are shown in Table 22.5. With regard to PDD, by far the largest study to date is by Emre *et al.* [50]. A total of 541 patients were enrolled, but 131 patients (24%) discontinued the study prematurely largely due to adverse events. After 24 weeks the total NPI scores did not change in the placebo group but improved by 2 points in the group on active drug. More patients in the rivastigmine group than in the placebo group had an improvement of at least 30% on the NPI-10 scores (45% vs. 35%).

With regard to DLB, there has been one 20-week RCT ($n$ = 120) using rivastigmine (mean dose 9.4 mg) [51]. Overall, rivastigmine reduced neuropsychiatric symptoms without exacerbating parkinsonism. At week 20, twice as many (63% vs. 30%) patients on rivastigmine vs. placebo showed at least a 30% improvement from baseline on the NPI-4. The symptoms which improved the most were apathy, followed by anxiety, delusions and hallucinations, with a tendency for symptoms to re-emerge during the 3-week discontinuation period at the end of the study.

#### *Memantine*

Memantine is licensed for moderate to severe AD and may have beneficial effects on behaviour and agitation in AD [52]. It is thought to have a neuroprotective effect by inhibiting the excitatory neurotoxic glutamate NMDA receptors. To date, its use in LBD has been too limited to draw any firm calculations. It may be well-tolerated with respect to the motor symptoms [53], and indeed may even offer some benefits [54], but case reports suggest it can increase psychosis and agitation [55, 56]. In one series 4 out of 11 subjects with DLB worsened or responded adversely when exposed to the drug [53].

**Table 22.5** Placebo controlled, double-blind, randomized trials using cholinesterase inhibitors in DLB and PDD

| *Study* | *Diagnosis* | *Study duration/ number of participants/ dropouts* | *Medication* | *Primary outcome measures* | *Efficacy: results non-cognitive symptoms* | *Efficacy: results cognitive function* | *Tolerability and safety* |
|---|---|---|---|---|---|---|---|
| McKeith *et al.* [51] | DL3 | 20 weeks<br>120 patients<br>28 dropouts | Rivastigmine 3–12 mg/day | NPI-4 (subscore of NPI-10)<br>Computerized cognitive assessment (speed of response score) | Significant improvement in NPI-4: apathy, anxiety delusions, hallucinations | Improvement in speed of response and attention [58]<br>Non-significant mean improvement in MMSE of 1.5 points vs. decline of 0.1 points on placebo | Increased nausea, vomiting, anorexia<br>Motor symptoms of PD – no worsening |
| Emre *et al.* [50] | PDD | 24 weeks<br>541 patients<br>131 dropouts | Rivastigmine 3–12 mg/day<br>Mean dose 8.4 mg/day) | ADAS-Cog<br>ADCS-CGIC | Significant improvement of at least 30% NPI-10 scores (45.4% vs. 34.6%) | Significant improvements in ADAS-Cog scores (2.1 points) at week 24 and significantly more favourable outcomes in 7 response categories of ADCS-CGIC<br>Improvement in attention [60] | Adverse events were the primary reason for discontinuation: approximately 17% of patients on rivastigmine and 8% of patients on placebo. This was despite a slow dose titration over 16 weeks of the 24-week study. Most frequent adverse events (all significantly more common in drug vs. placebo) were nausea (29% vs. 11.2%), vomiting (16.6% vs. 1.7%), and tremor (10.2% vs. 3.9%) |
| Aarsland *et al.* [72] | PDD | 10 weeks<br>14 patients<br>2 dropouts | Donepezil 5–10 mg/day | MMSE<br>CIBIC+ UPDRS-motor subscale | No effect on NPI scores | Drug: significant increase of MMSE score: 2.1 vs. 0.3 | PD – no worsening |

**Table 22.5** (Continued)

| | | | | | | | |
|---|---|---|---|---|---|---|---|
| Leroi *et al.* [73] | PDD | 15 weeks 16 patients 5 dropouts | Donepezil 2.5–10 mg/day – mean dose 6.2 mg/day | Neuropsychological test battery including assessments of global cognitive status, memory, attention, psychomotor speed, and visuospatial and executive function | No effect on NPI or Cornell Scale of Depression in Dementia | Significant improvement on memory subscale but not global measure of cognition | 4 of 7 patients on donepezil (57%) withdrew because of adverse side-effects including worsening of of motor symptoms, GI disturbance, hypersalivation, rhinorrhea, and urinary frequency |
| Ravina *et al.* [74] | PDD | 10 weeks 22 patients | Donepezil 5–10 mg/day | ADAS-Cog | No improvements on the Brief Psychiatric Rating Scale | Significant 2 point benefit on the MMSE. ADAS-Cog: non-significant trend of 1.9 point better scores on treatment vs. placebo. No change on the Mattis Dementia Rating Scale (MDRS) | Most adverse events were mild. No worsening of PD symptoms |

ADAS-Cog = Alzheimer's Disease Assessment Scale-Cognitive subscale; ADCS-CGIC = Alzheimer's Disease Cooperative Study-Clinician's Global Impression of change; CIBIC+ = clinician's interview based impression of change plus caregiver input; DLB = Dementia with Lewy bodies; MMSE = Mini-mental status examination; NPI = Neuropsychiatric Inventory; PD = Parkinson's disease; PDD = Parkinson's disease and dementia; UPDRS = Unified Parkinson's disease rating scale.

### *COGNITIVE IMPAIRMENT*

CHIs are the only medications which have proven beneficial effects on cognitive symptoms and as mentioned, rivastigmine is now licensed for the treatment of mild to moderately severe PDD.

#### *Cholinesterase inhibitors*

Case series and open-label studies have reported clinically significant improvements in cognition using donepezil, galantamine and rivastigmine in DLB and PDD [45, 47–49, 57, 58]. The benefits from RCTs tend to be more modest, as summarized in Table 22.5.

Returning to the largest study to date, Emre *et al.* [50] found the rivastigmine-treated patients with PDD had a mean improvement of 2.1 points in the score for the 70-point ADAS-Cog from a baseline, as compared with a 0.7-point worsening in the placebo group. The only RCT in DLB found no statistically significant effect of rivastigmine on MMSE (nor in the overall assessment of clinical global change), but there were differences in computerized measures of attention, particularly in those subjects with hallucinations [59, 60]. This may reflect the greater cholinergic deficits in areas of the brain responsible for visual hallucinations. Treatment of patients with PDD using CHIs also improves attention [61]. Further studies are required to determine whether the changes in cognitive function are associated with improvements in activities of daily living.

## OVERALL EFFICACY AND SAFETY OF CHIS IN LBD

In summary, the two larger RCTs in PDD and DLB have shown CHIs can be beneficial in the treatment of non-cognitive and cognitive symptoms in LBD and rivastigmine is now licensed for the treatment of PDD. However, the effect on measures of global cognition in the RCTs was modest, and at best appears to be similar to what is found for AD. There appears to be a more specific effect on attention, which could reflect the extensive loss in cholinergic function in LBD, but the full clinical relevance of these changes needs establishing.

Arguably CHIs have a more pronounced effect on non-cognitive symptoms, with the greatest benefit observed in treating apathy, anxiety, delusions and hallucinations. The effect on non-cognitive symptoms is possibly as good if not greater than that seen in AD. This may be due to relative preservation of post-synaptic cholinergic receptors.

Overall, response to CHIs is probably similar in DLB and PDD. There are pharmacological differences in the mode of action of the three CHIs which theoretically might yield different outcomes, but clinically these differences are not thought to be relevant [62].

Data from the RCTs would suggest the benefits from CHIs are unlikely to emerge early in the course of treatment, so their role in the acute management is less clear. In the long term, limited evidence indicates once patients have responded they will benefit from maintenance treatment [57]. Indeed, sudden withdrawal is usually detrimental and should be avoided [63].

As with AD, there are issues of tolerance, and patients can experience gastrointestinal upset and anorexia. Postural hypotension and falls in patients with DLB have also been reported [64]. Though CHIs may exacerbate the tremor associated with PD (possibly by increasing the imbalance between ACh and dopamine [DA] neurotransmission) this is relatively uncommon and generally the motor symptoms are not affected. It is possible that patients with PDD are more prone than those with DLB due to differences in nigrostriatal dopaminergic degeneration in DLB and PDD [62].

## MOTOR PARKINSONISM

Levodopa can be used for the motor disorder of both DLB and PDD [65], though individuals with DLB may be less responsive [1]. This could be because of intrinsic striatal degeneration in DLB [66]. Also, a proportion of the parkinsonian symptoms may be non-dopaminergic in origin [21]. It is advisable to 'start low, go slow' aiming for the minimum required dose to minimize disability without exacerbating psychiatric symptoms. Anti-cholinergics are best avoided.

## DESIGNING CLINICAL TRIALS IN PDD AND DLB

The relative lack of well-conducted, large-scale randomized placebo-controlled trials in PDD and DLB implies difficulties relating to trial design in these conditions, and McKeith *et al.* [67] propose combining these patient populations for future clinical trials (and using *post hoc* analysis as relevant).

The US Food and Drug Administration (FDA) has considered DLB as an indication for regulatory approval and suggested two primary outcome domains – a global and specific measure of cognition. However, measuring baseline and longitudinal outcome in LBD is confounded by the inherent fluctuations in attention and performance. Variability in the motor symptoms will also influence overall performance.

There are no validated tools to measure changes in global cognitive function in LBD. The MMSE may not be the most appropriate tool in trials in PDD and DLB, nor are tools designed for AD, such as the Alzheimer's Disease Assessment Scale – cognitive subscale (ADAS-Cog). These tools lack sensitivity in assessing processing speed and fluctuations in attention, and predominantly memory-based tools are not necessarily appropriate in LBD [69] Collins *et al.* [68] suggest that global mental status scales which are more sensitive in measuring deficits in attention and executive functioning might be a better screening tool in such cases.

In terms of specific cognitive outcomes, the Clinician Assessment of Fluctuation [69] and/or computerized test batteries might be better tools to use to assess the core feature of fluctuations. There also should be emphasis on other domains of cognitive functioning, such as visuospatial function and executive function.

Consideration also needs to be given to evaluating the impact of therapies on the non-cognitive symptoms. Not only are these symptoms prominent in LBD, behavioural and psychological symptoms of dementia are important determinants of patients' distress, carer burden, and outcome in general. Better methods to detect and measure these symptoms need to be developed and used in well-designed intervention trials in dementia [70].

## SUMMARY

The management of DLB and PDD is therapeutically challenging and will invariably require specialist advice and intervention. Within the framework of a bio-psycho-social approach, targeted and selective use of medication can offer benefits but needs careful consideration and monitoring. CHIs are increasingly viewed as first line intervention to treat the non-motor symptoms of LBD, though a proportion of patients will not be able to tolerate treatment. Clearly there is a need for further clinical trials so clinicians and patients can make more informed and hopefully effective treatment decisions. Ultimately, agents which can modify the underlying disease process such as alpha-synuclein accumulation will be a major advance.

## REFERENCES

1. McKeith IG, Dickson DW, Lowe J *et al.* Diagnosis and management of dementia with Lewy bodies. Third report of the DLB consortium. *Neurology* 2005; Oct 19.
2. Cummings JL. Managing psychosis in patients with Parkinson's disease. *N Engl J Med* 1999; 340:801–803.
3. Aarsland D, Perry R, Larsen JP *et al.* Neuroleptic sensitivity in Parkinson's disease and parkinsonian dementias. *J Clin Psychiatry* 2005; 66:633–637.

4. Barber R, Panikkar A, McKeith IG. Dementia with Lewy bodies: diagnosis and management. *Int J Geriatr Psychiatry* 2001; 16(suppl 1):S12–S18.
5. Cohen-Mansfield J. Nonpharmacological approaches to the care of dementia with Lewy bodies. In: O'Brien J, McKeith I, Ames D, Chiu E (eds). *Dementia with Lewy Bodies and Parkinson's Disease Dementia.* Taylor & Francis, London, 2005, pp 193–206.
6. Heyn P, Abreu BC, Ottenbacher KJ. The effects of exercise training on elderly persons with cognitive impairment and dementia: a meta-analysis. *Arch Phys Med Rehabil* 2004; 85:1694–1704.
7. Burn DJ, McKeith IG. Current treatment of dementia with Lewy bodies and dementia associated with Parkinson's disease. *Mov Disord* 2003; 18(suppl 6):S72–S79.
8. Movement Disorder Society Task Force. Treatment of depression in idiopathic Parkison's disease. *Mov Disord* 2002; 17(suppl 4):S112–S119.
9. Shabnam GN, Th C, Kho D *et al.* Therapies for depression in Parkinson's disease. *Cochrane Database Syst Rev* 2003; 3:CD003465.
10. Ghazi-Noori S, Chung TH, Deane KHO *et al.* Therapies for depression in Parkinson's disease. *The Cochrane Library*, vol. 1. John Wiley, Chichester, 2004.
11. Leentjens AF. Depression in Parkinson's disease: conceptual issues and clinical challenges. *J Geriatr Psychiatry Neurol* 2004; 17:120–126.
12. Andersen K, Balldin J, Gottfries CG *et al.* A double-blind evaluation of electroconvulsive therapy in Parkinson's disease with 'on-off' phenomena. *Acta Neurol Scand* 1987; 76:191–199.
13. Barone P, Amboni M, Vitale C *et al.* Treatment of nocturnal disturbances and excessive daytime sleepiness in Parkinson's disease. *Neurology* 2004; 63(suppl 3):S35–S38.
14. Morin CM, Colecchi C, Stone J *et al.* Behavioral and pharmacological therapies for late-life insomnia: a randomized controlled trial. *JAMA* 1999; 281:991–999.
15. Juri C, Chana P, Tapia J *et al.* Quetiapine for insomnia in Parkinson disease: results from an open-label trial. *Clin Neuropharmacol* 2005; 28:185–187.
16. Maclean LE, Collins CC, Byrne EJ. Dementia with Lewy bodies treated with rivastigmine: effects on cognition, neuropsychiatric symptoms, and sleep. *Int Psychogeriatr* 2001; 13:277–288.
17. McKeith I, Del Ser T, Spano P-F *et al.* Efficacy of rivastigmine in dementia with Lewy bodies: a randomized, double blind, placebo-controlled international study. *Lancet* 2000; 356:2031–2036.
18. Askenasy JJ. Sleep disturbances in Parkinsonism. *J Neural Transm* 2003; 110:125–150.
19. Boeve BF, Silber MH, Ferman TJ. REM sleep behavior disorder in Parkinson's disease and dementia with Lewy bodies. *J Geriatr Psychiatry Neurol* 2004;17:146–157.
20. Sinforiani E, Zangaglia R, Manni R *et al.* REM sleep behavior disorder, hallucinations, and cognitive impairment in Parkinson's disease. *Mov Disord* 2005; Oct 14.
21. McKeith IG, Gauthier S. Pharmacological treatment of dementia with lewy bodies. In: O'Brien J, McKeith I, Ames D, Chiu E (eds). *Dementia with Lewy Bodies and Parkinson's Disease Dementia.* Taylor & Francis, London, 2005, pp 183–192.
22. Friedman JH, Factor SA. Atypical antipsychotics in the treatment of drug-induced psychosis in Parkinson's disease. *Move Disord* 2000; 15:201–211.
23. Committee on Safety of Medicines. Atypical antipsychotic drugs and stroke. 2004. http://www.mca.gov.uk/ourwork/monitorsafequalmed/safetymessages/antipsystroke_9304.htm; http://www.mca.gov.uk/ourwork/monitorsafequalmed/safetymessages/atypicalantipsychotics_qa.htm
24. Schneider LS, Dagerman KS, Insel P. Risk of death with atypical antipsychotic drug treatment for dementia: meta-analysis of randomized placebo-controlled trials. *JAMA* 2005; 294:1934–1943.
25. US Food and Drug Administration. Public Health Advisory: deaths with antipsychotics in elderly patients with behavioral disturbances. Available at: http://www.fda.gov/cder/drug/advisory/antipsychotics.htm. April 2005.
26 Ballard C, Howard R. Neuroleptic drugs in dementia: benefits and harm. *Nat Rev Neurosci* 2006; 6:492–500.
27. The Parkinson Study Group. Low-dose of clozapine for the treatment of drug-induced psychosis in Parkinson's disease. *N Engl J Med* 1999; 340:757–763.
28. The French Parkinson Study Group. Clozapine in drug-induced psychosis in Parkinson's disease. *Lancet* 1999; 353:2041–2042.
29. Pollak P, Tison F, Rascol O *et al.* Clozapine in drug induced psychosis in Parkinson's disease: a randomized, placebo controlled study with open follow up. *J Neurol Neurosurg Psychiatry* 2004; 75:689–695.

30. Factor SA, Feustel PJ, Friedman JH *et al.* Parkinson Study Group Longitudinal outcome of Parkinson's disease patients with psychosis. *Neurology* 2003; 60:1756–1761.
31. Fernandez HH, Donnelly EM, Friedman JH. Long-term outcome of clozapine use for psychosis in parkinsonian patients. *Mov Disord* 2004; 19:831–833.
32. Burke WJ, Pfeiffer RF, McComb RD. Neuroleptic sensitivity to clozapine in dementia with Lewy bodies. *J Neuropsychiatry Clin Neurosci* 1998; 10:227–229.
33. Fernandez HH, Trieschmann ME, Friedman JH *et al.* Treatment of psychosis in Parkinson's disease: safety considerations. *Drug Saf* 2003; 26:643–659.
34. Cummings JL, Street J, Masterman D, Clark WS. Efficacy of olanzapine in the treatment of psychosis in dementia with lewy bodies. *Dement Geriatr Cogn Disord* 2003; 13:67–73.
35. Goetz CG, Blasucci LM, Leurgans S *et al.* Olanzapine and clozapine: comparative effects on motor function in hallucinating PD patients. *Neurology* 2000; 55:789–794.
36. Breier A, Sutton VK, Fedlman PD *et al.* Olanzapine in the treatment of dopamimetic-induced psychosis in patients with Parkinson's disease. *Biol Psychiatry* 2002; 52:438–445.
37. Fernandez HH, Friedman JH, Jacques C *et al.* Quetiapine for the treatment of drug-induced psychosis in Parkinson's disease. *Mov Disord* 1999; 14:484–487.
38. Fernandez HH, Trieschmann ME, Burke MA *et al.* Quetiapine for psychosis in Parkinson's disease versus dementia with Lewy bodies. *J Clin Psychiatry* 2002; 63:513–515.
39. Fernandez HH, Trieschmann ME, Burke MA *et al.* Long-term outcome of quetiapine use for psychosis among parkinsonian patients. *Mov Disord* 2003; 18:510–514.
40. Fernandez HH, Trieschmann ME, Friedman JH. Aripiprazole for drug-induced psychosis in Parkinson's disease: preliminary experience. *Clin Neuropharmacol* 2004; 27:4–5.
41. Tariot PN, Profenno LA, Ismail MS. Efficacy of atypical antipsychotics in elderly patients with dementia. *J Clin Psychiatry* 2004; 65(suppl 11):11–15.
42. Shea C, MacKnight C, Rockwood K. Donepezil for treatment of dementia with Lewy bodies: a case series of nine patients. *Int Psychogeriatr* 1998; 10:229–238.
43. Reading PJ, Luce AK, McKeith IG. Rivastigmine in the treatment of parkinsonian psychosis and cognitive impairment: preliminary findings from an open trial. *Mov Disord* 2001; 16:1171–1174.
44. Bullock R, Cameron A. Rivastigmine for the treatment of dementia and visual hallucinations associated with Parkinson's disease: a case series. *Curr Med Res Opin* 2002; 18:258–264.
45. Aarsland D, Hutchinson M, Larsen JP. Cognitive, psychiatric and motor response to galantamine in Parkinson's disease with dementia. *Int J Geriatr Psychiatry* 2003; 18:937–941.
46. Lanctot KL, Herrmann N. Donepezil for behavioural disorders associated with Lewy bodies: a case series. *Int J Geriatr Psychiatry* 2000; 15:338–345.
47. Samuel W, Caligiuri M, Galasko D *et al.* Better cognitive and psychopathologic response to donepezil in patients prospectivelydiagnosed as dementia with Lewy bodies: a preliminary study. *Int J Geriatr Psychiatry* 2000; 15:794–802.
48. Edwards KR, Hershey L, Wray L *et al.* Efficacy and safety of galantamine in patients with dementia with Lewy bodies: a 12-week interim analysis. *Dement Geriatr Cogn Disord* 2004; 17(suppl 1):40–48.
49. Thomas AJ, Burn DJ, Rowan EN *et al.* A comparison of the efficacy of donepezil in Parkinson's disease with dementia and dementia with Lewy bodies. *Int J Geriatr Psychiatry* 2005; 20:938–944.
50. Emre M, Aarsland D, Albanese A *et al.* Rivastigmine for dementia associated with Parkinson's disease. *N Engl J Med* 2004; 351:2509–2518.
51. McKeith I, Der Ser T, Spano P *et al.* Efficacy of rivastigmine in dementia with Lewy bodies: a randomized, double-blind, placebo-controlled international study. *Lancet* 2000; 356:2031–2036.
52. Areosa SA, Sherriff F, McShane R. Memantine for dementia. *Cochrane Database Syst Rev* 2005; 18; CD003154.
53. Sabbagh MN, Hake AM, Ahmed S *et al.* The use of memantine in dementia with Lewy bodies. *J Alzheimer's Dis* 2005; 7:285–289.
54. Merello M, Nouzeilles MI, Cammarota A *et al.* Effect of memantine (NMDA antagonist) on Parkinson's disease: a double-blind crossover randomized study. *Clin Neuropharmacol* 1999; 22:273–276.
55. Riederer P, Lange KW, Kornhuber J *et al.* Pharmacotoxic psychosis after memantine in Parkinson's disease. *Lancet* 1991; 19:1022–1023.
56. Ridha BH, Josephs KA, Rossor MN. Delusions and hallucinations in dementia with Lewy bodies: worsening with memantine. *Neurology* 2005; 65:481–482.

57. Grace J, Daniel S, Stevens T *et al.* Long-term use of rivastigmine in patients with dementia with Lewy bodies: an open-label trial. *Int Psychogeriatr* 2001; 13:199–205.
58. Giladi N, Shabtai H, Gurevich T *et al.* Rivastigmine (Exelon) for dementia in patients with Parkinson's disease. *Acta Neurol Scand* 2003; 108:368–373.
59. Wesnes KA, McKeith IG, Ferrara R *et al.* Effects of rivastigmine on cognitive function in dementia with Lewy bodies: a randomized placebo-controlled international study using the cognitive drug research computerized assessment system. *Dement Geriatr Cogn Disord* 2002; 13:183–192.
60. McKeith IG, Wesnes KA, Perry E *et al.* Hallucinations predict attentional improvements with rivastigmine in dementia with Lewy bodies. *Dement Geriatr Cogn Disord* 2004; 18:94–100.
61. Wesnes KA, McKeith I, Edgar C *et al.* Benefits of rivastigmine on attention in dementia associated with Parkinson's disease. *Neurology* 2005; 65:1654–1656.
62. Aarsland D, Mosimann UP, McKeith IG. Role of cholinesterase inhibitors in Parkinson's disease and dementia with Lewy bodies. *J Geriatr Psychiatry Neurol* 2004; 17:164–171 [Review].
63. Minett TS, Thomas A, Wilkinson LM *et al.* What happens with donepezil is suddenly withdrawn? An open label trial in dementia with Lewy bodies and Parkinson's disease with dementia. *Int J Geriatr Psychiatry* 2003; 18:988–993.
64. McLaren AT, Allen J, Murray A *et al.* Cardiovascular effects of donepezil in patients with dementia. *Dement Geriatr Cogn Disord* 2003; 15:183–188.
65. Bonelli SB, Ransmayr G, Steffelbauer M *et al.* L-dopa responsiveness in dementia with Lewy bodies, Parkinson's disease with and without dementia. *Neurology* 2004; 63:376–378.
66. Duda JE, Giasson BI, Mabon ME *et al.* Novel antibodies to synuclein show abundant striatal pathology in Lewy body diseases. *Ann Neurol* 2002; 52:205–210.
67. McKeith I, Mintzer J, Aarsland D *et al.* Dementia with Lewy bodies. *Lancet Neurol* 2004; 3:19–28 [Review].
68. Collins B, Constant J, Kaba S *et al.* Dementia with Lewy bodies: implications for clinical trials. *Clin Neuropharmacol* 2004; 27:281–292.
69. Walker MP, Ayre GA, Cummings JL *et al.* Quantifying fluctuation in dementia with Lewy bodies, Alzheimer's disease and vascular dementia. *Neurology* 2000; 54:1616–1625.
70. McKeith I, Cummings J. Behavioural changes and psychological symptoms in dementia disorders. *Lancet Neurol* 2005; 4:735–742.
71. Duda JE. Pathology and neurotransmitter abnormaliaties of dementia with Lewy bodies. *Dement Geriatr Cogn Disord* 2004; 17(suppl 1):3–14.
72. Aarsland D, Laake K, Larsen JP *et al.* Donepezil for cognitive impairment in Parkinson's disease: a randomized controlled study. *J Neurol Neurosurg Psychiatry* 2002; 72:708–712 [Erratum, *J Neurol Neurosurg Psychiatry* 2002; 73:354].
73. Leroi I, Brandt J, Reich SG *et al.* Randomized placebo-controlled trial of donepezil in cognitive impairment in Parkinson's disease. *Int J Geriatr Psychiatry* 2004; 19:1–8.
74. Ravina B, Putt M, Siderowf A *et al.* Donepezil for dementia in Parkinson's disease: a randomized, double blind, placebo controlled, crossover study. *J Neurol Neurosurg Psychiatry* 2005; 76:934–939.

# 23

# Mild cognitive impairment

*Y. E. Geda, S. Negash, R. C. Petersen*

## INTRODUCTION

The promotion of health and prevention of disease is a time honoured axiomatic truth [1]. This is particularly true of Alzheimer's disease (AD), a dementing illness that has increasingly become a global health problem [2]. Out of the estimated 25 million patients with dementia in 2000, about 13 million lived in the developing world [3]. In the US alone, AD is projected to afflict as many as 14 million people by the year 2050 [4]. Dementia has several devastatinag consequences including substantial socioeconomic burdens. Even though life is priceless, the economic impact of AD is quite alarming. In 1997, the average cost of care for a patient with AD in California was estimated to be over $40,000 per year [5]. For the above compelling reasons, the need to delay the onset of dementia is a global public health imperative. The prevention research is dependent upon identification of suitable targets for intervention; one such entity is mild cognitive impairment (MCI) [6].

MCI refers to the grey zone between the cognitive changes of normal ageing and very early dementia [7] (Figure 23.1). Individuals with MCI show memory impairment greater than expected for their age, but otherwise are functioning independently and do not meet the commonly accepted criteria for dementia [6]. As such, MCI serves as a useful clinical entity in that it provides a unique opportunity for therapeutic interventions aimed at earlier juncture in the cognitive decline.

## THE HISTORICAL GENESIS OF MCI

The discussion of MCI is not complete without reviewing the historical genesis of the research work that gave birth to the construct of MCI [1]. Reisberg and coworkers [8, 9] were perhaps the first to coin the term MCI. They used the Global Deterioration Scale (GDS) to define MCI. The GDS is an ordinal scale of one to seven with one being normal and seven signifying severe dementia. A GDS score of 3 is defined as MCI. This approach is in contrast with the Mayo Clinic definition, which uses clinical criteria to arrive at a diagnosis of MCI. The first attempt to characterize memory concerns with ageing dates back to the 1962 publication of VA Kral [10] who used the term *senescent forgetfulness* to describe this entity. This was followed by a pioneering initiative of the National Institute of Mental Health that

**Yonas Endale Geda**, MD, MSc, Consultant, Department of Psychiatry Mayo Clinic College of Medicine, Mayo Clinic College of Medicine, Alzheimer's Disease Research Centre, Rochester, Minnesota and Department of Psychiatry, Mayo Clinic College of Medicine, Mayo Clinic Jacksonville, Jacksonville, Florida, USA

**Selamawit Negash**, PhD, Cognitive Neuroscience, Research Fellow, Alzheimer's Disease Research Center, Mayo Clinic College of Medicine, Rochester, Minnesota, USA

**Ronald C. Petersen**, PhD, MD, Consultant, Department of Neurology, Alzheimer's Disease Research Center, Mayo Clinic College of Medicine, Rochester, Minnesota, USA

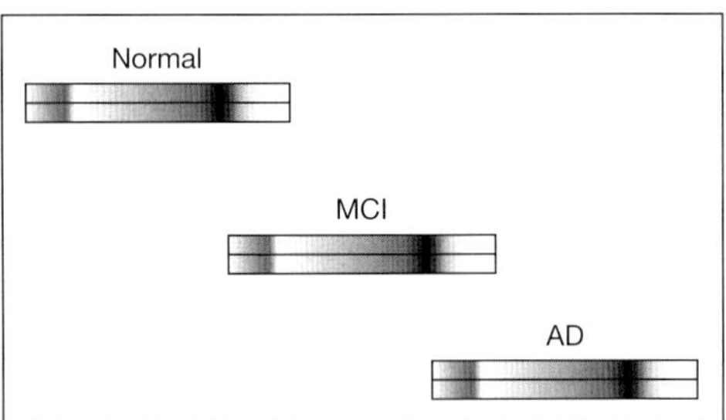


**Figure 23.1** Conceptual model of MCI.

proposed the term *age associated memory impairment* (AAMI) in 1986 [11]. The introduction of AAMI has spurred research work in the grey zone between ageing and dementia, however, the construct was noted to have its limitations such as restriction of impairment to memory domain only and comparison of memory function in older adults with that of young adults (at least 1 standard deviation below the mean for young adults) that led some to remark that depending on the memory test selected, up to 90% of those older than 50 would be labelled as impaired. This is a rather large proportion of the elderly population [12].

The International Psychogeriatric Association addressed these drawbacks by defining the term *age associated cognitive decline* (AACD) [13] hence, its operational criteria for AACD referenced a variety of cognitive domains presumed to decline in normal ageing, and included age- and education-adjusted normative values as well. In addition to AAMI and AACD there are several other terms suggested [14, 15] one of which is 'questionable dementia' [16] that is defined using the Clinical Dementia Rating (CDR) scale [17]. This severity scale designates individuals with a CDR of 0.5 to have 'questionable dementia'. While both GDS and CDR are useful scales for severity rating along the continuum of cognitive impairment, they do not necessarily coincide with various stages of impairment; in fact, many individuals with GDS 3 or CDR 0.5 may actually meet the criteria for mild dementia or AD.

The current widely used definition of MCI has incorporated advances made by theoretical constructs preceding it: additionally amnestic MCI was also empirically validated in a prospective study conducted in Rochester, Minnesota [6]. The Mayo criteria were also endorsed by the American Academy of Neurology that emphasized that patients with MCI are worthy of being followed as these patients develop dementia at 10–15% per year as compared to the general population of 1–2% per year [18].

## CLINICAL FEATURES

Physicians often encounter a clinical scenario in which an elderly person presents with memory concerns. Such a patient is often interested in finding out whether the memory concerns are indicative of AD. While such concerns could represent other states such as late-life depression or the patient being in the so-called 'worried well' state, they could also be suggestive of development of AD. Consider, e.g. a typical clinical scenario described below.

### *THE CASE RECORD OF PATIENT A*

A 68-year-old right-handed male patient presented with forgetfulness for recent events and future engagements. Family members and close friends had also noticed these changes. The patient had difficulty identifying the onset of these symptoms but felt that they had started insidiously and progressed gradually over a period of 2–3 years. Otherwise, he was living independently and had no difficulty carrying out activities of daily living, such as handling his own finances, cooking, and driving. He denied depression, stress, or other complicating medical issues. He requested an appointment with a physician in order to determine if this memory problem should be pursued further. The clinical evaluation, i.e. meticulous history and physical examination including bedside cognitive screening using the short test of mental status was suggestive of cognitive impairment, but not severe enough to warrant the diagnosis of dementia, hence a clinical diagnosis of MCI was made. Investigations including psychometric testing and magnetic resonance imaging (MRI) were ordered. The neuropsychological testing confirmed the clinical diagnosis. It revealed memory impairment, particularly on measures of learning and delayed recall beyond what was felt to be normal for age; but other cognitive domains such as language and visuospatial skills were relatively intact. MRI of head revealed mild hippocampal atrophy.

***Discussion***

This patient probably has amnestic MCI. He is becoming slightly more forgetful, and this is noticeable to his family and friends. The most salient feature of the history concerns forgetfulness of insidious onset that gradually progressed over a year or so. All other cognitive domains, i.e. language, comportment-executive function, visuospatial skills were intact. The individual did not have a decline in function. This likely represented an early disease process involving the medial temporal lobe since meaningful information could no longer be stored in an efficient manner, nor could it be recalled well.

## DIAGNOSTIC ALGORITHM FOR MCI SUBTYPES

MCI is essentially a clinical diagnosis that is based on detailed history, meticulous physical examination, and bedside cognitive screening such as the Mini-mental Status Examination (MMSE) [19] or equivalent scales [20]. The original Mayo criteria for amnestic MCI are: (1) a memory complaint, preferably corroborated by an informant; (2) impaired memory for age on psychometric testing; (3) normal general cognitive function; (4) intact activities of daily living; (5) not demented [18]. Even though amnestic MCI is the most widely studied and empirically validated construct, the first international consensus on MCI has indicated that there are three additional subtypes [21]. Figure 23.2 depicts the diagnostic algorithm that can be pursued to arrive at a diagnosis of a particular subtype of MCI. The process essentially boils down to two major steps, the first one being establishment of the diagnosis of MCI, while the second pertains to identification of the type and number of cognitive domains involved. The details of this process are discussed as follows. The algorithm is initiated when a patient or informant reports cognitive complaints, such as forgetfulness for recent events and future engagements. The clinician should then determine that the patient is neither demented nor normal for age. Once this is established, the next step is to make sure that there is no substantial decline in function; this can be accomplished *via* a careful history from the patient, preferably corroborated by a collateral source. If it is determined that the decline in function is not of sufficient magnitude to warrant the diagnosis of a very mild dementia, then the physician further assumes the diagnosis of MCI and proceeds to identify the number and types of cognitive domains impaired. A diagnosis of *amnestic MCI-single domain* is assumed if the impairment involves only memory domain, whereas *amnestic MCI-multiple domain* pertains to impairments in the memory domain plus at least one other cognitive domain, such as language, executive function or visuospatial skills. Likewise, a diagnosis of non-amnestic MCI-single domain is assumed if there is impairment in a single non-memory domain, whereas non-amnestic MCI-multiple domain refers to impairments in multiple non-memory domains.

This diagnostic algorithm may be helpful in gaining more insights into the prodromal forms of dementia, and this in turn may also have therapeutic implications insofar as medications for treatment of prodromal forms of dementia may very well be specific to the presumed

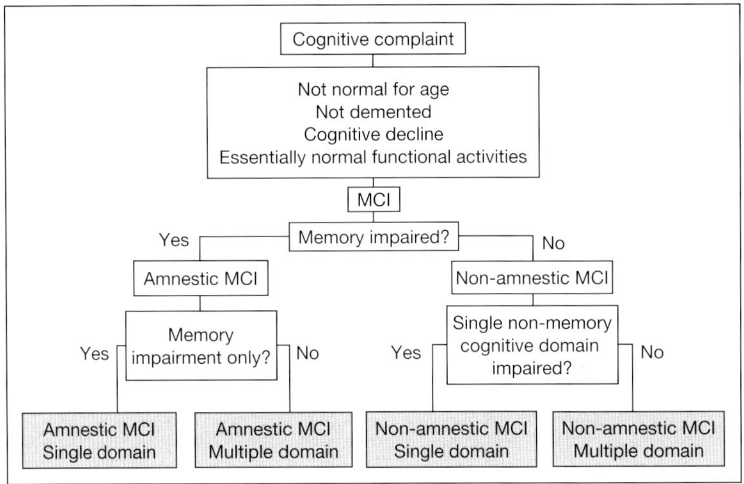


**Figure 23.2** Flow chart of decision process for making diagnosis of subtypes of MCI (with the kind permission of Ronald C. Petersen).

| Clinical classification | | Aetiology: Degenerative | Vascular | Psychiatric | Trauma |
|---|---|---|---|---|---|
| Amnestic MCI | Single domain | AD | | Depr | |
| | Multiple domain | AD | VaD | Depr | |
| Non-amnestic MCI | Single domain | FTD | | | |
| | Multiple domain | DLB | VaD | | |

**Figure 23.3** Classification of clinical subtypes of MCI with presumed aetiology. AD = Alzheimer's disease; DLB = dementia with Lewy bodies; Depr = depression; FTD = fronto-temporal dementia; VaD = vascular dementia (with the kind permission of Ronald C. Petersen).

underlying aetiology of the developing dementing disorder. Figure 23.3 depicts the presumed aetiologies along with clinical subtypes of MCI. The single- and multiple-domain amnestic MCI subtypes with presumed degenerative aetiology likely represent a prodromal form of AD [21]. The non-amnestic subtypes that emphasize impairments in the non-memory domains may have a higher likelihood of progressing to a non-AD dementia, such as dementia with Lewy bodies [21]. Therefore, the combination of clinical subtypes and putative aetiologies can be useful in predicting the ultimate type of dementia to which these diseases will evolve.

## THE EPIDEMIOLOGY OF MCI

The epidemiology of MCI is a broad topic that encompasses the design, conduct and analysis of various types of studies (case–control, cohort or clinical trials) pertinent to MCI. The main focus of this section, however, will be on three epidemiological indices derived from descriptive studies, i.e. the prevalence and incidence of MCI, as well as the conversion rate of MCI to dementia.

The incidence of MCI ranges from 1% to 6% per year while prevalence estimates range from 3% to 22% per year [22–27]. The factors that may account for this variability can be grouped under sampling, and measurement bias [28]. The former pertains to issues of study design and sampling, for instance recruiting research participants by using an advertisement can introduce non-respondent/volunteer bias [28] while the latter pertains to variability in the measurement of MCI. One good example to illustrate measurement bias would be studies that retrofit MCI criteria into a cohort. The ideal research design that is well suited to compute epidemiological indices such as prevalence and incidence would be a population-based study that prospectively employs the operational criteria of MCI in elderly individuals. The National Institute on Aging has recently funded such a study in Olmsted County, Minnesota to meet this specific need. This study is currently recruiting individuals, and preliminary results are expected to be reported at the 2006 annual conference of the American Academy of Neurology (personal communication, Ronald C. Petersen).

Perhaps the first population-based study that estimated the prevalence of MCI subtypes was that of the Cardiovascular Health Study. As the name implies this cohort was assembled to examine cardiovascular risk factors [29] hence the investigators retrofitted the criteria for amnestic and multi-domain MCI to the cohort and reported an overall prevalence of MCI to be 22%, with amnestic MCI accounting for 6% and multi-domain MCI representing 16% [27]. Recently, an Australian research group estimated prevalence in a probability sample of elderly individuals in the age range of 60–64 years old; they reported a much smaller prevalence rate than the Cardiovascular Health Study, i.e. 3.8% and 3.1% for MCI and AACD, respectively [30]. Even though their study design was optimal, limiting the sample to the relatively younger age group is likely to have biased their finding towards underestimation of the prevalence of MCI.

There are several studies that have estimated the progression rate of MCI to dementia [6, 7, 9, 31, 32]. Their findings vary depending upon the study design and measurement instrument utilized [33], e.g. researchers from Harvard University recruited study participants *via* advertisement, they then prospectively followed a cohort of subjects with MCI and reported a conversion rate of 6% per year [32] where as a recent multicentre randomized, double-blind, placebo-controlled clinical trial reported a conversion rate of 16% per year [7]. Prior to that, Mayo Clinic, and other researchers have reported a conversion rate in the range of 10–15%. Hence, the rather smaller rate reported by the Harvard group could be attributed to non-respondent/volunteer bias [28]. One important point that all studies point out is that individuals with MCI develop dementia at a higher rate than the general population. It is this consistent finding that makes MCI an optimal target for clinical trials.

One topic of debate and discussion is the 'instability' of the MCI construct [26, 34]. Larrieu and colleagues reported a reversion rate (i.e. from MCI back to normal) to be as high as 40% over 2–3 years follow-up. However, they defined MCI based on only one single memory measurement, i.e. Benton Visual Retention Test [35]. A recent international consensus panel on MCI did emphasize that the importance of progressive decline, rather than entirely relying on poor performance at any one given point in time, may help to minimize the 'instability' of the construct [21].

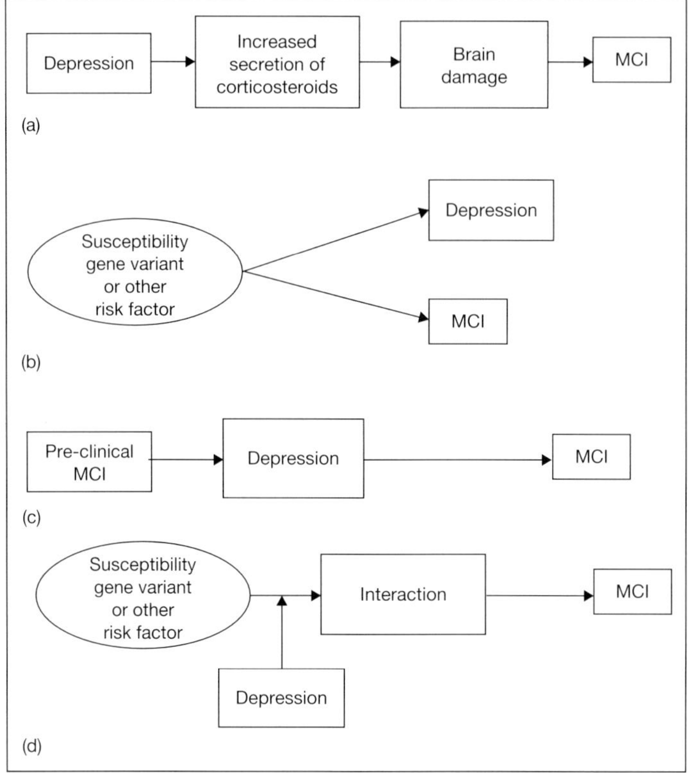


**Figure 23.4** Four hypotheses of the possible mechanisms linking depression to MCI.

## NEUROPSYCHIATRIC FEATURES

The neurological, psychometric and neuroimageing aspect of MCI have been reported [6, 36], however, there is little work done in the area of the neuropsychiatric aspect of MCI. It is quite logical to address this issue since the medial temporal lobe and its connections with prefrontal and other structures not only play a critical role in cognitive function but in emotional behaviour as well [37]. The first population based investigation of the neuropsychiatric symptoms of MCI was reported in 2002 [38] and since then there have been similar studies on this topic on samples largely derived from primary- or tertiary-care settings [39–41]. Psychiatric symptoms were also examined in prodromal AD [42] as well. Lyketsos and colleagues have postulated that if MCI is indeed a pre-Azheimer's state then the prevalence rate of neuropsychiatric symptoms in MCI should be intermediate between that of normal ageing and dementia [38]; indeed some have reported findings that substantiate this hypothesis [40, 41].

In a recent study, we prospectively followed a cohort of 840 elderly individuals, with neither depression nor cognitive impairment at baseline for a median period of 3.5 (1–15) years [43], to the outcome of incident MCI. We observed that depression, as measured by the short version of the Geriatric Depression Scale (GDS) [44] more than doubled the risk of transition from normal ageing to incident MCI. We also observed a synergistic interaction between depression and apolipoprotein E (ApoE) genotype.

**Table 23.1** Clinical trials in MCI

| *Sponsor* | *Duration* | *Endpoint* | *Treatments* |
|---|---|---|---|
| ADCS* | 3 years | AD | Vitamin E<br>Donepezil |
| Merck | 2–3 years | AD | Rofecoxib |
| Novartis | 3 years | AD | Rivastigmine |
| Janssen | 2 years | Symptoms | Galantamine |
| Pfizer | 6 months | Symptoms | Donepezil |
| UCB | 1 year | Symptoms | Piracetam |

*Alzheimer's Disease Cooperative Study supported by National Institute on Aging, Pfizer, Inc., Eisai, Inc., and Roche Vitamins.

We have proposed four hypotheses that can explain the association between depression and incident MCI (Figure 23.4). The first is *aetiologic pathway*, where depression is hypothesized to be in the chain of causality leading to MCI by virtue of its effect on a neurobiological pathway such as the neuroendocrine axis. This hypothesis assumes causality whereby depression causes an increased secretion of corticosteroids or other 'neurotoxic' biological factors that, in turn, lead to brain parenchymal damage. One implication of this hypothesis is that an intervention targeting depression may lead to the primary prevention of MCI. The second hypothesis pertains to *shared risk factor* or *confounding*, where depression is non-causally associated with a confounder [45]. The confounder at the same time is an independent risk factor for the outcome (incident MCI). The confounder could be genetic, environmental, or both. This hypothesis points to a susceptibility gene variant or another non-genetic risk factor that increases the risk of depression and MCI independently. The third hypothesis pertains to a *reverse causality*. Under this scenario, a person who is experiencing some degree of cognitive decline may first develop depression as a reaction to the symptoms. The depressive symptoms may then become early non-cognitive manifestations of dementia, which may 'unmask' the clinical manifestations of MCI in individuals with limited cognitive reserve. As such, depression is an early manifestation of pre-clinical MCI or is a reaction to the initial symptoms of MCI. Lastly, there could be an *interaction*, where depression is a risk factor for MCI only in the presence of a susceptibility gene variant or another non-genetic risk factor. We found evidence for a synergistic interaction between ApoE genotype and depression.

It is also important to note that these four mechanisms (and other possible mechanisms) are not mutually exclusive and may act in tandem as well. Future studies that further investigate these possible mechanisms could prove useful in understanding the psychiatric variables in MCI, and also in designing clinical trials that target psychiatric symptoms in the setting of MCI.

## TREATMENT

There is no standard treatment for MCI, however, as the focus of AD research moves towards prevention, numerous clinical trials are being undertaken since MCI is considered the optimum stage for interventional studies that aim to delay the onset of dementia [46]. Table 23.1 outlines the clinical trials targeting MCI currently underway or recently completed.

The reader is referred elsewhere for an extensive discussion of clinical trials in MCI [47]. The much awaited clinical trial involving 70 medical centres in North America, was recently reported [7]. The study was conducted by the Alzheimer's Disease Cooperative Study (ADCS) funded by the National Institute on Aging, with additional funding from Pfizer, Inc., Eisai, Inc., and Roche Vitamins. It was a randomized, double-blind, placebo-controlled study involving three arms to assess the safety and efficacy of high-dose vitamin E and donepezil. The objective was to assess the safety and efficacy of vitamin E (2000 IU per day) and donepezil (10 mg per day), and was powered to decrease the conversion rate of MCI to AD, from the anticipated 45% down to 30% over the course of three years. Seven hundred and sixty-nine subjects were randomized in the trial and the annual conversion rate from MCI to AD was approximately 16% per year. Over the course of the study donepezil reduced the risk of progressing to AD for the first 18 months of the trial. Vitamin E had no therapeutic effect. The secondary cognitive measures supported the overall group progression rates. No unexpected adverse events were observed. This was the first therapeutic trial to demonstrate an ability to delay the clinical diagnosis of AD using donepezil.

As such, while there are several clinical trials being conducted globally, currently, there are no pharmacological interventions demonstrated to be efficacious in MCI. Nonetheless, as MCI is a rapidly evolving area of investigation, more effective treatment options are likely to be forthcoming.

## ACKNOWLEDGMENTS

The authors would like to thank the superb assistance of Mrs Barbara Willimas, academic and research support service of Mayo Clinic Jacksonville. Preparation of this chapter was supported by KO1 MH68351 and in part by UO1 AG06786.

## REFERENCES

1. Geda YE, Negash S, Petersen RC. Memory disorders. In: Agronin M, Maletta G (eds). *Principles and Practice of Geriatric Psychiatry*, 1st edition. Lippincott Williams & Wilkins, Philadelphia, PA, 2006.
2. Chong MS, Sahadevan S. Preclinical Alzheimer's disease: diagnosis and prediction of progression. *Lancet Neurol* 2005; 4:576–579.
3. Wimo A, Winblad B, Aguero-Torres H, von Strauss E. The magnitude of dementia occurrence in the world. *Alzheimer's Dis Assoc Disord* 2003; 17:63–67.
4. Brookmeyer R, Grey S, Kawas C. Projections of Alzheimer's disease in the United States and the public health impact of delaying disease onset. *Am J Public Health* 1998; 88:1337–1342.
5. Rice DP, Fox PJ, Max W *et al.* The economic burden of Alzheimer's disease care. *Health Aff (Millwood).* 1993; 12:164–176.
6. Petersen RC, Smith GE, Waring SC *et al.* Mild cognitive impairment: clinical characterization and outcome [published erratum appears in *Arch Neurol* 1999 Jun;56(6):760]. *Arch Neurol* 1999; 56:303–308.
7. Petersen RC, Thomas RG, Grundman M *et al.* Vitamin E and donepezil for the treatment of mild cognitive impairment. *N Engl J Med* 2005; 352:2379–2388.
8. Reisberg B, Ferris SH, de Leon MJ, Crook T. The Global Deterioration Scale for assessment of primary degenerative dementia. *Am J Psychiatry* 1982; 139:1136–1139.
9. Flicker C, Ferris S, Reisberg B. Mild cognitive impairment in the elderly: predictors of dementia. *Neurology* 1991; 41:1006–1009.
10. Kral V. Senescent forgetfulness: benign and malignant. *Can Med Assoc J* 1962; 86:257–260.
11. Crook T, Bartus R, Ferris S *et al.* Age-associated memory impairment: Proposed diagnostic criteria and measures of clinical change – Report of a National Institute of Mental Health Work Group. *Dev Neuropsychol* 1986; 2:261–276.
12. Smith G, Ivnik RJ, Petersen RC *et al.* Age-associated memory impairment diagnoses: problems of reliability and concerns for terminology. *Psychol Ageing* 1991; 6:551–558.
13. Levy R. Ageing-associated cognitive decline. *Int Psychogeriatr* 1994; 6:63–68.
14. Blackford R, LaRue A. Criteria for diagnosing age associated memory impairment. *Dev Neuropsychol* 1989; 5:295–306.
15. Graham JE, Rockwood K, Beattie BL *et al.* Prevalence and severity of cognitive impairment with and without dementia in an elderly population. *Lancet* 1997; 349:1793–1796.

16. Devanand D, Folz M, Gorlyn M, Moeller J, Stern Y. Questionable dementia: clinical course and predictors of outcome. *J Am Geriatr Soc* 1997; 45:321–328.
17. Morris J. The Clinical Dementia Rating (CDR): current version and scoring rules [see comments]. *Neurology* 1993; 43:2412–2414.
18. Petersen RC, Stevens JC, Ganguli M *et al.* Practice parameter: early detection of dementia: mild cognitive impairment (an evidence-based review). Report of the Quality Standards Subcommittee of the American Academy of Neurology [see comments]. *Neurology* 2001; 56:1133–1142.
19. Folstein M, Folstein S, McHugh P. 'Mini-Mental State': a practical method for grading the cognitive state of patients for the clinician. *J Psychiat Res* 1975; 12:189–198.
20. Kokmen E, Naessens J, Offord K. A short test of mental status: descripton and preliminary results. *Mayo Clin Proc* 1987; 62:281–288.
21. Winblad B, Palmer K, Kivipelto M *et al.* Mild cognitive impairment – beyond controversies, towards a consensus: report of the International Working Group on Mild Cognitive Impairment. *J Intern Med* 2004; 256:240–246.
22. Ganguli M, Dodge HH, Shen C, DeKosky ST. Mild cognitive impairment, amnestic type: an epidemiologic study. *Neurology* 2004; 63:115–121.
23. Hanninen T, Hallikainen M, Tuomainen S, Vanhanen M, Soininen H. Prevalence of mild cognitive impairment: a population-based study in elderly subjects. *Acta Neurol Scand* 2002; 106:148–154.
24. Bennett DA, Wilson RS, Schneider JA *et al.* Natural history of mild cognitive impairment in older persons. *Neurology* 2002; 59:198–205.
25. DeCarli C. Mild cognitive impairment: prevalence, prognosis, aetiology, and treatment. *Lancet Neurol* 2003; 2:15–21.
26. Larrieu S, Letenneur L, Orgogozo JM *et al.* Incidence and outcome of mild cognitive impairment in a population-based prospective cohort. *Neurology* 2002; 59:1594–1599.
27. Lopez OL, Jagust WJ, DeKosky ST *et al.* Prevalence and classification of mild cognitive impairment in the Cardiovascular Health Study Cognition Study: part 1. *Arch Neurol* 2003; 60:1385–1389.
28. Sackett DL. Bias in analytic research. *J Chronic Dis* 1979; 32:51–63.
29. Fried LP, Borhani NO, Enright P *et al.* The Cardiovascular Health Study: design and rationale. *Ann Epidemiol* 1991; 1:263–276.
30. Kumar R, Dear KB, Christensen H *et al.* Prevalence of mild cognitive impairment in 60- to 64-year-old community-dwelling individuals: the Personality and Total Health through Life 60+ Study. *Dement Geriatr Cogn Disord* 2005; 29:67–74.
31. Tierney M, Szalai J, Snow W *et al.* A prospective study of the clinical utility of APOE genotype in the prediction of outcome in patients with memory impairment. *Neurology* 1996; 46:149–154.
32. Daly E, Zaitchik D, Copeland M *et al.* Predicting conversion to Alzheimer disease using standardized clinical information [see comments]. *Arch Neurol* 2000; 57:675–680.
33. Dawe B, Procter A, Philpot M. Concepts of mild memory impairment in the elderly and their relationship to dementia – a review. *Int J Geriatr Psychiatry* 1992; 7:473–479.
34. Ritchie K, Artero S, Touchon J. Classification criteria for mild cognitive impairment: a population-based validation study. *Neurology* 2001; 56:37–42.
35. Benton A, Hamsher K, Varney NR, Spreen O. *Contributions to Neuropsychological Assessment*. Oxford University Press, New York, NY, 1983.
36. Jack CR Jr, Petersen RC, Xu Y *et al.* Rates of hippocampal atrophy correlate with change in clinical status in ageing and AD. *Neurology* 2000; 55:484–489.
37. Mesulam M-M. From sensation to cognition. *Brain* 1998; 121:1013–1052.
38. Lyketsos CG, Lopez O, Jones B *et al.* Prevalence of neuropsychiatric symptoms in dementia and mild cognitive impairment: results from the cardiovascular health study. *JAMA* 2002; 288:1475–1483.
39. Feldman H, Scheltens P, Scarpini E *et al.* Behavioral symptoms in mild cognitive impairment. *Neurology* 2004; 62:1199–1201.
40. Geda YE, Smith GE, Knopman DS *et al.* De novo genesis of neuropsychiatric symptoms in mild cognitive impairment (MCI). *Intern Psychogeriatr* 2004; 16:51–60.
41. Hwang TJ, Masterman DL, Ortiz F, Fairbanks LA, Cummings JL. Mild cognitive impairment is associated with characteristic neuropsychiatric symptoms. *Alzheimer's Dis Assoc Disord* 2004; 18:17–21.
42. Copeland MP, Daly E, Hines V *et al.* Psychiatric symptomatology and prodromal Alzheimer's disease. *Alzheimer's Dis Assoc Disord* 2003; 17:1–8.
43. Geda YE, Knopman DS, Mrazek DM *et al.* Depression, ApoE genotype, and the incidence of mild cognitive impairment: a prospective cohort study. *Arch Neurol* 2006; 63:435–440.

44. Yesavage JA. Geriatric depression scale. *Psychopharmacol Bull* 1988; 24:709–711.
45. Szklo M, Nieto FJ. *Epidemiology: Beyond the Basics*. Aspen Publishers, Inc., Gaithersburg, MD, 2000.
46. Chertkow H. Mild cognitive impairment. *Curr Opin Neurol* 2002; 15:401–407.
47. Geda YE, Petersen RC. Clinical trials in mild cognitive impairment. In: Gauthier S, Cummings J (eds). *Alzheimer's Disease and Related Disorders*. 2nd edition. Martin Dunitz, London, 2001.

# 24

# Delirium

*E. Sampson*

## INTRODUCTION

Delirium (or acute confusional state) is a syndrome of abrupt onset with a range of varied and fluctuating symptoms including disturbance of consciousness and attention and global impairment of cognition. It is common in older people and the aetiology is often multifactorial. This chapter will review the clinical presentation and epidemiology of delirium before drawing together evidence implicating the cholinergic system in its pathophysiology and discussing the potential benefits of acetylcholinesterase inhibitors for prevention and treatment.

## CLINICAL PRESENTATION

The characteristic feature of delirium is the abrupt onset of global cognitive dysfunction. Typical symptoms fluctuate, with worsening in the early evening and at night when there are fewer external cues available to orientate the patient. Disturbance of consciousness is a key feature; this may range from mild drowsiness to coma. There is reduced ability to focus, sustain or shift attention [1]. There may be lack of awareness of the environment or patients may become hyperalert giving excessive indiscriminate attention to the environment and irrelevant visual stimuli.

Impairment of working and short-term memory is a cardinal feature, but long-term (remote) memory may be relatively well-preserved. This leads to disorientation in time and as severity increases, place and person. Initially, abstract thinking becomes impaired, then thought becomes muddled and disorganized; this is reflected by incoherent speech [2]. Poorly systematized transient delusions occur in a quarter of patients with delirium [3]. These are most commonly paranoid in nature and may be secondary to abnormal perceptions.

The sleep–wake cycle is disturbed with drowsiness during the day and wakefulness at night. In severe cases this may be completely reversed. Patients may experience disturbing dreams and nightmares which persist as hallucinations into wakefulness. In retrospect, many patients describe their experiences as 'dream-like' and some authors believe that delirium should be viewed as a disorder of wakefulness rather than a disorder of consciousness [4].

Visual perceptual disturbances occur in 27–51% of patients experiencing delirium [3, 5]. These range from distortions of normal visual perceptions (micropsia, macropsia and illusions) to florid and detailed visual hallucinations of people and animals. Auditory and tactile hallucinations are also reported but occur less frequently [3]. Emotional lability and changes

**Elizabeth Sampson**, MBChB, MRCPsych, MD, MSc, MRC Research Fellow, Department of Mental Health Sciences, Royal Free and University College Medical School, London, UK

**Table 24.1** DSM-IV diagnostic criteria for delirium*

| |
|---|
| A. Disturbance of consciousness (i.e. reduced clarity of awareness about the environment) with reduced ability to focus, sustain, or shift attention |
| B. A change in cognition (e.g. memory deficit, disorientation, language disturbance) or development of a perceptual disturbance that is not better accounted for by a pre-existing, established, or evolving dementia |
| C. The disturbance develops over a short period of time (usually hours to days) and tends to fluctuate during the course of a day |
| D. Evidence from the history, physical examination, or laboratory findings indicate that the disturbance is caused by direct physiologic consequences of a general medical condition |
| *Reprinted with permission from Diagnostic and Statistical Manual of Mental Disorders: DSM-IV-TR. Washington, DC, American Psychiatric Association, 2000, p 143. Copyright 2000, American Psychiatric Association. |

in mood are also common. These fluctuate and may be accompanied by flattened, fearful or perplexed affect, irritability and depressive symptoms. Up to 42% of acutely ill elderly inpatients thought to have depression actually have delirium [6].

As well as impairment of cognitive processes, behavioural disturbances also occur. Three clinical sub-syndromes of delirium have been described: agitated (hyperactive–hyperalert), somnolent (hypoactive–hypoalert) and mixed [7]. In older hospital inpatients, the hypoactive–hypoalert type is often under diagnosed but occurs in a third of cases [8]. Detection of hypoactive delirium is important as this form is associated with worse outcomes such as an increased risk of developing pressure sores, hospital acquired infections and increased length of hospital admission [9]. The pure hyperactive–hyperalert form is rarer occurring in a fifth of cases. Patients may have purposeless behaviours such as wandering, or display complex stereotypic movements. These symptoms are under-emphasized in diagnostic systems but are difficult to manage. These patients are more at risk of falls and experience more psychotic symptoms [8]. The most common subtype is the mixed form where patients are hypoactive and have periods of agitation, which accounts for 40% of cases [8].

The clinical identification of delirium can be improved by routine cognitive screening and the use of operationalized criteria and diagnostic instruments because these capture patients with this non-psychotic or hypoactive delirium[10]. The DSM-IV criteria for delirium are widely used in diagnosis and research [1] (Table 24.1). The Confusion Assessment Method (CAM), which is based on the DSM-IV criteria, has high sensitivity (90–95%), specificity of (94–100%) and good inter-rater reliability [11].

## EPIDEMIOLOGY

The prevalence of delirium varies widely, depending on the clinical setting. It is frequently under-diagnosed and 33–66% of cases are missed, often those with the hypoactive/hypoalert subtype [12]. Table 24.2 gives examples of the prevalence of delirium in a range of populations. It is of note that people with pre-existing dementia appear to be particularly vulnerable [13, 14], as are those undergoing surgical procedures.

The aetiology of delirium is usually complex and multifactorial with 2–6 factors identified per person [15]. These risk factors combine to have a multiplicative rather than additive effect on the risk of developing delirium [16]. The development of delirium is also very dependent on baseline risk. If this is low then precipitating factors may not be enough to cause delirium. If baseline risk is high, as is the case with people with dementia, then even minor exposures will precipitate a delirium episode [17]. Pre-disposing factors increasing this baseline risk of delirium include age, (being over 80 years increases the odds ratio [OR] of developing

**Table 24.2** Prevalence of delirium in a range of populations

| *Population studied* | *Prevalence of delirium* |
|---|---|
| Community sample [97] | 13.6% (over 85 years) |
| Nursing homes [98] | 58% |
| Emergency department [99] | 41% |
| Acute hospital wards [100] | 10–40% |
| People with dementia living in the community [101, 102] | 22–25% |
| Hospitalized people with dementia [13] | 56% |
| Hospitalized people with dementia admitted from the emergency department [14] | 76% |
| Post-operative elective abdominal aortic aneurysm repair [103] | 33% |
| Post-operative coronary artery bypass grafting [104] | 42% |
| Post-operative emergency total hip replacement [105] | 55% |

delirium by 5.2) [18], dementia (OR 5.2), medical comorbidity (OR 3.8) male gender (OR 1.9), alcohol abuse (OR 3.3) hearing (OR 1.9) and visual impairment (OR 1.7) [19].

These risk factors then interact with a wide range of precipitants. In the elderly, infection, alcohol withdrawal [20], metabolic disturbance (i.e. hypoxia, hypoglycaemia, renal or hepatic failure), dehydration, hypoalbuminaemia [19] and general anaesthesia [21] are most commonly cited. Medications, particularly those with anti-cholinergic properties, are implicated in 20–40% of delirium cases [22]. Commonly prescribed drugs with direct anti-cholinergic effects include prochlorperazine, oxybutinin, hyoscine and atropine [23]. Other drugs such as thioridazine, chlorpromazine, diphenhydramine and amitriptyline have anti-cholinergic side-effects and are frequently prescribed in the elderly [24].

## THE ASSOCIATION BETWEEN DELIRIUM AND DEMENTIA

Dementia is strongly implicated as a risk factor for delirium [19, 13] and a systematic review has found that delirium superimposed on dementia occurred in 22–89% of community and hospital populations over the age of 65 with dementia [25]. Delirium occurring in people with dementia is under-recognized [25], possibly because people with dementia are more likely to have the hypoactive/hypoalert form [26]. Many studies have also found that delirium is associated with an increased risk for the subsequent development of dementia. It is not clear whether delirium 'unmasks' a pre-existing dementia [25] or whether delirium precipitates cognitive decline and the development of dementia. One study found a trend for greater cognitive impairment being associated with longer duration of delirium [27], but there is a lack of prospective studies in this field and therefore it has been difficult to establish the direction of causality of these associations. Clinically the presentation of delirium in the setting of concurrent dementia is very similar to delirium without dementia [28].

## COURSE AND OUTCOMES

The symptoms of delirium frequently persist beyond the acute phase; in half of cases this may be for a year after onset. Impairment of attention and orientation appear to be particularly persistent [29–31]. The prognosis is worse if the delirium is undetected [32] and hyper active delirium has a better outcome than the hypoactive form which is associated with an increased risk of developing pressure sores, hospital acquired infections [8] and increased length of hospital admission [33]. Delirium inflates the cost of hospital care and cases have a higher risk of subsequent nursing home placement [34, 35]. The risk of in-hospital mortality and subsequent death for the 12 months following discharge is also raised. This shows a dose–response relationship with more severe delirium leading to a higher risk of mortality at 1 year [36].

## THE NEUROPHYSIOLOGICAL BASIS OF DELIRIUM – THE ROLE OF THE CHOLINERGIC SYSTEM

The range of symptoms associated with delirium suggests that there is widespread disruption of neural pathways and transmitter systems. This is reflected by the EEG, which shows abnormal generalized diffuse slowing of background activity in 80–90% of patients with delirium [37]. Many neurotransmitters have been implicated in the genesis of delirium. Dopamine excess can cause delirium and psychosis [38] and the dopaminergic and cholinergic systems interact reciprocally; excess of dopamine may result in a hypocholinergic state [39]. The dopaminergic and cholinergic systems modulate and interact *via* the cortex, striatum and thalamus with glutaminergic, GABA (γ-aminobutyric acid) and serotonergic systems (for a comprehensive review of these complex pathways, see [40]). There is consistent evidence that the cholinergic system acts a final common pathway downstream from alterations in other neurotransmitters and disruption of the cholinergic pathway has a pivotal role in the development of delirium.

It is also possible to measure peripheral acetylcholine activity. Since the early 1980s, a radio receptor assay has been available to quantify a person's overall anti-cholinergic burden caused by endogenous substances, drugs and their metabolites – referred to as serum anti-cholinergic activity or serum anti-cholinergicity (SA) [41, 42]. This has been shown to correlate with the measurable anti-cholinergic effects of specific drugs [43, 44]. SA has consistently been shown to be associated with cognitive impairment [23] or frank delirium in older patients [45, 46]. Many of the characteristic symptoms of delirium have been associated with specific brain regions and disruption of the cholinergic system that innervates them.

Acetylcholine plays a critical role in attentional processing. Attention has been defined as 'the ability to maintain a coherent line of thought or action' [47]. Attentional deficits are important as they will impair performance in all other domains of cognitive functioning. Two neural networks have been recognized as mediating attentional function, a diffuse system comprising the thalamus and cerebral hemispheres and a more localized system located in the right hemisphere. The diffuse system maintains a baseline level of attention and monitors internal and external sensory events. Important areas of this system include the white-matter tracts connecting the thalamus with the cortex and the frontal lobes which have a specific role in selective and sustained attention. The right hemisphere localized system narrows the focus of attention to focal spatial stimuli. It is localized in the posterior parietal cortex (sensory surveillance and stimulus selection), dorsolateral pre-frontal cortex including the frontal eye fields and the anterior cingulate gyrus (maintaining motivation and effort) [48]. Disruption of this system in delirium has been demonstrated by imaging [49] and EEG [50] studies. Scopolamine, a muscarinic receptor antagonist causes deficits in attention, learning and memory [51, 52]. Nicotine improves performance, particularly on attentional tasks, possibly by activating nicotinic acetylcholine receptors in the pre-frontal cortex [53]. Acetylcholine has a role in neuromodulation, increasing the 'signal to noise' ratio improving the discrimination of and responsiveness to incoming stimuli thus enhancing attentional processes [54].

The brain areas thought to be the neural correlates of consciousness are principally integrated by the intralaminar nuclei of the thalamus. These receive inputs from the brain stem, mainly the reticular formation, the cingulate cortex, and midbrain structures such as the superior colliculus. The intralaminar nuclei then provide diffuse thalamocorticol projections that spread neuronal activity across many brain areas [55]. The dorsal thalamus is thought to generate the synchronized oscillatory activity generated by the brain and altered states of consciousness such as delirium are reflected by characteristic changes in the EEG [56]. The thalamus is vital in non-selective attention and general corticol arousal which is a cholinergic function mediated through nicotinic and muscarinic M2 receptors. The majority of brainstem projections to the thalamus are cholinergic suggesting that the cholinergic system has an important role in conscious awareness [57, 58].

The hippocampus, cingulate cortex, amygdala and neocortex receive cholinergic innervation from the basal forebrain (Nucleus Basalis of Meynert). Lesions of the cholinergic pathways leading to the hippocampus have significant effects on learning and memory as demonstrated in animal models [59] and by the degeneration of the basal cholinergic system that occurs in Alzheimer's disease [60] where impairment of episodic memory is a major clinical feature [61]. Scopolamine, a muscarinic receptor antagonist induces amnesia in young healthy subjects which is similar to that seen in older subjects [62] or in patients with Alzheimer's disease [63].

The psychotic and behavioural symptoms that occur in delirium may also be associated with disturbance in the cholinergic system. Some authors have described Lewy body dementia as a prolonged delirious state; the fluctuating course, delusions and hallucinations, and abnormalities of the sleep–wake cycle are similar to some of the core clinical features of delirium [64]. In dementia with Lewy Bodies (DLB) there is a profound deficit of neocorticol cholinergic activity [65]. Hallucinations can be induced by cholinergic antagonists acting on muscarinic receptors [56]. Specifically visual hallucinations and delusional misidentification may be associated with lower $\alpha_7$ nicotinic receptor binding in the temporal cortex of individuals with DLB [66]. This supports previous work linking hallucinations to cholinergic deficits in DLB patients and patients with schizophrenia who under-express the $\alpha7$ nicotinic receptor gene [67]. Reduced cholinergic activity in Alzheimer's disease patients has also been associated with some behavioural disturbances including motor over-activity [68].

The final common pathway through which infection, toxins and metabolic disturbances lead to the disruption of neurotransmission and the cholinergic deficit of delirium has not been clearly elucidated. Endogenous cytokines are released from cells following an inflammatory insult and may be involved in the pathogenesis of delirium. Following systemic infection, cytokines generated by the systemic inflammatory response signal across the blood–brain barrier to generate cytokines in the brain [69]. This has an amplifying effect, activating microglia which then synthesize further pro-inflammatory cytokines [70]. Raised levels of cytokines are associated with other common causes of delirium such as infection, and cardiac failure [71]. Cytokines such as interleukin-2 can precipitate delirium in patients undergoing treatment for cancer [72]. Insulin-like growth factor (IGF)-I and IGF-II are potent modulators of acetylcholine release, IGF-I inhibiting release while IGF-II is a potent stimulant [73]. The primary deficit in delirium may be associated with a lack of protective cytokines such as IGF-I which inhibits cytotoxic cytokines and low levels of IGF-I are a risk factor for delirium [74]. Animal studies have demonstrated that cytokines are associated with reduced acetylcholine activity similar to that observed in delirium [75]. Some therapeutic efficacy for IGF-I has been demonstrated in animal models [76] and in the future, cytokines may have a role in the prevention and treatment of delirium in humans [77].

## THE CLINICAL MANAGEMENT OF DELIRIUM

To date, the management of delirium has focused on early identification and treatment of the underlying cause, environmental modifications (i.e. a well lit, quiet environment), and good nursing care (reassurance, reorientation to time and place, consistency of staff and the presence of a relative [20, 78]. Pharmacological interventions may become necessary if the patient is severely disturbed or distressed, or if their behavioural and psychiatric symptoms become dangerous to others. The most commonly used agents are the typical anti-psychotics such as haloperidol or droperidol. Their mode of action is thought to be *via* blockade of $D_2$ receptors which reciprocally increases acetylcholine release [38]. These are effective in both hyper and hypoactive delirium [79, 80] but must be used with caution as older people are at high risk of developing extra-pyramidal side-effects. Atypical anti-psychotics such as risperidone and olanzapine may be effective and have a preferable side-effect profile [81, 82] but there is no randomized controlled trial evidence for their efficacy compared to placebo for patients with delirium. Benzodiazepines may be useful in delirium caused by alcohol or benzodiazepine withdrawal, or in severely agitated patients who are unable to tolerate typical anti-psychotics [20]. Their mode of action is primarily one of sedation.

The use of neuroleptics and sedatives may complicate the ongoing assessment of the patient's mental state, impairs the patient's ability to understand and cooperate with treatment and increases the risk of falls. These strategies, however, only relieve the symptoms of delirium and have little impact on prevention or treatment of the underlying cholinergic deficit. Low-dose haloperidol prophylactic treatment demonstrates no efficacy in reducing the incidence of postoperative delirium [83]. A meta-analysis found that, on average, non-pharmacological interventions reduce the absolute risk of delirium by only 13% [84]. Therefore, given the morbidity and mortality associated with delirium, other preventative and treatment strategies are urgently required.

## THE ROLE OF CHOLINESTERASE INHIBITORS FOR THE TREATMENT OF DELIRIUM

Cholinergic systems are involved in cognition, arousal and sensory gating. Deficits of cholinergic transmission have been demonstrated in delirium and therefore cholinergic stimulation may be a target for intervention with a view to reducing both the incidence and severity of delirium. Cholinesterase inhibitors such as donepezil (DPZ) are of proven efficacy in the treatment of moderately severe Alzheimer's disease [85].Through inhibition of the metabolic enzyme acetylcholinesterase, DPZ increases the synaptic availability of acetylcholine. The mechanism through which cholinesterase inhibitors may treat delirium is multifactorial and it is likely that they would act on a variety of symptoms associated with this cholinergic deficit. They have been shown to improve working memory in cognitively intact subjects [86] probably by enhancing attention and concentration [87] (both of which are severely impaired in delirium). DLB shares core clinical features such as hallucinations and fluctuating level of confusion with delirium. Rivastigmine has been demonstrated to improve visual hallucinations [88] and sleep pattern [89] in DLB suggesting that it may improve similar symptoms seen in delirium.

The evidence base for the use of cholinesterase inhibitors in delirium has developed from a number of single patient case reports (Table 24.3). DPZ is the most commonly used compound followed by rivastigmine. Single patient studies suggest that cholinesterase inhibitors are effective in treating delirium caused by a variety of aetiologies including opioid, lithium and anti-cholinergic drug intoxication, haemorrhagic cerebral infarct, and post-operative delirium. It is of note that they may be of particular benefit in treating delirium in patients with underlying dementia. These case reports are promising but liable to publication bias.

There have been two retrospective case note studies examining the efficacy of rivastigmine in preventing and treating delirium in patients over the age of 60 years admitted with acute medical or surgical disease to a general hospital. Eleven patients who were 'chronic' users of rivastigmine were compared to randomly selected controls who did not take the drug. In the group that used rivastigmine 45% developed delirium compared to 89% in the control group [90]. The authors concluded that chronic rivastigmine use may have a preventative effect on the development of delirium but this was a small sample size with limited recording and analysis of potential confounders such as concomitant psychotropic drug use. The second study examined the efficacy of rivastigmine in treating patients with chronic delirium who have not responded to anti-psychotics. The authors reported that 71%

**Table 24.3** Search of the English language literature: cholinesterase inhibitors for the treatment of delirium

| *Title* | *Methodology* | *Intervention* | *Findings* |
|---|---|---|---|
| *Systematic review/meta-analysis* | | | |
| Cholinesterase inhibitors for delirium [101] | Cochrane protocol | Cholinesterase inhibitors | Work in progress |
| *RCTs* | | | |
| Donepezil in the prevention and treatment of post-surgical delirium [100] | Double-blind placebo-controlled randomized trial, 40 in each arm | Donepezil | No effect demonstrated |
| Donepezil hydrochloride for reducing symptoms of post-operative delirium (Sampson *et al.*, unpublished) | Double-blind placebo-controlled randomized trial (19 on DPZ, 14 on placebo) | Donepezil | No effect demonstrated |
| *Open-label studies* | | | |
| Delirium in vascular dementia [99] | Controlled open 24-month study of 246 patients | Rivastigmine | 40% on rivastigmine had delirium compared to 62% on aspirin. Duration of delirium was shorter in rivastigmine group |
| *Retrospective case note studies* | | | |
| Adding rivastigmine to anti-psychotics in the treatment of chronic delirium [98] | 21 patients with chronic delirium given rivastigmine compared to those not given rivastigmine | Rivastigmine | 71.4% of those given rivastigmine recovered, no information available on recovery in the control group |
| Delirium in elderly hospitalized patients: protective effect of chronic rivastigmine usage [97] | Retrospective cohort study of patients with dementia admitted to acute hospital | Rivastigmine | 45% of those on rivastigmine developed delirium compared to 89% in the control group |
| *Case reports* | | | |
| Treatment of opioid-induced delirium with Ach inhibitors [106] | 1 patient with terminal illness | Physostigmine iv then donepezil | 'Dramatic improvement' in clinical condition |
| Donepezil for anti-cholinergic drug intoxication [107] | 1 patient who took an amitriptyline o.d. | Donepezil | 'Dramatic response' |
| Rivastigmine in prevention of delirium in a 65-year-old man with Parkinson's disease [108] | 1 patient with Parkinson's disease | Rivastigmine | Successful treatment of two delirious episodes |

**Table 24.3** (Continued)

| | | | |
|---|---|---|---|
| Donepezil improves symptoms of delirium in dementia [109] | 1 patient with dementia | Donepezil | Delirium 'resolved rapidly' |
| Severe delirium due to basal forebrain vascular lesion and efficacy of donepezil [110] | 1 patient with haemorrhagic infarct | Donepezil | Resolution of delirium |
| Treatment of typical Charles Bonnet syndrome with donepezil [111] | 1 patient with complex visual hallucinations | Donepezil | Improvement of hallucinations |
| Donepezil-responsive alcohol related prolonged delirium [112] | 2 patients | Donepezil | Both patients showed a marked improvement |
| Donepezil for postoperative delirium | 1 patient post hip arthroplasty | Donepezil | Improved after 2 days |
| Successful treatment of non-anti-cholinergic delirium with a cholinesterase inhibitor [113] | 1 patient with bipolar affective disorder and lithium toxicity | Rivastigmine | Clinical improvement |
| Donepezil for postoperative delirium associated with Alzheimer's disease [114] | 1 post-operative patient | Donepezil | Delirium resolved |

of those patients given rivastigmine 'improved' but acknowledge that there were considerable methodological problems with their retrospective study [91].

The open-label study by Moretti *et al.* [92] involved 246 patients with probable vascular dementia as defined by the National Institute of Neurological Disorders and Stroke–Association Internationale pour la Recherche et L'Enseignement en Neuroscience (NINDS-AIREN) criteria. Patients were divided into two groups (matched on age, level of education, concomitant medication and medical morbidity) and given rivastigmine titrated up to a dose of 6 mg per day or aspirin 100 mg once daily for 24 months. Of those on rivastigmine, 40% presented with at least one episode of delirium, as diagnosed on the CAM, compared to 62% of those taking aspirin (this difference was reported to be significant at the $P < 0.001$ level). The mean duration of delirium was shorter in those taking rivastigmine (4 days vs. 8 days for those on aspirin; $P < 0.01$). This study showed promising results for cholinesterase inhibitors in the prevention of delirium but the authors were not blind to the treatment group allocation and thus there is the possibility of significant bias in the results. No information is given regarding adverse events or tolerability.

Liptzin *et al.* [93] have published a randomized double-blind, placebo-controlled pilot study of DPZ for the prevention and treatment of post-surgical delirium. There were 39 subjects in the DPZ group and 41 in the placebo group. The mean age of the cohort was 67 years. Subjects were given the trial medication for 14 days before surgery and 14 days post-operatively. The authors found no significant differences between the placebo and DPZ groups in terms of the occurrence or duration of delirium as diagnosed using the DSM-IV criteria. However, only 58 patients completed the full study and adherence to the study medication was poor. The drug was well-tolerated and side-effect rates were comparable between the two groups.

Another pilot randomized double-blind, placebo-controlled trial of DPZ for the prevention of postoperative delirium has been completed on a cohort of 31 patients undergoing elective total hip replacement surgery (Sampson *et al.*, submitted for publication). Subjects received 5 mg of DPZ daily for four days after surgery. The mean age of patients in this cohort was 68 years and there were 19 subjects in the DPZ group and 14 in the placebo group. The drug was well-tolerated with no serious adverse events. The authors found no significant effect for DPZ on the incidence or severity of delirium. Again, it is likely that this study was underpowered and the authors estimated from their results that a sample size of 104 per arm would be required per treatment arm to achieve 99% power in a similar patient population.

This research is in an early phase but there is a developing evidence base for the use of cholinesterase inhibitors for the prevention of delirium, particularly in patients undergoing elective orthopaedic surgery. It is likely that both of the double-blind, randomized placebo-controlled trials were underpowered to demonstrate a preventative effect for DPZ and methodological issues may need to be refined before a definitive trial is completed. In particular it is not clear what the optimum dose should be, whether treatment should start pre, peri or postoperatively and how long the cholinesterase inhibitor should be continued after surgery.

Both of these trials used subjects undergoing elective surgery and may be biased towards healthier populations. These patients (who were relatively young) have a much lower baseline risk of developing delirium compared to frail older people with multiple medical problems who are more likely to develop delirium and subsequently suffer greater adverse consequences. These trials excluded people with pre-existing dementia who are known to be at higher risk of delirium. There is no randomized double-blind, placebo-controlled data currently available on the use of cholinesterase inhibitors for the treatment of acute delirium. Although this population may derive the greatest benefit from such a treatment, these studies present significant logistical challenges in terms of ethical and methodological complexity, particularly regarding the issues surrounding informed consent. A systematic review is currently in progress and aims to assess both the efficacy and safety of cholinesterase inhibitors for delirium. Outcomes under investigation will include the length of delirium and hospital stay, behavioural disturbance and mortality [94].

## SUMMARY

Delirium is a common problem with a multitude of causes; however, the symptomatology suggests that the syndrome is underpinned by a profound cholinergic deficit. Delirium has serious sequelae, increasing the length of hospital stay and leading to complications such as pressure sores, functional deterioration, increased risk of subsequent dementia and mortality. The development and widespread use of cholinesterase inhibitors for the treatment of dementia has prompted interest in their use for the prevention and treatment of delirium.

Delirium is a marker for severe medical illness [95]. Inouye *et al.* [96] have noted that delirium may serve as a 'window' to the hospital care of elderly patients as it is frequently iatrogenic, closely linked with the process of care and as such serves as a useful outcome measure of quality of care. It is hoped that now there is the possibility of a treatment which is specifically targeted at the underlying neurochemical deficit, clinicians will become less nihilistic about the condition and more active in seeking and treating it.

## REFERENCES


1. American Psychiatric Association. *Diagnostic Statistical Manual of Mental Disorders*, 4th edition, text revision ed. American Psychiatric Association, Washington, DC, 1994.
2. Burns A, Gallagley A, Byrne J. Delirium. *J Neurol Neurosurg Psychiatry* 2004; 75:362–367.
3. Webster R, Holroyd S. Prevalence of psychotic symptoms in delirium. *Psychosomatics* 2000; 41:519–522.
4. Fleminger S. Remembering delirium. *Br J Psychiatry* 2002; 180:4–5.
5. Cutting J. The phenomenology of acute organic psychosis. Comparison with acute schizophrenia. *Br J Psychiatry* 1987; 151:324–332.
6. Farrell KR, Ganzini L. Misdiagnosing delirium as depression in medically ill elderly patients. *Arch Intern Med* 1995; 155:2459–2464.
7. Lipowski ZJ. *Delirium: Acute Confusional States*. Oxford University Press, New York, 1990.
8. O'Keeffe ST. Clinical subtypes of delirium in the elderly. *Dement Geriatr Cogn Disord* 1999; 10:380–385.
9. Levkoff SE, Evans DA, Liptzin B *et al.* Delirium. The occurrence and persistence of symptoms among elderly hospitalized patients. *Arch Intern Med* 1992; 152:334–340.
10. Camus V, Burtin B, Simeone I, Schwed P, Gonthier R, Dubos G. Factor analysis supports the evidence of existing hyperactive and hypoactive subtypes of delirium. *Int J Geriatr Psychiatry* 2000; 15:313–316.
11. Inouye SK, van Dyck CH, Alessi CA, Balkin S, Siegal AP, Horwitz RI. Clarifying confusion: the confusion assessment method. A new method for detection of delirium. *Ann Intern Med* 1990; 113:941–948.
12. Inouye SK. The dilemma of delirium: clinical and research controversies regarding diagnosis and evaluation of delirium in hospitalized elderly medical patients. *Am J Med* 1994; 97:278–288.
13. Rockwood K, Cosway S, Carver D, Jarrett P, Stadnyk K. The risk of dementia and death after delirium. *Age Ageing* 1999; 28:551–556.
14. McCusker J, Cole M, Dendukuri N, Belzile E, Primeau F. Delirium in older medical inpatients and subsequent cognitive and functional status: a prospective study. *Can Med Assoc J* 2001; 165:575–583.
15. Pompei P, Foreman M, Rudberg MA, Inouye SK, Braund V, Cassel CK. Delirium in hospitalized older persons: outcomes and predictors. *J Am Geriatr Soc* 1994; 42:809–815.
16. Inouye SK. Predisposing and precipitating factors for delirium in hospitalized older patients. *Dement Geriatr Cogn Disord* 1999; 10:393–400.
17. Inouye SK, Charpentier PA. Precipitating factors for delirium in hospitalized elderly persons. Predictive model and interrelationship with baseline vulnerability. *JAMA* 1996; 275:852–857.
18. Schor JD, Levkoff SE, Lipsitz LA *et al.* Risk factors for delirium in hospitalized elderly. *JAMA* 1992; 267:827–831.
19. Elie M, Cole MG, Primeau FJ, Bellavance F. Delirium risk factors in elderly hospitalized patients. *J Gen Intern Med* 1998; 13:204–212.

20. Meagher DJ. Delirium: optimizing management. *BMJ* 2001; 322:144–149.
21. Moller JT, Cluitmans P, Rasmussen LS *et al.* Long-term postoperative cognitive dysfunction in the elderly ISPOCD1 study. ISPOCD investigators. International Study of Post-Operative Cognitive Dysfunction. *Lancet* 1998; 351:857–861.
22. Tune L, Carr S, Hoag E, Cooper T. Anticholinergic effects of drugs commonly prescribed for the elderly: potential means for assessing risk of delirium. *Am J Psychiatry* 1992; 149:1393–1394.
23. Mintzer J, Burns A. Anticholinergic side-effects of drugs in elderly people. *J R Soc Med* 2000; 93:457–462.
24. Blazer DG, Federspiel CF, Ray WA, Schaffner W. The risk of anticholinergic toxicity in the elderly: a study of prescribing practices in two populations. *J Gerontol* 1983; 38:31–35.
25. Fick DM, Agostini JV, Inouye SK. Delirium superimposed on dementia: a systematic review. *J Am Geriatr Soc* 2002; 50:1723–1732.
26. Sandberg O, Gustafson Y, Brannstrom B, Bucht G. Clinical profile of delirium in older patients. *J Am Geriatr Soc* 1999; 47:1300–1306.
27. Jackson JC, Hart RP, Gordon SM *et al.* Six-month neuropsychological outcome of medical intensive care unit patients. *Crit Care Med* 2003; 31:1226–1234.
28. Trzepacz PT, Mulsant BH, Amanda DM, Pasternak R, Sweet RA, Zubenko GS. Is delirium different when it occurs in dementia? A study using the delirium rating scale. *J Neuropsychiatry Clin Neurosci* 1998; 10:199–204.
29. Rockwood K. The occurrence and duration of symptoms in elderly patients with delirium. *J Gerontol* 1993; 48:M162–M166.
30. McCusker J, Cole MG, Dendukuri N, Belzile E. Does delirium increase hospital stay? *J Am Geriatr Soc* 2003; 51:1539–1546.
31. Levkoff SE, Marcantonio ER. Delirium: a major diagnostic and therapeutic challenge for clinicians caring for the elderly. *Compr Ther* 1994; 20:550–557.
32. Rockwood K, Cosway S, Stolee P *et al.* Increasing the recognition of delirium in elderly patients. *J Am Geriatr Soc* 1994; 42:252–256.
33. Liptzin B, Levkoff SE. An empirical study of delirium subtypes. *Br J Psychiatry* 1992; 161:843–845.
34. Cole MG, Primeau FJ. Prognosis of delirium in elderly hospital patients. *Can Med Assoc J* 1993; 149:41–46.
35. Inouye SK, Rushing JT, Foreman MD, Palmer RM, Pompei P. Does delirium contribute to poor hospital outcomes? A three-site epidemiologic study. *J Gen Intern Med* 1998; 13:234–242.
36. Leslie DL, Zhang Y, Holford TR, Bogardus ST, Leo-Summers LS, Inouye SK. Premature death associated with delirium at 1-year follow-up. *Arch Int Med* 2005; 165:1657–1662.
37. Jacobson S, Jerrier H. EEG in delirium. *Semin Clin Neuropsychiatry* 2000; 5:86–92.
38. Trzepacz PT. Update on the neuropathogenesis of delirium. *Dement Geriatr Cogn Disord* 1999; 10:330–334.
39. Trzepacz PT. Is there a final common neural pathway in delirium? Focus on acetylcholine and dopamine. *Semin Clin Neuropsychiatry* 2000; 5:132–148.
40. Gaudreau JD, Gagnon P. Psychotogenic drugs and delirium pathogenesis: the central role of the thalamus. *Med Hypotheses* 2005; 64:471–475.
41. Tune L, Coyle JT. Serum levels of anticholinergic drugs in treatment of acute extrapyramidal side effects. *Arch Gen Psychiatry* 1980; 37:293–297.
42. Tune LE, Damlouji NF, Holland A, Gardner TJ, Folstein MF, Coyle JT. Association of postoperative delirium with raised serum levels of anticholinergic drugs. *Lancet* 1981; 2:651–653.
43. Tune LE, Egeli S. Acetylcholine and delirium. *Dement Geriatr Cogn Disord* 1999; 10:342–344.
44. Thienhaus OJ, Thoene J, Allen A, Zemlan FP. Plasma anticholinergic activity and cognitive function in geriatric patients. *Psychiatry Neurol Med Psychol (Leipz)* 1990; 42:275–281.
45. Rovner BW, David A, Lucas-Blaustein MJ, Conklin B, Filipp L, Tune L. Self-care capacity and anticholinergic drug levels in nursing home patients. *Am J Psychiatry* 1988; 145:107–109.
46. Tune L, Brandt J, Frost JJ *et al.* Physostigmine in Alzheimer's disease: effects on cognitive functioning, cerebral glucose metabolism analyzed by positron emission tomography and cerebral blood flow analyzed by single photon emission tomography. *Acta Psychiatr Scand Suppl* 1991; 366:61–65.
47. Geschwind N. Disorders of attention: a frontier in neuropsychology. *Philos Trans R Soc Lond B Biol Sci* 1982; 298:173–185.
48. Posner MI, Dehaene S. Attentional networks. *Trends Neurosci* 1994; 17:75–79.
49. Doyle M, Warden D. Use of SPECT to evaluate postcardiotomy delirium. *Am J Psychiatry* 1996; 153:838–839.

50. Reischies FM, Neuhaus AH, Hansen ML, Mientus S, Mullert C, Gallinat J. Electrophysiological and neuropsychological analysis of a delirious state: the role of the anterior cingulate gyrus. *Psychiatry Res* 2005; 138:171–181.
51. Dunne MP, Hartley LR. Scopolamine and the control of attention in humans. *Psychopharmacology* 1986; 89:94–97.
52. Warburton DM, Rusted JM. Cholinergic control of cognitive resources. *Neuropsychobiology* 1993; 28:43–46.
53. Mansvelder HD, van Aerde KI, Couey JJ, Brussaard AB. Nicotinic modulation of neuronal networks: from receptors to cognition. *Psychopharmacology (Berl)* 2006; 184:292–305.
54. Muir JL. Attention and stimulus processing in the rat. *Brain Res Cogn Brain Res* 1996; 3:215–225.
55. Jones EG. Viewpoint: the core and matrix of thalamic organization. *Neuroscience* 1998; 85:331–345.
56. Perry EK, Perry RH. Acetylcholine and hallucinations: disease-related compared to drug-induced alterations in human consciousness. *Brain Cogn* 1995; 28:240–258.
57. Perry E, Walker M, Grace J, Perry R. Acetylcholine in mind: a neurotransmitter correlate of consciousness? *Trends Neurosci* 1999; 22:273–280.
58. Ballard CG, Court JA, Piggott M *et al*. Disturbances of consciousness in dementia with Lewy bodies associated with alteration in nicotinic receptor binding in the temporal cortex. *Conscious Cogn* 2002; 11:461–474.
59. Hagan JJ, Salamone JD, Simpson J, Iversen SD, Morris RG. Place navigation in rats is impaired by lesions of medial septum and diagonal band but not nucleus basalis magnocellularis. *Behav Brain Res* 1988; 27:9–20.
60. Perry EK, Perry RH, Blessed G, Tomlinson BE. Changes in brain cholinesterases in senile dementia of Alzheimer type. *Neuropathol Appl Neurobiol* 1978; 4:273–277.
61. Muir JL. Acetylcholine, aging, and Alzheimer's disease. *Pharmacol Biochem Behav* 1997; 56:687–696.
62. Drachman DA, Leavitt J. Human memory and the cholinergic system. A relationship to aging? *Arch Neurol* 1974; 30:113–121.
63. Koller G, Satzger W, Adam M *et al*. Effects of scopolamine on matching to sample paradigm and related tests in human subjects. *Neuropsychobiol* 2003; 48:87–94.
64. Kaufer DI, Catt KE, Lopez OL, DeKosky ST. Dementia with Lewy bodies: response of delirium-like features to donepezil. *Neurology* 1998; 51:1512.
65. Perry EK, Haroutunian V, Davis KL *et al*. Neocortical cholinergic activities differentiate Lewy body dementia from classical Alzheimer's disease. *Neuroreport* 1994; 5:747–749.
66. Court JA, Ballard CG, Piggott MA *et al*. Visual hallucinations are associated with lower alpha bungarotoxin binding in dementia with Lewy bodies. *Pharmacol Biochem Behav* 2001; 70:571–579.
67. Freedman R, Olincy A, Ross RG *et al*. The genetics of sensory gating deficits in schizophrenia. *Curr Psychiatry Rep* 2003; 5:155–161.
68. Minger SL, Esiri MM, McDonald B *et al*. Cholinergic deficits contribute to behavioral disturbance in patients with dementia. *Neurology* 2000; 55:1460–1467.
69. Holmes C, El Okl M, Williams AL, Cunningham C, Wilcockson D, Perry VH. Systemic infection, interleukin 1beta, and cognitive decline in Alzheimer's disease. *J Neurol Neurosurg Psychiatry* 2003; 74:788–789.
70. Konsman JP, Parnet P, Dantzer R. Cytokine-induced sickness behaviour: mechanisms and implications. *Trends Neurosci* 2002; 25:154–159.
71. Niebauer J, Volk HD, Kemp M *et al*. Endotoxin and immune activation in chronic heart failure: a prospective cohort study. *Lancet* 1999; 353:1838–1842.
72. Rosenberg SA, Lotze MT, Yang JC *et al*. Experience with the use of high-dose interleukin-2 in the treatment of 652 cancer patients. *Ann Surg* 1989; 210:474–484.
73. Kar S, Seto D, Dore S, Hanisch U, Quirion R. Insulin-like growth factors-I and -II differentially regulate endogenous acetylcholine release from the rat hippocampal formation. *Proc Natl Acad Sci USA* 1997; 94:14054–14059.
74. Wilson K, Broadhurst C, Diver M, Jackson M, Mottram P. Plasma insulin growth factor-1 and incident delirium in older people. *Int J Geriatr Psychiatry* 2005; 20:154–159.
75. Seto D, Zheng WH, McNicoll A, Collier B, Quirion R, Kar S. Insulin-like growth factor-I inhibits endogenous acetylcholine release from the rat hippocampal formation: possible involvement of GABA in mediating the effects. *Neuroscience* 2002; 115:603–612.

76. Saatman KE, Contreras PC, Smith DH *et al.* Insulin-like growth factor-1 (IGF-1) improves both neurological motor and cognitive outcome following experimental brain injury. *Exp Neurol* 1997; 147:418–427.
77. Broadhurst C, Wilson K. Immunology of delirium: new opportunities for treatment and research. *Br J Psychiatry* 2001; 179:288–289.
78. Schofield I. A small exploratory study of the reaction of older people to an episode of delirium. *J Adv Nurs* 1997; 25:942–952.
79. Breitbart W, Marotta R, Platt MM *et al.* A double-blind trial of haloperidol, chlorpromazine, and lorazepam in the treatment of delirium in hospitalized AIDS patients. *Am J Psychiatry* 1996; 153:231–237.
80. Platt MM, Breitbart W, Smith M, Marotta R, Weisman H, Jacobsen PB. Efficacy of neuroleptics for hypoactive delirium. *J Neuropsychiatry Clin Neurosci* 1994; 6:66–67.
81. Skrobik YK, Bergeron N, Dumont M, Gottfried SB. Olanzapine vs haloperidol: treating delirium in a critical care setting. *Intensive Care Med* 2004; 30:444–449.
82. Breitbart W, Tremblay A, Gibson C. An open trial of olanzapine for the treatment of delirium in hospitalized cancer patients. *Psychosomatics* 2002; 43:175–182.
83. Kalisvaart KJ, de Jonghe JF, Bogaards MJ *et al.* Haloperidol prophylaxis for elderly hip-surgery patients at risk for delirium: a randomized placebo-controlled study. *J Am Geriatr Soc* 2005; 53:1658–1666.
84. Cole MG, Primeau F, McCusker J. Effectiveness of interventions to prevent delirium in hospitalized patients: a systematic review. *Can Med Assoc J* 1996; 155:1263–1268.
85. Feldman H, Gauthier S, Hecker J, Vellas B, Subbiah P, Whalen E. A 24-week, randomized, double-blind study of donepezil in moderate to severe Alzheimer's disease. *Neurology* 2001; 57:613–620.
86. Yesavage JA, Mumenthaler MS, Taylor JL *et al.* Donepezil and flight simulator performance: effects on retention of complex skills. *Neurology* 2002; 59:123–125.
87. Furey ML, Pietrini P, Haxby JV. Cholinergic enhancement and increased selectivity of perceptual processing during working memory. *Science* 2000; 290:2315–2319.
88. McKeith I, Del Ser T, Spano P *et al.* Efficacy of rivastigmine in dementia with Lewy bodies: a randomized, double-blind, placebo-controlled international study. *Lancet* 2000; 356:2031–2036.
89. Grace JB, Walker MP, McKeith IG. A comparison of sleep profiles in patients with dementia with lewy bodies and Alzheimer's dizease. *Int J Geriatr Psychiatry* 2000; 15:1028–1033.
90. Dautzenberg PL, Mulder LJ, Olde Rikkert MG, Wouters CJ, Loonen AJ. Delirium in elderly hospitalized patients: protective effects of chronic rivastigmine usage. *Int J Geriatr Psychiatry* 2004; 19:641–644.
91. Dautzenberg PL, Mulder LJ, Olde Rikkert MG, Wouters CJ, Loonen AJ. Adding rivastigmine to antipsychotics in the treatment of a chronic delirium. *Age Ageing* 2004; 33:516–517.
92. Moretti R, Torre P, Antonello RM, Cattaruzza T, Cazzato G. Cholinesterase inhibition as a possible therapy for delirium in vascular dementia: a controlled, open 24-month study of 246 patients. *Am J Alzheimer Dis Other Dement* 2004; 19:333–339.
93. Liptzin B, Laki A, Garb JL, Fingeroth R, Krushell R. Donepezil in the prevention and treatment of post-surgical delirium. *Am J Geriatr Psychiatry* 2005; 13:1100–1106.
94. Overshott R, Burns A, Karim S. Cholinesterase inhibitiors for delirium (protocol). *Cochrane Database Syst Rev* 2005.
95. Johnson J. Identifying and recognizing delirium. *Dement Geriatr Cogn Disord* 1999; 10:353–358.
96. Inouye SK, Schlesinger MJ, Lydon TJ. Delirium: a symptom of how hospital care is failing older persons and a window to improve quality of hospital care. *Am J Med* 1999; 106:565–573.
97. Folstein MF, Bassett SS, Romanoski AJ, Nestadt G. The epidemiology of delirium in the community: the Eastern Baltimore Mental Health Survey. *Int Psychogeriatr* 1991; 3:169–176.
98. Sandberg O, Gustafson Y, Brannstrom B, Bucht G. Prevalence of dementia, delirium and psychiatric symptoms in various care settings for the elderly. *Scand J Soc Med* 1998; 26:56–62.
99. Naughton BJ, Saltzman S, Ramadan F, Chadha N, Priore R, Mylotte JM. A multifactorial intervention to reduce prevalence of delirium and shorten hospital length of stay. *J Am Geriatr Soc* 2005; 53:18–23.
100. Fann JR. The epidemiology of delirium: a review of studies and methodological issues. *Semin Clin Neuropsychiatry* 2000; 5:64–74.
101. Baker FM, Wiley C, Kokmen E, Chandra V, Schoenberg BS. Delirium episodes during the course of clinically diagnosed Alzheimer's disease. *J Nat Med Assoc* 1999; 91:625–630.
102. Lerner AJ, Hedera P, Koss E, Stuckey J, Friedland RP. Delirium in Alzheimer disease. *Alzheimer Dis Assoc Disord* 1997; 11:16–20.

103. Benoit AG, Campbell BI, Tanner JR *et al.* Risk factors and prevalence of perioperative cognitive dysfunction in abdominal aneurysm patients. *J Vasc Surg* 2005; 42:884–890.
104. Rudolph JL, Babikian VL, Birjiniuk V *et al.* Atherosclerosis is associated with delirium after coronary artery bypass graft surgery. *J Am Geriatr Soc* 2005; 53:462–466.
105. Santana SF, Wahlund LO, Varli F, Tadeu V, I, Eriksdotter JM. Incidence, clinical features and subtypes of delirium in elderly patients treated for hip fractures. *Dement Geriatr Cogn Disord* 2005; 20:231–237.
106. Slatkin N, Rhiner M. Treatment of opioid-induced delirium with acetylcholinesterase inhibitors: a case report. *J Pain Symptom Manage* 2004; 27:268–273.
107. Noyan MA, Elbi H, Aksu H. Donepezil for anticholinergic drug intoxication: a case report. *Prog Neuropsychopharmacol Biol Psychiatry* 2003; 27:885–887.
108. Dautzenberg PL, Wouters CJ, Oudejans I, Samson MM. Rivastigmine in prevention of delirium in a 65 year old man with Parkinson's disease. *Int J Geriatr Psychiatry* 2003; 18:555–556.
109. Wengel SP, Roccaforte WH, Burke WJ. Donepezil improves symptoms of delirium in dementia: implications for future research. *J Geriatr Psychiatry Neurol* 1998; 11:159–161.
110. Kobayashi K, Higashima M, Mutou K *et al.* Severe delirium due to basal forebrain vascular lesion and efficacy of donepezil. *Prog Neuropsychopharmacol Biol Psychiatry* 2004; 28:1189–1194.
111. Ukai S, Yamamoto M, Tanaka M, Takeda M. Treatment of typical Charles Bonnet syndrome with donepezil. *Int Clin Psychopharmacol* 2004; 19:355–357.
112. Hori K, Tominaga I, Inada T *et al.* Donepezil-responsive alcohol-related prolonged delirium. *Psychiatry Clin Neurosci* 2003; 57:603–604.
113. Fischer P. Successful treatment of nonanticholinergic delirium with a cholinesterase inhibitor. *J Clin Psychopharmacol* 2001; 21:118.
114. Wengel SP, Burke WJ, Roccaforte WH. Donepezil for postoperative delirium associated with Alzheimer's disease. *J Am Geriatr Soc* 1999; 47:379–380.

# Abbreviations

| | |
|---|---|
| 3-APS | 3-amino-1-propansulfonic acid |
| 3MS | modified MMSE |
| AACD | age associated cognitive decline |
| AAMI | age associated memory impairment |
| ACE | angiotensin-converting enzyme |
| ACES | Agitation-Calmness Evaluation Scale |
| Ach | acetylcholine |
| AchE | acetylcholinesterase |
| AchEI | acetylcholinesterase inhibitor |
| AD | Alzheimer's disease |
| ADAPT | Alzheimer's Disease Anti-inflammatory Prevention Trial |
| ADAS-Cog | Alzheimer's Disease Assessment Scale – cognitive subscale |
| ADAS-Noncog | Alzheimer's Disease Assessment Scale – non-cognitive subscale |
| ADCS | Alzheimer's Disease Cooperation Study |
| ADCS-ADL | Alzheimer's Disease Cooperative Study – Activity of Daily Living Scale |
| ADFACS | Alzheimer's Disease Functional Assessment and Change Scale |
| ADL | activities of daily living |
| ADMT | Alzheimer's disease-modifying treatment |
| AE | adverse event |
| AHEAD | Assessment of Health Economics in AD |
| AMPA | alpha-amino-3-hydroxy-5-methyl-4-isoxazolepropionic acid |
| ANCOVA | analysis of covariance model |
| APL | allosteric potentiating ligand |
| ApoE | apolipoprotein E |
| APP | amyloid precursor protein |
| Aβ | amyloid-β |
| BADL | Bristol ADL scale |
| BEHAVE-AD | Behavioural Pathology in Alzheimer's Disease Rating scale |
| BGP | behavioural rating scale for geriatric patients |
| BLT | bright light therapy |
| BMI | body mass index |
| BPRS | Brief Psychiatric Rating Scale |
| BPSD | behavioural and psychological symptoms of dementia |
| BuChE | butyrylcholinesterase |
| CADASIL | cerebral autosomal dominant arteriopathy |
| CAD-DTC | California Alzheimer's Disease Diagnostic and Treatment Centres |
| CAM | complementary and alternative medicine |
| CAM | Confusion Assessment Method |
| CAMCOG | Cambridge Cognitive Examination |
| CANDID | Counselling and Diagnosis in Dementia |
| CASI | Cognitive Abilities Screening Instrument |

| | |
|---|---|
| CAT | choline acetyl transferase |
| CBD | corticobasal degeneration |
| CDR | Clinical Dementia Rating |
| CDR | Clinical Dementia Rating Scale |
| CDR-SB | Clinical Dementia Rating – Sum of Boxes |
| CERAD | Consortium to Establish a Registry in Alzheimer's Disease |
| CGI | clinical global impression |
| CGIC | Clinical Global Impression of Change |
| ChAT | choline acetyltransferase |
| ChEI | cholinesterase inhibitor |
| CHI | cholinesterase inhibitor |
| CI | confidence interval |
| CIBIC+ | Clinicians' Interview-Based Impression of Change-Plus |
| CIR | Clinical Insight Rating scale |
| CMAI | Cohen-Mansfield Agitation Inventory |
| CNTB | Computerised Neuropsychological Test Battery |
| COX | cyclo-oxygenase |
| CPMC | Commission for Medicinal and Pharmaceutical Compounds |
| CSDD | Cornell Scale for Depression in Dementia |
| CSF | cerebrospinal fluid |
| CSM | Committee of Safety of Medicines |
| CT | computed tomography |
| CVAE | cerebrovascular adverse event |
| CVD | cerebrovascular disease |
| DAD | Disability Assessment for Dementia |
| DASNI | Dementia Advocacy and Support Network International |
| DIADS | Depression in AD Study |
| DLB | Dewy body dementia |
| DLB | dementia with Lewy bodies |
| DPZ | donepezil |
| DS | Down's syndrome |
| DSS | Digit Symbol Substitution test |
| DSM-IIIR | Diagnostic and Statistical Manual of Mental Disorders, Third Edition, Revised |
| ECG | electrocardiogram |
| ECT | electroconvulsive therapy |
| EEG | electroencephalogram |
| ELISA | enzyme-linked immunosorbent assay |
| EP | evaluable patient |
| EPS | extrapyrimidal symptoms |
| EPSP | excitatory post-synaptic potential |
| ES | effect size |
| FAST | functional assessment staging tool |
| FCA | Family Caregiver Alliance |
| FDA | Food and Drug Administration |
| FDDNP | aminonaphthalene |
| fMRI | functional MRI |
| FSH | follicle stimulating hormone |
| FTC | full-time-care |
| FTD | fronto-temporal dementia |
| FTLD | fronto-temporal lobar degeneration |
| GABA | gamma-aminobutyrinic acid |
| GAG | glycosaminoglycan |

| | |
|---|---|
| GAP | growth-associated protein |
| GBS | Gottfries-Brane-Steen scale |
| GDS | Global Deterioration Scale |
| GDS | Geriatric Depression Scale |
| GERRI | Geriatric Evaluation by Relative's Rating Instrument |
| GnRH | gonadotrophin-releasing hormone |
| GPI | glycosyl phosphatidylinositol |
| HAMD | Hamilton rating scale for Depression |
| HARS | Hamilton Anxiety Rating Scale |
| HDRS | Hamilton Depression Rating Scale |
| HIS | Hachinski Ischaemic Score |
| HNARS | human nAChR sensitizer |
| HOPE | Heart Outcomes Prevention Evaluation |
| HOPE-TOO | HOPE-The Ongoing Outcomes |
| HPG | hypothalamic-pituitary-gonadal |
| HR | hazard ratio |
| HRQL | health-related quality of life |
| HRT | hormone replacement therapy |
| HUI | Health Utility Index |
| IADL | instrumental ADL |
| IDE | insulin degrading enzyme |
| IGF | insulin-like growth factor |
| IL | interleukin |
| IP | isoprostane |
| ITT | intention to treat |
| LB | Lewy bodies |
| LBD | Lewy body disease |
| LH | luteinizing hormone |
| LN | Lewy neuritis |
| LOCF | last observation carried forward |
| LP | lumbar puncture |
| LPAC | lipid-protein attenuating compound |
| LTP | long-term potentiation |
| MA | meta-analysis |
| MADRS | Montgomery Asberg Depression Rating Scale |
| MAO-A | monoamine oxidase type A |
| MCI | mild cognitive impairment |
| m-CPP | meta-chlorophenyl-piperazine |
| MDRS | Mattis Dementia Rating Scale |
| MIBG | iodine-131-meta-iodobenzylguanidine |
| MID | multi-infarct dementia |
| MMSE | Mini-mental State Examination |
| MPAC | metal-protein attenuating compound |
| MRC | Medical Research Council |
| MRI | magnetic resonance imaging |
| NAB | Nürnberger Alters-Beobachtungskala |
| nAChR | nicotinic acetylcholine receptor |
| NBRS | Neurobehavioural Rating Scale |
| NCCAM | National Centre for Complementary and Alternative Medicine |
| NFT | neurofibrillary tangle |
| NGF | nerve growth factor |
| NHS | National Health Service |

| | |
|---|---|
| NIA | National Institute of Aging |
| NICE | National Institute for Clinical Excellence |
| NIH | National Institutes of Health |
| NINCDS-ADRDA | National Institute of Neurological and Communicative Diseases and Stroke/Alzheimer's Disease and Related Disorders Association |
| NINDS-AIREN | National Institute of Neurological Disorders and Stroke and the Association Internationale pour la Reserche et l'Enseignement on Neurosciences |
| NMDA | *N*-methyl-D-aspartate |
| NNT | number needed to treat |
| NOSGER | nurses geriatric observation (scale) |
| NOSIE | Nurses Observation Scale for Inpatient Behaviour |
| NPE | neprilysin |
| NPI | Neuropsychiatric Inventory |
| NSAID | non-steroidal anti-inflammatory drug |
| OAS | Overt Aggression Scale |
| OC | observed case |
| OPTIMA | Oxford Project To Investigate Memory and Ageing |
| OR | odds ratio |
| PA | progressive non-fluent aphasia |
| PANSS | Positive and Negative Symptoms Scale |
| PD | Parkinson's disease |
| PDD | Parkinson's disease and dementia |
| PET | positron emission tomography |
| PIB | Pittsburgh Compound-B |
| PPAC | protein-protein attenuating compound |
| PPAR-γ | peroxisome proliferators-activated receptor-gamma |
| PROGRESS | Perindopril Protection Against Recurrent Stroke Study |
| PS | presenilin |
| PSP | progressive supranuclear palsy |
| p-tau | phophorylated tau |
| QALY | quality-adjusted life-year |
| QOL | quality of life |
| RBD | REM sleep behaviour disorder |
| rCBF | regional cortical blood flow |
| RCT | randomized controlled trial |
| REM | rapid eye-movement |
| RMA | regression meta-analysis |
| RNAi | RNA interference |
| ROS | reactive oxygen species |
| SA | serum anti-cholinergicity |
| SANS-AD | Scale for Assessment of Negative Symptoms in Alzheimer's Disease |
| SCAG | Sandoz Clinical Assessment-Geriatric |
| SCGB | Screen for Caregiver Burden |
| SCOPE | Study in Cognition and Prognosis in the Elderly |
| SD | semantic dementia |
| SHEP | Systolic Hypertension in Elderly Program |
| SHTAC | Southampton Health Technology Assessments Centre |
| SIB | Severe Impairment Battery |
| siRNA | small interfering RNA |
| SIVD | subcortical ischaemic VaD |
| SKT | Syndrom-Kurztest (*or* Short Syndrome Test) |

| | |
|---|---|
| SPECT | single proton emission computed tomography |
| SR | systematic review |
| SRI | Stereotyping Rating Inventory |
| SSRI | selective serotonin reuptake inhibitor |
| Syst-Eur | Systolic Hypertension in Europe trial |
| TCA | tricyclic anti-depressant |
| TIA | transient ischaemic attack |
| VaD | vascular dementia |
| VaDAS-Cog | Vascular Dementia Assessment Scale – cognitive subscale |
| VCI | vascular cognitive impairment |
| WHIMS | Women's Health Initiative Memory Study |
| ZnT3 | neuronal zinc-transporter |

# Index